Fulfilling the Potential of Cancer Prevention and Early Detection

Susan J. Curry, Tim Byers, and Maria Hewitt,
Editors

National Cancer Policy Board

INSTITUTE OF MEDICINE
NATIONAL RESEARCH COUNCIL
OF THE NATIONAL ACADEMIES

THE NATIONAL ACADEMIES PRESS
Washington, D.C.
www.nap.edu

THE NATIONAL ACADEMIES PRESS • 500 Fifth Street, N.W. • Washington, DC 20001

NOTICE: The project that is the subject of this report was approved by the Governing Board of the National Research Council, whose members are drawn from the councils of the National Academy of Sciences, the National Academy of Engineering, and the Institute of Medicine. The members of the committee responsible for the report were chosen for their special competences and with regard for appropriate balance.

Support for this project was provided by the National Cancer Institute; the Centers for Disease Control and Prevention; the American Cancer Society; Abbott Laboratories; the American Society of Clinical Oncology; Amgen, Inc.; Aventis; and the United Health Care Foundation. The views presented in this report are those of the Institute of Medicine and the National Research Council National Cancer Policy Board and are not necessarily those of the funding agencies.

Library of Congress Cataloging-in-Publication Data

Fulfilling the potential of cancer prevention and early detection /
Susan J. Curry, Tim Byers, and Maria Hewitt, editors ; National Cancer
Policy Board.
p. ; cm.
Includes bibliographical references and index.
ISBN 0-309-08254-4 (hardcover)
ISBN 0-309-50619-0 (PDF Full Book)
1. Cancer—United States—Prevention.
[DNLM: 1. Neoplasms—prevention & control—United States. 2. Health
Behavior—United States. 3. Health Policy—United States. 4. Health
Promotion—methods—United States. 5. Mass Screening—United States.
QZ 200 F962 2003] I. Curry, Susan J. II. Byers, Tim. III. Hewitt, Maria
Elizabeth. IV. National Cancer Policy Board (U.S.)

RC268.F85 2003
616.99'4052—dc21

2003000742

Additional copies of this report are available from the National Academies Press, 500 Fifth Street, N.W., Lockbox 285, Washington, DC 20055; (800) 624-6242 or (202) 334-3313 (in the Washington metropolitan area); Internet, http://www.nap.edu.

For more information about the Institute of Medicine, visit the IOM home page at: **www.iom.edu.**

Printed in the United States of America.

THE NATIONAL ACADEMIES

Advisers to the Nation on Science, Engineering, and Medicine

The **National Academy of Sciences** is a private, nonprofit, self-perpetuating society of distinguished scholars engaged in scientific and engineering research, dedicated to the furtherance of science and technology and to their use for the general welfare. Upon the authority of the charter granted to it by the Congress in 1863, the Academy has a mandate that requires it to advise the federal government on scientific and technical matters. Dr. Bruce M. Alberts is president of the National Academy of Sciences.

The **National Academy of Engineering** was established in 1964, under the charter of the National Academy of Sciences, as a parallel organization of outstanding engineers. It is autonomous in its administration and in the selection of its members, sharing with the National Academy of Sciences the responsibility for advising the federal government. The National Academy of Engineering also sponsors engineering programs aimed at meeting national needs, encourages education and research, and recognizes the superior achievements of engineers. Dr. Wm. A. Wulf is president of the National Academy of Engineering.

The **Institute of Medicine** was established in 1970 by the National Academy of Sciences to secure the services of eminent members of appropriate professions in the examination of policy matters pertaining to the health of the public. The Institute acts under the responsibility given to the National Academy of Sciences by its congressional charter to be an adviser to the federal government and, upon its own initiative, to identify issues of medical care, research, and education. Dr. Harvey V. Fineberg is president of the Institute of Medicine.

The **National Research Council** was organized by the National Academy of Sciences in 1916 to associate the broad community of science and technology with the Academy's purposes of furthering knowledge and advising the federal government. Functioning in accordance with general policies determined by the Academy, the Council has become the principal operating agency of both the National Academy of Sciences and the National Academy of Engineering in providing services to the government, the public, and the scientific and engineering communities. The Council is administered jointly by both Academies and the Institute of Medicine. Dr. Bruce M. Alberts and Dr. Wm. A. Wulf are chair and vice chair, respectively, of the National Research Council.

www.national-academies.org

CECIL B. PICKETT, Executive Vice President, Discovery Research, Schering-Plough Research Institute, Kenilworth, NJ
LOUISE RUSSELL, Professor, Rutgers University, New Brunswick, NJ
JOHN SEFFRIN, Chief Executive Officer, American Cancer Society, Atlanta, GA (member through March 2002)
THOMAS J. SMITH, Professor, Virginia Commonwealth University, Richmond, VA
SANDRA UNDERWOOD, ACS Oncology Nursing Professor, University of Wisconsin School of Nursing, Milwaukee, WI (member through March 2002)
SUSAN WEINER, President, The Children's Cause, Silver Spring, MD
ROBERT C. YOUNG, President, American Cancer Society and the Fox Chase Cancer Center, Philadelphia, PA

Consultants

Graham A. Colditz, Catherine Tomeo Ryan, Charles H. Dart, III, Geetanjali Datta, Laurie Fisher, and Beverly Rockhill, Channing Laboratory, Boston, MA
Steven H. Woolf, Department of Family Practice, Virginia Commonwealth University
Parthiv J. Mahadevia, Farin Kamangar, and Jonathan M. Samet, Bloomberg School of Public Health, Johns Hopkins University
Edwin B. Fisher and Mario Schootman, Washington University School of Medicine, and Ross C. Brownson, Amy A. Eyler, and Debra L. Haire-Joshu, St. Louis University
Judith Ockene, Jane Zapka, Lori Pbert, Suzanne Brodney, and Stephenie Lemon, University of Massachusetts Medical School
Suzanne Phelan and Rena R. Wing, Weight Control and Diabetes Research Center, Brown University

Study Staff

Maria Hewitt, Study Director
Mary Joy Ballantyne, Research Assistant
Gelsey Lynn, Research Assistant
Timothy K. Brennan, Research Assistant
Michael K. Hayes, Editor

NCPB Staff

Roger Herdman, Director, National Cancer Policy Board
Nicci T. Dowd, Administrator
Jennifer Cangco, Financial Associate
Rosa Pommier, Financial Associate

REVIEWERS

This report has been reviewed in draft form by individuals chosen for their diverse perspectives and technical expertise, in accordance with procedures approved by the National Research Council's Report Review Committee. The purpose of this independent review is to provide candid and critical comments that will assist the institution in making its published report as sound as possible and to ensure that the report meets institutional standards for objectivity, evidence, and responsiveness to the study charge. The review comments and draft manuscript remain confidential to protect the integrity of the deliberative process. We wish to thank the following individuals for their review of this report:

Timothy B. Baker, University of Wisconsin, Madison
Dileep G. Bal, Cancer Control Branch, California Department of Health, Sacramento, CA
Moon S. Chen, Jr., Ohio State University, Dublin, OH
Wendy Demark-Wahnefried, Duke University Medical Center, Durham, NC
Paul Frame, Tri-County Family Medicine, Cohoctin, NY
Carolyn Gotay, Cancer Research Center of Hawaii, Honolulu
Kathy Helzlsouer, Bloomberg School of Public Health, Johns Hopkins University
Arthur Levin, Center for Medical Consumers, New York, NY
Anne McTiernan, Cancer Prevention Research Program, Fred Hutchinson Cancer Research Center, Seattle, WA
Duncan B. Neuhauser, Department of Epidemiology & Biostatistics, Case Western Reserve University Medical School, Cleveland, OH
Malcom C. Pike, USC/Norris Cancer Center, Los Angeles, CA
Helen Halpin Schauffler, Center for Health and Public Policy Studies, University of California, Berkeley
David Schottenfeld, Department of Epidemiology, University of Michigan School of Public Health, Ann Arbor, MI
Steve Taplin, Center for Health Studies, Group Health Cooperative of Puget Sound, Seattle, WA
Beti Thompson, Cancer Prevention Research Program, Fred Hutchinson Cancer Research Center, Seattle, WA

Although the reviewers listed above have provided many constructive comments and suggestions, they were not asked to endorse the conclusions or recommendations, nor did they see the final draft of the report before its release. The review of this report was overseen by **Maureen M. Henderson,**

M.D., D.P.H., Professor Emeritus of Epidemiology and Medicine, University of Washington. Appointed by the National Research Council, she was responsible for making certain that an independent examination of this report was carried out in accordance with institutional procedures and that all review comments were carefully considered. Responsibility for the final content of this report rests entirely with the authoring committee and the institution.

Acknowledgments

The National Cancer Policy Board first and foremost acknowledges the contribution of the Board's prevention subgroup. These Board members provided leadership and spent many hours shaping the study plan, reviewing drafts, discussing recommendations, and offering assistance to staff throughout the report's production.

Board Prevention Subgroup

- Susan Curry, (*Group leader*), University of Illinois at Chicago
- Diana Petitti, (*Board Vice Chair)*, Kaiser Permanente of Southern California
- Tim Byers, University of Colorado Health Sciences Center
- Vivien W. Chen, Louisiana State University Medical Center
- William McGuire, UnitedHealth Group
- Nancy Mueller, Harvard School of Public Health
- Louise Russell, Rutgers University
- John Seffrin, American Cancer Society
- Sandra Underwood, University of Wisconsin School of Nursing

Former Board members Robert Day, Fred Hutchinson Cancer Research Center, and Ellen Gritz, M.D. Anderson Cancer Center, helped plan the report.

The Board also acknowledges the tremendous contribution made by authors of background papers that formed the basis of several of the report's chapters.

• Graham A. Colditz and his colleagues Catherine Tomeo Ryan, Charles H. Dart, III, Geetanjali Datta, Laurie Fisher, and Beverly Rockhill wrote "Quantifying the Contribution of Risk Factors to Cancer Incidence and the Estimated Reduction in Cancer Burden Through Selected Risk Factor Modifications."

• Edwin B. Fisher and his colleagues Ross C. Brownson, Amy A. Eyler, Debra L. Haire-Joshu, and Mario Schootman wrote "Interventions to Promote Key Behaviors in Cancer Prevention and Early Detection."

• Parthiv J. Mahadevia, Farin Kamangar, and Jonathan M. Samet wrote "Fulfilling the Potential of Lung Cancer Prevention and Early Detection: What Are the Implications of Adopting New Technologies in the Face of Uncertain Science?"

• Judith Ockene and her colleagues Jane Zapka, Lori Pbert, Suzanne Brodney, and Stephenie Lemon wrote "Provider, System, and Policy Strategies to Enhance the Delivery of Cancer Prevention and Control Activities in Primary Care."

• Suzanne Phelan and Rena R. Wing wrote "Interventions to Reduce Obesity and Maintain a Healthy Weight."

• Steven H. Woolf wrote "The Effectiveness of Screening for Cancer and Its Unfulfilled Potential in the United States: A Review of the Evidence."

Several other individuals addressed the Board at their quarterly meetings providing important information and perspectives:

• Ralph Coates and Kevin Brady, National Center for Chronic Disease Prevention and Health Promotion, Division of Cancer Prevention and Control, Centers for Disease Control and Prevention

• Barbara Rimer and Robert Croyle, Division of Cancer Control and Population Sciences, National Cancer Institute (NCI)

Several individuals met with or corresponded with Board staff to provide information about their programs and activities.

• Carol Ashton, Houston Veterans Administration Center for Quality of Care and Utilization Studies

• Kevin Brady, Division of Cancer Prevention and Control, Centers for Disease Control and Prevention

• Mary Burdick, Veterans Administration National Center for Health Promotion and Disease Prevention (NCHPDP)

• Leslie Given, Division of Cancer Prevention and Control, Centers for Disease Control and Prevention

• Peter Greenwald, Division of Cancer Prevention, NCI

• Brian Kimes, Office of Centers, Training, and Resources, NCI

• Wendy Perry, Office of the Director, Agency for Healthcare Research and Quality

• Stacey Vandor, Office of the Director, Division of Cancer Control and Population Sciences, NCI

Many individuals made important contributions by reviewing sections of the report for accuracy

• Jean K. Brown, University at Buffalo School of Nursing, State University of New York
• Sachiko St. Jeor, Nutrition Education and Research Program, University of Nevada
• Helen Meissner, Applied Cancer Screening Research Branch, Behavioral Research Program, DCCPS, NCI
• John D. Potter, Fred Hutchinson Cancer Research Center
• Linda Meyers and Paula Trumbo, Food and Nutrition Board, Institute of Medicine
• Nancy Riese Daly, American Society for Therapeutic Radiology and Oncology (ASTRO)
• William T. Sause, Department of Radiation Oncology, LDS Hospital, Salt Lake City, Utah
• Michael Whitcomb, Division of Medical Education, Association of American Medical Colleges

The Board also wishes to thank David Berrigan, NCI Cancer Prevention Fellow, who followed the progress of the report and reviewed commissioned papers and report drafts.

The Board thanks high school students Ben Markwell and Alex Del Pinal for their contribution in checking references.

Acronyms and Abbreviations

AACE	American Association for Cancer Education
AAHP	American Association of Health Plans
AAMC	Association of American Medical Colleges
ACRIN	American College of Radiology Imaging Network
ACS	American Cancer Society
ACSM	American College of Sports Medicine
ACT	Activity Counseling Trial
AHCPR	Agency for Health Care Policy and Research
AHEC	Area Health Education Center
AHRQ	Agency for Healthcare Research and Quality
ALA	American Lung Association
ASPO	American Society of Preventive Oncology
ATBC	Alpha-Tocopherol Beta-Carotene Cancer Prevention Study Group
ATPM	Association of Teachers of Preventive Medicine
BED	binge eating disorder
BMI	body mass index
BPHC	Bureau of Primary Health Care (HRSA)
CAD	computer-aided diagnosis
CARET	Beta-Carotene and Retinol Efficacy Trial
CATCH	Child and Adolescent Trial for Cardiovascular Health
CDC	Centers for Disease Control and Prevention
CDMRP	Congressionally Directed Medical Research Programs
CHC	Community Health Center Program

CI	confidence interval
CME	continuing medical education
CMS	Centers for Medicare and Medicaid Services (formerly the Health Care Financing Administration)
CONQUEST	Computerized Needs-Oriented Quality Measurement Evaluation System
CQI	continuous quality improvement
CSP	Cooperative Studies Program (VA)
CT	computed tomography
DCCPS	Division of Cancer Control and Population Sciences (NCI)
DCIS	ductal carcinoma in situ
DHHS	U.S. Department of Health and Human Services
DoD	U.S. Department of Defense
ELCAP	Early Lung Cancer Action Project
FDA	Food and Drug Administration
FFS	fee for service
FOBT	fecal occult blood test
FQHC	federally qualified health centers
FY	fiscal year
GM	General Motors
HCFA	Health Care Financing Administration (now the Centers for Medicare and Medicaid Services)
HEDIS	Health Plan Employer Data and Information Set
HMO	health maintenance organization
HPV	human papillomavirus
HRA	health risk appraisal
HRSA	Health Resources and Services Administration
IARC	International Agency for Research on Cancer
IHS	Indian Health Service
IOM	Institute of Medicine
kcal/day	kilocalories per day
kg	kilogram
kg/m^2	kilogram per square meter
lb	pound (1 pound = 0.45 kilogram)
LCD	low-calorie diet
mA	milliangstroms
MCO	managed care organization
mg	milligram
MHC	Migrant Health Center Program

mm	millimeter
mrad	millirad
MTCP	Massachusetts Tobacco Control Program
NBCCEDP	National Breast and Cervical Cancer Early Detection Program
NCI	National Cancer Institute
NDC	National Dialogue on Cancer
ng/dl	nanograms per deciliter
NHANES	National Health and Nutrition Examination Survey
NHLBI	National Heart, Lung, and Blood Institute
NIH	National Institutes of Health
NNS	number needed to screen
NNT	number needed to treat
NRT	nicotine replacement therapy
NSAID	nonsteroidal anti-inflammatory drug
NTAO	National Technical Assistance Office
OTC	over the counter (nonprescription)
PACE	Physician-Based Assessment and Counseling for Exercise
PBGH	Pacific Business Group on Health
PCAP	Prevention Curriculum Assistance Program
PDQ	Physician Data Query
PLCO study	Prostate, Lung, Colorectal, and Ovarian study
PPIP	Put Prevention into Practice
PPV	positive predictive value
PSA	prostate-specific antigen
QALY	quality-adjusted life year
QUERI	Quality Enhancement Research Initiative
QuIC	Quality Interagency Coordination
RADIUS	Research and Development in the United States (database)
RWJF	Robert Wood Johnson Foundation
SCHIP	State Children's Health Insurance Program
SEER	Surveillance, Epidemiology, and End Results Program
SPN	Special Populations Networks for Cancer Awareness, Research, and Training
TRCBSs	Translational Research Centers in Behavioral Science
TRIP	Translating Research into Practice
USPSTF	U.S. Preventive Services Task Force
VA	U.S. Department of Veterans Affairs
VANAC	VA Nurses Against Cancer
VBG	vertical banded gastroplasty

VHA	Veterans Health Administration
VISN	Veterans Integrated Service Networks
VLCD	very low-calorie diet
WHO	World Health Organization
WIC	Special Supplemental Food Program for Women, Infants, and Children

Contents

List of Boxes, Figures, and Tables

BOXES

FIGURES

TABLES

Fulfilling the Potential of Cancer Prevention and Early Detection

Executive Summary

The nation needs new strategies to prevent cancer and, when cancer occurs, to catch it at its earliest stages. Smoking, unhealthy diet, obesity, sedentary lifestyles, and failure to get screened all contribute to the excess burden of cancer. Failure to implement proven methods of cancer prevention leads to avoidable disease and death. A 19 percent decline in the rate at which new cancer cases occur and a 29 percent decline in the rate of cancer deaths could potentially be achieved by 2015 if efforts to help people change their behaviors that put them at risk were stepped up and if behavioral change were sustained. This would equate to the prevention of approximately 100,000 cancer cases and 60,000 cancer deaths each year by the year 2015 (Byers et al., 1999). The possible reductions in cancer incidence are particularly striking for certain cancers: accelerated changes in risk behavior could halve the number of smoking-related cancers such as lung cancer and reduce the numbers of cases of colorectal cancer by up to one-third.

To save the most lives from cancer, health care providers, health plans, insurers, employers, policy makers, and researchers should be concentrating their resources on helping people to stop smoking, maintain a healthy weight and diet, exercise regularly, keep alcohol consumption at low to moderate levels, and get screened for breast, cervical, and colorectal cancer. The health benefits of such behavioral changes extend beyond cancer to cardiovascular disease and diabetes as well. Such efforts may also help alleviate the disproportionate burden of cancer borne by members of racial and ethnic minority groups.

Many of the behaviors that place individuals at risk for cancer are well recognized, and calls for behavioral change are not new. What is new is the growing body of evidence confirming the effectiveness of interventions to help people improve their health-related behaviors. Health care providers can boost quit rates among their patients who smoke by adhering to smoking cessation guidelines. Administrators can improve the use of screening tests among health plan members by having systems in place to remind physicians and patients of needed tests. Communities can enact policies to curb exposure to secondhand smoke, limit access to tobacco products by teenagers, and create safe places for physical activity. Each of these strategies works, but especially effective in bringing about behavioral change is the simultaneous action of several parties: health care providers, administrators, educators, and policy makers.

Although personal experience illustrates for most people the great difficulty of achieving sustained behavioral change, Americans have made substantial improvements in their health habits in the past few decades. There has been, for example, a steep decline in the number of Americans who smoke; there have been some improvements in diet; and screening for some cancers is widespread. Investment in the effective clinical and public health tools at hand can produce much greater improvements.

In this report, the National Cancer Policy Board reviews the evidence that cancer incidence rates can be dramatically reduced and outlines a national strategy to realize the promise of cancer prevention and early detection. The report examines

- the extent to which the burden of cancer could be reduced through cancer prevention and early detection;
- the effectiveness of cancer screening methods and interventions to alter smoking, eating, and exercise habits;[1]
- approaches to enhancing the potential benefits of proven interventions;
- a case study of screening for lung cancer, illustrating the problem of adopting new technology when the science is uncertain;
- professional education and training needs;
- federal and state programs that support cancer prevention and early detection; and

---

[1]The Board recognized that a number of personal and health care behaviors are known to contribute to the burden of cancer but limited its review to tobacco use, obesity, physical activity, diet, alcohol use, and the use of screening tests. Examples of behaviors known to contribute to cancer risk but not considered in this review include exposure to sun and exposure to cancer-causing viruses through sexual activity (e.g., human papillomavirus) and blood contact such as through intravenous drug use (e.g., hepatitis B virus). Behaviors were selected based on their contribution to cancer and to other chronic illnesses such as cardiovascular disease and diabetes.

- research trends and opportunities.

The Board recommends that the following steps be taken to increase the rates of adoption, the reach, and the impacts of evidence-based cancer prevention and early detection interventions.

Recommendation 1: The U.S. Congress and state legislatures should enact and provide funding for enforcement of laws to substantially reduce and ultimately eliminate the adverse public health consequences of tobacco use and exposure.

Tobacco is the greatest contributor to deaths from cancer, and reduction in tobacco use offers the greatest opportunity to reduce the incidence, morbidity, and mortality of cancer. Specific actions that would be effective include the following:

- Taxation is the single most effective method of reducing the demand for tobacco. States should set sufficiently high levels of excise taxation on tobacco products to discourage tobacco use, but levels should not be so high that they encourage significant tax avoidance activities.
- States should allocate sufficient funds from the Tobacco Master Settlement Agreement and tobacco excise taxes to support comprehensive, state-based tobacco control efforts consistent with guidelines of the Centers for Disease Control and Prevention.
- States should improve compliance with the provisions of the 1992 Synar amendment, which requires that states have sales-to-minor rates of no greater than 20 percent in order to receive federal Substance Abuse Prevention and Treatment Block Grant awards. By 2000, only 25 states had achieved this level of compliance.
- States should impose tobacco-licensing requirements for merchants selling tobacco products, as recommended in the 2000 report of the Surgeon General (U.S. Department of Health and Human Services and Office of Disease Prevention and Health Promotion, 2000). The threat of revocation of the license as a consequence of selling tobacco products to minors could provide a strong incentive for merchants to comply with existing laws. Further, requiring that merchants pay for a license to sell tobacco could provide needed funds for monitoring and enforcement.
- Internet sales of tobacco products are not covered by the Synar amendment, which leaves a significant opening for minors to have access to tobacco. More than 90 websites sell cigarettes in the United States, and the number is expected to grow. Congress should therefore act to prohibit the promotion, sale, and distribution of tobacco products over the Internet to individuals under the age of 18.
- Regulations at the state level vary greatly across the country. Until the passage of federal legislation, state and local legislatures should increase

their regulatory efforts related to environmental tobacco smoke by establishing smoke-free indoor workplaces, public buildings, and restaurants.

• Further restrictions are needed to reduce tobacco promotion and advertising, which compromises youth tobacco prevention efforts. Restrictions now in place include a mix of voluntary agreements, restrictions resulting from settlements of lawsuits, and prohibitions defined by state or local ordinances, but some efforts have been hampered by protection of commercial speech. The Board urges renewed national consideration of how to address the practices of placing advertising at convenience stores and in magazines that are particularly attractive to minors, and tobacco sponsorship of youth-oriented events.

Recommendation 2: A national strategy should be developed and coordinated by the U.S. Department of Health and Human Services to address the epidemic of obesity, unhealthy diet, and physical inactivity in America, which are all significant risk factors for cancer and other diseases. Effective interventions need to be identified and broadly applied to reduce cancer risk among the general population and among populations at higher risk.

Dietary interventions to prevent cancer have, to date, focused primarily on particular components such as the consumption of fruits and vegetables, fiber, and fats. Obesity and physical inactivity have recently joined unhealthy diet as leading risk factors for cancer.

Efforts to maintain a healthy weight that start early in childhood and continue throughout adulthood are likely to be more successful than efforts to achieve and maintain weight loss once obesity is established. Over time, even a small decrease in the numbers of calories consumed and a small increase in physical activity can help prevent weight gain or facilitate weight loss.

Worksite fitness programs have resulted in increased levels of physical activity among employees, and it is recognized that environmental policies related to zoning, land use, safety, and transportation greatly affect opportunities for exercise. Among youth, school policies regarding healthy school lunches, physical education requirements, and the availability of after-school recreational programs improve nutrition and affect rates of participation in exercise.

The National Cancer Policy Board endorses the comprehensive Recommendations for Public Health Action on Weight Control and Physical Activity to Promote Cancer Prevention proposed by the International Agency for Research on Cancer, an agency within the World Health Organization (International Agency for Research on Cancer, 2000) (see Box 11.3 in Chapter 11). These recommendations could serve as a basis for the formulation of a national strategy through the Office of Disease Prevention and Health Promotion.

Recommendation 3: The U.S. Congress should provide sufficient appropriations to the Centers for Disease Control and Prevention to support innovative public and private partnerships to develop, implement, and evaluate comprehensive community-based programs in cancer prevention and early detection. Every state should have and implement a comprehensive cancer control plan.

The Centers for Disease Control and Prevention (CDC) is the federal link to the nation's public health infrastructure, principally through state and local health departments. State efforts in cancer prevention and early detection are in many cases piecemeal and are organized around categorically funded programs. CDC needs to build the capacities of states—and, in turn, their local partners—to develop and implement comprehensive cancer control plans.

CDC's National Comprehensive Cancer Control Program defines cancer control plans as those with an integrated and coordinated approach to reduce the rates of incidence, morbidity, and mortality of cancer through prevention, early detection, treatment, rehabilitation, and palliation (www.cdc.gov/cancer/ncccp/index.htm). Roughly half of the states (27 states) report having a comprehensive cancer control plan, but the plans are in various stages of implementation. CDC supports states in developing and implementing such plans, but the available support has been modest (approximately $37 million since 1998). The CDC estimates that $30 million per year would be needed for states to have plans developed and implementation in progress by 2005 (Leslie Given, Division of Cancer Prevention and Control, CDC, personal communication to Maria Hewitt, IOM, September 9, 2002).

State and local health departments, in partnership with private organizations, can play important roles in instituting and coordinating comprehensive cancer prevention programs. Health departments can, for example:

- monitor and publicize state trends in cancer and cancer-related behaviors;
- support media campaigns to promote healthy behaviors;
- target interventions to low income and racial/ethnic groups at high risk for cancer, e.g., by providing breast, cervical, and colorectal cancer screening services to medically uninsured and medically underserved populations;
- develop and distribute best-practice guidelines to major employer human resources departments to encourage smoking cessation programs, wellness programs, on-site healthy eating and exercise facilities, flexible time for employees to allow alternative means of commuting (e.g., by bicycle or foot), and use of preventive health services (e.g., screening and smoking cessation programs);
- collaborate with school systems to develop cancer prevention-related educational curricula and programs;

- collaborate with public and private organizations to provide incentives for physical activity, healthy eating, and participation in weight loss programs (e.g., reduced fees for fitness clubs, on-site weight control groups, employer nonautomotive commuting programs);
- track state use of funds available through the 1998 Transportation Equity Act for the 21st Century (Public Law 105-178), which provides federal funds to construct sidewalks and bicycle trails and to integrate mass transit, roads, and pedestrian and bicycle facilities into a comprehensive transportation plan;
- support free and reduced-fee health clinics organized through local health departments and other community-based programs; and
- evaluate the effectiveness of services and programs.

Recommendation 4: Public and private insurers and providers should consider evidence-based cancer prevention and early detection services to be essential benefits and should provide coverage for them. These services at a minimum should include interventions recommended in the 2000 U.S. Public Health Service's clinical practice guideline on treating tobacco use and dependence, screening for breast cancer among women age 50 and older, screening for cervical cancer among all sexually active women with an intact cervix, and screening for colorectal cancer among adults age 50 and older.

Public and private health insurers and providers who want to improve the health of their beneficiaries should include in their benefit packages coverage for evidence-based interventions for cancer prevention and early detection. Nicotine replacement therapy, treatment with certain antidepressants (e.g., Bupropion SR), and counseling, for example, are effective in helping individuals quit smoking. Very few insurers or health maintenance organizations cover the cost of pharmaceutical treatment for smoking cessation, and health education and preventive counseling are usually not defined benefits.

For insurers that offer coverage for preventive services, the reduction or elimination of cost sharing (e.g., coinsurance and copayments) can address a financial deterrent to seeking services and can improve the rate of service use (Solanki and Schauffler, 1999; Solanki et al., 2000). Employer benefits managers informed of the effectiveness of cancer prevention services might be motivated to obtain more comprehensive coverage for their employees.

Just as preventive services of proven effectiveness should be covered under insurance plans, services for which evidence of benefit is lacking should be excluded from coverage. Population-based or routine screening of smokers for lung cancer using spiral or helical computed tomography (CT) scans, for example, does not presently meet standards of evidence to support their coverage under health insurance plans.

Employers can provide coverage for preventive services as part of their insurance benefit packages, give discounts to employees who choose plans with more extensive prevention services, and can create financial incentives for health plans to meet performance goals. Employers can also support wellness and physical fitness programs either through on-site facilities or through employee discounts to local gymnasiums or fitness programs.

Recommendation 5: The U.S. Congress should increase support for programs that provide primary care to uninsured and low-income people (e.g., Community and Migrant Health Centers and family planning programs of Title X of the Public Health Service Act). These programs increase the use of cancer prevention and early detection services among medically underserved populations.

A pervasive problem in the United States is poor access to health care because of a lack of health insurance. People with health insurance are more likely to have a primary care provider and to have received appropriate preventive care such as recent cancer screening tests. In 2001, an estimated 15 percent of the U.S. population (41.2 million individuals) was uninsured during the entire year (U.S. Census Bureau, 2002). Many others are underinsured, with poor coverage for interventions that have been proven to be effective, such as smoking cessation counseling and products.

Individuals who are uninsured (or underinsured) rely on a patchwork of public and private programs for primary care (IOM, 2000d). Community and Migrant Health Centers and Title X family planning clinics are vital sources of primary health care and are important providers of cancer prevention and early detection services. Full support for these programs enhances the nation's health care safety net and at the same time extends the availability of cancer prevention and early detection services to vulnerable populations. Even with increased program support, however, many people would likely remain underserved, given the fragmented and limited nature of the nation's health care safety net.

Recommendation 6: Support for the Centers for Disease Control and Prevention's National Breast and Cervical Cancer Early Detection Program should be increased so that the program can reach all uninsured women using innovative delivery strategies. Support is also needed for a similar program at the CDC to provide screening for colorectal cancer for uninsured and low-income men and women.

Underfunding of CDC's National Breast and Cervical Cancer Early Detection Program (NBCCEDP) contributes to lost opportunities for prevention. NBCCEDP has succeeded in improving screening rates among medically underserved populations, but the program reaches only 15 percent of eligible women because of limited financial support. This is especially unfortunate insofar as racial, ethnic, and socioeconomic disparities in cancer mortality can often be traced to under-use of screening services.

Because screening for colorectal cancer is also a proven strategy for reducing cancer mortality in people over 50 years of age, a similar program is needed to provide colorectal cancer screening to people who are uninsured and underinsured. The majority of individuals eligible for colorectal screening have not been screened, and screening rates are particularly low among minority and low-income populations.

Recommendation 7: The U.S. Department of Health and Human Services should complete a comprehensive review to assess whether evidence-based prevention services are being offered and successfully delivered in federal health programs.

The federal government administers or funds Medicare; Medicaid; the Health Resources and Services Administration's Community and Migrant Health Centers; Title X family planning clinics; the U.S. Department of Agriculture's programs such as the Special Supplemental Nutrition Program for Women, Infants, and Children; the Indian Health Service; U.S. Department of Defense health programs; and Federal Employees Health Benefits Program. These programs do not always reflect best practices in cancer prevention and early detection.

The Medicare program, for example, does not cover any costs for smoking cessation treatment, and two-thirds of state Medicaid programs cover such treatments (Schauffler et al., 2001a). The lack of coverage for effective prevention services in public programs introduces a significant barrier to those most burdened by cancer: the uninsured population and members of racial and ethnic minority groups who often depend on federal programs for care.

Evidence-based prevention services should be available in these and other public programs. Therefore, a comprehensive review of the benefits being offered and the effectiveness of delivery systems is needed to identify opportunities to improve access to cancer prevention and early detection services in federal programs.

Recommendation 8: Programs are needed for health care providers to improve their education and training, monitor their adherence to evidence-based guidelines, and enhance their practice environments to support their provision of cancer prevention and early detection services.

Primary care providers in health care settings are effective agents of behavioral change. When counseled about smoking in clinical settings, 5 to 10 percent of individuals are able to quit. Evidence suggests, however, that physicians and other practitioners are not providing effective clinical interventions such as counseling and screening tests as often as would be beneficial. Fewer than half of adults who smoke cigarettes, for example, report that at their last visit the physician inquired whether they smoked.

Shortcomings in providers' delivery of clinical preventive services can, in part, be traced to a lack of education and training. Strategies for improving education and training include:

- Professional education and training programs should adequately cover cancer prevention and early detection in their curricula.
- Training institutions and professional organizations should provide continuing education in cancer prevention and early detection. Continuing medical education programs can be made more accessible by applying new learning technologies (e.g., distance learning and online continuing medical education).
- Professional organizations representing primary care providers should promote their members' adherence to evidence-based cancer prevention and early detection guidelines.

Systems of health care depend on supportive management structures; efficient patient-flow procedures; and information systems that support reminder systems, documentation of services, timely follow-up and referrals, and coordinated communication with providers and institutions across the community. Evidence consistently shows that such support systems improve physician and patient compliance with recommended preventive practices.

- Health systems should support the infrastructure needed to identify patients in need of intervention (e.g., smokers or those who are due for screening), remind providers to intervene, and track progress toward clinical goals.

Efforts to improve the quality of health care delivery have increasingly relied on monitoring the performance of health care providers and systems of care. There are many opportunities to monitor performance and assist providers in improving their practices:

- CMS could examine provider performance regarding adherence to recommended cancer prevention and early detection recommendations. CMS has specified in the most recent scope of work for Quality Improvement Organizations that the quality of breast cancer services is a priority area. Assessments of provider adherence to mammography guidelines could be undertaken.
- State health departments could use data from cancer registries to examine regions and population subgroups characterized by high rates of late-stage diagnoses of breast, cervical, and colorectal cancer, for which screening programs are available, to identify where to target outreach efforts.

- The National Committee for Quality Assurance could expand efforts to monitor preventive practices of managed care plans through its Health Plan Employer Data and Information Set system.
- Employers and other group benefit managers could define performance targets for health education and preventive counseling to hold health plans accountable for the provision of these services (Schauffler et al., 1999; Schauffler and Rodriguez, 1996).
- The Joint Commission on the Accreditation of Healthcare Organizations could evaluate the availability of services to promote risk behavior change as part of its accreditation process.

The aging of the nation's population will sharply increase the demand for certain cancer prevention services such as colorectal screening and mammography, and impending shortages of trained personnel have been predicted. If such shortages are anticipated, policies to address them will need to be identified.

- The Health Resources and Services Administration should assess the adequacy of the future supply of providers of cancer prevention and early detection services.

There is convincing evidence that nonphysician providers are just as effective as physician providers in delivering certain smoking cessation and screening services, but research is needed on how to integrate provision of prevention services by such providers into routine primary care.

- The Agency for Healthcare Research and Quality and other research sponsors should support demonstration programs to evaluate innovative models of prevention service delivery.

Recommendation 9: The U.S. Congress should provide sufficient support to the U.S. Department of Health and Human Services for the U.S. Preventive Services Task Force and the U.S. Task Force on Community Preventive Services to conduct timely assessments of the benefits, harms, and costs associated with screening tests and other preventive interventions. Summaries of recommendations should be made widely available to the public, health care providers, and state and local public health officials and policy makers.

Evidence-based guidelines for clinical and community practice provide maps for action. Two task forces provide rigorous assessments of the effectiveness of preventive services.

The U.S. Preventive Services Task Force, overseen by the Agency for Healthcare Research and Quality, has provided comprehensive assessments of clinical prevention services. Until recently, it has been convened only periodically. In 2001 the task force published selected updates of recommendations made in 1996 (U.S. Preventive Services Task Force, 2001a,b, 2002). Assessments of prevention services are needed on a continual basis to ensure that public health recommendations incorporate the latest scientific evidence.

The U.S. Community Services Task Force, overseen by CDC, is relatively new and has the responsibility to identify interventions that work for communities. As state efforts to implement comprehensive cancer control plans gain momentum, guidance on the effectiveness of public health interventions will be critically needed.

The Board recommends that support for both task forces be sufficient for systematic syntheses and meta-analyses of data from the literature and to keep abreast of developments in both clinical and community disease prevention and health promotion. Greater investments in dissemination activities are also needed to reach health providers and the general public, both about areas of consensus among public health scientists regarding interventions that work, and about the areas of controversy that remain.

There are examples of screening and other prevention interventions that were quickly adopted before adequate research had been completed to fully understand their potential benefits and harms. Screening for prostate cancer by prostate-specific antigen testing, for example, for which there is comparatively little evidence of effectiveness, is more commonly used than colorectal cancer screening, for which there is strong evidence of effectiveness. More recently, low-dose computed tomography scanning has been promoted as a screening test for lung cancer among high-risk individuals, with the scientific community divided on the merits of its effectiveness. It will be years before the results of clinical trials are available to answer questions about the test's effectiveness. These two task forces can provide clear information on the potential benefits, harms, and costs of new technologies so that consumers and health care providers can make informed judgments.

Recommendation 10: Public and private organizations (e.g., the National Cancer Institute, the American Cancer Society) should take steps to improve the public's understanding of cancer prevention and early detection with a focus on promoting healthy lifestyles and informed decision making about health behaviors and cancer screening.

Raising public awareness of the benefits of cancer prevention and early detection is central to reducing the cancer burden. One barrier to effective communication is the contradictory and sometimes questionable research reported by the media.

The public's thirst for quick medical "miracles" and simple impatience also pose significant barriers to progress in cancer prevention and early detection. It can take many years to reap the benefits of behavioral change like smoking cessation. Significant reductions in breast cancer mortality rates as a result of screening programs have only recently been observed in the general population. The fascination of the American public with advanced technology and "getting tested," the commercial and marketing interests in servicing this demand, and the sense of urgency to take action in combating cancer set the stage for the premature adoption of interventions that are potentially ineffective or harmful.

Increasingly, cancer screening guidelines incorporate the tenets of informed decision making. Rather than issuing prescriptive recommendations regarding prostate-specific antigen testing, for example, most organizations are suggesting that individuals discuss the relative benefits and harms of screening, weigh these factors according to their individual values and preferences, and decide whether or not to proceed with screening. Although this shared decision-making approach tends to be embraced by the well-educated health consumer, little is known regarding its acceptance among the general public and how best to incorporate it into the delivery of preventive services.

Improved understanding of cancer prevention by the general public is also critical to support for research in this area. Although the public is generally supportive of clinical medical innovation, it has less of an appreciation of the potential of public health interventions.

Recommendation 11: Public and private initiatives to reduce disparities in the cancer burden (e.g., initiatives of the National Cancer Institute and the American Cancer Society) should be supported.

There are glaring disparities in rates of morbidity and mortality from cancer among socioeconomic groups, insured and uninsured populations, and certain racial and ethnic groups (IOM, 1999b). The differences among these groups present both a challenge to understand the reasons and an opportunity to reduce the burden of cancer (U.S. Department of Health and Human Services and Office of Disease Prevention and Health Promotion, 2000). Lack of health insurance coverage is a key predictor of lower rates of use of cancer screening tests. Personal barriers can include cultural differences, language barriers, not knowing how or when to seek care, or concerns about confidentiality or discrimination (U.S. Department of Health and Human Services and Office of Disease Prevention and Health Promotion, 2000). In a nation of increasing diversity, interventions to improve cancer prevention and early detection must accommodate different languages, cultural values, and beliefs.

The elimination of racial and ethnic disparities in health is an overarching goal of *Healthy People 2010* (U.S. Department of Health and Human Services and Office of Disease Prevention and Health Promotion, 2000), and cancer screening and management is one of six focus areas of an ongoing initiative involving agencies of the U.S. Department of Health and Human Services (http://raceandhealth.hhs.gov/sidebars/sbinitOver.htm). The National Institutes of Health (NIH) has drafted a trans-NIH, 5-year Strategic Research Plan to Reduce and Ultimately Eliminate Health Disparities (www.nih.gov/about/hd/strategicplan.pdf), and in December 2000 the National Cancer Institute (NCI) established the Center to Reduce Cancer Health Disparities (http://crchd.nci.nih.gov) to implement the NCI Strategic Plan to Reduce Health Disparities. The Board fully supports this NCI initiative and encourages NCI to collaborate with other private and public efforts to achieve success. Also needed are effective methods to evaluate and track the success of this and other initiatives.

Recommendation 12: Public and private sponsors of research including the National Institutes of Health, the Agency for Healthcare Research and Quality, the Centers for Medicare and Medicaid Services, the Centers for Disease Control and Prevention, the U.S. Department of Defense, and the American Cancer Society should expand their support of applied behavioral research and how best to disseminate evidence-based prevention interventions. Effective strategies are especially needed to encourage healthy behaviors among children and their families, medically underserved populations, and the public at large through multicomponent interventions.

The United States is at a crossroads in cancer prevention research. Basic science and epidemiology are advancing knowledge in a number of areas, from the relationship between cancer and modifiable behavioral risk factors all the way down to the molecular pathways that mediate the actions of those risk factors. At the same time applied research is illustrating how the already vast amount of available evidence can be better used to more rapidly reduce cancer rates. To effectively reduce the cancer burden in the United States, however, there needs to be greater emphasis on action-oriented research (Colditz, 1997, 2001; Wegman, 1992). Knowledge about health problems and their causes does not automatically guarantee that appropriate actions are taken. Only when etiological knowledge is linked to evidence on the sustained effectiveness of behavioral change strategies, and in turn to public awareness and policy support, can the potential to reduce the burden of cancer be realized.

1

Introduction

Imagine opening your morning paper and seeing the headline "Interventions Succeed in Preventing 100,000 Cancer Cases and 60,000 Cancer Deaths Each Year." Reading further, you learn not only that lives had been saved from cancer but also that remarkable gains had been made in reducing heart disease, diabetes, and other major health threats. Such a promising headline is within reach because prevention interventions are available today that can sharply reduce the future burden of cancer and, at the same time, reduce the risk for other chronic diseases. This report of the National Cancer Policy Board reviews the evidence that such a dramatic impact is possible and calls for a national strategy to ensure that the promise of cancer prevention and early detection is realized.

The National Cancer Policy Board was established in March 1997, at the Institute of Medicine (IOM) and National Research Council to address issues that arise in the prevention, control, diagnosis, treatment, and palliation of cancer. The 21-member Board includes consumers, health care providers, and investigators in several disciplines. In this report, the Board addresses four questions:

1. What lifestyle and health care behaviors contribute to the burden of cancer?
2. What share of new cases of cancer and cancer deaths could be prevented with changes in lifestyle and health care behaviors?
3. What interventions work to bring about health-enhancing behavioral change?

4. What steps can be taken to overcome barriers to using effective interventions and to improve what is known about cancer prevention and early detection?

In the preparation of this report, the Board listened to presentations made by representatives of federal agencies at its quarterly meetings and commissioned six background papers on cancer prevention and early detection.[1] Several of the report's chapters were based on these commissioned papers. The six papers and their authors are as follows:

- Quantifying the Contribution of Risk Factors to Cancer Incidence and the Estimated Reduction in Cancer Burden Through Selected Risk Factor Modifications, Graham A. Colditz, Catherine Tomeo Ryan, Charles H. Dart III, Geetanjali Datta, Laurie Fisher, and Beverly Rockhill
- Interventions to Promote Key Behaviors in Cancer Prevention and Early Detection, Edwin B. Fisher, Ross C. Brownson, Amy A. Eyler, Debra L. Haire-Joshu, and Mario Schootman
- Interventions to Reduce Obesity and Maintain a Healthy Weight, Suzanne Phelan and Rena R. Wing
- The Effectiveness of Screening for Cancer and Its Unfulfilled Potential in the United States: A Review of the Evidence, Steven H. Woolf
- Fulfilling the Potential of Lung Cancer Prevention and Early Detection. What Are the Implications of Adopting New Technologies in the Face of Uncertain Science? Parthiv J. Mahadevia, Farin Kamangar, and Jonathan M. Samet
- Provider, System, and Policy Strategies to Enhance the Delivery of Cancer Prevention and Control Activities in Primary Care, Judith Ockene, Jane Zapka, Lori Pbert, Suzanne Brodney, and Stephenie Lemon

The Board has also drawn on its previous work on tobacco control (IOM, 1998, 2000a) and has benefited from other recent IOM reports relating to behavior and health (IOM, 2001a,b, 2000b,c, 1999a,b) and by prevention-related reports of the President's Cancer Panel (President's Cancer Panel, 1998, 1994).

FRAMEWORK OF THE REPORT

The Board chose to focus its attention on opportunities to fulfill the potential of cancer prevention and early detection in light of current epidemiological knowledge and evidence regarding the effectiveness of interven-

[1]Copies of the commissioned papers are available at the National Cancer Policy Board website, www.IOM.edu/ncpb.

tions to reduce cancer risk. The Board recognized that a number of personal behaviors are known to contribute to the burden of cancer but limited its review of primary prevention to tobacco use, physical activity, obesity, diet, and alcohol use. Examples of behaviors known to contribute to cancer risk but not considered in this review include exposure to sun, and exposure to cancer-causing viruses through sexual activity (e.g., human papillomavirus) and blood contacts such as intravenous drug use (e.g., hepatitis B virus). The Board elected to focus on factors that are risks for common cancers and that also have a large impact on the incidence of other major diseases, including cardiovascular disease, stroke, diabetes, and osteoporosis. Other important areas of prevention, for example, chemoprevention, were excluded from this report, but will likely be the subject of future Board work. Cancer screening modalities are reviewed in some detail and a case study on lung cancer screening is presented to illustrate issues related to adoption of new, yet unproven, technology. As described in detail below, the report's chapters provide reviews of the evidence regarding the associations between the selected health behaviors and cancer, interventions to bring about improvements in health behaviors, and opportunities to improve the delivery of preventive services and improve population health.

Chapter 2 examines estimates of the reductions of cancer incidence and mortality rates that are achievable through major favorable shifts in the distribution of modifiable risk factors in the U.S. population such as smoking, physical activity, and dietary practices and through increased rates of adherence to cancer screening recommendations.

Chapter 3 summarizes evidence regarding the links between the following five lifestyle behaviors and cancer: tobacco use, physical inactivity, overweight and obesity, poor diet, and alcohol use.

Chapter 4 examines how individual behaviors can be changed through direct services or via community-based approaches such as worksite- or school-based programs or public education campaigns. The chapter also reviews current evidence on the effectiveness of behavioral and educational interventions to promote four key behaviors in cancer prevention: nonsmoking, healthy diet, physical activity, and healthy weight.

Chapter 5 reviews the principles of assessing the effectiveness of screening for cancer and summarizes evidence of the effectiveness of screening for colorectal cancer, breast cancer, prostate cancer, and cervical cancer.

Chapter 6 identifies challenges inherent in systems of care and interventions to improve the rates of participation in cancer screening programs.

Chapter 7 presents a case study on screening for lung cancer to illustrate the dilemma of decision making in the face of uncertain science.

Chapter 8 reviews the status of professional education and training in cancer prevention and early detection with a focus on primary care providers.

Chapter 9 describes selected federal programs that support cancer prevention and early detection through the development of national objectives and guidelines, information dissemination, surveillance, facilitation of statewide program planning and evaluation, and provision and payment for services.

Chapter 10 surveys ongoing health services research that addresses cancer prevention and early detection and that is sponsored by selected federal agencies and private organizations.

Chapter 11 summarizes the key findings and presents the Board's recommendations for action by the U.S. Congress, the states, health care providers and systems of care, and the public at large.

This chapter provides background information on the burden of cancer and defines the terms cancer prevention and early detection as used in this report.

THE BURDEN OF CANCER

Cancer ranks second only to heart disease as the leading cause of death in the United States (Table 1.1) (Anderson, 2001). The rates of death from cancer began to fall in the U.S. about 10 years ago (Figures 1.1 and 1.2), but

TABLE 1.1 Deaths and Percent of Total Deaths for Leading Causes of Death by Sex: United States, 1999

	Males			Females		
Cause of death	Rank[a]	Deaths	% of total deaths	Rank[a]	Deaths	% of total deaths
All causes	—	1,175,460	100.0	—	1,215,939	100.0
Diseases of heart	1	351,617	29.9	1	373,575	30.7
Malignant neoplasms	2	285,832	24.3	2	264,006	21.7
Cerebrovascular diseases	3	64,485	5.5	3	102,881	8.5
Accidents (unintentional injuries)	4	63,535	5.4	7	34,325	2.8
Chronic lower respiratory diseases	5	62,415	5.3	4	61,766	5.1
Diabetes mellitus	6	31,150	2.7	5	37,249	3.1
Influenza and pneumonia	7	27,718	2.4	6	36,012	3.0
Intentional self-harm (suicide)	8	23,458	2.0	—	5,741	0.5
Chronic liver disease and cirrhosis	9	17,115	1.5	—	9,144	0.8
Nephritis, nephrotic syndrome and nephrosis	10	17,016	1.4	9	18,509	1.5
Alzheimer's disease	—	13,391	1.1	8	31,145	2.6
Septicemia	—	13,395	1.1	10	17,285	1.4

[a]Rank based on number of deaths.
— Category not applicable.
SOURCE: Anderson (2001).

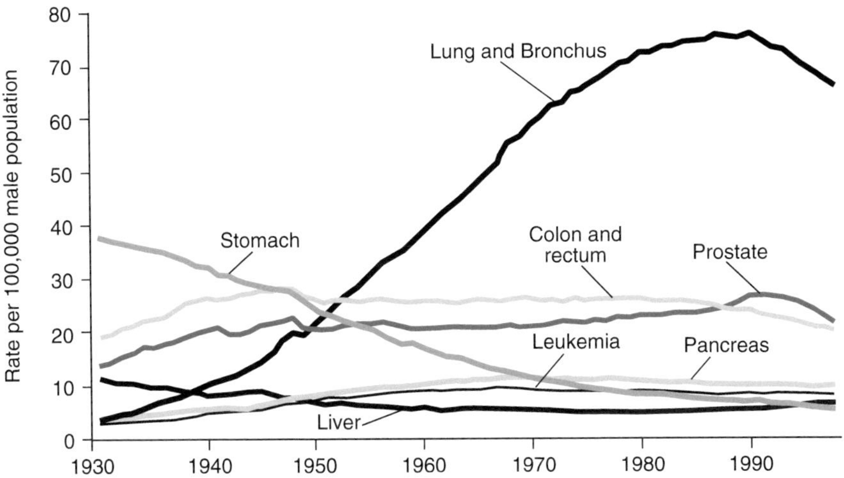

FIGURE 1.1 Age-adjusted cancer death rates,* for males by site, U.S. 1930–1997.
*Per 100,000, age-adjusted to the 1970 standard population.
NOTE: Due to changes in ICD coding, numerator information has changed over time. Rates for cancers of the liver, lung and bronchus, and colon and rectum are affected by these coding changes. Data obtained from U.S. Mortality Public Use Data Tapes 1960–1968, U.S. Mortality Volumes 1930–1959, National Center for Health Statistics, Centers for Disease Control and Prevention, 2000.
SOURCE: ACS, 2002a.

cancers still account for 23 percent of all deaths in this country (Anderson, 2001). In 2002 cancers claimed the lives of an estimated 555,500 Americans (ACS, 2002a) (Table 1.2). For every 100,000 persons in the United States, cancer claims an estimated 1,747 years of life before age 75 (National Center for Health Statistics, 2001). Estimates are that, on average, each individual who dies of cancer loses 15 years of expected life (Ries et al., 2002).

As demonstrated in Table 1.2, in 2002 lung, breast, prostate, and colon cancer accounted for roughly half of all new cancer cases and half of all deaths due to cancer (ACS, 2002a). Accordingly, the burden due to these four cancers must be reduced if total cancer incidence and mortality rates are to be affected.

The lifetime probability[2] of developing cancer is 43 percent for males

[2]Lifetime probability is a statistical estimate of being diagnosed with a specified cancer during an individual's lifetime, expressed as percent. It is derived by summing all cancer cases from age 0 through 95+ and dividing by 100,000 × 100 (expressed as percent) (ACS, 2002a).

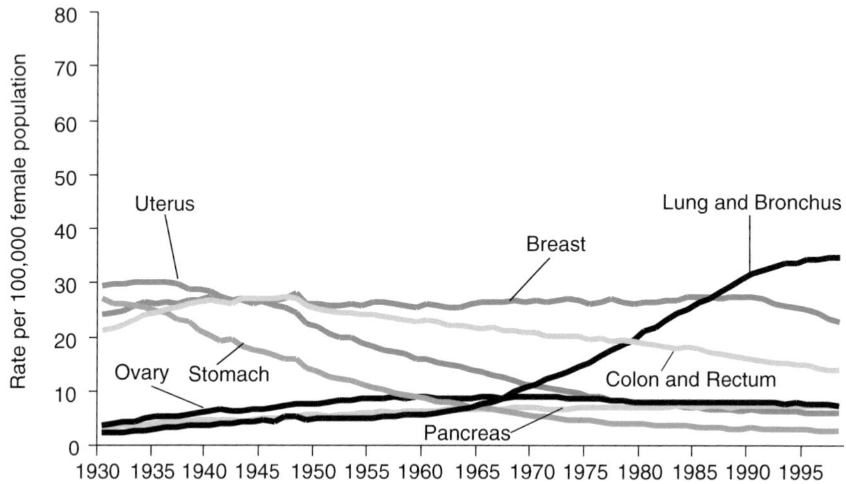

FIGURE 1.2 Age-adjusted cancer death rates,* for females by site, U.S. 1930–1997.
*Per 100,000, age-adjusted to the 1970 standard population.
NOTE: Due to changes in ICD coding, numerator information has changed over time. Rates for cancers of the liver, lung and bronchus, and colon and rectum are affected by these coding changes. Data obtained from U.S. Mortality Public Use Data Tapes 1960–1968, U.S. Mortality Volumes 1930–1959, National Center for Health Statistics, Centers for Disease Control and Prevention, 2000.
SOURCE: ACS, 2002a.

and 38 percent for females (ACS, 2002a). The stresses that cancer imposes on society and the health care system are formidable. The American Cancer Society estimates that 1.3 million new cases of invasive cancer were diagnosed in 2002 (Table 1.2) (ACS, 2002a). Each year, the United States spends an estimated $56.4 billion in direct medical costs caring for patients with this disease. In addition, there is an estimated $100.3 billion cost associated with lost productivity due to illness or premature death (ACS, 2002a).

The estimated 8.9 million Americans alive today with cancer (Ries et al., 2000b) suffer considerable morbidity as well as risk for premature mortality. Both the disease itself and its treatment can diminish quality of life. Patients may be burdened with pain and other physical symptoms, anxiety and depression, decreased functional status, disrupted life routines, impaired well-being, disability, overwhelming medical bills, and the many ordeals of obtaining treatment. Family members, friends, and other caregivers who aid in the coping process may also suffer from the disease. Cancer is thus an affliction that touches the lives of most Americans.

Certain members of the population face a disproportionate burden

TABLE 1.2 Estimated Number of New Cancer Cases and Cancer Deaths in the United States, 2002

Cancer Site or Type	New Cases	Deaths
Total	1,284,900	555,500
Lung and bronchus	169,400	154,900
Colon and rectum	148,300	56,600
Breast	205,000	40,000
Prostate	189,000	30,200
Pancreas	30,300	29,700
Non-Hodgkin's lymphoma	53,900	24,400
Leukemia	30,800	21,700
Liver and intrahepatic duct	16,600	14,100
Ovary	23,300	13,900
Brain and other nervous system	17,000	13,100
Stomach	21,600	12,400
Esophagus	13,100	12,600
Urinary bladder	56,500	12,600
Kidney and renal pelvis	31,800	11,600
Multiple myeloma	14,600	10,800
Melanoma, skin	53,600	7,400
Uterine corpus	39,300	6,600
Uterine cervix	13,000	4,100
Soft tissue (including heart)	8,300	3,900
Larynx	8,900	3,700
Gallbladder and other biliary tract	7,100	3,500
Mouth	9,800	2,000
Pharynx	8,600	2,100
Other nonepithelial skin	4,700	2,200
Tongue	7,100	1,700
Other oral cavity	3,400	1,600
Other digestive organs	4,400	1,800
Bones and joints	2,400	1,300
Thyroid	20,700	1,300
Hodgkin's disease	7,000	1,400
Small intestine	5,300	1,100
Other respiratory organs	4,900	2,800
Other endocrine system	2,000	1,000
Vulva	3,800	800
Vagina and other genital, female	2,000	800
Anus, anal canal, anorectum	3,900	500
Ureter and other urinary organs	2,400	700
Testis	7,500	400
Penis and other genital, male	1,200	200
Eye and orbit	2,200	200
Other and unspecified primary sites	30,200	43,700

NOTE: Data obtained from NCI's SEER program, 1979–1998. Incidence mortality data obtained from the National Center for Health Statistics.
SOURCE: Adapted from ACS, 2002a.

from cancer. The incidence of most cancers increases with age, making elderly individuals the group most burdened by cancer. The majority (58 percent) of new cases of cancer occur among those age 65 and older (Ries et al., 2002). For women the risk of dying from cancer is increasing, mainly because of the increasing incidence of lung cancer among women.

Cancer is the leading cause of death among women ages 35 to 64 (National Center for Health Statistics, 2001). Like age and sex, family history is another risk factor that cannot be modified but that is an important indicator of increased susceptibility.

Cancer incidence is correlated with adverse socioeconomic conditions, which affect the lives of many Americans. In the United States, people are more likely to die from cancer if they are poor, have limited education, or both. For example, the probability that a 65-year-old man will die from lung cancer is 547.9/100,000 if his annual family income is less than $10,000, but the risk decreases to 273.6/100,000 if his annual family income exceeds $25,000 (National Center for Health Statistics, 1998). Certain racial and ethnic groups in the United States, African Americans in particular, are at substantially higher risk for cancer (Table 1.3).

There are many differences in host susceptibility, lifestyle, the environment, and health modifiers that are independently associated with each of these demographic factors, and the complex interrelationships among these factors have not been fully described to account for the racial and ethnic disparities in cancer risk (Berkman and Kawachi, 2000).

African Americans are more likely than the rest of the population to suffer morbidity and die from cancer (Table 1.3). The rate of mortality from cancer among African Americans is 33 percent greater than that among whites (218.2/100,000 and 164.5/100,000, respectively) (ACS, 2002a). The fact that health outcomes are worse in certain populations also has multifaceted explanations, some of which include documented disparities in access to and the quality of health care (Berkman and Kawachi, 2000; Smith, 1998). For certain populations cancers are more advanced at diagnosis, partly because the individuals in those populations have less exposure to screening services, as documented later in this report. African Americans are less likely than whites to be diagnosed with cancer at a localized stage and, for each stage of diagnosis for almost every cancer, African Americans have lower 5-year survival rates than whites (Table 1.4) (Greenlee et al., 2001; Ries et al., 2000a). The failings of the health care system are only part of the explanation for these disparities. Personal health behaviors, biological factors, adherence to treatment, and a complex sociological and environmental milieu are interwoven factors contributing to morbidity and death from cancer.

Cancer is characterized by abnormal cell growth; but it is really more than 100 different diseases, each with a unique profile in terms of the

TABLE 1.3 Incidence and Mortality Rates[a] by Site, Race, and Ethnicity, United States, 1992–1998

Incidence	White	Black	Asian/Pacific Islander	American Indian	Hispanic[b]
All Sites					
Males	470.4	596.8	327.7	227.7	319.7
Females	354.4	337.6	252.1	186.3	237.7
Total	401.4	445.3	283.4	202.7	270.0
Breast (female)	115.5	101.5	78.1	50.5	68.5
Colon & rectum					
Males	51.4	57.7	47.3	33.5	35.2
Females	36.3	44.7	31.0	24.6	23.2
Total	42.9	50.1	38.2	28.6	28.4
Lung & Bronchus					
Males	69.6	107/2	51.9	44.3	36.0
Females	43.6	45.7	22.7	20.6	18.7
Total	54.7	71.6	35.5	31.0	26.0
Prostate	144.6	234.0	82.8	47.8	103.4

Mortality	White	Black	Asian/Pacific Islander	American Indian	Hispanic[b]
All Sites					
Males	203.2	297.7	125.6	125.3	128.8
Females	138.0	166.6	82.4	90.8	84.3
Total	164.5	218.2	101.2	105.4	102.6
Breast (female)	24.3	31.0	11.0	12.4	14.8
Colon & rectum					
Males	20.6	27.3	12.9	11.9	13.0
Females	13.9	19.6	8.9	8.9	8.0
Total	16.8	22.8	10.7	10.3	10.2
Lung & Bronchus					
Males	67.8	96.2	33.8	41.8	30.5
Females	34.6	33.6	15.1	20.9	10.9
Total	48.8	59.1	23.3	30.1	19.3
Prostate	22.4	53.1	9.8	14.0	15.9

[a]Per 100,000, age-adjusted to the 1970 U.S. standard population.
[b]Hispanic is not mutually exclusive from white, black, Asian/Pacific Islanders, and American Indian.
NOTE: Incidence data are from NCIS 11 SEER areas; mortality data are from the National Cancer Center for Health Statistics and include all states, except data for Hispanics. Data for Hispanics include deaths that occurred in all states except Connecticut, Louisiana, New Hampshire, and Oklahoma.
SOURCE: ACS, 2002a.

population at risk, symptoms, and prognosis. As cancers of the lung, breast, prostate, and colon together make up more than half of all new cancer cases, they are important targets for prevention. Invasive cervical cancer is a less common cancer among women, in large part because of the application of effective screening programs (NIH, 1996).

TABLE 1.4 Five-Year Relative Survival Rates, by Racial or Ethnic Group and Stage at Diagnosis, United States, 1989–1996

Cancer Site or Type and Racial or Ethnic Group	Five-Year Relative Survival Rate (percent) for the Following Stage at Diagnosis: Localized	Regional	Distant
Breast (female)			
White	97	79	22
African American	89	64	15
Colon and rectum			
White	91	66	9
African American	84	59	7
Esophagus			
White	28	12	2
African American	14	12	2
Lung and bronchus			
White	49	21	2
African American	42	16	2
Melanoma of the skin			
White	96	59	13
African American	95	35	Not calculated
Oral cavity and pharynx			
White	82	45	23
African American	73	29	16
Ovary			
White	95	79	28
African American	91	76	25
Pancreas			
White	17	7	1
African American	17	6	1
Prostate			
White	100	Not calculated	32
African American	98	Not calculated	30
Stomach			
White	56	19	2
African American	58	25	3
Urinary bladder			
White	94	49	7
African American	87	41	0
Uterine cervix			
White	92	50	15
African American	86	37	7
Uterine corpus			
White	97	66	29
African American	81	41	13

NOTE: Based on data from cancer registries of NCI's SEER program.
SOURCE: Greenlee et al. (2001).

Lung Cancer

After deaths due to heart disease and stroke, cancer of the lung and bronchus is the third leading cause of death in the United States and is the leading cause of cancer deaths (National Center for Health Statistics, 1998), estimated to claim 154,900 lives in 2002 (ACS, 2002a). With 169,400 new cases expected in 2002, cancer of the lung and bronchus is also the third most common cancer, following prostate cancer in men and breast cancer in women. Lung cancer has one of the poorest prognoses of all cancers, with a 5-year survival rate of only 14 percent (Ries et al., 2000a). The lifetime probability of developing lung cancer is 1 in 12 for males and 1 in 17 for females. Lung cancer trends have followed tobacco use trends by 10 to 20 years. The incidence of lung cancer in males began to decline in the 1980s, but the rate has been increasing in females, only recently beginning to stabilize, a trend attributed to past increased rates of tobacco use by women. These tragic consequences of tobacco use among women were first manifest in 1987, when lung cancer replaced breast cancer as the leading cause of cancer deaths in women, now accounting for an estimated 25 percent of cancer deaths in females (ACS, 2002a). Most lung cancer deaths (87 percent) can be attributed to tobacco use (ACS, 2002b).

As noted earlier, the rate of mortality from lung cancer is higher in low-income persons (National Center for Health Statistics, 1998). The incidence of cancer of the lung and bronchus is considerably higher in African Americans (71.6/100,000) than in whites (54.7/100,000), as are mortality rates from cancer of the lung and bronchus (59.1/100,000 versus 48.8/100,000, respectively). Hispanics, Asians and Pacific Islanders, and American Indians have lower incidences of lung cancer and lower rates of mortality from lung cancer than African Americans and whites (Table 1.3) (ACS, 2002a).

Breast Cancer

Breast cancer is the most commonly diagnosed cancer in women, accounting for an estimated 203,500 new cases in 2002, or about 31 percent of all new cancers in women. The lifetime probability of developing breast cancer is 1 in 8. An estimated 39,600 women died of breast cancer in 2002 (ACS, 2002a).

The risk of breast cancer increases with age and a family history of breast cancer. Up to 20 percent of women in the general population have a family history of breast cancer, but less than 5 percent of women are at high risk for hereditary breast cancer syndromes (Warner et al., 1999). A variety of susceptibility genes, the most well known being *BRCA1* and *BRCA2*, substantially increase the risk of developing breast cancer, but such mutations occur in a relatively small proportion of the general population.

Women who carry mutations in these genes face a 48 to 74 percent probability of developing breast cancer by age 80 (Anglian Breast Cancer Study Group, 2000). Other risk factors include a personal history of breast cancer, biopsy-confirmed atypical hyperplasia, a long menstrual history (menstrual periods that started early and ended late in life), nulliparity or having a first child after age 30, postmenopausal obesity, and higher socioeconomic status. Use of oral contraceptives, prolonged use of hormone replacement therapy, and increased alcohol intake have also been suggested as risk factors for breast cancer. Although breast cancer is more common in white women (115.5/100,000) than in African-American women (101.5/100,000), the mortality rate is lower for white women (24.3/100,000) than for African-American women (31.0/100,000) (Table 1.3) (ACS, 2002a).

Prostate Cancer

Prostate cancer is the most common cancer among men in the United States (excluding basal and squamous cell skin cancer), accounting for 189,000 new cases in 2002, or approximately 30 percent of all newly diagnosed cancers in men. The lifetime probability of developing prostate cancer is 1 in 6. The incidence of prostate cancer increased sharply from 1988 to 1992, a phenomenon attributed to increased rates of screening (Potosky et al., 1995), but the incidence has declined in subsequent years (ACS, 2002a). An estimated 30,200 men are expected to die of prostate cancer in 2002, making it the second most common cause of death from cancer in men (ACS, 2002a).

The risk of prostate cancer increases with age. More than 70 percent of diagnoses occur after age 65. A family history of prostate cancer modestly increases risk (ACS, 2002a). Prostate cancer is considerably more common in African-American men (234.2/100,000) than in white men (144.6/100,000), and is less common in Hispanics (103.4/100,000), Asians and Pacific Islanders (82.8/100,000), and Native Americans (47.8/100,000) (Table 1.3). African Americans have the highest prostate cancer incidence rates and death rates in the world (Parkin et al., 1997). Similar disparities exist with regard to the rate of mortality from prostate cancer (Table 1.3) (ACS, 2002a).

Colorectal Cancer

Colorectal cancer is the third most common cancer in the United States, accounting for an estimated 148,300 new cases in 2002. The lifetime probability of developing colorectal cancer is 1 in 17 for men and 1 in 18 for women. The disease is more common in African Americans than whites. Between 1992 and 1998, the incidence rate of colon cancer was approximately 42.9/100,000 in whites and 50.1/100,000 in African Americans (ACS, 2002a).

The American Cancer Society estimates that 56,600 Americans died of colorectal cancer in 2002, making it the second most common cause of death from cancer. Rates of mortality from colorectal cancer are higher for African Americans (22.8/100,000) and whites (16.8/100,00) than for Hispanics, Asians and Pacific Islanders, and Native Americans (10.2 to 10.7/100,000) (Table 1.3) (Greenlee et al., 2001).

A personal history of colorectal polyps, or chronic inflammatory bowel disease, or a family history of hereditary colorectal cancer syndrome place individuals at higher risk for colorectal cancer (ACS, 2002a). Approximately 90 percent of all colorectal cancer cases and deaths are thought to be preventable, through dietary or other lifestyle changes in conjunction with screening (ACS, 2002a).

Cervical Cancer

Decades ago, cervical cancer was a common cause of death from cancer, but the mortality rate has fallen significantly: 40 percent since 1973 (Agency for Health Care Policy and Research, 1999), a trend largely attributed to routine screening for cervical cancer by cytological examination (Pap smear). Nonetheless, an estimate of 13,000 new cases of invasive cervical cancer occurred in 2002 (ACS, 2002a). The lifetime probability of developing cervical cancer is 1 in 117. Largely through successes in early detection and treatment, cervical cancer currently accounts for only 2 percent of cancer deaths in women, with 4,100 deaths from cervical cancer estimated to occur in 2002 (ACS, 2002a). Cervical cancer is now considered a sexually transmitted disease, mediated by exposure to human papillomavirus. Infection with this virus is the most important risk factor for the disease. Other risk factors include onset of sexual intercourse at an early age, multiple sexual partners (or sex with individuals who have had multiple sexual partners), and cigarette smoking.

DEFINITIONS OF CANCER PREVENTION AND EARLY DETECTION

Primary Prevention

The most desirable strategy for the amelioration of suffering from cancer is *primary prevention*, a public health approach which keeps people from acquiring cancer in the first place. Unfortunately, the fundamental etiologies of cancer are not fully understood, making a definitive strategy for primary prevention elusive. Epidemiological data shed insights on potentially modifiable risk factors associated with certain cancers (e.g., exposure to tobacco, obesity, a diet low in fruits and vegetables, excessive alcohol intake, workplace carcinogens), but the quality and consistency of the evidence regarding the precise causal roles of these factors in carcinogenesis are mixed (see Chapter 3). Nonetheless, healthier lifestyles and reduced levels of exposure to carcinogens offer great promise as effective means of reducing the incidence of cancer.

Chief among these is avoiding the use of tobacco, which accounts for an estimated 30 percent of cancer deaths in the United States (ACS, 2002b). Helping the 23.5 percent of adults who smoke cigarettes (ACS, 2002b) discontinue their habit and preventing youth from adopting the habit of tobacco use will save more lives than the sum of all the incremental benefits of improving cancer screening rates or cancer treatments. Other primary preventive strategies also offer promise. One-third of cancer deaths are thought to be related to nutrition and other lifestyle factors including body weight, physical activity, and food choices (Byers et al., 2002).

Secondary Prevention

Until the ability to prevent the occurrence of cancer (primary prevention) becomes a reality, a complementary strategy is *secondary prevention*, the early detection of cancer through screening. The fundamental tenet of screening for cancer is that detection of the disease before symptoms develop enables detection at a less advanced stage and that the institution of treatment before symptoms develop will produce improved health outcomes. Although this syllogism seems intuitive and is widely assumed to be true by both health professionals and the lay public, the value of early detection is not proven for many cancers (see Chapter 5).

Tertiary Prevention

While not the topic of this report, tertiary prevention involves limiting disability and providing rehabilitation when disease has already occurred and left residual damage (Mausner and Kramer, 1985). The National Cancer Policy Board has a study in progress, Cancer Survivorship: Improving Care and Quality of Life After Treatment, that will address issues related to tertiary prevention. The Board addressed issues related to symptom control and end-of-life care in its report, *Improving Palliative Care for Cancer* (Institute of Medicine, 2001d).

Health Promotion

Major stages in the evolution of public health have been described as addressing first, communicable diseases, and second, chronic, noncommunicable diseases. Some suggest that society has entered a third "public health revolution" with a focus on advancing health, with health defined following the World Health Organization's formulation, as "physical, mental and social well-being, not merely the absence of disease and infirmity" (Breslow, 1999, p. 1031). The term health promotion is often coupled with that of disease prevention and has been defined as "the process of enabling people to increase control over, and to improve their health" (Breslow, 1999, p. 1030). The concept of health promotion has emerged, in part, because of increases in longevity and time spent without significant disability. Health promotion then "seeks the development of community and individual measures which can help people to develop lifestyles that can maintain and enhance the state of well-being" (Breslow, 1999, p. 1030). The concept of health promotion underlies many of the approaches to reducing the risk of cancer among individuals and populations.

SUMMARY AND CONCLUSIONS

In 2002 an estimated 1.3 million new cases of cancer were diagnosed and over half a million deaths were due to cancer. Cancer is a diverse set of conditions, but just four cancers contribute disproportionately to cancer's toll, accounting for half of all newly diagnosed cases and deaths: cancers of the lung and bronchus, breast, prostate, and colon and rectum. Especially burdened by cancer are individuals who are elderly and socially and economically disadvantaged. Members of certain minority groups including African Americans are also more likely than others to suffer morbidity and die from cancer. Primary prevention through elimination of risk factors such as smoking and poor nutrition is the most effective way to reduce the burden of cancer. Secondary prevention, the early detection of cancer at its most treatable stage, can also be effective for selected cancers. The remainder of this report reviews recent progress and current opportunities for primary and secondary prevention of cancer in the United States.

2

Potential to Reduce the Cancer Burden Through Cancer Prevention and Early Detection[1]

Several attempts have been made to estimate the potential reduction in cancer incidence and mortality rates that could be achieved with major favorable shifts in the distribution of modifiable risk factors in the U.S. population. The four analyses described in this chapter apply different methods and underlying assumptions in making their projections but arrive at a similar conclusion: that major reductions in the cancer burden are achievable by sharply reducing rates of tobacco use, increasing levels of physical activity, decreasing the prevalence of obesity, improving dietary practices, keeping alcohol consumption at low to moderate levels, and getting screened for cancer at recommended intervals. How rapidly such changes can occur will largely depend upon social investments and political will.

The methods, key assumptions, and strengths and limitations of each of the selected analyses are described in the following sections. Many of the assumptions used to develop the predictive models vary and are uncertain (Rockhill et al., 1998). There is uncertainty, for example, regarding biological latency, the strength of causal associations, and the prevalence of risk factors. Nevertheless, such models provide a useful mechanism that can be used to gauge what is achievable under various social conditions.

---

[1]This chapter is based on the background paper prepared by Graham A. Colditz, Catherine Tomeo Ryan, Charles H. Dart III, Geetanjali Datta, Laurie Fisher, and Beverly Rockhill (www.iom.edu/ncpb).

DESCRIPTIONS OF THE FOUR ANALYSES

Doll and Peto, 1981

In 1981 Doll and Peto examined the degree to which cancer incidence and mortality rates could be reduced in the United States. Their approach did not attempt to project the level of reduction in the rate of mortality from cancer within a defined time frame. Rather, Doll and Peto estimated the reduction theoretically possible by comparing the rates in the United States with those in other countries. Their choice of method stemmed from the observation that the cancer incidence rate among migrants tends to be that found in the country to which they migrated, indicating that differential cancer incidence rates are due in part to environmental factors such as diet, exercise, occupational exposures, and smoking habits, and that cancer does not arise exclusively because of genetic factors.

Doll and Peto included in their estimates only information for people who were younger than age 65 because data on the incidence of cancer among older individuals were considered unreliable. Furthermore, they omitted cases of nonmelanoma skin cancers from their analysis because data on the incidence of these cancers were unreliable and also because these cancers are easily treated and are rarely fatal. Doll and Peto's analysis was conducted by comparing the site-specific cancer incidence rates among male and female residents in Connecticut (the most complete U.S. cancer registry at that time) with the lowest reliable international site-specific cancer incidence rates available. Age-adjusted rates were collected from 1968 to 1972 from registries selected by the International Agency for Research on Cancer (IARC) (International Agency for Research on Cancer, 1976). The analysis used data from the United Kingdom, New Mexico, Japan, East Germany, Norway, Israel, Nigeria, Iowa, Puerto Rico, Finland, and New Zealand. The results of the analysis suggested that in 1970, 75 to 80 percent of all cancers in the United States could have theoretically been avoided if the population of the United States could be like that of the countries with the lowest incidences. This figure of 75 to 80 percent can thus be thought of as a crude estimate of the proportion of cancer in the United States that was (in 1970) due to "environmental" factors that made the U.S. population different from low-risk populations. The "environmental" factors that differ between the United States and low-risk populations are many and diverse and include birth weight; age at puberty; and lifelong patterns of tobacco use, diet, physical activity, alcohol consumption, use of pharmacological agents, and reproduction.

Of course, the more traditional and limited definition of "environmental" exposure fits in here, as the U.S. population and the populations of other countries also experience different levels of exposure to contaminants in air, water, and food. Occupational and environmental exposures are estimated to be less important than lifestyle factors as contributors to cancer in the United States today (Monson and Christiani, 1997). Given the major shift toward the regulation of occupational exposures to known carcinogens and the active surveillance of workers previously exposed to many of these carcinogens, the most modifiable component of cancer risk remains lifestyle factors.

Doll and Peto acknowledged that although their estimates were theoretical maximums, it would take a great amount of time to effect social change and that the large amount of change necessary to decrease the cancer incidence rate 75 to 80 percent was unlikely. Although Doll and Peto's methods might seem rudimentary by today's methodological standards, they provided a foundation for later, similar work.

Willett et al., 1996

In 1996 Willett and colleagues used an international comparison approach at the ecological level similar to that used by Doll and Peto (1981) to assess the degree to which cancer mortality could be reduced in the United States. They limited their data on rates of mortality from cancer to those for the United States, Japan, and China because they were considered to be the most reliable data available. They used age-adjusted data from the Surveillance, Epidemiology, and End Results (SEER) Program and from Cancer Incidence in Five Continents, an IARC publication (Parkin et al., 1992). The country with the lowest site-specific cancer incidence rate was considered to have the "baseline" rate. The difference between the highest and the baseline incidence rates was calculated to indicate the maximum degree of cancer reduction possible.

To provide information on behavior-specific reductions in the rate of mortality from cancer, the investigators considered data for unique populations in the United States such as those from the Adventist Health Study, which indicated the magnitude of change possible within the context of the current U.S. culture. Neither Willett and colleagues nor Doll and Peto provided a time frame for the reduction of the cancer mortality rate estimated in their analyses; that is, they did not specify the latency of effects.

Willett and colleagues reported the degree of reduction in the incidence of cancer possible by making specific behavioral changes, considering not only the theoretically greatest possible reduction but also more realistic reductions based on the amount of behavioral change that would likely occur in the U.S. population. Considering the downward trend in cigarette smoking, they suggested that a two-thirds reduction in the number of individuals who smoked and, thus, a similar eventual reduction in tobacco-related cancer mortality rates would be possible. If a percentage of those who consumed more than two drinks per day reduced their intakes, they estimated that alcohol-related cancer mortality rates could be reduced by a third. Another 10 percent decrease in cancer mortality rates could be achieved if a majority of the U.S. population made important diet- and exercise-related changes, such as exercising vigorously for 20 minutes a day, eating one additional serving of leafy vegetables each day, or consuming no more than one serving of red meat a week. The investigators acknowledged that not everyone could or would make behavioral changes and thus stated that although the comparisons of international rates of cancer incidence would suggest that cancer risk could theoretically be reduced by 60 percent, a more realistic estimate of future reduction would be closer to 33 percent.

National Cancer Institute, 1986

Using another approach, the National Cancer Institute (NCI) estimated in 1986 the likely consequences of reductions in specific cancer-related risk factors from 1980 to 2000 in an effort to set national cancer control objectives. NCI considered prevention, screening, and treatment in modeling future cancer mortality rates and in setting objectives for 2000. NCI set a goal of a 50 percent reduction in the total cancer mortality rate between 1980 and 2000. The corresponding risk factor reduction goals determined by NCI to allow achievement of this goal are listed in Table 2.1.

The NCI goal of a 50 percent reduction in the rate of mortality was, in retrospect, overly optimistic. Cancer mortality rates in the United States (for both sexes combined) actually rose through the 1980s and reached their highest levels ever from 1990 to 1992. Since the early 1990s, however, mortality rates have declined somewhat, and mortality rates in 1997 were approximately 7 percent lower than they were in 1980 (Ries et al., 2000b). Although NCI modeled the effects of reductions in various risk factors with a sophisticated computer program (called Can*trol), to arrive at their goal of a 50 percent reduction in total cancer mortality rates, they underestimated the latencies of the social and political changes that would be needed to bring about large changes in the behavior of the population.

Byers et al., 1999

In 1996, the American Cancer Society (ACS) set an ambitious "challenge goal" for a 25 percent reduction in cancer incidence and a 50 percent reduction in the rate of mortality from cancer by 2015. Thereafter, Byers and colleagues (1999) examined the feasibility of reaching the ACS challenge goals by 2015 on the basis of possible reductions in selected major risk factors. For that analysis, the researchers used the 1990 cancer incidence and mortality rates as the baseline rates.

Byers and colleagues used data on cancer incidence and survival rates from the SEER Program, cancer mortality statistics from the National Cen-

TABLE 2.1 Risk Factors, Goals, and Assumptions Used by NCI Working Group and ACS in Predictions for the United States

Risk Factor	NCI Goals for Reduction
Tobacco	By 1990, rate of decline of smoking should be 4% or more per year; by 2000, proportion of all persons 21 years and older who smoke should be ≤15%; by 2000, proportion of youth who begin to smoke should be ≤15% (proportion of youth ages 12–18 years who begin to smoke should be <3%).
Diet	By 1990, per capita consumption of fiber from grains, fruits, and vegetables should be increased to ≥15 g/day; per capita consumption of fat should be below 35% of total daily calories. By 2000, per capita consumption of fiber should increase to 20–30 g/day; per capita consumption of fat should be 30% of total daily calories.
Alcohol	No goals
Antiestrogen use (e.g., Tamoxifen)	No goals
Screening	By 1990, 70% of women aged 50–70 years should have clinical breast exam each year; 45% of these women should have a mammogram every year; 85% of women aged 20–39 years should have a Papanicolaou (Pap) smear every 3 years; 70% of women aged 40–70 years should have a Pap smear every 3 years. By 2000, 80% of women aged 50–70 years should have clinical breast exam each year; 80% of these women should have a mammogram every year; 90% of women aged 20–39 years should have a Pap smear every 3 years; 80% of women aged 40–70 years should have a Pap smear every 3 years.
Treatment	By 2000, increase the rate of adoption of state-of-the-art treatment; continue to advance treatment, as reflected in increasing cancer survival rates; cancer-specific objectives defined in terms of desired increase in 5-year survival rates.

ter for Health Statistics, the prevalence of cancer risk factors from the Behavioral Risk Factor Surveillance System of the Centers for Disease Control and Prevention, and information on cancer treatment from the American College of Surgeons' National Cancer Database.

Byers and colleagues made projections for cancer incidence and mortality rates for each cancer site separately and for all cancers combined, con-

ACS Risk Factor Reduction Assumptions	Biological Latency Assumptions NCI	ACS
Smoking prevalence reduced to: 16–20% by 2005 (18–22% among men, 14–18% among women)	15 years	10 years
Prevalence of low levels of fruit and vegetable consumption reduced to 47–58% by 2010; Prevalence of high fat intake reduced to 9–15% by 2010	not explicitly stated	5 years
Prevalence of frequent alcohol intake reduced among women to 12–14% by 2010; Prevalence of frequent and heavy alcohol intake reduced to 1–4% by 2010	—	5 years
Prevalence of nonuse reduced to 23–35% by 2010	—	5 years
Prevalence of failure to get sigmoidoscopy every 5 years reduced to 45–55% by 2010; Prevalence of failure to get mammography every 2 years reduced to 10–15% by 2010; Prevalence of failure to get PSA test every 2 years reduced to 20–30% by 2010	not explicitly stated	5 years
Prevalence of failure to get best therapy reduced to 14–16% by 2010	not explicitly stated	5 years

sidering major cancer risk factors that had been changing over time (see Table 2.1). They assumed a 10-year latency for the effects of tobacco and a 5-year latency for the effects of other factors. They reported two sets of calculations: (1) calculations in which the current trends in the reductions of risk factor prevalence continued, and (2) calculations in which the trend in the reduction of risk factor prevalence accelerated because of increased

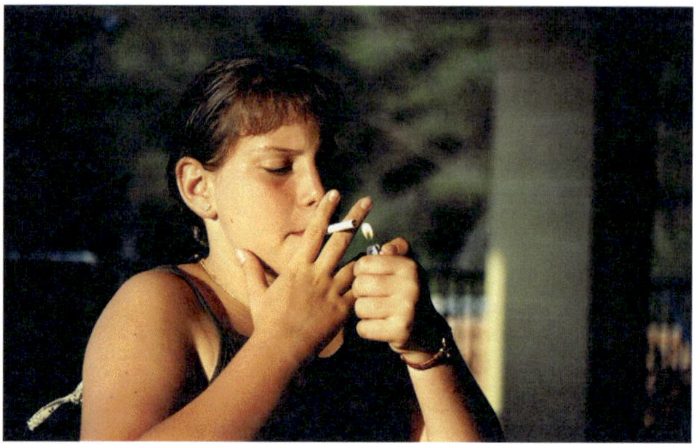

SOURCE: PhotoDisc, Inc.

public health efforts. The future rates of cancer were calculated by the following formula: (1990 population attributable risk[2]) × (projected reduction after the period of latency in the prevalence of the risk factor). The total reduction in cancer incidence and mortality rates was calculated as a weighted average of the rates of cancer of the lung, other tobacco-related sites, colon-rectum, breast, prostate, and other sites.

Byers and colleagues found that past and future reductions in rates of tobacco use were the single largest contributor to the projected future declines in overall cancer incidence and mortality rates. Other risk factors for which declines in prevalence were projected to be important contributors to declines in cancer incidence and mortality rates were poor dietary practices (low levels of consumption of fruits and vegetables), especially for colorectal and lung cancers; levels of alcohol intake; and failure to be screened, especially for colorectal cancer and, to a lesser extent, breast and prostate cancer.

Byers and colleagues estimated that if the reductions in the prevalence of risk factors continued at the 1990 rate, the total reduction in the cancer incidence rate would be 13 percent from 1990 to 2015 and the reduction in the cancer mortality rate would be 21 percent from 1990 to 2015. If the declines in the prevalence of these risk factors accelerated, however, the cancer incidence rate could decline by 19 percent and the cancer mortality rate could decline by 29 percent. When specific cancers are considered, some of the projections based on accelerated declines in risk factor prevalence were

---

[2] The population attributable risk is the proportion of all cancers in the population due to a particular risk factor. Its calculation is derived from estimates of the relative risk for each risk factor (the ratio of the cancer incidence rate among those exposed to a risk factor divided by the rate among those not exposed) and the proportion of the population exposed to that risk factor (Byers et al., 1999).

striking: they calculated that up to 33 percent of deaths from colorectal and breast cancer could be eliminated and that up to 50 percent of the occurrences of and deaths from tobacco-related cancers could be eliminated by 2015 if the prevalence of each of the specified risk factors was to decline at an accelerated pace. Although these projections apply to the entire population, if the rates of decline in risk factors vary by race, ethnic group, or income, disparities in cancer incidence and mortality rates may increase.

It is possible that the estimates of Byers and colleagues are overly optimistic. They assume in their model that current rates of decline in risk factor prevalence will continue or even accelerate, but such declines may not occur. It is possible that persons who have not adopted behavioral changes to date (e.g., those who continue to smoke, avoid dietary change, or avoid screening recommendations) may be more resistant to change, so that it may be difficult to sustain the pace of change over time as "resistors" become a larger proportion of the remaining "unchanged" population (Rogers, 1993). In addition, Byers and colleagues did not estimate future increases in obesity-related cancers (e.g., postmenopausal breast cancer and colon cancer) due to the adverse trends in obesity in the United States. They stated that they assumed the obesity epidemic would be turned around in the coming years, thus negating the past adverse trends, but this turnaround is far from certain. If the obesity trends continue, adverse effects will be seen on breast and colon cancer by the year 2015.

Presentation and analysis of historical trend data would be useful in an evaluation of the feasibility of achieving estimated cancer mortality rate reductions as a result of increased screening. For instance, since the late 1980s a decline in the rate of mortality from breast cancer has been observed in the United States. There is debate about how much, if any, of this decline is attributable to increased rates of screening and earlier detection of invasive disease as compared to improved treatment. This debate is especially active for prostate cancer, for which the certainty of screening benefit is less, but which has shown a sharp mortality decline since 1990. Despite the lack of scientific consensus on the explanations for cancer mortality declines, it seems reasonable to state that the detectable favorable changes in incidence or mortality rates that occur as a result of population-wide shifts in risk factors usually take at least several years to become manifest.

Byers and colleagues discuss the value of well-reasoned predictions with respect to achievable reductions in cancer incidence and mortality rates, noting that such predictions are far better than guesses. They state that although all causes of cancer are not known, many of the major population-level determinants have been identified and that over the next decade expanded efforts to reduce the prevalence of these known, major risk factors could have a substantial impact on the population burden of cancer.

SUMMARY AND CONCLUSIONS

The models reviewed in this chapter illustrate the promise of stepped up efforts to assist individuals and communities in reducing the prevalence of modifiable risk factors but also suggest the difficulties of achieving large reductions in risk factor prevalence. The earliest models estimated the potential of reducing cancer incidence and mortality rates in the best of all possible worlds. When attempts were made to translate the available evidence into national goals, overly optimistic projections of behavioral change were incorporated into the models, leading to unrealistic expectations. Later models have generated more realistic projections by incorporating historical trends in rates of change in risk factor modification and participation in screening programs.

In the earliest of these analyses, Peto and Doll concluded that 75 to 80 percent of all cancers in the United States in 1970 could have theoretically been avoided if the population of the United States could be like those of the countries in which the incidence of cancer was the lowest. Those investigators did not distinguish the contributions of environmental and occupational exposures to carcinogens from individual risk behaviors and noted that realistic and practical reductions in the cancer burden would be substantially lower than 75 to 80 percent. The analysis by Willett and colleagues (1996) found that the cancer mortality rate could theoretically be reduced by 60 percent but that a more realistic reduction based on trends in risk behaviors would be 33 percent. The model developed by NCI in 1986 relied on overly optimistic assumptions regarding population-level changes in risk behaviors that resulted in setting an unrealistic national goal to halve the total cancer mortality rate between 1980 and 2000 (in fact, the mortality rate was reduced by only 7 percent for 1980 to 1997). In the last analysis reviewed, Byers and colleagues estimated that by 2015 there would be a 13 percent total reduction in the cancer incidence rate and a 21 percent reduction in the cancer mortality rate if the prevalence of the major modifiable risk factors continued to decline at the 1990 rate; but if there were accelerated declines in these risk factors, they estimated that the cancer incidence rate could decline by 19 percent and that the cancer mortality rate could decline by 29 percent Using very different methods, the estimates of Willett et al. and Byers et al. are quite similar—that about a one-third reduction in cancer mortality is feasible with the concerted application of current knowledge.

Improvements in the ability to project the impacts of interventions such as primary prevention and screening on observed trends in cancer incidence and mortality rates are likely with further development of analytic modeling techniques. One important initiative is the NCI-sponsored Cancer Intervention and Surveillance Modeling Network, through which a network of investigators has evaluated the impacts of population-level changes in smoking, diet, physical activity, weight status, and the use of screening tests on the rates of cancer incidence and mortality (http://www-dccps.ims.nci.nih.gov/SRAB/cisnet.html).

To date, scientific estimates of the proportion of the cancer burden that can be eliminated if the population distributions of major risk factors were to be shifted in a positive direction have focused on the important but relatively narrow issues of strength of risk factor-disease associations and biological latency. The issue of social or political latency to support behavioral change has gone unaddressed. More research needs to be done on these issues, perhaps through historical case studies of previous successes and failures in encouraging widespread changes in the health of the population. For example, a recent publication of population-level trends in the mortality rate over the 15 years after the tobacco tax was implemented in California shows a substantial lag from the passage of the proposition to the implementation of programs, to reductions in tobacco use, and finally to reductions in lung cancer mortality rates (Fichtenberg and Glantz, 2000). Likewise, the estimate of the rate of decline in tobacco smoking will reflect the level of government and community commitment, as indicated by the experience in California and Massachusetts, where the rate of decline after the implementation of comprehensive programs was faster than that observed in other states (Biener et al., 2000; Pierce et al., 1998; Siegel et al., 2000). Since the introduction of a comprehensive tobacco control program in Massachusetts in 1992 and 1993, the prevalence of smoking among adults has decreased annually by 0.43 percent, whereas in other states there has been an increase of 0.03 percent (Biener et al., 2000). Another important area of research is how observed disparities in cancer incidence and mortality rates might be affected by divergent patterns of risk behaviors observed within certain racial and ethnic and socioeconomic groups.

Goal-setting philosophies vary across individuals and organizations. Goals usually incorporate an element of challenge to improve prevention practice and an element of hope that new research will lead to favorable outcomes. Although setting lofty goals may be intended to provide extra motivation to individuals and institutions, goals that are unrealistic can have the opposite effect. If year after year goals are largely unmet, credibility may begin to wane, affecting both individual and political motivation. Consistently unmet goals may be construed as organizational failures and may therefore threaten future cancer prevention funding and undermine the potential value of public health more broadly. Challenge goals that are set to motivate the application of current knowledge and the research for new knowledge must be accompanied by the attention and resources needed to move toward success. National cancer-related objectives set as part of the *Healthy People 2010* initiative are described in Chapter 9. These objectives differ from the projections reviewed in this chapter, but they have important implications for public health programs.

In reviewing the models of potential reductions in rates of cancer incidence and mortality examined in this chapter, it is important to recognize that the benefits of primary prevention strategies against cancer (as distinguished from secondary prevention, i.e., screening) will lead to improvements in public health that go well beyond cancer alone, and these improvements may occur quite rapidly (Colditz and Gortmaker, 1995). A person who stops smoking today or who is prevented from starting smoking instantaneously reduces his or her risk of respiratory and cardiovascular problems, although the effect on the lung cancer risk may not be seen for many years (US DHHS, 1990). Similarly, a person who adopts a healthier diet and a more active lifestyle will reduce his or her risk of heart disease, stroke, diabetes (Knowler et al., 2002) and many other health problems that may have shorter latency periods than cancer.

3

Lifestyle Behaviors Contributing to the Burden of Cancer[1]

Much of the burden of cancer in the United States can be traced to modifiable health behaviors that increase one's risk of disease. This chapter reviews evidence on the contributions of five major risk factors to cancer incidence and mortality: tobacco use, physical inactivity, overweight and obesity, poor diet, and alcohol use. Although other lifestyle factors such as sun exposure, sexual practices, and exposure to infected blood also contribute substantially to cancer incidence, this chapter focuses only on the factors that are risks for common cancers and that also have large impacts on the incidences of other major diseases such as cardiovascular disease, stroke, diabetes, and osteoporosis. The benefits of intervention are far greater when reductions in the incidence of other chronic diseases add to reductions in the incidence of cancer achieved through lifestyle changes (Colditz and Gortmaker, 1995).

This chapter summarizes the epidemiological evidence with respect to cancer incidence for each of the five selected risk factors by using the criteria outlined by the World Cancer Research Fund and the American Institute of Cancer Research. For each epidemiological association the level of evidence is categorized as convincing, probable, or possible (Box 3.1).

Much of the literature reviewed in this chapter has been published from research conducted with data from one of the several large prospective cohort studies described in Box 3.2. Such studies involve the identification

[1]The chapter is based on the background paper prepared by Graham A. Colditz, Catherine Tomeo Ryan, Charles H. Dart III, Geetanjali Datta, Laurie Fisher, and Beverly Rockhill (www.iom.edu/ncpb).

BOX 3.1 Definition of Levels of Evidence for Epidemiological Associations

Level of Evidence	Criteria
Convincing	• Epidemiological findings across a large number of well-designed studies are consistent. • A dose-response relationship has been demonstrated. • Mechanisms are biologically plausible. • Laboratory evidence is supportive.
Probable	• Epidemiological evidence is either inconsistent or not extensive enough to make definitive judgment. • Laboratory or mechanistic evidence is supportive.
Possible	• Epidemiological findings are supportive but limited in quantity, quality, or consistency. • Supportive mechanistic or laboratory evidence may or may not be available. • Supportive evidence from other disciplines may be available.

SOURCE: Adapted from (World Cancer Research Fund and American Institute for Cancer Research, 1997).

of a group of individuals who share a common experience within a defined time period and monitoring of those individuals forward in time for the development of disease (Mausner and Kramer, 1985). These studies have been essential to providing an understanding of the links between health-related behaviors and health outcomes. Other evidence comes from case-control studies in which investigators identify a group of patients with a particular cancer (cases) and a group of patients without cancer (controls) and then compare the histories of the cases and controls to determine the extent to which each was exposed to the intervention of interest.

TOBACCO

Tobacco is the scourge of public health. In the United States alone, tobacco use, primarily in the form of cigarette smoking, causes more than 440,000 premature deaths from cancer and other causes each year and is responsible for approximately 30 percent of all cancer-related deaths (ACS, 2002b). Worldwide, the numbers are even more staggering. The World Health Organization estimated that in 1998 there would be approximately 4 million deaths linked to tobacco use worldwide (World Health Organization, 1999). By 2020, this number is expected to at least double.

BOX 3.2 Frequently Referenced Prospective Cohort Studies

American Cancer Society's Cancer Prevention Studies

Cancer Prevention Study I (CPS I)

A prospective study of approximately one million men and women. Enrollment started in 1959 and follow-up ran through 1972, with mortality being the primary outcome measure (ACS, 2001). Enrollment was household-based, and all members of a household age 30 or older were included in the study if at least one household member was age 45 or older. Upon entering the study, participants completed questionnaires assessing lifestyle factors (e.g., occupation, diet, and tobacco use), reproductive factors (in women), personal and family history of cancer, as well as anthropometric and demographic information. After this, questionnaires were sent to participants at regular intervals to update tobacco use and assess vital status.

Cancer Prevention Study II (CPS II)

A prospective study of approximately 1.2 million men and women (ACS, 2001). Started in 1982 and still ongoing, the primary aim of CPS II is to assess the effect that lifestyle and environmental factors have on cancer development. As with CPS I, enrollment in CPS II was household-based and included all household members age 30 or older if at least one member was age 45 or older. A range of lifestyle and other factors were assessed by questionnaire at study enrollment. The study's main outcome measure is mortality, which is assessed biennially through links with the National Death Index.

Health Professionals Follow-Up Study

A prospective study of approximately 52,000 male health professionals—including dentists, optometrists, osteopaths, podiatrists, pharmacists, and veterinarians (Harvard School of Public Health, 2001). Started in 1986 in men ages 40–75, it is still ongoing. The primary aim of the Health Professionals Follow-Up Study is to assess the effect of lifestyle on the risk of chronic disease, particularly cancer and cardiovascular disease. Data are gathered largely through biennial questionnaires that ask participants detailed questions about their disease status as well as about their lifestyle and personal characteristics.

Male British Doctors Study

A prospective mortality study of 34,000 male British doctors, which started in 1951 and is still ongoing (Doll et al., 1994). The study's initial aim was to build a body of evidence linking tobacco use to chronic disease. While the questionnaire at enrollment focused largely on tobacco use, subsequent follow-up questionnaires added questions related to alcohol use, aspirin use, disease status, and certain personal characteristics.

Nurses' Health Study

A prospective study of approximately 120,000 female registered nurses, which is primarily designed to assess the effect of lifestyle on the risk of chronic disease, particularly cancer and cardiovascular disease (Colditz, 1995). Started in 1976 in women ages 30–55, the Nurses' Health Study is still ongoing. Data are gathered primarily through biennial questionnaires that ask participants detailed questions about their disease status as well as their lifestyle and personal characteristics. To provide a more accurate accounting of the intake of certain minerals, participants provided toenail samples in 1982. In 1989, participants provided blood samples to allow the study of potential disease biomarkers.

Since the first Surgeon General's report on smoking and health was released in 1964, a causal link has been confirmed between smoking and several cancers (U.S. Department of Health, Education, and Welfare, 1964). The data available at that time were able to support a causal link between smoking and only two cancers: lung cancer and laryngeal cancer. Over the following 35 years, however, enough evidence has accrued to now support smoking as a cause of eight cancers: lung, oral, pharyngeal, laryngeal, esophageal, bladder, kidney, and pancreatic cancer. A review of the current literature provides sufficient evidence to also implicate tobacco as a cause of additional cancers, including cancers of the colon, stomach, and cervix, and leukemia. Smoking has also been identified as a probable cause of liver cancer and has been associated with an increase in the risk of developing aggressive, more deadly forms of prostate cancer (Table 3.1). Smoking is not causally related to several types of cancer, such as breast or brain cancer.

Impact of Cessation of Tobacco Use on Cancer Incidence

Although the prevention of smoking is the best approach to avoiding tobacco-related diseases, there are substantial health benefits for smokers who quit. Scientific data on the benefits of smoking cessation were reviewed in detail in a 1990 Surgeon General's report (US DHHS, 1990). In the last quarter century, half of all living Americans who have ever smoked have now quit. The 1990 Surgeon General's report concluded that smoking cessation has major and immediate health benefits for men and women of all ages. Former smokers live longer than continuing smokers; for instance, persons who quit smoking before age 50 have, on average, half the risk of dying in the next 15 years than continuing smokers. This reduction in mortality comes from a reduction in the risk of nearly all smoking-related

TABLE 3.1 Increase in Risk of Incident Cancer Associated with Smoking

	Relative Risk (RR)	
Level of Evidence	Moderate (RR 1.35–1.99)	Large (RR 2.0+)
Convincing	Colon Stomach Leukemia Cervical	Lung Oral Pharyngeal Laryngeal Esophageal Bladder Kidney Pancreatic
Probable	Prostate (mortality)	Liver

diseases. Among former smokers, the decline in the risk of death compared with that for individuals who continue smoking begins shortly after quitting and continues for at least 10 to 15 years. The health benefits of smoking cessation far exceed the risk from the weight gain, which is approximately 2.3 kilograms (kg) (5 pounds [lb]), on average, that may follow quitting.

Tobacco Use and Lung Cancer

Voluminous and convincing epidemiological evidence links smoking to lung cancer, the leading cause of cancer death in both men and women in the United States. An estimated 169,400 new cases of lung cancer are diagnosed annually, with an estimated 154,900 deaths each year (ACS, 2002a). More than 80 percent of lung cancer cases are attributable to smoking. As outlined in detail in the Surgeon General's reports on smoking and health, cigarette smoking is the strongest risk factor for lung cancer, increasing the risk of the disease by at least 10-fold and as much as 20-fold, depending on smoking habits and history (US DHHS, 1989; Thun, Dally-Lally et al., 1997). There is a consistent, strong, and specific link between smoking and lung cancer, with a dose-response relationship seen with the number of cigarettes smoked, the deepness of inhalation of cigarette smoke, and the duration of smoking (US DHHS, 1989).

There is convincing evidence from numerous case-control and cohort studies that former smokers have a lower risk of lung cancer than current smokers (US DHHS, 1990). The benefits begin 2 to 3 years after quitting, and the risk steadily drops over the next 10 years. Although the risk of lung cancer is drastically reduced after quitting, the risk of lung cancer in former smokers never quite returns to the risk for those who have never smoked.

The overall pattern seen in the study of U.S. veterans mimics that of most other large cohort studies of smoking cessation and lung cancer risk (Rogot and Murray, 1980; US DHHS, 1990). In the U.S. Veterans Study, the lung cancer mortality rate in current smokers divided by the rate in nonsmokers (i.e., the mortality rate ratio) was 11.3. In the first 4 years after quitting, this ratio increased to nearly 19 for former smokers and then slowly decreased: 7.7 after 5 to 9 years, 4.7 after 10 to 14 years, 4.8 after 15 to 19 years, and 2.1 after 20 or more years. The increase in lung cancer risk in the first few years after quitting seen in many studies likely reflects the tendency of smokers to quit because of symptoms of disease rather than a true increase in risk linked to cessation per se.

Numerous studies have also found that smoking cessation benefits nearly all smokers, regardless of sex, age, and level of habit. The American Cancer Society's Cancer Prevention Study I and Cancer Prevention Study II have demonstrated that both men and women benefit from cessation, as do both light smokers (those who smoke 1 to 20 cigarettes/day) and heavy smokers (those who smoke 21 or more cigarettes/day). In addition, an analysis of national smoking trends in the United Kingdom found substantial benefits for smokers who stopped at a wide range of ages (Peto et al., 2000). Those smokers who stopped before middle age benefited the most, avoiding 90 percent of the excess risk of lung cancer linked to tobacco use. However, those who stopped at ages 50 and 60 years also benefited substantially.

Tobacco Use and Oral, Pharyngeal, Laryngeal, and Esophageal Cancers

Tobacco use is a well-established cause of cancer of the oral cavity, pharynx, larynx, and esophagus (US DHHS, 1989). Oropharyngeal cancer alone—including cancer of the lip, tongue, oral cavity, and oropharynx—is diagnosed in approximately 28,900 people each year in the United States and accounts for about 7,400 deaths annually (ACS, 2002a). Once oropharyngeal cancer was as much as six times more common in men than in women, but men are now only about twice as likely as women to develop the disease. This is due in large part to the disappearing disparity in smoking rates between the two sexes (CDC, 1999b). Although disparity in the incidence of oropharyngeal cancer by sex is waning, the disparity in the incidence by race or ethnicity persists. African Americans not only have a greater risk than whites of developing oropharyngeal cancer, but they also have a much less favorable prognosis after they receive a diagnosis. Only about a third of African Americans survive 5 years after diagnosis, compared to more than half of whites (Ries et al., 2000a).

Numerous cohort and case-control studies have found that the risks of both the incidence of and the mortality from these types of cancers are significantly increased in smokers compared with those in nonsmokers, and many studies have demonstrated a dose-response relationship. The long-running cohort study of British male doctors found rates of mortality from esophageal cancer among the heaviest smokers to be 15 times that among nonsmokers (Doll et al., 1994). Among all current smokers combined, the increased rate of mortality was over seven times that among nonsmokers. In a study of U.S. veterans, current smokers experienced 10 times the risk of mortality from laryngeal cancer than those who never smoked, a risk similar to that seen in the American Cancer Society's Cancer Prevention Study II (Kahn, 1966; US DHHS, 1990). In addition, a case-control study conducted by the National Cancer Institute found that the risk of oropharyngeal cancer was increased two to three times among those who ever smoked compared with that among those who never smoked, and the risk increased with the amount and duration of smoking. Women who smoked 40 or more cigarettes per day had six times the risk of oropharyngeal cancer as someone who never smoked. Men who smoked 40 or more cigarettes per day had three times the risk. Overall, the increased incidence of oropharyngeal cancer in smokers compared with that in nonsmokers across studies ranges from 3 to 13 (Schottenfeld and Fraumeni, 1996).

The most likely causal pathway between tobacco use and these cancers is the direct contact of the carcinogens in tobacco and its smoke with the tissues of the oral cavity, larynx, and esophagus. Yet, although smoking alone is an independent risk factor for oral, laryngeal, and esophageal cancer, alcohol consumption greatly exacerbates smoking's effect on risk (Blot et al., 1988). It is estimated that alcohol and tobacco use together account for approximately 75 percent of oral cancers in the United States (Blot et al., 1988).

There is convincing evidence that former smokers have lower risks of cancers of the oral cavity, pharynx, larynx, and esophagus than current smokers. For oropharyngeal cancer, the risk for former smokers compared with that for current smokers decreases steadily with the number of years since cessation (after the first few years), with some studies demonstrating that the risk of oropharyngeal cancer actually returns to that for never smokers 10 or more years after quitting (Blot et al., 1988). As with lung cancer and smoking cessation, there is also good evidence that the excess risk of oropharyngeal cancer decreases with younger age at cessation (US DHHS, 1990). For laryngeal and esophageal cancer, numerous studies have demonstrated significant drops in risk for former smokers compared with that for current smokers beginning 3 to 4 years after cessation (US DHHS, 1990).

Tobacco Use and Bladder Cancer

Approximately 56,500 cases of bladder cancer are diagnosed each year (ACS, 2002a). Whites have the highest incidence rates, about twice the rate of Hispanics and African Americans (Miller et al., 1996). Significant disparity in the incidence of bladder cancer also exists by sex, as men are about three to four times more likely to develop the disease than women (Miller et al., 1996).

There is convincing evidence that smoking is a cause of bladder cancer. More than 30 case-control and 10 prospective cohort studies support a strong link between smoking and the disease (Silverman et al., 1992). Overall, moderate to heavy smokers tend to have two to five times the risk of nonsmokers, and there is a strong dose-response relationship between smoking and the risk of bladder cancer, with the risk increasing with the duration and amount of smoking. Specifically, the 40-year analysis of British male doctors found that the rate of mortality from bladder cancer was three times greater among heavy smokers (those who smoke 25 or more cigarettes a day) than among nonsmokers (Doll et al., 1994). The most likely causal pathway between tobacco smoking and bladder cancer is the exposure of bladder tissue to the carcinogenic by-products of tobacco metabolism that are excreted in urine. It is estimated that a third of all bladder cancers in women and half of all bladder cancers in men are caused by cigarette smoking (Silverman et al., 1992).

There is convincing evidence that smoking cessation can lower the risk of bladder cancer in former smokers compared with that in current smokers. A recent pooled analysis of 11 case-control studies conducted by the International Agency for Research on Cancer found that the risk of bladder cancer in former smokers compared with that in current smokers began to decrease almost immediately after smoking cessation and continued to do so with the duration of cessation (Brennan et al., 2000). The risk dropped 35 percent 1 to 4 years after quitting and dropped more than 60 percent 25 years after quitting, but it never reached that for someone who had never smoked.

Tobacco Use and Kidney Cancer

Although kidney cancer is less common than bladder cancer, there is convincing evidence from case-control and prospective cohort studies that smoking causes kidney cancer. Approximately 31,800 cases of kidney cancer are diagnosed each year (ACS, 2002a). Men are approximately twice as likely as women to develop the disease (Miller et al., 1996) African Americans, whites, and Hispanics each appear to develop kidney cancer at similar rates (Miller et al., 1996). As reviewed in the 1989 Surgeon General's report, the relative risk for kidney cancer associated with smoking ranges from one to five and exhibits a dose-response relationship with the number of cigarettes smoked (U.S Department of Health and Human Services, 1989). More recent studies bolster these results. A large study with a cohort of U.S. veterans found that men who smoked more than 40 cigarettes a day had double the risk of kidney cancer compared with that for nonsmokers (McLaughlin et al. 1995a). The International Renal Cell Cancer Study, a large case-control study, also found that the risk increased with both the number of cigarettes smoked and the duration of smoking (McLaughlin et al. 1995b). The causal pathway is likely similar to that for bladder cancer: exposure of kidney tissue to the carcinogenic by-products of tobacco metabolism that end up in urine.

For kidney cancer (including cancer of the renal pelvis), smoking cessation does not seem to provide as much of a benefit as it does for bladder cancer. The study of U.S. veterans found only slight differences in the risk of kidney cancer between former and current smokers (Kahn, 1966), and the International Renal Cell Cancer Study found that after more than 15 years of cessation, the risk of kidney cancer in former smokers was only 15 to 25 percent lower than among current smokers (McLaughlin et al., 1995b).

Tobacco Use and Pancreatic Cancer

Pancreatic cancer is the most deadly of the major cancers, with 5-year survival rates after diagnosis only about 5 percent (ACS, 2002a). Approximately 30,300 cases are diagnosed each year in the United States (ACS, 2002a). The disease is more common in men than in women and is about 50 percent more common in African Americans than in whites (Miller et al., 1996). Smoking was described as a contributory factor to pancreatic cancer in the 1989 Surgeon General's report, but the evidence now supports smoking as a cause of the disease (US DHHS, 1989). Both case-control and prospective cohort studies have not only linked smoking to an increased risk of pancreatic cancer but also demonstrated a dose-response relationship. Overall, smokers appear to have two to three times the risk of getting pancreatic cancer as nonsmokers. Although the causal pathway between smoking and pancreatic cancer is unknown, it has been proposed that tobacco carcinogens or their by-products cause mutations in pancreatic cells linked to carcinogenesis.

There is convincing evidence that individuals who quit smoking experience significantly decreased risks of pancreatic cancer. Unlike many other cancers linked to smoking, the risk of pancreatic cancer in former smokers begins to drop in the first couple of years after cessation (Anderson et al., 1996). A large prospective study of men found that the risk of the disease dropped nearly 50 percent within 2 years of stopping, and after less than 10 years, the risk nearly returned to that for someone who had never smoked (Fuchs et al., 1996).

Tobacco Use and Colon Cancer

The American Cancer Society estimates that there were 148,300 new cases of colorectal cancer in 2002 and that 56,600 Americans died of the disease (ACS, 2002a). An association between smoking and colorectal cancer was not discussed in previous Surgeon General's reports on smoking and health because of a lack of data, but there is now convincing new evidence for a causal association between smoking and an increased risk of colon cancer, as well as colon polyps, among both men and women (Giovannucci and Martinez, 1996). A Swedish prospective study of nearly 57,000 men and women found a 60 percent increased risk of colon cancer in smokers compared with that in nonsmokers after 11 to 20 years of follow-up (Knekt et al., 1998). The Nurses' Health Study and the Health Professionals Follow-Up Study demonstrated significant elevations in risk in long-term smokers as well (Giovannucci et al., 1994a,b). Men who had been smoking for at least 35 years had nearly double the risk of colon cancer compared with that for nonsmokers, as did women who had smoked for 45 years. The long latency period between the initiation of smoking and the elevation in risk, coupled with the consistent relationship seen between smoking and colorectal polyps, suggests that tobacco may be an initiator of colorectal carcinogenesis.

There is an increasing amount of evidence that smoking cessation can lower the risk of colon cancer, although this evidence was not included in the 1990 Surgeon General's report mentioned above. Data from the American Cancer Society's Cancer Prevention Study II indicate that the risk of colon cancer drops with the number of years of smoking cessation as well as a younger age at the time of cessation (Chao et al., 2000).

Tobacco Use and Stomach Cancer

Stomach cancer is one of the most common cancers worldwide. Although it is much less common in the United States, nearly 21,600 cases of stomach cancer are diagnosed and there are approximately 12,400 deaths from stomach cancer each year (ACS, 2002a). In general, Asian populations in the United States have the highest rates of incidence of the disease; the exception, however, is Filipinos, who, along with whites, have the lowest rates of stomach cancer (Miller et al., 1996). African Americans and Hispanics tend to have higher rates than whites but lower rates than most Asian groups.

As early as 1982, the Surgeon General's reports on smoking and health have documented a positive association between smoking and stomach cancer (US DHHS, 1982). Both prospective and case-control studies have found a link between the two, with a number demonstrating a dose-response relationship (Tredaniel et al., 1997). Although the results of case-control studies have been somewhat variable, prospective cohort studies have consistently found an increased risk of stomach cancer linked to smoking. One meta-analysis of 40 studies—case-control and cohort studies combined—found that, overall, smoking increased the risk of stomach cancer by 50 to 60 percent (Tredaniel et al., 1997). When men and women were assessed separately, male smokers had a greater risk of stomach cancer from smoking than female smokers. A number of possible causal pathways exist between smoking and stomach cancer. Smoking has been linked to *Helicobacter pylori* infection, a major risk factor for stomach cancer worldwide, as well as decreased levels in serum of certain micronutrients such as carotenoids and vitamin C that may help protect against the disease. It is estimated that 11 percent of stomach cancers worldwide can be attributed to tobacco smoking (Tredaniel et al., 1997).

A growing body of evidence supports a lower risk of stomach cancer in former smokers compared with that in current smokers. The risk of stomach cancer decreases with increasing years of cessation, with the risk nearing that for those who have never smoked after approximately 20 years of cessation (Tredaniel et al., 1997).

Tobacco Use and Cervical Cancer

Worldwide, cervical cancer is one of the most common cancers in women. In the United States, both the incidence of cervical cancer and the rate of mortality from the disease have been declining steadily since the middle of the last century. Since the early 1970s alone, the incidence and mortality for cervical cancer have dropped by approximately 40 percent (Miller et al., 1996), a decrease most likely due to increased screening by Pap tests and the use of effective treatment. Cervical cancer is now known to be caused in large part by chronic infection of the cervix by some subtypes of human papilloma virus (HPV). Cervical cancer is more common in African-American women than white women. Between 1988 and 1992, incidence rates according to the Surveillance, Epidemiology, and End Results (SEER) Program were 13.2/100,000 for African-American women and 8.7/100,000 for white women. Vietnamese women had the highest rates in the United States (43/100,000), and Japanese women had the lowest (5.8/100,000) (Miller et al., 1996).

One challenge with studying smoking and cervical cancer is potential confounding by other risk factors linked with low socioeconomic status. In particular, human papillomavirus (HPV) infection and high levels of sexual activity each increase the risk of cervical cancer and are each also more common in smokers than in nonsmokers. Separation of the effect of smoking from these other risk factors is key to uncovering the true relationship between smoking and cervical cancer.

The Surgeon General's report *Women and Smoking* summarizes the evidence linking smoking with cervical cancer (US DHHS, 2001a). Overall, case-control studies that have not controlled for HPV infection status demonstrate a twofold increase in the risk of cervical cancer in smokers compared with that in those who have never smoked, and the risk increases with the duration of smoking. For women who have smoked for more than 20 years, the risk of cervical cancer is threefold that for women who have never smoked (Daling et al., 1996). Results have been mixed in studies that have controlled for HPV infection status. Some have found that smoking raises the risk of cervical cancer, regardless of HPV infection status (Ylitalo et al., 1999; Daling et al., 1996), and others have found that smoking increases the risk of cervical cancer only among women who are not infected with HPV (Bosch et al., 1992; Eluf-Neto et al., 1994; Munoz et al., 1993).

There is evidence of a probable inverse association between smoking cessation and cervical cancer. Taken as a whole, there are good data that former smokers experience a lower risk of cervical cancer than current smokers (US DHHS, 1990). It is unclear how the amount of time since quitting affects the risk of cervical cancer in former smokers.

Tobacco Use and Liver Cancer

Approximately 16,600 cases of liver cancer (including cancer of the bile ducts) are diagnosed each year in the United States (ACS, 2002a). Men have about twice the incidence rate of women, and African Americans and Hispanics have about twice the incidence rate of whites (Miller et al., 1996).

There is evidence of a probable positive association between smoking and liver cancer. Although some studies on this topic have not adequately controlled for alcohol intake and viral hepatitis infection—two key factors that can potentially confound the relationship—the evidence supports a positive relationship with cigarette smoking and suggests a dose-response association. Overall, the relative risk of liver cancer associated with smoking appears to range from 1.5 to 7, with the highest association observed among those without hepatitis (Trichopoulos et al. 1980; Lam et al., 1982; Tu et al., 1985; Trichopoulos et al., 1987; Hsing et al., 1990a; Tanaka et al., 1992; McLaughlin et al., 1995a). However, the results of all studies have not been consistent (Doll et al., 1994). There is only limited evidence that the risk of liver cancer is lower in former smokers than in current smokers (US DHHS, 1990).

Tobacco Use and Leukemia

Approximately 30,800 cases of leukemia are diagnosed each year in the United States, half of which are classified as acute leukemia and half of which are classified as chronic (ACS, 2002a). The large majority of leukemias occur in adults, and men are about 50 percent more likely to develop the disease than women. Whites have the highest rates in the United States, with certain Asian populations—Chinese, Japanese, and Koreans—having the lowest rates (Miller et al., 1996).

The current weight of evidence supports a causal association between smoking and acute leukemia, mainly of the myeloid type. A 1993 meta-analysis of 15 studies found that the data accumulated from prospective and case-control studies support relative risks of 1.3 and 1.1, respectively (Brownson et al., 1993). A dose-response was also seen with the number of cigarettes smoked. Overall, having ever smoked seems to increase the risk of leukemia by 30 to 50 percent. For smokers who smoke more than a pack a day, risk appears to increase about twofold. The chemical benzene is one of the likely causal links between cigarettes and leukemia. In experiments with both humans and animals, benzene has been shown to promote cancerous changes in white blood cells (Korte, Hertz-Picciotto et al., 2000). It has been estimated that 14 percent of all leukemia cases in the United States may be attributable to cigarette smoking (Brownson et al., 1993).

The results of studies on the benefits of smoking cessation on the risk of leukemia are mixed. The American Cancer Society's Cancer Prevention

Study I and Cancer Prevention Study II both found small decreases in the risk of leukemia in former smokers compared with that in current smokers (Garfinkel and Boffetta, 1990), but other studies did not (Doll et al., 1994; McLaughlin et al., 1995a).

Tobacco Use and Prostate Cancer

More than 189,000 men are diagnosed with prostate cancer each year in the United States, making it the most common cancer in men (ACS, 2002a). Although studies do not currently support a link between smoking and the incidence of prostate cancer, a growing body of evidence links smoking with mortality from prostate cancer. A number of large, prospective cohort studies have documented a link between smoking and mortality from prostate cancer, with some demonstrating a dose-response relationship with the amount smoked (Hsing et al., 1990b; Hsing et al., 1991; Coughlin et al., 1996; Rodriguez et al., 1997; Giovannucci et al., 1999). Overall, relative risks for mortality from prostate cancer seem to range from 1.3 to 2.0 for smokers compared with nonsmokers. Unlike many other cancers, however, recent smoking seems to be more important than total lifetime exposure to cigarette smoke. Although the exact causal pathway between smoking and mortality from prostate cancer is unknown, it may be that the increased levels of testosterone (and other adrenal hormones) seen in the serum of smokers may stimulate the growth of prostate cancer cells (Gann et al., 1996).

Tobacco and Endometrial Cancer

Endometrial cancer is a common cancer in U.S. women, with approximately 39,300 cases diagnosed each year (ACS, 2002a). Current evidence documents that smokers have a lower risk of endometrial cancer compared with the risk for nonsmokers, most likely mediated through weight and hormone levels (US DHHS, 1989). Increased serum estrogen levels and overweight (primarily postmenopause) are linked to an increased risk of endometrial cancer. On average, smokers weigh less than nonsmokers and so have lower serum estrogen levels, which may reduce the risk of endometrial cancer. Although this one inverse association with smoking is well documented, the decreased risk of endometrial cancer is far outweighed by the increased risk of the many other more common cancers as well as other common chronic diseases.

Environmental Tobacco Smoke

In 1993 environmental tobacco smoke was categorized as a Group A carcinogen by the Environmental Protection Agency. Exposure to environmental tobacco smoke significantly increases the risk of lung cancer and other diseases, such as heart disease and respiratory illness in children. One meta-analysis of 5 cohort and 34 case-control studies found that non-smoking women who lived with a smoker had an approximately 25 percent greater risk of developing lung cancer than non-smoking women who lived with a nonsmoker (Hackshaw et al., 1997). A dose-response relationship with the number of cigarettes that the husband smoked per day was also seen. Passive exposure to tobacco smoke has also been defined as a cause of heart disease among women (US DHHS, 2001a).

Cigars and Pipes

Cigarettes are by far the most common delivery device for tobacco in the United States. However, a substantial number of people also use tobacco in pipes and cigars. Although they are seemingly less dangerous and less addictive than cigarettes, an analysis of the large cohort in the American Cancer Society's Cancer Prevention Study II found that cigar smoking by men substantially increases their risk of lung, oral, and laryngeal cancer. Lung cancer risk was increased about fivefold, and the risk of pancreas and bladder cancers about threefold (Shapiro et al., 2000). An analysis of a large cohort of U.S. veterans found that cigar and pipe use increased the risk of liver cancer approximately threefold (Hsing et al., 1990b). In addition, pipe smoking is causally related to lip cancer and increases the risk of lung cancer, although to a lesser degree than cigarette smoking (U.S. Department of Health, Education, and Welfare, 1964; Lange et al., 1992; Boffetta et al., 1999).

Smokeless Tobacco

Although the rate of use of smokeless tobacco is generally low nationwide, it is quite common in certain subpopulations, especially young adult males of low socioeconomic status living in rural areas (Nelson et al., 1996; Bell et al., 2000). The relationship between the use of smokeless tobacco and cancer of the oral cavity was reviewed in detail in a 1986 Surgeon General's Report, *The Health Consequences of Using Smokeless Tobacco* (Advisory Committee to the Surgeon General, 1986). There is convincing evidence that smokeless tobacco causes cancer of the oral cavity.

Disparities in Use of Tobacco

Nearly one-quarter (23.5 percent) of the US population are current cigarette smokers (Table 3.2). Of the 46.5 million Americans who are, the percentage of users varies by age, race, ethnicity, gender, and education (Table 3.2). Younger adults are more likely to smoke than adults 65 years

TABLE 3.2 Current Cigarette Use, Adults 18 Years or Older, United States, 1999

Characteristic	% Men	% Women	% Total
Age group (years)			
18 to 24	29.5	26.3	27.9
25 to 44	29.6	25.1	27.3
45 to 64	25.8	21.0	23.3
65 or older	10.5	10.7	10.6
Race/Ethnicity			
White (non-Hispanic)	25.5	23.1	24.3
Black (non-Hispanic)	28.7	20.8	24.3
Hispanic	24.1	12.3	18.1
American Indian/Alaska Native[a]	40.9	40.8	40.8
Asian/Pacific Islander	24.3	7.1	15.1
Education (Years)[b]			
8 or fewer	24.7	12.8	18.3
9 to 11	42.4	33.5	37.7
12	30.2	23.2	26.3
13 to 15	27.6	23.3	25.3
16	14.0	11.9	13.0
More than 16	9.1	7.8	8.5
Total	25.7	21.5	23.5

[a]Estimates should be interpreted with caution because of the small sample sizes.
[b]Persons aged 25 years or older.
NOTE: Data from the National Health Interview Survey, 1999.
(Cigarette use is defined as having reported smoking at least 100 cigarettes during a lifetime or having smoked every day or some days at the time of the interview.)
SOURCE: ACS, 2002b.

or older. More than a third of high school students are current smokers (Table 3.3). Although cigarette smoking increased among high school students in the 1990s and is the most prevalent form of tobacco use among this age group, smokeless tobacco and cigars are becoming more commonly used (Table 3.3) (ACS, 2002b).

Among racial and ethnic groups, American Indians and Alaska Natives are most likely to use cigarettes (41 percent) and Asian and Pacific Islanders are the least likely to use cigarettes (15 percent). Whites, African Americans, and Hispanics fell in between and had similar smoking rates (approximately 18–24 percent). Once quite pronounced, the disparity in smoking rates by sex is now relatively small. In 1999, 26 percent of men were current smokers, as compared to 21 percent of women (Table 3.2) (ACS, 2002b).

Smoking rates are also closely tied to income. By both sex and race or ethnicity, people with lower incomes are more likely to smoke than people

TABLE 3.3 Tobacco Use, High School Students, United States, 1999

Characteristic	Cigarette use: Current[a] %	Cigarette use: Frequent[b] %	Current Smokeless Tobacco[c] %	Current Cigar Use[d] %
Gender				
Male	34.7	17.9	14.2	25.4
Female	34.9	15.6	1.3	9.9
Race/Ethnicity				
White, non-Hispanic	38.6	20.2	10.4	18.8
Male	38.2	20.9	18.8	28.3
Female	39.1	19.4	1.5	8.6
Black, non-Hispanic	19.7	7.0	1.3	13.7
Male	21.8	9.1	2.5	16.0
Female	17.7	5.0	0.2	11.6
Hispanic	32.7	10.4	3.9	16.7
Male	34.0	12.5	6.1	21.9
Female	31.5	8.5	1.8	11.6
Grade				
9	27.6	11.2	6.8	13.7
10	34.7	15.2	7.1	17.8
11	36.0	18.7	8.4	18.2
12	42.8	23.1	8.9	22.0
Total	34.8	16.8	7.8	17.7

[a]Smoked cigarettes on one or more of the 30 days preceding the survey.
[b]Smoked cigarettes on 20 or more of the 30 days preceding the survey.
[c]Used chewing tobacco or snuff on one or more of the 30 days preceding the survey.
[d]Smoked cigars on one or more of the 30 days preceding the survey.
NOTE: Data from the Youth Risk Behavior Surveillance System, 1999.
(A current user has smoked cigarettes, cigars, or used tobacco respectively, on one or more of the 30 days preceding the survey. A frequent smoker has smoked at least 20 of the 30 days preceding the survey.)
SOURCE: ACS, 2002b.

with higher incomes (National Center for Health Statistics, 1998). Low-income African-American men and women are about twice as likely to be smokers as African Americans with middle or high incomes. A similar, although slightly lower, disparity in smoking rates exists between income groups among whites. In addition to income level, overall socioeconomic status is associated with smoking among adults, adolescents, and children (Choiniere et al., 2000; Lewis et al., 2001; Lowry et al., 1996; Ross, 2000; Samet et al., 1992; Zhu et al., 1996; Whitlock et al., 1997b; Sussman and Dent, 2000). This relationship is especially apparent among vulnerable populations. For example, pregnant women of lower socioeconomic status are much more likely (3.7 times) to smoke than their counterparts of higher socioeconomic status (King et al., 1993b; Najman et al., 1998). When education level alone is examined, individuals with only 9 to 11 years of education are about three times more likely to smoke than those with a college education (Table 3.2).

Occupation is strongly linked to rates of smoking as well, even after controlling for age, income, gender, and race or ethnicity (Nelson et al., 1994; Leigh, 1996; Bang and Kim, 2001). According to analyses of smoking by occupation and industry using the third National Health and Nutrition Examination Survey (1988 to 1994), the prevalence of cigarette smoking was highest among material-moving occupations, construction laborers, and vehicle mechanics and repairers. The lowest smoking prevalence was found among teachers. Among industry groups, the construction industry had the highest prevalence of cigarette smoking (Bang and Kim, 2001). Although disparities by occupation have persisted for many years, recent data suggest that the gap in smoking rates may be widening between blue-collar workers and white-collar workers (Nelson et al., 1994). Blue-collar workers tend to be heavier smokers and, therefore, more nicotine-dependent (Covey et al., 1992; Bang and Kim, 2001). Data from the 1997 National Health Interview Survey show that 27.5 percent of blue-collar smokers smoke 25 or more cigarettes per day, whereas only 18 percent of white-collar smokers do (Bang and Kim, 2001).

As with tobacco use, there are disparities in smoking cessation by race or ethnicity as well as other socio-demographic characteristics. When the disparity is assessed by race or ethnicity, whites have a higher rate of smoking cessation than African Americans. The 1989 Behavioral Risk Factor Surveillance System found that whites had a quit rate of 47 percent and African Americans had a quit rate of 39 percent (US DHHS, 1998). In 1994–1995, the percentage of adult African-American ever smokers who had quit was 35.4 percent (US DHHS, 1998). These numbers, however, do not reflect an aversion to quitting. The 1999 Behavioral Risk Factor Surveillance System found that about 59 percent of African Americans and Hispanics had quit for at least 1 day in the previous 12 months, as compared to 49 percent of whites (CDC, Division of Adult and Community Health, 1999). That African Americans have a harder time successfully quitting smoking may reflect a number of issues, such as a lack of access to appropriate smoking cessation programs as well as heightened nicotine dependence (US DHHS, 1990; Caraballo et al., 1998).

Education level is closely tied to rates of cessation of tobacco use. Typically, the higher the level of education that is attained, the higher the rate of smoking cessation (US DHHS, 1990). The quit rate for individuals with less than 12 years of education was 35 percent; for those with 12 years of education, it was 38 percent; for those with 13 to 15 years of education, it was 44 percent; and for those with 16 or more years of education, it was 57 percent.

PHYSICAL ACTIVITY

Physical activity has numerous mental and physical health benefits, including reductions in the risks of premature mortality, cardiovascular diseases, hypertension, diabetes, depression, osteoporosis, and cancer (US DHHS, 1996). Important health benefits include a reduced risk of colon, breast, and endometrial cancer (Table 3.4). In addition, physical activity is an important complement to dietary management for the avoidance of weight gain, and is essential for weight maintenance after intentional weight loss (National Heart, Lung, and Blood Institute, 1998). The International Agency for Research on Cancer (IARC) has estimated that at least 11 to 15 percent of breast and colorectal cancer may be attributable to inadequate physical activity (International Agency for Research on Cancer, 2002). Overall, sedentary lifestyles have been linked to 23 percent of deaths from major chronic diseases (Hahn et al., 1990), including 5 percent of deaths from cancer (Colditz et al., 1996). Fortunately, the negative effects of a sedentary lifestyle are reversible: evidence shows that increasing one's level of physical activity, even after years of inactivity, can reduce the risk of mortality (Paffenbarger et al., 1993). In addition, the level of activity necessary to reduce risk is not necessarily vigorous. Moderate activity, for example, walking briskly for 30 minutes a day, will lower an individual's risk of premature death, heart disease, stroke, diabetes, and colon cancer (US DHHS, 1996; Hu et al., 1999; Manson et al., 1999; Hu et al., 2000; International Agency for Research on Cancer, 2002). Because more than half of American adults do not participate in moderate or vigorous leisure-time physical activity (40 percent are not active at all) and because physical activity levels continue to decline in the United States (ACS, 2002b; US DHHS, 1996), the message that significant health benefits are achievable with moderate amounts of physical activity is especially important.

A large number of epidemiological studies have examined the relationship between physical activity and various types of cancers (US DHHS, 1996; McTiernan, et al. 1998; Marrett et al., 2000; International Agency

TABLE 3.4 Reduction in Risk of Incident Cancer Associated with Physical Activity

	Relative Risk (RR)	
Level of Evidence	Small (RR 0.76–0.90)	Moderate (RR 0.51–0.75)
Convincing	Breast	Colon
Probable	Endometrium	
Possible		

for research on Cancer, 2002). Over time, the designs of these studies have become progressively more sophisticated in terms of the measurement of physical activity and accounting for potential confounding factors. The studies summarized below were able to remove people with preexisting disease from the analysis and then examine the effect of physical activity over time in healthy populations.

Physical Activity and Colon Cancer

Among both men and women, high levels of physical activity may decrease the risk of colon cancer by as much as 50 percent (Colditz et al., 1997; Marrett et al., 2000). Although studies have not consistently used a standard measure of activity or similarly defined a "high" level of activity, a dose-response relationship between physical activity and colon cancer has consistently been observed across studies with a variety of designs and in many different populations (Garabrant et al., 1984; Slattery et al., 1988; Gerhardsson de Verdier et al., 1990; Whittemore et al., 1990; Giovannucci et al., 1995a; Martinez et al., 1997). In addition, physical activity appears to lower the risk of large adenomatous polyps, which suggests that it may act early in the adenoma-carcinoma sequence (Giovannucci et al., 1995a; Giovannucci et al., 1996; Kahn et al., 1998). The relation is seen across levels of obesity, suggesting a benefit of physical activity for reduction in cancer incidence in addition to weight reduction.

Maintaining high levels of physical activity throughout life appears to impart the greatest protection (Lee et al., 1989; Kune et al., 1990). In a study of Harvard alumni, men who were at least moderately active at two assessments were 48 percent less likely to develop colon cancer than men who were inactive at both assessments (Lee et al., 1991). However, this does not mean that those who have been sedentary in the past cannot reap the benefits if they become active. The same study showed that among men who were sedentary at the initial assessment, those who increased their activity during the 11- to 15-year follow-up period were 13 percent less likely to develop colon cancer than those who remained sedentary during the same time period (Lee et al., 1991). Data from at least two prospective studies indicated that both men and women can lower their risk of colon cancer simply by engaging in moderate physical activity such as brisk walking or stair climbing for an hour a day (Giovannucci et al., 1995a; Martinez et al., 1997). In those studies the risk decreased with increasing walking pace among those whose only recreational activity was walking.

Several mechanisms have been proposed to explain this. Physical activity may decrease gastrointestinal transit time, thereby minimizing contact of the gastrointestinal tract with potential carcinogens in the stool (McTiernan et al., 1998), and it may also reduce circulating levels of insulin, a growth factor for colonic epithelial cells (McKeown-Eyssen, 1994; Giovannucci, 1995b). Additional hypotheses suggest that physical activity alters prostaglandin levels, improves immune function, and modifies bile acid metabolism (Martinez et al., 1999).

Physical Activity and Breast Cancer

A woman's risk of breast cancer depends largely on the amount of estrogen circulating in her body (Willett et al., 2000; Hankinson et al., 1995). Because physical activity is thought to lower the cumulative level of lifetime exposure to circulating estrogens, researchers have long speculated that it might lower the risk of breast cancer. Numerous studies have examined this possibility, and although their results are not entirely consistent, the majority of studies support an inverse relationship between physical activity and breast cancer (Gammon et al., 1998; McTiernan et al., 1998; Marrett et al., 2000). Just as with colon cancer, the physical activity benefit for breast cancer is mediated both by its effect on body weight and by other mechanisms independent of bodyweight.

Physical activity in childhood may also affect breast cancer risk (Frisch et al., 1985; Bernstein et al., 1994; Colditz and Frazier, 1995). By interacting with the adrenaline system to reduce levels of circulating estrogens, physical activity may result in delayed menarche or a delay in the onset of regular ovulatory menstrual cycles, factors known to be associated with lower lifelong risk for breast cancer (Willett et al., 2000).

Physical Activity and Lung Cancer

Several studies have examined the impact of physical activity on lung cancer risk, and most have suggested a protective effect (World Cancer Research Fund and American Institute for Cancer Research, 1997). Researchers cannot completely control for the confounding effects of cigarette smoking, however. Since active people are less likely to smoke than inactive people and nonsmokers are far less likely to develop lung cancer than smokers, it is not clear whether active people are at lower risk of the disease because they are physically active or because they do not smoke. Most studies have attempted to control for smoking, but the potential for residual confounding cannot be ruled out, as smoking is such a strong causal factor in lung cancer and is associated with many health behaviors, including physical activity (International Agency for Research on Cancer, 2002).

Physical Activity and Prostate Cancer

As with breast cancer, physical activity has been hypothesized to lower the risk of prostate cancer by altering hormone levels. Despite this clear biological hypothesis and a number of studies on the topic, the relationship between physical activity and prostate cancer has remained unclear (World Cancer Research Fund and American Institute for Cancer Research, 1997; International Agency for Research on Cancer, 2002). Some studies have produced null results, whereas others report an inverse association and still others a positive association. Of the studies that have reported an inverse association, most have shown only a modest protective effect and no dose-response (Paffenbarger et al., 1987; Albanes et al., 1989; Paffenbarger et al., 1992). In addition, several of these studies showed significant relationships only among certain subgroups of men, defined by either age (Lee et al., 1992; Oliveria et al., 1996) or very high levels of activity (Lee et al., 1992; Giovannucci et al., 1998a).

OBESITY

Excess body fat causes numerous medical conditions, including cardiovascular diseases and some major cancers (U. S. Department of Agriculture and U. S. Department of Health and Human Services, 1995; International Agency for Research on Cancer, 2002), and is a growing problem in many countries. A linear relation exists between adiposity and most health conditions, although for mortality the shape of the relations has been debated, in part because of excess mortality among the leanest individuals. This relation between mortality and leanness is confounded in part by cigarette smoking and in part by reverse causation: the major illnesses such as cancer that predispose an individual to death first lead to weight loss and the artifactual appearance of increased mortality risk among lean individuals.

Consistent with the mortality burden described above, the study of cancer incidence shows many of the relations relating increasing adiposity or obesity to the onset of cancer (Table 3.5). Follow-up of 28,129 men and women in Sweden showed a 33 percent excess risk of cancer among obese individuals than among nonobese individuals (Wolk et al., 2001). Obesity contributes to the incidence of cancers through several possible mecha-

TABLE 3.5 Increase in Risk of Incident Cancer Associated with Obesity

	Relative Risk (RR)	
Level of Evidence	Moderate (RR 1.35–1.99)	Large (RR 2.0+)
Convincing	Colon	Breast Endometrial Kidney Esophageal
Possible	Prostate (mortality)	

nisms. These may include female hormones for breast and uterine cancer, insulin pathways for colon cancer, and various other explanations for cancer at other sites. The IARC estimates that about 10 percent of breast cancer and colorectal cancer may be attributable to overweight and obesity, and between 25 and 40 percent of kidney, esophageal, and endometrial cancer may be attributed to obesity.

Obesity and Breast Cancer

Consistent relationships have been seen between obesity and postmenopausal breast cancer, reflecting the role of adipose cells in the production of estrogen after menopause (Hunter and Willett, 1993; Hankinson et al., 1995; World Cancer Research Fund and American Institute for Cancer Research, 1997). The strongest relation may be seen among women who have never used postmenopausal hormones (Huang et al., 1997). This may be due in part to the predisposition of lean women and those with low circulating hormone levels to use postmenopausal hormones at the time of menopause, or it may be due to the fact that elevations in estrogen, regardless of the source, increase breast cancer risk similarly. Obesity has been associated with reduced risk for premenopausal breast cancer (International Agency for Research on Cancer, 2002), a relationship likely due to the adverse effects of obesity on ovarian function in premenopausal women.

Obesity and Endometrial Cancer

Women who are overweight are at increased risk of developing endometrial cancer. The risk is two to three times higher in obese women than in lean women, and the risk is more clearly evident in older women (Tornberg and Carstensen, 1994). This association is likely due to higher circulating estrogen levels after menopause among women who are obese.

Obesity and Prostate Cancer

The evidence for an association between obesity and prostate cancer is quite mixed. Although obesity may not increase risk of prostate cancer incidence, there is some evidence to suggest a higher risk of death after the diagnosis of prostate cancer among obese men (Andersson et al., 1997). Obesity may predispose an individual to more aggressive tumors or, alternatively, may stimulate growth or metastases of prostate cancer after it has developed. Several possible mechanisms through which obesity may influence the prostate gland involve hormones, including the insulin-like growth factor pathway, insulin itself, and, potentially, androgens.

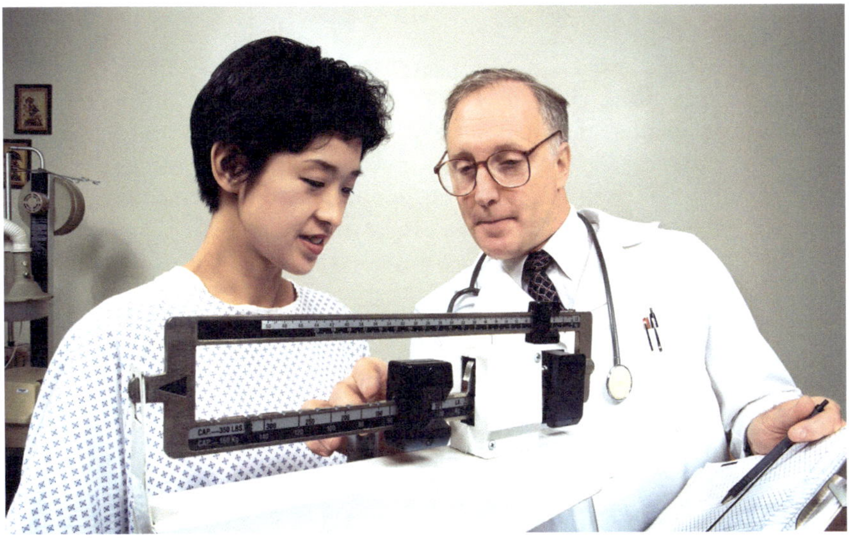

SOURCE: Corbis Corporation.

Obesity and Kidney Cancer

Obesity is directly related to the risk of kidney cancer among both men and women (McLaughlin et al., 1996). Virtually every study that has examined this relation has observed a positive association, although it is usually stronger among women than among men. The mechanism for the effect of obesity on the risk of kidney cancer is not clear, though insulin or insulin-like growth factors may be involved.

Obesity and Colon Cancer

Obesity and central adiposity have been related to colon cancer in numerous studies. The association is seen in both sexes, although it has usually been observed to be weaker among women. The mechanism by which obesity contributes to the development of colon cancer has not been fully documented. However, strong evidence supports a relation between excess weight, glycemic control, and colon cancer. Obesity is related to increased insulin resistance and hyperinsulinemia, which in turn are related to proliferation of colon cells in laboratory studies (McKeown-Eyssen, 1994; Giovannucci, 1995b; Kono et al., 1998). Further evidence supporting this mechanism comes from studies of the insulin-like growth factor pathway, which have demonstrated that insulin-like growth factor is directly related to colon cancer risk (Ma et al., 1999). Higher levels of estrogen in obese women after menopause may serve to lower colon cancer risk somewhat, which could explain the weaker association with obesity among women.

Obesity and Esophageal Cancer

Obesity is a known cause of gastroesophageal reflux, a risk factor for esophageal adenocarcinoma. In a population-based case-control study performed in Sweden, a strong direct relation between obesity and esophageal cancer was observed, with a relative risk of esophageal cancer of 16 for obese adults compared with the risk for lean adults. Other studies have observed relative risks of about 3–5 (Brown et al., 1995; Vaughan et al., 1995; Ji et al., 1997; Chow et al., 1998).

Trends in Obesity

In the United States, the age-adjusted prevalence of obesity increased from 15 percent in the late 1970s to 27 percent in 1999. The most recent estimates (1999) from the National Health and Nutrition Examination Survey (NHANES) show that 61 percent of the adult population (20–74 years) exceed the healthy weight range (BMI > 25 kg/m^2), 34 percent are overweight (BMI 25–29 kg/m^2), and 27 percent are obese (BMI ≥ 30 kg/m^2) (Figure 3.1) (US DHHS, 2001b).

According to the NHANES III (1988–1994) men are more likely than women to be either overweight or obese (59 vs. 51 percent), but women are

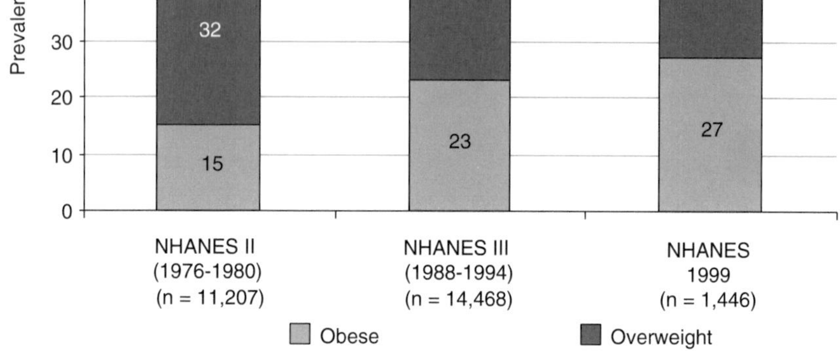

FIGURE 3.1 Age-adjusted prevalence of overweight (BMI 25–29 kg/m^2) and obesity (BMI ≥ 30 kg/m^2) in U.S. adults aged 20–74.
SOURCE: US DHHS, 2001b.

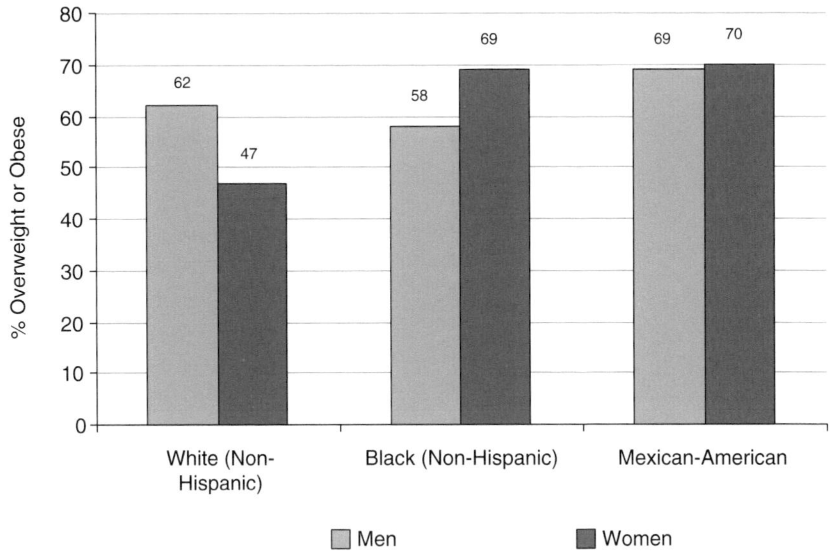

FIGURE 3.2 Age-adjusted prevalence of overweight or obesity (BMI ≥ 25 kg/m^2) by sex and race/ethnicity.
SOURCE: US DHHS, 2001b.

more likely than men to be obese (25 vs. 20 percent) (Flegal et al., 1998; ACS, 2001).

Obesity or overweight is higher among non-Hispanic African-American women and Mexican-American women than among non-Hispanic white women. Among men, the prevalence of obesity or overweight is somewhat higher among Mexican-Americans (Figure 3.2).

Setting Weight Guidelines

One essential part of effective policy planning is basing action on consistent messages. Yet, despite solid epidemiological evidence that weight affects the risk of cancer and other chronic diseases—including heart disease, stroke, and diabetes—setting weight guidelines has long been problematic, and recommendations have varied over time.

BMI is used in all these guidelines as a measure of adiposity. It is calculated as weight divided by height squared. Growing evidence suggests that BMI reflects adiposity well through middle age but may be less clearly related to adiposity at older ages, when lean muscle mass may decrease and mass is redistributed to the abdomen.

Debate continues regarding the possible use of waist circumference or waist circumference-to-hip-circumference ratio as a measure of adiposity.

Neither is yet standard clinical practice, and use of a ratio of two measures (the waist circumference-to-hip-circumference ratio) has additional problems, as it includes more complex measurements and the possibility of errors in both measures. "Girth grow," or increasing waist circumference with age, appears to predict the risk of diabetes, heart disease, and stroke.

In setting the 1995 weight guidelines (U.S. Department of Agriculture and US DHHS, 1995), the Dietary Guidelines Advisory Committee concluded that mortality risk increased significantly among persons with BMIs of 25 kg/m^2 or higher (Lee and Paffenbarger, 1992; Rimm et al., 1995; Willett et al., 1995), whereas a linear increase in the risk of being diagnosed with diabetes, hypertension, and coronary heart disease was observed with increasing BMI, even among individuals with BMIs well below 25 kg/m^2 (Chan et al., 1994; Colditz et al., 1995; Willett et al., 1995). Because of the importance of total mortality as a summary measure of the public health impact of obesity, the Dietary Guidelines Advisory Committee concluded that a BMI of 25 kg/m^2 represents a reasonable upper limit for healthy weight. This cutoff point is consistent with those recommended by a steering committee of the American Institute of Nutrition (Kuller et al., 1993) and an expert committee of the World Health Organization (World Health Organization, 1995).

DIET

There has been an explosion of prospective studies on diet and chronic disease in recent years, and this has greatly furthered understanding of the etiology of cancer (Willett, 1998). Building on international correlation studies and retrospective case-control studies, prospective cohort studies offer the potential to evaluate diet-disease relationships free from recall bias and to correct for measurement error. This section summarizes major areas of advance according to components of the American diet.

Fruits and Vegetables

The strongest evidence of a relationship between diet and cancer has long been related to the benefit of the consumption of least five servings of fruits and vegetables per day. The majority of this evidence has arisen from case-control studies, while the prospective data have been less consistent (Table 3.6). Fruits and vegetables lower the risk of hypertension, coronary heart disease, and ischemic stroke, in addition to containing vitamins and minerals that may protect against cancer and a host of other conditions (World Cancer Research Fund and American Institute for Cancer Research, 1997).

Numerous mechanisms have been proposed to explain the possible

TABLE 3.6 Reduction in Risk of Incident Cancer Associated with Fruit and Vegetable Intake

	Relative Risk (RR)		
Level of Evidence	Small (RR 0.76–0.90)	Moderate (RR 0.51–0.75)	Large (RR < 0.50)
Convincing			
Probable		Pancreas Bladder Lung Colon	Mouth Pharynx Larynx Esophagus Stomach
Possible	Breast Prostate Endometrium Ovary	Thyroid Cervical Liver Kidney	

inverse relationship between fruit and vegetable consumption and the risk of various cancers. Most have focused on the effects of specific agents contained in fruits and vegetables, such as carotenoids, selenium, folic acid, fiber, and vitamins C and E. However, Steinmetz and Potter (1991) have suggested that fruits and vegetables contain an anticarcinogenic cocktail of substances, including both recognized nutrients and nonnutritive constituents. Together, these substances inhibit the formation of carcinogens, act as substrates for the endogenous production of anticarcinogens, reduce the capacity of transformed cells to proliferate, and act as antioxidants.

Fruit and Vegetable Consumption and Cancers of the Mouth, Pharynx, Larynx, and Esophagus

Cancers of the mouth, pharnyx, larynx, and esophagus are caused primarily by alcohol and tobacco smoking. To a lesser extent, they may also be influenced by fruit and vegetable consumption. Most of the evidence for this comes from case-control studies, which have consistently shown a moderate to large reduction in risk among those who consume at least one serving of fruits and vegetables a day (World Cancer Research Fund and American Institute for Cancer Research, 1997). Very few prospective data support these findings, however; and the possibility of residual confounding by tobacco and alcohol use and/or recall bias cannot be eliminated.

Fruit and Vegetable Consumption and Stomach Cancer

Of the many cancers that have been studied in association with fruit and vegetable consumption, stomach cancer has been examined most extensively. More than 30 case-control studies have been conducted, with the majority supporting an inverse relationship (World Cancer Research Fund and American Institute for Cancer Research, 1997). However, as with most cancers, the data from prospective studies are less consistent. Although 8 of the 11 prospective studies suggested that the consumption of fruits and vegetables (either total intake or specific groups) might protect against stomach cancer (Chyou et al., 1990; Hirayama, 1990; Nomura et al., 1990; Zheng et al., 1995; Galanis et al., 1998; Terry et al., 1998; Botterweck et al., 1998; Dorant et al., 1996), only 5 reported a statistically significant association (Chyou et al., 1990; Hirayama, 1990; Galanis et al., 1998; Terry et al., 1998; Dorant et al., 1996). Two additional studies reported null findings (Kneller et al., 1991; Guo et al., 1994), and one suggested a nonsignificant positive relationship (Kato et al., 1992).

Fruit and Vegetable Consumption and Pancreatic Cancer

Of the 15 case-control studies that have been conducted on fruit and vegetable consumption and the risk of pancreatic cancer, 14 have provided evidence of an inverse association (Ohba et al., 1996; World Cancer Research Fund and American Institute for Cancer Research,1997; Mori et al., 1999). These studies, including those that controlled for smoking, consistently suggest a moderate protective effect for both fruits and vegetables. However, data from the four cohort studies on the topic have been far less consistent (Howe and Burch, 1996; World Cancer Research Fund and American Institute for Cancer Research, 1997). Although none of the findings have been statistically significant, they have suggested both inverse and positive associations (World Cancer Research Fund and American Institute for Cancer Research, 1997).

Although case-control studies typically yield less conclusive evidence than cohort studies because of the greater potential for recall bias and residual confounding, cohort studies on this topic are also limited because of the rarity of the disease. Three of the four cohort studies on fruit and vegetable consumption and pancreatic cancer included only 40 to 65 incident cases or deaths, and so their results must be interpreted cautiously (Howe and Burch, 1996).

Fruit and Vegetable Consumption and Bladder Cancer

There is evidence of a probable inverse association between fruit and vegetable consumption and the risk of bladder cancer. Nearly all studies on the topic have adequately controlled for smoking, the primary cause of bladder cancer, and most suggest that both fruits and vegetables offer some degree of protection against bladder cancer (World Cancer Research Fund and American Institute for Cancer Research, 1997).

A recent meta-analysis suggests that fruits might have a greater impact on risk than vegetables (Steinmaus et al., 2000). In that analysis, the risk of bladder cancer was increased 40 percent among those with low levels of consumption of fruits and 16 percent among those with low levels of consumption of vegetables.

Fruit and Vegetable Consumption and Lung Cancer

An inverse association between high levels of consumption of fruits and vegetables and the risk of lung cancer has been observed in both case-control studies and large cohort studies (World Cancer Research Fund and American Institute for Cancer Research, 1997). Most cohort studies have shown, after controlling for smoking status, that a high level of consumption of fruits and vegetables is associated with substantially lower risk of lung cancer (World Cancer Research Fund and American Institute for Cancer Research, 1997; Yong et al., 1997; Knekt et al., 1999; Voorrips et al., 2000b). However, one analysis, which combines data from two large cohort studies, suggests only a weak association (Feskanich et al., 2000).

Much effort has been expended to identify the specific components of fruits and vegetables that might be responsible for the possible reduction in lung cancer risk. The majority of studies have focused on provitamin A carotenoids, particularly beta-carotene, because of their antioxidant properties and the importance of vitamin A in cell differentiation. However, clinical trials of high-dose beta-carotene supplements failed to produce the expected reduction in lung cancer risk (Alpha-Tocopherol Beta-Carotene Prevention Study Group, 1994; Hennekens et al., 1996; Omenn et al., 1996).

Fruit and Vegetable Consumption and Breast Cancer

The relationship between fruit and vegetable consumption and the risk of breast cancer has been evaluated extensively in case-control studies, with the majority suggesting either no association or a modest inverse association. However, in a large reanalysis combining the primary data from eight cohort studies, Smith-Warner et al. (2001) found no association between total levels of fruit and vegetable consumption and the risk of breast cancer. Similar null results were observed both for individual fruits and vegetables and for various botanical groups.

Fruit and Vegetable Consumption and Colon Cancer

The relationship between fruit and vegetable consumption and the risk of colon cancer has been examined in many case-control studies, most of which have suggested a protective effect for higher levels of vegetable intake (World Cancer Research Fund and American Institute for Cancer Research, 1997). In those studies, green vegetables and cruciferous vegetables (any of a family of vegetables including cabbage, turnip, and mustard) seemed particularly beneficial. However, the prospective cohort studies to examine this relationship have yielded less conclusive findings (Phillips and Snowdon, 1985; Singh and Fraser, 1998; Thun et al., 1992; Voorrips et al., 2000a).

In one study with a large cohort, Thun and colleagues (1992) compared the risk of fatal colon cancer among those in the quintile with the highest levels of vegetable consumption and those in the quintile with the lowest levels of vegetable consumption. Statistically significant reductions were observed for women but not men. In another prospective study, overall fruit and vegetable intake was weakly associated with colon cancer risk, but raw vegetables, green leafy vegetables, and cruciferous vegetables appeared to be more protective for both men and women (Steinmetz et al., 1994). Michels and colleagues (2000) combined data from two large cohort studies and observed no association between overall levels of fruit and vegetable consumption and the risk of colon cancer. Similar null findings were observed for various categories of fruits and vegetables, including green leafy vegetables, citrus fruits, and cruciferous vegetables.

Vegetables contain so many beneficial vitamins and nutrients that it is difficult to identify which ones might be responsible for the possible association with colon cancer. Fiber has received the most attention so far, mainly because the proposed mechanism is so intuitive: fiber can help push waste through the colon more quickly, so that the colon is less likely to come into contact with any carcinogens. However, data from two randomized controlled trials recently failed to support a link between increased fiber intake over three years and the risk of recurrence of colon polyps, the precursor lesion for colon cancer (Alberts et al., 2000; Schatzkin et al., 2000).

Fruit and Vegetable Consumption and Ovarian Cancer

A high level of consumption of vegetables may reduce the risk of ovarian cancer, although few studies have addressed the issue (World Cancer Research Fund and American Institute for Cancer Research, 1997). In the only two cohort studies conducted on this topic to date, researchers did not observe an association between the overall levels of fruit and vegetable consumption and the risk of ovarian cancer (Kushi et al., 1999; Fairfield et al., 2001). In both of those studies, however, and in a large case-control study (Risch et al., 1994), there was a suggestion of modest reduction in risk with higher levels of vegetable consumption.

Fruit and Vegetable Consumption and Endometrial Cancer

The association between fruit and vegetable consumption and the risk of endometrial cancer has been evaluated in several case-control studies, with results suggesting the possibility of a modest inverse association (World Cancer Research Fund and American Institute for Cancer Research, 1997). In the only cohort study to address this relationship to date, researchers found the suggestion of an increased risk of endometrial cancer among those with very low levels of vegetable consumption (Terry et al., 1999).

Fruit and Vegetable Consumption and Prostate Cancer

Although the effects of fruit and vegetable consumption on the risk of prostate cancer have been examined in nearly 20 studies, the data are quite inconsistent. The majority of studies suggest that overall levels of fruit and vegetable consumption have little effect, if any, on the risk of prostate cancer. However, individual fruits and vegetables may provide a greater reduction of risk, with tomatoes being the most promising (Giovannucci, 1999). Four cohort studies have reported on tomato consumption and prostate cancer risk, and all of them demonstrated a 40 to 50 percent reduction in risk among men who consumed large amounts of tomatoes. The carotenoid lycopene is hypothesized to be responsible for a protective effect.

Fruit and Vegetable Consumption and Thyroid Cancer

Several case-control studies have reported an inverse association between fruit and vegetable consumption and the risk of thyroid cancer (World Cancer Research Fund and American Institute for Cancer Research, 1997). In all of the studies, cruciferous vegetables appeared to be particularly beneficial. However, this has not been examined in cohort studies, given the rarity of the disease.

Fruit and Vegetable Consumption and Cervical Cancer

There is evidence of a possible inverse relationship between fruit and vegetable consumption and the risk of cervical cancer. Of the five studies published on the topic, four reported a reduced risk with one or more measures of fruit and vegetable intake (World Cancer Research Fund and American Institute for Cancer Research, 1997). Despite this consistency, few conclusions can be drawn about the relationship because of the potential for confounding. Most of the identified risk factors for cervical cancer—including human papillomavirus infection, cigarette smoking, and infrequent use of Pap screening—are closely related to socioeconomic status, which is in turn related to dietary intake (Potischman and Brinton, 1996; World Cancer Research Fund and American Institute for Cancer Research, 1997).

Fruit and Vegetable Consumption and Liver Cancer

A high level of consumption of vegetables may lower the risk of liver cancer. In the two cohort studies that have examined this relationship, one demonstrated a sevenfold increase in risk among those who consumed small amounts of fresh vegetables, and the other suggested a protective effect for green-yellow vegetables. Five case-control studies have also been conducted on the topic, three of which suggested a moderate to large inverse association with the consumption of certain types of vegetables.

Fruit and Vegetable Consumption and Kidney Cancer

A number of case-control studies have demonstrated an inverse association between fruit and vegetable consumption and the risk of kidney cancer (Mellemgaard et al., 1996; Wolk et al., 1996; Lindblad et al., 1997; World Cancer Research Fund and American Institute for Cancer Research, 1997; Yuan et al., 1998). In the largest of these studies, the International Renal Cell Cancer Study, Wolk and colleagues (1996) reported a protective effect for several groups of fruits and vegetables, with the strongest association observed for orange and dark green vegetables.

Red Meat

The levels of consumption of red meats such as beef, pork, and lamb have declined dramatically in the United States in the past 40 years, in part because of increasing concern about the effects of meat on health. Although red meat is an excellent source of protein and iron, it also contains large amounts of saturated fat, which can raise the level of cholesterol in the blood. In addition, when cooked at high temperatures, high-protein foods such as red meat may generate carcinogens. Evidence linking the consumption of red meat to a higher incidence of cancer is not yet convincing (Table 3.7).

Red Meat Consumption and Colorectal Cancer

There is probable evidence that the consumption of large amounts of red meat increases the risk of colorectal cancer among both men and women. Although not entirely consistent, numerous studies with both cohort and case-control designs have reported a positive association between the consumption of red meat and colon cancer (World Cancer Research

TABLE 3.7 Increase in Risk of Incident Cancer Associated with High Intakes of Red Meat

	Relative Risk (RR)	
Level of Evidence	Moderate (RR 1.35–1.99)	Large (RR ≥2.0)
Convincing		
Probable		Colon and rectum
Possible	Kidney Prostate Pancreas	

Fund and American Institute for Cancer Research, 1997). For most studies showing an association, the median relative risk between the categories of high and low levels of red meat consumption is about 2, with the majority falling between 1.5 and 2.5 (Giovannucci and Goldin, 1997).

Several mechanisms have been proposed to explain the relationship between red meat consumption and colon cancer. First, the specific fatty acid content of red meat may be particularly harmful (Giovannucci, 1995a). However, the fatty acids in beef are not unique and overlap substantially with those in dairy fat, which is not related to colon cancer. Second, fat from red meat may be less readily digested or absorbed in the small intestine than fat from other sources; therefore, more of it may reach the large bowel (Giovannucci and Willett, 1994). Third, initiators or promoters may be formed when red meat is cooked, particularly at high temperatures (Schiffman et al., 1989; Gerhardsson de Verdier et al., 1991). Finally, high levels of consumption of red meat may increase the concentrations of fecal iron, which could influence the risk of colon cancer via the generation of hydroxyl radicals (Giovannucci and Willett, 1994; Sesink et al., 1999; Sesink et al., 2000).

Red Meat Consumption and Prostate Cancer

The relationship between red meat consumption and the risk of prostate cancer has been examined in a number of cohort and case-control studies, with results suggesting a positive association (World Cancer Research Fund and American Institute for Cancer Research, 1997). In the largest cohort study to address this issue, the risk of advanced prostate cancer was more than twice as high among men who consumed red meat frequently than among those who consumed it rarely (Giovannucci et al., 1993a). Other studies have shown similar results, although positive findings have generally been limited to populations whose diets include large amounts of red meat (World Cancer Research Fund and American Institute for Cancer Research, 1997).

Red Meat Consumption and Pancreatic Cancer

The overall evidence on red meat consumption and the risk of pancreatic cancer is somewhat inconsistent but generally suggestive of a positive relationship. Although three cohort studies have demonstrated an increased risk for those with higher levels of meat consumption (World Cancer Research Fund and American Institute for Cancer Research 1997), only one examined the specific effects of red meat. That study reported a twofold increase among men with higher levels of red meat consumption (Zheng et al., 1993).

Case-control studies have gone one step further by evaluating the effects of specific types of red meat, including beef and pork, as well as processed meats, like bacon and sausage. Those studies have consistently shown a positive association between pork consumption and pancreatic cancer risk, although they have yielded inconsistent results for other meats (World Cancer Research Fund and American Institute for Cancer Research, 1997).

Red Meat Consumption and Kidney Cancer

The association between red meat consumption and the risk of kidney cancer has been evaluated in several case-control studies, with results suggesting the possibility of a positive association (World Cancer Research Fund and American Institute for Cancer Research, 1997). In the largest case-control study conducted to date, Wolk and colleagues (1996) reported no association between red meat consumption and the risk of kidney cancer. However, the means of meat preparation and the degree of "doneness" were both related to risk. Compared with baked and roasted meats, the consumption of fried and sautéed meats was associated with a 44 percent increase in risk, and the consumption of meats that are cooked well done, charred, or burnt was associated with a 24 percent increase in risk.

Whole-Grain Foods

Grains such as wheat, rice, corn, barley, and rye form the basis of most diets worldwide. Some grain products, like wheat bread or brown rice, remain in the whole-grain form, whereas others, like white bread or white rice, are more refined. Because most of the fiber, vitamins, and minerals are removed from grains during the refining process, whole-grain foods tend to be more nutrient-rich than refined foods (World Cancer Research Fund and American Institute for Cancer Research, 1997). The relationship between dietary whole-grain and cancer should be placed in context of the established cardiovascular benefits of whole-grain foods, which have been shown to lower the risk of both coronary heart disease and ischemic stroke (World Cancer Research Fund and American Institute for Cancer Research, 1997).

Whole-Grain Food Consumption and Stomach Cancer

The data on overall levels of grain consumption and the risk of stomach cancer are too inconsistent to judge the nature of the relationship. However, studies that have isolated the effects of whole-grain foods (compared with the effects of both whole grains and refined grains) suggest that whole-grain foods offer moderate levels of protection. In a summary of seven case-control studies, Jacobs and colleagues (1995) reported an inverse association for all but one study. In three of the studies, the relative risk was 0.4 for a high level of consumption compared with that for a low level of consumption. In addition, several of the studies showed either no association or a positive association between the consumption of refined grains and stomach cancer. Taken collectively, these studies suggest that the effect of grains depends on the extent to which the grains have been refined (World Cancer Research Fund and American Institute for Cancer Research, 1997).

Fiber Consumption and Colon Cancer

Recent trials of the effects of increased levels of fiber consumption on the prevention of polyp recurrence among patients who have had polyps removed have shown no reduction in the recurrence of polyps during follow-up of some 3 years. In one trial, a supplement with wheat bran with high levels of fiber (13.5 grams [g]/day) was compared with a supplement with low levels of fiber (2 g/day) (Alberts et al., 2000). In the other study participants were counseled to increase their levels of fiber, fruit, and vegetable consumption, and the comparison group received usual care in the form of a standard brochure on healthy eating (Schatzkin et al., 2000). In both randomized trials the percentage of subjects with recurrent polyps was almost identical in each group. Although the three-year time frame for the preventive intervention may not be long enough, parallel data from the prospective Nurses' Health Study also showed no relation between fiber intake and the risk of colon cancer during 16 years of follow-up (Fuchs et al., 1999).

Milk and Dairy Products

The effects of dairy products on cancer risk have not been well studied, and most links between the two have been made only indirectly (World Cancer Research Fund and American Institute for Cancer Research, 1997).

The available evidence suggests that milk and other dairy products may raise the risk of prostate cancer, kidney, and ovarian cancer, but may lower the risk of colon cancer.

Milk and Dairy Product Consumption and Prostate Cancer

Case-control studies generally support a positive association between the consumption of dairy products and prostate cancer risk, whereas cohort studies are less consistent (World Cancer Research Fund and American Institute for Cancer Research 1997). A higher level of milk consumption was related to an increased risk of prostate cancer in three of the seven cohort studies on dairy products (Snowdon et al., 1984; Le Marchand et al., 1994; Schuurman et al., 1999). In addition, one study suggested an increased risk with higher levels of consumption of butter, margarine, and cheese (Severson et al., 1989). Taken collectively, the evidence suggests the possibility of a moderate positive association between the consumption of dairy products and prostate cancer risk. Although this relationship has been attributed to the high fat contents of many dairy products, recent evidence suggests that calcium may be the responsible agent (Chan et al., 1998). Calcium has been shown to cause a compensatory decrease in circulating levels of 1,25-dihydroxy vitamin D, which may in turn raise the risk of prostate cancer (Giovannucci, 1998).

Milk and Dairy Product Consumption and Kidney Cancer

Evidence of a possible relationship between the consumption of dairy products and kidney cancer comes entirely from case-control studies (World Cancer Research Fund and American Institute for Cancer Research, 1997). Of nine such studies, seven have shown an increased risk among those with high levels of milk consumption (Mellemgaard et al., 1996; Wolk et al., 1996; World Cancer Research Fund and American Institute for Cancer Research, 1997). Odds ratios tend to be in the range of 1.3 to 1.8, with some studies suggesting even larger effects. Proposed mechanisms involve both animal protein and animal fat (World Cancer Research Fund and American Institute for Cancer Research, 1997).

Milk and Dairy Product Consumption and Ovarian Cancer

Lactose is the primary sugar found in milk and other dairy products. When lactose is consumed and digested, it is broken down into two components, galactose and glucose, which are then broken down even further. If galactose is not metabolized properly, it can accumulate in the ovaries, affecting ovarian function and hormone levels. This may, in turn, contribute to the development of ovarian tumors. Two large cohort studies, the Nurses' Health

Study and the Iowa Women's Health Study, have examined the association of lactose consumption on ovarian cancer. Both studies found a modest increase in risk among women who consume large amounts of lactose.

NUTRIENTS

The link between whole foods and cancer is only one aspect of the diet-cancer relationship, but it is generally the most practical link when it comes to policy decisions and consumer action. Overall, people buy, prepare, and eat whole foods rather than specific nutrients. For this reason, this report focuses on the whole-food aspects of diet and their impact on cancer risk. There is a growing body of evidence that specific macronutrients or micronutrients could explain the associations between foods and cancer risk.

Macronutrients

Fat, carbohydrates, fiber, and protein have each been linked with cancer in some way (Table 3.8). A number of studies support a possible association between a high total fat intake and an increased risk of lung, colorectal, and prostate cancer (World Cancer Research Fund and American Institute for Cancer Research, 1997). The findings across studies are not consistent, however. Analyses based on prospective data tend to show very little, if any, association between total fat intake and cancer risk when total energy intake and other potential confounders are controlled for. A large combined analysis of breast cancer and dietary fats showed no association across a wide range of fat intakes (Hunter et al., 1996). The hypothesis that reducing intake of fats will reduce breast cancer risk is now being tested in the Women's Health Initiative, a large intervention study in the United States (http://www.nhlbi.nih.gov/whi/). More plausible is a link between different types of fat and certain cancers. Saturated or animal fat, *trans*-unsaturated fat, and cholesterol have been found in some studies to increase the risk of cancer, whereas monounsaturated fat has been found in some studies to lower the risk of breast cancer (World Cancer Research Fund and American Institute for Cancer Research, 1997; Chiu et al., 1996; Willett, 1999; Zhang et al., 1999b). The consumption of large amounts of starch has been linked to a possible increase in stomach cancer risk and a possible decrease in colorectal cancer risk (World Cancer Research Fund and American Institute for Cancer Research, 1997).

Micronutrients

The link between micronutrients and cancer has been studied extensively, and although a number of possible associations have been identified, only a few have enough evidence to qualify as probable associations (Table

TABLE 3.8 Risk of Incident Cancer Associated with Selected Macronutrients

	Association of Type of Cancer for the Following Level of Evidence:		
Macronutrients	Convincing	Probable	Possible
Fat and cholesterol			
Total fat			Positive association: • Lung cancer • Colorectal cancer • Prostate cancer
Saturated/animal fat			Positive association: • Endometrial cancer • Lung cancer • Colorectal cancer • Prostate cancer • Non-Hodgkin's lymphoma
trans-Unsaturated fat			Positive association: • Non-Hodgkin's lymphoma
Monounsaturated fat			Inverse association: • Breast cancer
Cholesterol			Positive association: • Lung cancer • Pancreatic cancer
Carbohydrates			
Starch			Inverse association: • Colorectal cancer Positive association: • Stomach cancer
Fiber			Inverse association: • Endometrial cancer • Pancreatic cancer • Colorectal cancer
Protein			Inverse association: • Breast cancer (survival)
Total energy intake			Positive association: • Pancreatic cancer

3.9). The most well-established link is between folate and colorectal cancer. A number of studies have found that as the level of folate consumption increases, the risk of colorectal cancer (as well as polyps) decreases (Freudenheim et al., 1991; Giovannucci et al., 1993b; Giovannucci et al., 1998b; Willett, 2000). The Nurses' Health Study found that the consumption of large amounts of folate from fruits and vegetables was sufficient to lower

TABLE 3.9 Risk of Incident Cancer Associated with Selected Micronutrients

	Association of Type of Cancer for the Following Level of Evidence:		
Macronutrients	Convincing	Probable	Possible
Vitamin A and carotenoids		Inverse association: • Lung cancer	Inverse association: • Breast cancer • Esophageal cancer • Stomach cancer • Colorectal cancer • Cervical cancer
Folate		Inverse association: • Colorectal cancer	Inverse association: • Breast cancer
Vitamin D		Inverse association: • Colorectal cancer	
Vitamin E			Inverse association: • Lung cancer • Cervical cancer • Colorectal cancer
Calcium			Inverse association: • Colorectal cancer Positive association: • Prostate cancer • Kidney cancer • Ovary cancer
Selenium			Inverse association: • Lung cancer • Prostate cancer • Colorectal cancer

the colorectal cancer risk and that supplementation with a multivitamin that contained folate offered additional reductions (Giovannucci et al., 1998b). The underlying biological role of folate and its interaction with the *MTHFR* gene offers a plausible biological pathway for a causal relation between low levels of folate consumption and colon cancer.

The association of vitamin A and carotenoids with cancer risk has also been studied extensively, with the strongest evidence supporting a probable inverse relation with breast and lung cancers. Currently, however, it seems at most only a small reduction in the risk of breast cancer is associated with the consumption of large amounts of carotenoids from food sources (Zhang et al., 1999a). In addition, a number of observational studies support an association between the consumption of large amounts of carotenoids from food and a lower risk of lung cancer. Randomized trials of beta-carotene supplements found either no effect or an increased risk of lung cancer (Alpha-Tocopherol Beta Carotene Cancer Prevention Study Group, 1994;

Hennekens et al., 1996; Omenn et al., 1996), suggesting that a protective effect of fruits and vegetables is not explained by beta carotene alone. A surprise finding of the ATBC study was the lower prostate cancer risk observed in the vitamin E arm. Whether supplemental vitamin E might reduce prostate cancer risk is now being tested in the SELECT trial (http://www.cancer.gov/newscenter/SELECT).

Studies with animals have suggested that the consumption of larger amounts of selenium reduces the risk of various tumors, and ecological studies show an inverse relation between selenium and cancers of the breast and colon (Clark, 1985). A randomized trial to test the ability of a selenium supplement to reduce skin cancer risk showed no effect for skin cancer, but a significant reduction in the rates of mortality from cancers of the lung, colon, and prostate (Clark et al., 1996). Evidence against a large and rapid impact of selenium on cancer risk comes from a fortification intervention that was implemented in Finland. Because of the low selenium content of the soil in Finland (leading to low food selenium levels), selenium was applied with fertilizer in the mid-1980s. Blood selenium levels rose rapidly following this ecological intervention, but there has been no apparent decline in incidence or mortality rates for prostate or colon cancer (Willett, 1999). Whether supplemental selenium might reduce prostate cancer risk is now being tested, along with vitamin E, in the SELECT trial (http://www.cancer.gov/newscenter/SELECT).

Glycemic Index

The relation between macronutrients in diet and the physiological response to foods is complex. During digestion, the body breaks down dietary glucose into either sugar or starch so that it can be absorbed into the bloodstream. The resulting spike in blood glucose levels leads to a compensatory increase in blood insulin levels. Because insulin allows glucose to be taken up by the tissues, the blood glucose level drops in response to the high insulin levels. Once the blood glucose levels return to normal, insulin is released into the blood at a much lower rate.

The impact that a food has on these patterns of circulating blood glucose and insulin is estimated by its glycemic index. Foods with high glycemic indices are digested and absorbed more quickly, causing a rapid influx of glucose into the bloodstream, causing the insulin level to rise rapidly, while foods with a low glycemic index are converted to glucose more slowly and thus lead to a smaller spike in insulin levels. Foods with high glycemic indices may increase the risk of diabetes and coronary heart disease (Salmeron et al., 1997a; Salmeron et al., 1997b; Liu et al., 2000).

Whether foods with a high glycemic index also have an impact on the risk of cancer is unclear. If hyperinsulinemia is important in carcinogenesis in the colon, however, then the glycemic load from foods may be an important risk factor for colon cancer. An increasing number of epidemiological studies have found that the consumption of large amounts of sugar and foods with a high glycemic index is associated with an increased risk of colon cancer (Giovannucci, 1995b). On the basis of this growing evidence relating insulin, glycemic load, and colon cancer risk, further research is needed to determine if the insulin pathway might also contribute to other major malignancies.

Disparities in Dietary Intake

The proportion of adults consuming the recommended five servings of fruits and vegetables a day has been estimated to be no more than 32 percent (Krebs-Smith et al., 1995a; Krebs-Smith et al., 1995b; Thompson et al., 1999; Li et al., 2000). Although these estimates are clearly low for the entire population, there is also considerable variation across subgroups defined by sex, race or ethnicity, education, and income. The levels of fruit and vegetable consumption are lower among men than among women (Subar et al., 1995; Kamimoto et al., 1999). One study showed that the level of fruit and vegetable consumption was lowest among Hispanics (Thompson et al., 1999), another found higher levels of consumption among whites than African Americans ages 55 and older (Kamimoto et al., 1999), and other studies have found lower levels of consumption of fruits and vegetables among individuals with lower incomes and lower levels of educational attainment (Subar et al., 1995; Thompson et al., 1999).

Although the level of consumption of red meat has decreased substantially in the population as a whole (U.S. Department of Agriculture, 1999), lower-income households have experienced less of a reduction than higher-income households (Interagency Board for Nutrition Monitoring and Related Research, 1993). In general, dietary trends in the last 60 years in the United States have shown a complex relationship with social class. Among those with higher socioeconomic status, diets have improved in regards to cancer and heart disease risk, whereas among those at lower socioeconomic classes, diets have worsened in the last half of the 20th century (Popkin et al., 1996).

ALCOHOL

Alcohol consumption has both beneficial and harmful effects on health. A U-shaped relationship between mortality and consumption of alcohol was described as early as 1926 (Pearl, 1926). A number of studies since then have shown that persons who drink heavily have higher rates of death from certain types of acute death, such as poisoning (Anderson, 1995), injuries (Andreasson et al., 1988; CDC, 1995), violence (Andreasson et al., 1988), and suicide (Andreasson et al., 1988), whereas the long-term use of alcohol increases the risk of death from cirrhosis (Norton et al., 1987), hemorrhagic stroke (Donahue et al., 1986), and certain cancers (International Agency for Research on Cancer, 1988). Alcohol is listed as one of the top identifiable contributors to death in the United States (McGinnis and Foege, 1993), after tobacco and diet and activity patterns; and of all the threats to human health, alcohol probably causes the widest range of diseases and injuries (Rose, 1992).

In 1990, approximately 5 percent of all deaths (about 100,000 deaths) were attributable to alcohol consumption, as were 15 percent of potential years of life lost before age 65 (Rose, 1992). The consequences of alcohol consumption extend beyond death rates. Alcohol affects nerve cells in the brain and impairs cognitive function, both temporarily and permanently, over the long term (Meyer, Terayama et al., 1998), and it contributes to the destruction of personal and social relationships (Brookoff et al., 1997). An estimated 18 million people in the United States suffer from alcohol dependence, and an estimated 76 million people are affected by the consequences of alcohol abuse through either their own habit or that of someone close to them (McGinnis and Foege, 1993). Nearly a third of all U.S. adults engage in risky drinking patterns and thus need some kind of intervention, whether it is advice to cut down or referral for further evaluation and treatment for suspected abuse or dependence (Dawson, 2002).

In contrast to these harmful effects, however, there is substantial evidence for a beneficial effect of the consumption of moderate amounts of alcohol on the risk of coronary heart disease and thrombotic stroke. The risk of death from these cardiovascular causes is reduced, on average, by about 20 to 40 percent by the consumption of moderate amounts of alcohol (Doll, 1997; Thun et al., 1997). Because cardiovascular disease is the leading cause of death among those of middle and old ages, a reduction in the risk of mortality from cardiovascular disease with moderate alcohol use will translate into a reduction in the total risk of mortality in many populations. Clearly, there is a need to balance the many risks and benefits of alcohol use.

The Impact of Alcohol on Cancer Incidence

Because alcohol use tends to be associated with cigarette use and other high-risk behaviors, its independent effects on cancer have long been questioned. However, in 1988, on the basis of abundant epidemiological evidence, the International Agency for Research on Cancer concluded that alcohol is, in fact, a Group A carcinogen and an independent risk factor for cancers of the upper aerodigestive tract and liver (World Cancer Research Fund and American Institute for Cancer Research, 1997). Since publication of that report, a large body of evidence has confirmed that alcohol use also increases the risk of breast cancer (Longnecker et al., 1988; Willett et al., 2000) and, probably, colon cancer (Tomeo et al., 1999) (Table 3.10).

Although numerous studies have compared the effects of beer, wine,

TABLE 3.10 Increase in Risk of Incident Cancer Associated with Alcohol Use

	Relative Risk (RR)	
Level of Evidence	Moderate (RR 1.35–1.99)	Large (RR >2.0)
Convincing	Breast	Mouth Pharynx Larynx Esophagus Liver[a]
Probable	Colon and rectum	

[a]Although light and moderate levels of alcohol consumption do not increase the risk of liver cancer, heavy drinking increases the risk substantially.

and liquor, the type of alcohol consumed does not appear to influence the cancer risk as much as does the amount consumed (World Cancer Research Fund and American Institute for Cancer Research, 1997). For cancers of the upper aerodigestive tract, breast, colon, and rectum, there is a dose-response relationship, such that even low or moderate levels of consumption increase risk slightly. For liver cancer, the most important factor is heavy and persistent use, such as that defined by alcoholism, which can cause chronic liver injury.

Alcohol Consumption and Cancers of the Mouth, Pharynx, Larynx, and Esophagus

There is convincing epidemiological evidence from both cohort and case-control studies that alcohol consumption increases the risk of cancers of the mouth, pharynx, larynx, and esophagus (World Cancer Research Fund and American Institute for Cancer Research, 1997; Kjaerheim et al., 1998). All of the cohort studies that have examined this association, including those that controlled for smoking, have demonstrated a substantially increased risk. In addition, a dose-response relationship has been observed in the majority of case-control studies, including most of those that controlled for smoking. Alcohol also appears to act synergistically with tobacco in causing these cancers (World Cancer Research Fund and American Institute for Cancer Research, 1997).

Several mechanisms have been proposed to explain the carcinogenic effect of alcohol on cancers of the upper aerodigestive tracts, although none are proven (World Cancer Research Fund and American Institute for Cancer Research, 1997). Alcohol may directly influence carcinogenesis in the cells that it touches; it may alter the permeabilities of cell membranes or modify cellular metabolism, thus making these cells more vulnerable to chemical carcinogens;

it may contain toxic substances, such as nitrosamines and polycyclic aromatic hydrocarbons, that alter DNA; and alcohol may in other ways compromise nutritional status and increase susceptibility to cancer (World Cancer Research Fund and American Institute for Cancer Research, 1997).

Alcohol Consumption and Liver Cancer

More than 40 studies have evaluated the relationship between high levels of alcohol intake and liver cancer. Although these studies did not use a standard definition of heavy drinking or even the same reference groups (nondrinkers versus the entire population), a positive association has been observed across a variety of study designs and populations (World Cancer Research Fund and American Institute for Cancer Research, 1997). Unlike most other cancers, liver cancer is associated only with the heavy persistent type of drinking characteristic of alcoholism, with its related chronic liver damage. Neither light nor moderate drinking increases liver cancer risk.

Alcohol Consumption and Breast Cancer

More than 25 studies have shown that alcohol increases breast cancer risk, most likely by raising the level of estrogen in the bloodstream or making the breast more vulnerable to carcinogens (Smith-Warner et al., 1998). A randomized feeding trial indicated that estrogen levels are increased when women consume even low levels of alcohol on a regular basis (Reichman et al., 1993).

The dose-response relationship between alcohol and breast cancer risk is best demonstrated in results from an analysis of data pooled from six prospective studies (Smith-Warner et al., 1998). In that analysis, women's risk of breast cancer rose by 7 percent for every 10-g increase in daily alcohol consumption. The association did not differ substantially by type of alcoholic beverage consumed. Because breast tissue may be particularly vulnerable during adolescence and early adulthood, researchers have speculated that alcohol consumption during these time periods might be more harmful than alcohol consumption later in life (Colditz and Frazier, 1995), but to date, studies on this topic have been inconsistent (Harvey et al., 1987; Young, 1989; Garland et al., 1999).

Alcohol Consumption and Colorectal Cancer

Although the results are not entirely consistent, the majority of studies support an association between alcohol intake and an increased risk of colorectal cancer in both men and women (Giovannucci and Willett, 1994). Moreover, alcohol consumption is related to an increased risk of colorectal adenomas (Giovannucci et al., 1993b; Kahn et al., 1998). A dose-response relationship has been observed across several studies, and some evidence suggests that even moderate drinkers (those who consume one drink a day) are at higher risk of colorectal cancer than nondrinkers (World Cancer Research Fund and American Institute for Cancer Research, 1997).

The effects of alcohol may be exacerbated by low levels of folate (Freudenheim et al., 1991). In the Health Professionals Follow-Up Study, an increased risk of colon cancer was observed only among those current and past drinkers who consumed lower levels of methionine or folate in their diets (Giovannucci et al., 1995b). Because alcohol is an antagonist of folate-related methyl group metabolism, it may cause an imbalance in DNA methylation, which may then contribute to colorectal carcinogenesis.

Alcohol Consumption and Lung Cancer

Although a number of cohort studies have examined the association between alcohol consumption and lung cancer, few have adequately adjusted for the effects of smoking. Those that have adjusted adequately have yielded inconsistent findings. Four cohort studies have shown a positive association (Klatsky et al., 1981; Kvåle et al., 1983; Pollack et al., 1984; Potter et al., 1992), and four have yielded null results (Gordon and Kannel, 1984; Bandera et al., 1997; Woodson et al., 1999; Breslow et al., 2000).

Disparities in Alcohol Use

Data on alcohol consumption in the United States indicate that the top 20 percent of drinkers consume more than 85 percent of all alcohol consumed (Greenfield and Rogers, 1999). Men and young adults ages 18 to 29 years are disproportionately represented among those with the highest alcohol consumption levels. The National Health Interview Survey (1998) indicates that at each age, the proportion of current drinkers is highest among non-Hispanic white men, followed by African-American men, and then Hispanic men (National Center for Health Statistics, 2000). Among women, the proportion of current drinkers is also highest among non-Hispanic white women at each age.

SUMMARY AND CONCLUSIONS

There is overwhelming evidence that lifestyle factors affect cancer risk. As detailed throughout this chapter, current epidemiological evidence links the major behavioral risk factors with several major cancers. Tobacco use causes cancers of the lung, oropharynx, larynx, esophagus, bladder, kidney, and pancreas and contributes to the risk of leukemia as well as cancers of the colon, stomach, cervix, and liver. Recent declines in the rates of lung cancer in the United States among men—first among those who are younger and then among those who are older successively over time—and among women ages 40 to 59 reflect past declines in the use of cigarettes (Wingo et al., 1999). The cessation of tobacco use reduces the excess risk of nearly all of these cancers over time. Obesity increases the risk of breast, endometrial, colorectal, kidney, and esophageal cancer. Regular physical activity lowers the risk of cancers of the colon and breast cancer, and, possibly, endometrial cancer as well. Regular alcohol intake increases the risk of cancers of the oropharynx, larynx, esophagus, breast, liver, colon, and rectum. Diet has been linked to several cancers, with the most consistent evidence linking the consumption of large amounts fruits and vegetables with a lower risk cancer.

Numerous researchers have also estimated that positive changes in these lifestyle factors can reduce a good proportion of the national cancer burden (see Chapter 2). Although the specific methods and the results of these analyses vary, they are all remarkably consistent in pointing to the potential benefits of reducing tobacco use, improving diet, increasing physical activity, maintaining a healthy body weight, keeping alcohol consumption at low to moderate levels, and getting screened regularly for cancer.

4

Modifying Health Risk Behaviors[1]

Significant reductions in the burden of cancer are possible through changes in health behaviors. This chapter reviews current evidence of the effectiveness of interventions to promote three key behaviors in cancer prevention: nonsmoking, healthy diet, and physical activity. Although alcohol consumption was identified as a risk factor for cancer (Chapter 3), interventions to reduce alcohol consumption are not reviewed because of the cardiovascular health benefits associated with moderate consumption. The focus in this chapter is on changing individual behaviors through the provision of direct services (e.g., one-on-one counseling), contacts with health care providers or systems of care, and via community-based approaches such as worksite or school-based programs and public education media campaigns. Research on interventions to improve use of screening services is summarized in Chapter 6.

Interventions to modify behavioral risk factors can be implemented at several levels, for example, at the individual (e.g., group nutrition, exercise, or smoking cessation programs), interpersonal (e.g., advice and support from one's physician for smoking cessation), organizational (e.g., worksite cafeteria menu changes, health care benefit policies, mass media programs),

[1]This chapter is based on three background papers: (1) Interventions to Promote Key Behaviors in Cancer Prevention and Early Detection, by Edwin B. Fisher, Ross C. Brownson, Amy A. Eyler, Debra L. Haire-Joshu, and Mario Schootman; (2) The Effectiveness of Interventions to Assist in Weight Loss, by Suzanne Phelan and Rena Wing; and (3) Provider, System and Policy Strategies to Enhance the Delivery of Cancer Prevention and Control Activities in Primary Care, by Judy Ockene, Jane Zapka, Lori Pebert, Suzanne Brodney, and Stephanie Leman (www.iom.edu/ncpb).

and societal level (e.g., tobacco control legislation, changes in standards for school nutrition programs) (Winett et al., 1989; McLeroy et al., 1988). These levels are not mutually exclusive, and reflect an evolution in prevention research from a primary focus on determinants of behavior within the individual to broader perspectives that encompass interpersonal, organizational, and community influences.

This chapter begins with a description of the many opportunities to deliver behavioral interventions, from clinical settings to public health programs. An overview is then provided of conceptual frameworks and intervention paradigms that underlie much of the reviewed behavioral research. Next, treatment-outcome research is summarized for tobacco cessation and prevention, physical activity, and diet (weight loss interventions and modification of eating patterns). Lastly, the challenges faced by health care providers in delivering effective interventions are reviewed.

THE DELIVERY OF BEHAVIORAL INTERVENTIONS

The delivery of health behaviorial interventions can take place in the context of a clinical setting or be more broadly applied to public health practice (Lichtenstein and Glasgow, 1992). Clinical programs include group and individual counseling offered through a variety of channels, including private, non-profit agencies, commercial programs, community organizations such as schools, health care centers, churches or other religious institutions, and worksites. The target population for clinical interventions is usually individuals who are motivated (or who can be motivated) to actively seek treatment. Interventions may be delivered by medical or allied health professionals or by non-medical professionals with specialty training. Behavioral interventions are often intensive, involving multiple sessions.

The target population for public health interventions is usually an unselected group of individuals or members of specific high-risk groups, regardless of their motivation to change their behavior. Interventions are delivered in natural settings, and the providers of interventions are not necessarily specialists. Public health interventions can include translating intensive behavioral programs into formats that can be delivered on a wide scale, such as self-help guides, computer-generated messages or reminders, and outreach telephone counseling. Advances in information technology have made it possible to create customized or tailored materials and to deliver them via the Internet. Also in the realm of public health interventions are large-scale efforts such as mass media programs (which can be paired with written self-help materials that are disseminated, for example, through community retail outlets) and legislative or regulatory approaches (e.g., excise taxes, school lunch policies).

Related to the clinical-public health continuum of intervention is the construct of "program impact." The impact of an intervention is a product of its reach into the target population (i.e., the proportion of individuals who access the intervention) and the effectiveness (or rate of behavior change) associated with the interventions offered (Abrams et al., 1995). Because of their greater intensity and personal contact, clinical interventions have higher rates of individual change relative to public health interventions. However, intensive clinical programs may actually have less impact because of their lower reach in to the population. Modest changes in a large segment of the population can result in meaningful reductions in cancer incidence and mortality.

Clearly, clinical and public health approaches are not mutually exclusive. The potential for cancer prevention through modification of health risk behaviors is optimized by a combination of the two approaches. In fact, strategies and interventions are needed on multiple levels to overcome barriers to the delivery of and access to cancer prevention and control interventions (Rimer et al., 2001). A general consensus has emerged that efforts to change social and behavioral risk factors are most successful if they link multiple levels of influence, for example, at the individual, interpersonal, institutional, community, and policy levels (Institute of Medicine, 2000b).

CONCEPTUAL FRAMEWORKS GUIDING BEHAVIORAL RESEARCH

Behavioral research is driven by theoretical models of the determinants of the target behavior. This section describes three models that guide assessments of behavioral interventions relating to tobacco use, diet, and physical activity: value expectancy theories, the social cognitive theory, and the transtheoretical or stages of change model.

Value Expectancy Theories

Value expectancy theories emphasize cognitive factors that are associated with motivation for behavior change. Motivation is viewed as a rational, decision-making process that results from an individual's subjective value of an outcome and of the subjective probability or expectation that a particular behavior will attain the desired outcome. Two prominent value expectancy theories are the Health Belief Model (HBM) and the Theory of Reasoned Action (TRA).

Health Belief Model

First developed in the 1950s, the HBM has evolved into a psychosocial model that proposes three main determinants of motivation for health behavior change (Rosenstock, 1974):

1. perceived susceptibility to a disease or the subjective risks of contracting a serious illness;
2. perceived seriousness of an illness, in terms of both medical and lifestyle consequences; and
3. belief that particular behaviors will reduce the perceived threat, and that the associated benefits of those behaviors will outweigh the perceived costs and barriers.

Perceived susceptibility and severity are based largely on an individual's knowledge of a disease and its potential outcome. The HBM also recognizes the potential importance of "cues to action" in starting the process of behavior change. These cues can be internal (e.g., physical symptoms that suggest disease risk or vulnerability such as "smoker's cough") or external (e.g., strong advice from a physician to quit smoking). More recently, the concept of self-efficacy, the belief in one's capability to organize and execute the courses of action required to manage prospective situations, was added to the HBM (Janz and Becker, 1984). Self-efficacy can affect initiation of behavior, motivation to change behavior, and maintenance of behavior changes. The addition of self-efficacy into the model acknowledges the importance of individuals needing to believe they have the skills and abilities to implement the change.

Theory of Reasoned Action

The Theory of Reasoned Action (TRA) is another value expectancy theory that provides a mathematical description of the relationship among beliefs, attitudes, intention, and behavior (Fishbein and Ajzen, 1975). According to this model, behavioral intentions are the best single predictor of behavior. Behavioral intentions are influenced by two factors: the individual's attitude towards the behavior (i.e., whether the person has positive or negative feelings about engaging in the behavior), and subjective norms regarding the behavior (i.e., the individual's perception of the social pressures to engage or not engage in the behavior and one's motivation to comply with these normative influences). Although both the HBM and TRA focus on attitudes and beliefs, the TRA goes beyond the focus of the HBM on assessment of risk to also include assessment of the social normative context. The TRA has been expanded and renamed the Theory of Planned Behavior to incorporate the self-efficacy concept.

There are potential limitations of exclusive use of value-expectancy models to guide intervention development and evaluation. First, these models assume a rational decision-making process, which is not always operative. Second, they focus primarily on health concerns as motivators. While necessary, health concerns may not be sufficient to motivate behavior change. Finally, the emphasis of these models on cognitive factors needs to be augmented by models that take into account behavioral (e.g., skills) and environmental (e.g., situational determinants of behavior) components of the behavior change process.

Social Cognitive Theory

The cognitive-behavioral model on which most state-of-the art behavior change interventions are built has its conceptual roots in Social Cognitive Theory (SCT) (Bandura, 1989). This model extends the primarily cognitive focus of value expectancy theories and incorporates both behavioral and environmental components as equally important determinants of behavior. SCT highlights the influence of three factors: behavioral, cognitive, and environmental. Behavioral factors comprise an individual's experiences with the target behavior (e.g., eating patterns, participation in preventive health care, prior attempts to quit smoking) and their general repertoire of behavioral skills (e.g., interpersonal skills, coping strategies, problem solving abilities). Cognitive factors include knowledge, attitudes and beliefs as outlined in the value-expectancy models plus more specific cognitive representations of situational factors relevant to the target behavior (e.g., the perception of high-fat meals as "comfort" food). Environmental factors refer to influences that are external to the person such as the actions of family members, physicians, and peer groups. Also included are more global environmental influences such as advertising and mass media, regulations and restrictions on behaviors (e.g., clean indoor air legislation), and availability of health-promoting alternatives (e.g., fruit and vegetable availability in supermarkets).

Central to social cognitive theory is the concept of reciprocal determinism to indicate that cognitive, behavioral, and environmental factors are continually interacting in an open system. An intervention could, for example, start by teaching new skills in preparing lower-fat foods (behavioral) which leads to more positive attitudes towards dietary modification (cognitive), which then results in changes in food purchases and the availability of healthy food in the home (environmental).

Social cognitive theory also introduced the concept of self-efficacy, described earlier.

Transtheoretical Model

The transtheoretical model is widely applied in studies of the determinants of behavioral risk factor modification as well as in randomized intervention trials in the areas of smoking cessation, dietary change, and physical activity (Velicer et al., 1999; Kristal et al., 2000a; Peterson and Aldana,

1999). The model describes five stages of change along a continuum of intentions and actions to modify behaviors (Prochaska and DiClemente, 1982):

1. precontemplation (not considering change in the near future);
2. contemplation (planning to change in the near future, but not taking any immediate actions);
3. preparation (taking early steps to change in the immediate future or having tried to change in the past);
4. action (made the target behavior change within the past six months); and
5. maintenance (maintained the target behavior change for more than six months).

The transtheoretical model, in addition to laying out these stages of change, describes processes that are hypothesized to result in movement through the stages of change (e.g., stimulus control, reinforcement management, social liberation). The model also assumes that the decision-making process is rational, where individuals weigh the pros and cons associated with the target behavior (Janis and Mann, 1977).

All of the models reviewed suggest that two fundamental processes must occur for successful adoption or modification of behaviors:

1. individuals must be sufficiently motivated to attempt to change their behavior, and
2. they must have the requisite skills and supports to initiate and maintain those changes.

A counseling technique called motivational interviewing facilitates these processes by providing Feedback, enhancing personal Responsibility, giving Advice along with a Menu of options, and supporting self-Efficacy by using the success of others as encouragement in a non-confrontational and Supportive context (Miller and Rollnick, 1991). A FRAMES acronym summarizes these components. Brief motivational interviewing can be applied during routine medical encounters (Rollnick, Heather and Bell, 1992).

Another strategy to bring about behavioral change is cognitive-behavioral skill-training. This approach is targeted to individuals who are actively working to change their behavior. Core components of skill-training interventions are listed in Box 4.1.

The theoretic models and intervention strategies described are often applied in the context of assessments of efforts to promote behaviors to reduce the burden of cancer.

BOX 4.1 Core Components of Skill-Training Interventions

Self-Monitoring	• The systematic observation and recording of behavior.
Stimulus Control	• Eliminating or minimizing environmental cues for the behavior that are identified through self-monitoring.
Cognitive Restructuring	• The systematic identification and alteration of distorted thoughts and beliefs that may undermine behavior change efforts.
Goal Setting	• Setting specific, quantifiable, and reasonable goals. Focus is on setting both short-term (i.e., 1 to 2 weeks) and long-term (i.e., 6 months) goals.
Problem Solving	• Used to identify and cope with high-risk situations that may lead to relapse. The problem solving method for coping with high-risk situations involves: (a) specifying a situation; (b) generating several possible strategies for coping with it; (c) evaluating the possible coping strategies; (d) planning and implementing the best coping strategy(ies); (e) evaluating the effectiveness of the chosen strategy; and (f) reevaluating and selecting another solution if necessary.
Social Support	• Seeking support from others and informing others of the types of support desired.

TOBACCO CESSATION INTERVENTIONS

There is general agreement regarding the value of several approaches to smoking cessation (Task Force on Community Preventive Services, 2001; Hopkins et al., 2001a,b; US DHHS, 2000a; Fiore et al., 1996; US Preventive Services Task Force, 1996; http://www.cochrane.org/cochrane/revabstr/g160index.htm):

- individual treatment including behavioral change procedures and medication;
- advice to quit from physicians and other credible professionals;
- programs implemented through community channels such as worksites, churches, and health care settings; and
- broad, multicomponent, multichannel programs such as statewide programs to prevent smoking and encourage smoking cessation.

Smoking cessation has the advantage of a well-defined, single outcome measure (abstinence from tobacco) that lends itself well to outcomes assessment. A central conclusion from the literature on smoking cessation is that the more comprehensive and varied the treatment and the longer it is sustained, the more likely cessation will be achieved.

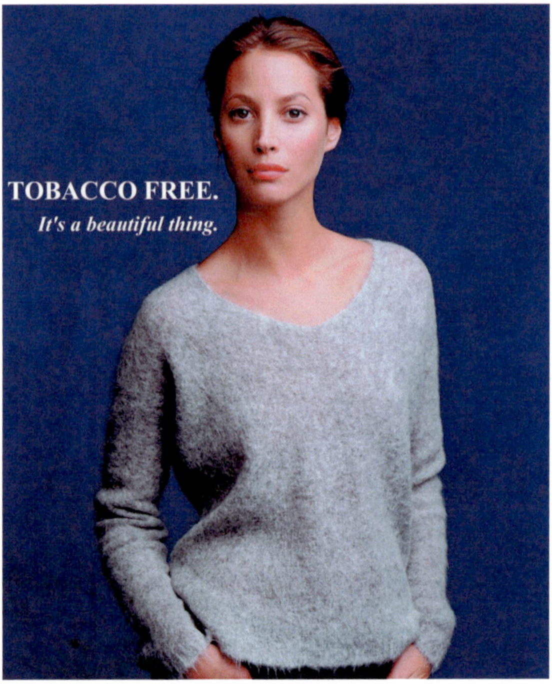

SOURCE: Centers for Disease Control and Prevention. Christy Turlington.

The 2000 Public Health Service Guideline presents the results of meta-analyses assessing the impact of various elements of treatments. As summarized in Table 4.1, increases in cessation rates and in the odds of quitting are parallel to increased amount of time and individualized personal contact. There is a similar trend when the data are disaggregated by the number of formats used.

These analyses demonstrate an important feature of smoking cessation: the number of different formats used in cessation interventions may be more important than the nature of the formats used. There is no one "magic bullet" in smoking cessation. Similar trends for increased rates of cessation are found for duration of contacts, duration of programs, and intervention providers. Compared to no treatment, even contact as brief as three minutes improves the odds of quitting smoking by as much as 20%. The greatest benefit (OR = 2.4) occurs for contacts above 10 minutes. Interventions that are sustained beyond 8 weeks increase the odds of quitting nearly threefold (OR = 2.7) compared to those that last less than two weeks. Receiving interventions from either nonphysician (OR = 1.7) or physician providers (OR = 2.2) improves quit rates over no treatment. Quit rates also increase with the number of clinician types involved in treatment

TABLE 4.1 Summary of Treating Tobacco Uses and Dependence (TTUD) Meta-Analysis Assessing the Impact of Various Elements of Treatment Structure

Structure variable	Number of Study arms	Estimated OR for abstinence (95% CI)	Estimated abstinence rate (95% CI)
Level of contact (43 studies)			
No contact	30	1.0	10.9
Minimal counseling (<3 min)	19	1.3 (1.01, 1.6)	13.4 (10.9–16.1)
Low-intensity counseling (3–10 min)	16	1.6 (1.2, 2.0)	16.0 (12.8–19.2)
Higher-intensity counseling (>10 min)	55	2.3 (2.0, 2.7)	22.1 (19.4–24.7)
Total amount of contact time (35 studies)			
None	16	1.0	11.0
1–3 min	12	1.4 (1.1, 1.8)	14.4 (11.3, 17.5)
4–30 min	20	1.9 (1.5, 2.3)	18.8 (15.6, 22.0)
31–90 min	16	3.0 (2.3, 3.8)	26.5 (21.5, 31.4)
91–300 min	16	3.2 (2.3, 4.6)	28.4 (21.3, 35.5)
>300 min	15	2.8 (2.0, 3.9)	25.5 (19.2, 31.7)
Number of person-to-person sessions (45 studies)			
0–1 session	43	1.0	12.4
2–3 sessions	17	1.4 (1.1, 1.7)	16.3 (13.7, 19.0)
4–8 sessions	23	1.9 (1.6, 2.2)	20.9 (18.1, 23.6)
>8 sessions	51	2.3 (2.1, 3.0)	24.7 (21.0, 28.4)
Type of clinician (29 studies)			
No clinician	16	1.0	10.2
Self-help	47	1.1 (0.9, 1.3)	10.9 (9.1, 12.7)
Non-physician	39	1.7 (1.3, 2.1)	15.8 (12.8, 18.8)
Physician	11	2.2 (1.5, 3.2)	19.9 (13.7, 26.2)
Number of clinician types (37 studies)			
No clinician	30	1.0	10.8
One type	50	1.8 (1.5, 2.2)	18.3 (15.4, 21.1)
Two types	16	2.5 (1.9, 3.4)	23.6 (18.4, 28.7)
Three or more types	7	2.4 (2.1, 2.9)	23.0 (20.0, 25.9)
Format (58 studies)			
No format	20	1.0	10.8
Self-help	93	1.2 (1.02, 1.3)	12.3 (10.9, 13.6)
Proactive telephone counseling	26	1.2 (1.1, 1.4)	13.1 (11.4, 14.8)
Group counseling	52	1.3 (1.1, 1.6)	13.9 (11.6, 16.1)
Individual counseling	67	1.7 (1.4, 2.0)	16.8 (14.7, 19.1)
Number of formats (54 studies)			
No format	20	1.0	10.8
One format	51	1.5 (1.2, 1.8)	15.1 (12.8, 17.4)
Two formats	55	1.9 (1.6, 2.2)	18.5 (15.8, 21.1)
Three or four formats	19	2.5 (2.1, 3.0)	23.2 (19.9, 26.6)

OR, odds ratio; CI, confidence interval. Odds ratios and abstinence rates refer to long-term (>5-month) follow-up.

SOURCE: Adapted from US DHHS (2000a), Tables 12–18. Reprinted from Piasecki and Baker (2001) (www.tandf.co.uk/journals).

delivery. The consistency in findings across different intervention characteristics reflects the importance of intensity and duration of interventions.

The Effectiveness of Behavioral Interventions

Cognitive-behavioral treatment components can be delivered in a variety of formats, ranging from minimal counseling and advice from medical providers to intensive, inpatient clinical programs.

Self-Help Programs

A variety of self-help pamphlets, books, videotapes, and resources on the World Wide Web are available commercially and through volunteer agencies, including the American Lung Association, the American Heart Association, and the American Cancer Society. In a review of 24 studies that used randomization in the research design, Curry (1993) found that self-help methods achieved long-term results comparable to those achieved by intensive interventions. She attributed this to the tendency of the success rates of the self-help interventions to increase over time. As opposed to a scheduled group program, self-help materials remain available for the smoker to use again as readiness to quit increases.

Several studies have evaluated self-help programs that are tailored to individual characteristics, such as readiness to change, specific motives for quitting, or the reasons for a previous relapse. Preparation and dissemination of tailored materials may be automated to reach large numbers of smokers. Among the successful tailored approaches are individualized mailings based on participants' answers to initial questionnaires about their smoking (Strecher et al., 1994; Prochaska et al., 1993, 2001), individualized mailings based on initial questionnaires and provided as supplements to use of over-the-counter (OTC) nicotine gum (Shiffman et al., 2000), and personalized feedback added to a self-help manual (Curry et al., 1991; Becona and Vazquez, 2001).

Physician Advice

A physician's advice or brief counseling for smoking cessation often includes a presentation of the risks individualized by symptoms or family history, provision of accompanying cessation materials, and follow-up (Kottke et al., 1988; Ockene et al., 1991a; Rose and Hamilton, 1978; Russell et al., 1979). A recent meta-analysis (Silagy and Ketteridge, 1998) reviewed 31 studies of brief advice, defined as consisting of advice delivered in less than 20 minutes with the possibility of one follow-up contact. Smokers who received such advice were 1.7 times more likely to quit than were those who received usual care. On the basis of a review of such research, the

PHS Guidelines for Smoking Cessation (US DHHS, 2000a) emphasize the five A's, "Ask, Advise, Assess, Assist, Arrange," as a structure for organizing smoking cessation interventions. Adding a video on how to quit, counseling by a nurse, follow-up phone calls, referral to self-help materials, referral to group treatment, or giving patients a choice between self-help and group treatment all increased smoking cessation rates (Hollis et al., 1993; Whitlock et al., 1997a).

The national *Healthy People 2010* objectives set a goal of increasing to at least 85 percent the proportion of primary care providers who routinely identify their patients' smoking status and offer smoking cessation advice, assistance, and follow-up for all their patients who smoke (US DHHS and Office of Disease Prevention and Health Promotion, 2000).

Telephone Counseling

Another channel for delivery of brief advice as well as repeated and more extended counseling and follow-up is the telephone. A review of this literature (Lichtenstein et al., 1996) found that reactive telephone services (those that users must call) are effective for those who do access them but are not used by many quitters. Proactive services provide outreach telephone counseling to smokers, usually in conjunction with written self-help materials. The 2000 PHS Clinical Practice Guidelines concluded that telephone counseling is an effective approach to smoking cessation counseling (US DHHS, 2000a, p. 63).

Group Programs or Classes

Group smoking cessation classes have long been offered by many hospitals and at many worksites as well as by volunteer agencies such as the American Lung Association. An analysis of 494 participants in 42 of the American Lung Association's Freedom from Smoking clinics showed a long-term abstinence rate of 29 percent (Rosenbaum and O'Shea, 1992), relative to a benchmark of 20 percent suggested by a contemporary review of published studies (Glasgow and Lichtenstein, 1987). Group programs generally include multiple components. Study designs preclude assessment of the efficacy of individual components, but their aggregate impacts are appreciable (Compas et al., 1998; Stevens and Hollis, 1989). Overall, smoking cessation rates among groups across a wide array of multicomponent group programs are quite similar.

Intensive Interventions for Individuals

In 1992, Lichtenstein and Glasgow noted the popularity in the preceding decade of public health approaches to smoking that sought to disseminate brief, inexpensive interventions to large numbers of smokers, thereby achieving a greater benefit to the population than intensive interventions implemented with quite small numbers. However, they also noted that the growing proportion of heavy smokers who found it difficult to quit suggested a renewed role for intensive interventions directed to small numbers of high-risk or difficult cases.

Using models for intensive inpatient treatment of drug dependence, researchers at the Mayo Clinic have developed an intensive residential treatment for smoking cessation. The evaluation compared participants in this program with smokers treated as outpatients and matched by age, sex, year treated, number of cigarettes smoked per day, longest previous abstinence, education, and marital status (but not psychological distress or psychopathology) (Hays et al., 2001). On the basis of self-reports of smoking status, those who received residential treatment reported rates of abstinence of 45 percent at both 6- and 12-month follow-ups, relative to abstinence rates of 26 and 23 percent in the matched comparison patients at the two times of follow-up, respectively.

Pharmacological Interventions

Pharmacotherapies for smoking cessation that have been approved by the Food and Drug Administration (FDA) and recommended in the PHS Guidelines include several forms of nicotine replacement (gum, patch, nasal spray, and inhaler) and bupropion SR, currently available as the trademarked Zyban™. Two other medications, nortriptyline and clonidine, although not approved to be marketed for smoking cessation by the FDA, are recommended as second-line medications if nicotine replacement and/or bupropion SR are not effective.

Two nicotine replacement treatment (NRT) products, gum (2 mg and 4 mg) and patch (21 mg, 14 mg, and 7 mg) are available for purchase over the counter. Nicotine patches are also available by prescription; bupropion SR can only be obtained by prescription. NRT works by partially replacing nicotine that was previously obtained by smoking. The availability of NRT in different dosages and forms allows individuals to tailor their initial dose to their baseline levels of smoking (i.e., higher-dose gum and patches and more frequent use of the nasal spray and inhaler are recommended for persons who smoke more than 25 cigarettes a day) as well as to taper their use of NRT over time. Sustained-release bupropion is an antidepressant medication that has evidence of effectiveness for smoking cessation. The mechanism of action for this medication is unknown although it is likely through its inhibitive effect on the neuronal uptake of norepinephrine and dopamine.

Results of meta-analyses of randomized trials of pharmacotherapies are summarized in Table 4.2. Overall, rates of cessation are doubled for active

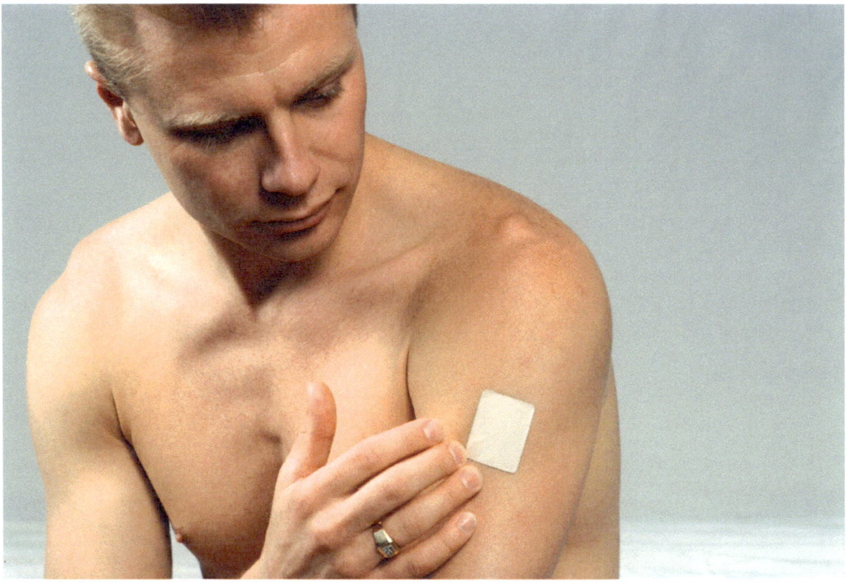

SOURCE: Corbis Corporation.

versus placebo medication. As indicated in Table 4.2, recent research has examined the combination of nicotine replacement therapies. Combinations of NRT reflect recognition of the utility of augmenting steady levels of nicotine replacement obtained with the nicotine patch, with more flexible forms of dosing (e.g., nicotine gum) to cope with transient urges. A recent study also evaluated the efficacy of combining the nicotine patch with bupropion SR. In this study, the combined drugs did not significantly outperform either therapy alone. Still unanswered is whether combining bupropion SR with NRT that has a more flexible dosing regimen (e.g., gum, nasal spray, or inhaler) would enhance cessation.

The 1988 Surgeon General's report on smoking as nicotine addiction (US DHHS, 1988) concluded that nicotine replacement is best viewed as an adjunct to counseling or other smoking cessation programs and efforts. The 1996 Agency for Health Care Policy and Research (AHCPR) Guidelines were unable to reach a clear conclusion as to whether nicotine replacement without any behavioral counseling was no better than placebo (AHCPR, 1996). Other reviews found little evidence for nicotine replacement in isolation. For example, a meta-analysis found an odds ratio of 1.91 for continued smoking cessation for those who receive nicotine gum plus a brief intervention versus those who receive only nicotine gum (Baillie et al., 1994). The 2000 PHS Guidelines emphasized the importance of at least brief counseling for all smokers interested in quitting and concluded that, except in special circumstances, all individuals interested in quitting smok-

TABLE 4.2 Summary of TTUD Meta-Analyses Evaluating First-Line Pharmacotherapies

Condition	Number of study arms	Estimated OR (95% CI)	Estimated abstinence rate (95% CI)
Bupropion (2 studies)			
Placebo	2	1.0	17.3
Bupropion	4	2.1 (1.5, 3.0)	30.5 (23.2, 37.8)
Nicotine gum (13 studies)			
Placebo	16	1.0	17.1
Nicotine gum	18	1.5 (1.3, 1.8)	23.7 (20.6, 26.7)
Nicotine inhaler (4 studies)			
Placebo	4	1.0	10.5
Nicotine inhaler	4	2.5 (1.7, 3.6)	22.8 (16.4, 29.2)
Nicotine nasal spray (3 studies)			
Placebo	3	1.0	13.9
Nicotine nasal spray	3	2.7 (1.8, 4.1)	30.5 (21.8, 39.2)
Nicotine patch (27 studies)			
Placebo	28	1.0	10.0
Nicotine patch	32	1.9 (1.7, 2.2)	17.7 (16.0, 19.5)
Combination nicotine replacement (3 studies)			
One NRT	3	1.0	17.4
Two NRTs	3	1.9 (1.3, 2.6)	28.6 (21.7, 35.4)

OR, odds ratio; CI, confidence interval. Odds ratios and abstinence rates refer to long-term (>5-month) follow-up.
SOURCE: Adapted from US DHHS (2000a), Tables 12–18. Reprinted from Piasecki and Baker (2001) (www.tandf.co.uk/journals).

ing should be offered medication to assist them in their efforts (US DHHS 2000a, pp. 3–5).

Worksite Programs

Worksites are an attractive channel through which to disseminate interventions because of their reach into the adult population. Reductions in smoking have been reported through workplace programs aimed at smoking alone or at multiple risk factors (Gomel et al., 1993, 1997; Emmons et al., 1999). A recent meta-analysis (Chapman et al., 1999) found that 17 of 19 studies reported reductions in the prevalence of smoking through workplace programs. However, the Working Healthy Project, a large study of multiple risk factor interventions in 26 manufacturing worksites, found benefits for reported activity levels and reported levels of consumption of fruits and vegetables but no impacts on smoking (Emmons et al., 1999). Programs aimed at worksite norms and general support for nonsmoking have reported substantial cessation rates, even among smokers who did not formally join smoking cessation clinics (Fisher et al., 1994). Effective also are worksite restrictions on smoking, which led 18 percent of smokers in one study to quit (Sorensen et al., 1991). The meta-analysis on workplace programs (Chapman et al., 1999) estimated that 12.7 percent of the decrease in cigarette consumption in the United States between 1988 and 1994 was attributable to workplace restrictions and interventions.

Insurance Coverage of Smoking Cessation Interventions

The provision and acceptance of smoking prevention services are enabled when they are covered insurance benefits. A lack of reimbursement affects both patients and physicians (Frame, 1992; Jaen et al., 1994; Kottke et al., 1993). Smoking cessation counseling and pharmacotherapies are not consistently covered as paid services by Medicaid, health insurance plans, and managed care organizations (MCOs) and are not covered at all by Medicare (Professional Assisted Cessation Therapy, 2001; Schauffler and Parkinson, 1993). Cost may be a barrier even among individuals who are insured because of significant cost sharing (e.g., through deductibles and copayments).

Despite the higher rates of smoking among adults in the Medicaid population compared with those among insured adults (for example, 31 versus 19 percent in 1999 in California [Schauffer and Brown, 2000]), Medicaid coverage for smoking cessation services is limited. In 2000, the Medicaid programs of only 33 states and the District of Columbia covered one or more treatments for tobacco dependence, and those of 17 covered no treatments at all (CDC, 2001e). State Medicaid programs were most likely to cover some form of pharmacotherapy, but the programs of only 11 states covered at least one type of pharmacotherapy and one type of counseling, despite clear evidence that quit rates are doubled when counseling and pharmacotherapy are combined (US DHHS, 2000a). Only one state offered coverage for all treatments recommended by the Public Health Service clinical practice guidelines.

Medicare does not require coverage for smoking cessation counseling, nor does it provide reimbursements for pharmacotherapy, although a pilot program for elders has been initiated (Health Care Financing Administration, undated).

Only four states mandate that private health insurers or managed care providers offer a smoking cessation treatment benefit (Professional Assisted Cessation Therapy, 2001). However, a growing number of health insurers and MCOs are offering some form of treatment for smoking cessation (Halpin Schauffler et al., 2001; Pickett et al, 2001; Zapka et al., 1997). Results from the first annual national survey of managed health care plans conducted in 1997 (McPhillips-Tangum, 1998) showed that 75 percent of MCOs report the availability of full coverage for some smoking cessation interventions.

Unfortunately, this often consists of self-help materials, which have been found to be less effective than counseling and the use of pharmacotherapy. A survey of employers conducted in 1997 regarding their single highest-enrolled health plan indicated that 23 percent of employers provided coverage for smoking cessation devices and drugs and 22 percent provided coverage for smoking cessation counseling (Partnership for Prevention, 1997).

Thus, although there is a growing trend toward increasing coverage and reimbursement for tobacco services, it is not adequate or consistently provided through Medicaid, Medicare, health insurers, or MCOs. Several states have programs that provide tobacco treatment services to low-income, high-risk populations (see Box 4.2). In addition, the Tobacco Master Settlement Agreement in some states is providing opportunities to fund counseling or for pharmacotherapy to be available to tobacco users in those states (Professional Assisted Cessation Therapy, 2001).

Effects of Costs of Care

Costs have complex roles in discouraging or encouraging healthy behavior and the use of preventive services. This was examined in a study by Curry and colleagues (1998) at Group Health Cooperative of Puget Sound. Among participants in smoking cessation services, those who had to pay for some portion of costs achieved higher quit rates than those who received them at no cost. This reflects the commonly expressed opinion that offering services for free is counterproductive because recipients will not value services for which they do not have to pay. However, offering services at no charge resulted in participation in cessation services by a greater percentage of smokers. The benefit of increased volume outweighed the difference in efficacy among participants. As a result, when quit rates were examined as a percentage not just of participants but of all smokers in a plan, the quit rates were higher when the services were free (quit rate, 2.8 percent of all smokers) than when reduced coverage was available (quit rates, 0.7 percent of all smokers).

In another randomized controlled trial, full coverage of a tobacco dependence treatment benefit implemented in two IPA model HMOs in California was an effective and relatively low-cost strategy for significantly increasing quit rates, quit attempts, and use of nicotine gum and patch in adult smokers (Schauffler et al., 2001b). In this study, 1,204 eligible smokers were randomly assigned either to the control group, which received a self-help kit (video and pamphlet), or to the treatment group, which received the self-help kit and fully covered benefits for over-the-counter nicotine replacement therapy gum and patch, and participation in a group behavioral cessation program with no patient cost sharing. The quit rates after one year of follow-up were 18 percent in the treatment group and 13 percent in the control group (adjusted odds ratio 1.6).

BOX 4.2 Selected State Tobacco Control Initiatives

Arizona

Twenty-three percent of the revenues from a 40-cent Arizona state cigarette excise tax increase in 1992 were dedicated to programs to prevent and reduce tobacco use. Five percent was dedicated to research on prevention and treatment of tobacco-related disease and addiction. However, until 1997, multiple programmatic restrictions were placed on use of the funds, not allowing the Arizona Tobacco Education and Prevention Program (AzTEPP) to be as comprehensive as was initially proposed. By 1998, AzTEPP had a $28.2 million budget and program efforts were able to extend to youth and adult cessation activities. Surveillance systems and program evaluation studies have been implemented to assess the success of the program. Results from baseline surveys of adults show a 21 percent decline in smoking prevalence from 1996 to 1999.

California

California's Tobacco Control Program was developed following the passage of state legislation in 1988. In 1989 and 1994, the cigarette excise tax was increased. By 1999, the budget for California's program, housed within the Department of Education and the Department of Health Services, had grown to $126.8 million. The program is the largest and most comprehensive program in the United States to reduce tobacco use. It is focused on getting resources to local communities through grants to local health departments and community organizations. A major media campaign was launched to change public opinions regarding tobacco use. Resources have also been allocated to treatment programs and to adopting clean indoor air policies. This comprehensive multi-component program has been a success according to program evaluations. The rate of decline in cigarette consumption between 1993 and 1996 was steeper in California than in the rest of the country.

Florida

Florida was able to fund the Florida Tobacco Pilot Program with $70 million from its 1997 individual settlement with the tobacco industry. The comprehensive program began in 1998 to accomplish the main goals of changing young people's attitudes towards tobacco use, increasing youth empowerment through community involvement, reducing young people's access to tobacco products, and reducing youth exposure to environmental tobacco smoke. With an obvious focus on youth, the Florida State Department of Health directly involved youth in the development of the program. From 1998 to 2000, smoking rates have declined 47 percent among middle school students and 30 percent among high school students. In 2001, funding for the program was cut by nearly one-third, and perhaps as a result more recent surveys show no statistically significant declines in smoking rates.

Maine

In 1997, legislation in Maine increased the cigarette excise tax by 37 cents and established the Tobacco Prevention and Control Program with an initial annual budget of $4.35 million. The program became an expansion of the already existing ASSIST program. The expansion met the 1997 legislative requirements of providing an ongoing major media campaign, grants for funding community-based programs, program surveillance and evaluation, and law enforcement efforts regarding transportation, distribution, and sale of tobacco products. In 2000, the program was expanded and budgeted $18.3 million. A large portion of the budget ($8.35 million) was used for community and school-based grants, and another large portion ($6.75 million) was used for cessation and statewide multimedia campaigns. Since 1997, smoking among high school students in Maine has declined by 36 percent.

Massachusetts

The 25-cent increase in Massachusetts' cigarette excise tax in 1992 produced enough revenue to fund the Massachusetts Tobacco Control Program. The program began with a large media campaign and then moved on to support community-based education and prevention activities. The state's regional primary care Prevention Centers provided ongoing educa-

continued on next page

BOX 4.2 (*continued*)

tion, technical assistance, and training to local community programs and initiatives. Efforts were also aimed at increasing community awareness, promoting smoke-free workplaces, and enforcing regulation about tobacco use. The per capita consumption of cigarettes in Massachusetts declined by 32 percent between 1992 and 1999, in comparison to an 8 percent decline in the rest of the United States. Relative to the U.S. population in 1999, 25 percent more of Massachusetts' residents lived in a town with a complete ban on smoking in restaurants.

Minnesota

Minnesota was one of the first states to pass statewide legislation for clean indoor air in 1975. In 1983, the Center for Nonsmoking and Health developed The Minnesota Plan for Nonsmoking and Health. By 1986, increased attention was drawn to the relationship between smoking and health, stimulating legislation to increase the state cigarette excise tax and launch a major statewide initiative, The Minnesota Tobacco Use Prevention Initiative. The initiative focused on changing the social climate surrounding the use of tobacco through school-based programs and a mass media campaign. An evaluation of the programs suggests that the initiative was successful in changing attitudes towards smoking, and in increasing school curricula dedicated to smoking prevention. However, there was not a significant decline in smoking rates in Minnesota between 1986 and 1990. Receipt of tobacco settlement money enabled the state in 2000 to support a new tobacco prevention initiative with the ambitious legislative goal of reducing tobacco use among young people by 30 percent by 2005. The initiative, called Target Market, has a large public awareness and advertising component, as well as a grassroots movement among Minnesota youth. After one year, the program has been associated with a change in teen attitudes and also reductions in tobacco use.

Mississippi

The Partnership for a Healthy Mississippi is a nonprofit corporation that manages a pilot program dedicated to fostering a healthier Mississippi and eliminating tobacco use among Mississippi youth. In 1997, the program's first year budget amounted to $23.7 million, funded by an individual state settlement with the tobacco industry. Twenty-five community and youth partnership coalitions were formed during the program's first year, with the requirement that a quarter of membership must be young people. Since 1998, the program has flourished through major youth initiatives, an increase in the number of school and community programs, numerous grants for law enforcement activities, the Mississippi Tobacco Quitline, a tobacco treatment center, and a public awareness campaign. Before 1997, smoking rates among Mississippi high school students were increasing, whereas between 1997 and 1999 smoking rates within this age group leveled off. Since the program's expansion in 1999, smoking among public high school students in Mississippi has declined by 25 percent and the youth advocacy movement, Frontline, has helped enact state legislation banning tobacco use on school grounds and at all school events.

Oregon

In 1996, the Oregon state cigarette excise tax was raised by 30 cents and 10 percent of the revenue was designated for a statewide Tobacco Education and Prevention Program (TEPP). The budget totaled $17 million and was spent on five categories: (1) local coalitions; (2) public awareness and education; (3) statewide and regional projects; (4) schools; and (5) statewide coordination and evaluation. An evaluation of the program found that community-based coalitions were in place in each of the state's counties and school projects reached 30 percent of the state's schools. In the first year of the program, per capita cigarette consumption declined by 11.3 percent in Oregon as opposed to the 1 percent decline seen in the rest of the nation that year. From 1996 to 2000 adult smoking decreased by 9 percent in Oregon.

SOURCE: USDHHS, 2000b; http://www.tobaccofreekids.org/research/factsheets/pdf/0045.pdf.

Cost-Effectiveness of Smoking Cessation

Compared with other preventive interventions, smoking cessation is extremely cost effective (Coffield et al., 2001; Warner, 1997; Cromwell et al., 1997; Croghan et al., 1997; Elixhauser, 1990). According to a recent systematic assessment of the value of clinical preventive services, providing tobacco cessation counseling to adults should be a highly prioritized service because it is both cost-effective and likely to reduce disease burden (Coffield et al., 2001). Implementation of the 1996 Agency for Health Care Policy and Research (now the Agency for Healthcare Research and Quality) smoking cessation guideline was estimated to gain 1.7 million new quitters in the first year at an average cost of $3,779 per quitter, or $2,587 per life-year saved (Cromwell et al., 1997).

Programs for Entire Communities

As noted above, the more varied the means of encouragement of nonsmoking are, the greater the rates of abstinence that are achieved. This fact and the desirability of reaching large numbers of smokers have fueled efforts to promote nonsmoking across entire communities.

Among community-based programs, mass media programs achieve effects that are modest in terms of the percentage of smokers who quit (Flay, 1987), but that are quite substantial when one considers the numbers of smokers they may reach. The pattern of results from mass media approaches to smoking cessation shows a striking parallel to the pattern of results from clinical approaches: the more channels of influence that support cessation, the greater the impact (Kottke et al., 1988). Thus, televised programs achieve greater impacts when they are accompanied by printed materials distributed to viewers (Flay, 1987; Warnecke et al., 1992) or by group activities that provide local support for cessation (Flay, 1987; Korhonen et al., 1992).

The National Cancer Institute sponsored the Community Intervention Trial for Smoking Cessation (COMMIT), a large clinical trial that evaluated community-based programs for smoking cessation. COMMIT achieved appreciable impacts among light and moderate smokers but did not significantly increase smoking cessation among heavy smokers (Lichtenstein et al., 1995). The COMMIT program centered on a set of activities and curricula developed centrally and implemented through communities. Community involvement and ownership of the activities occurred through community boards with representatives from major community sectors such as media, health care, and education. This approach, in which the program was implemented through community boards, can be differentiated from approaches that place priority on the authority of community-based organization leadership to plan and direct programs (Fisher, 1995).

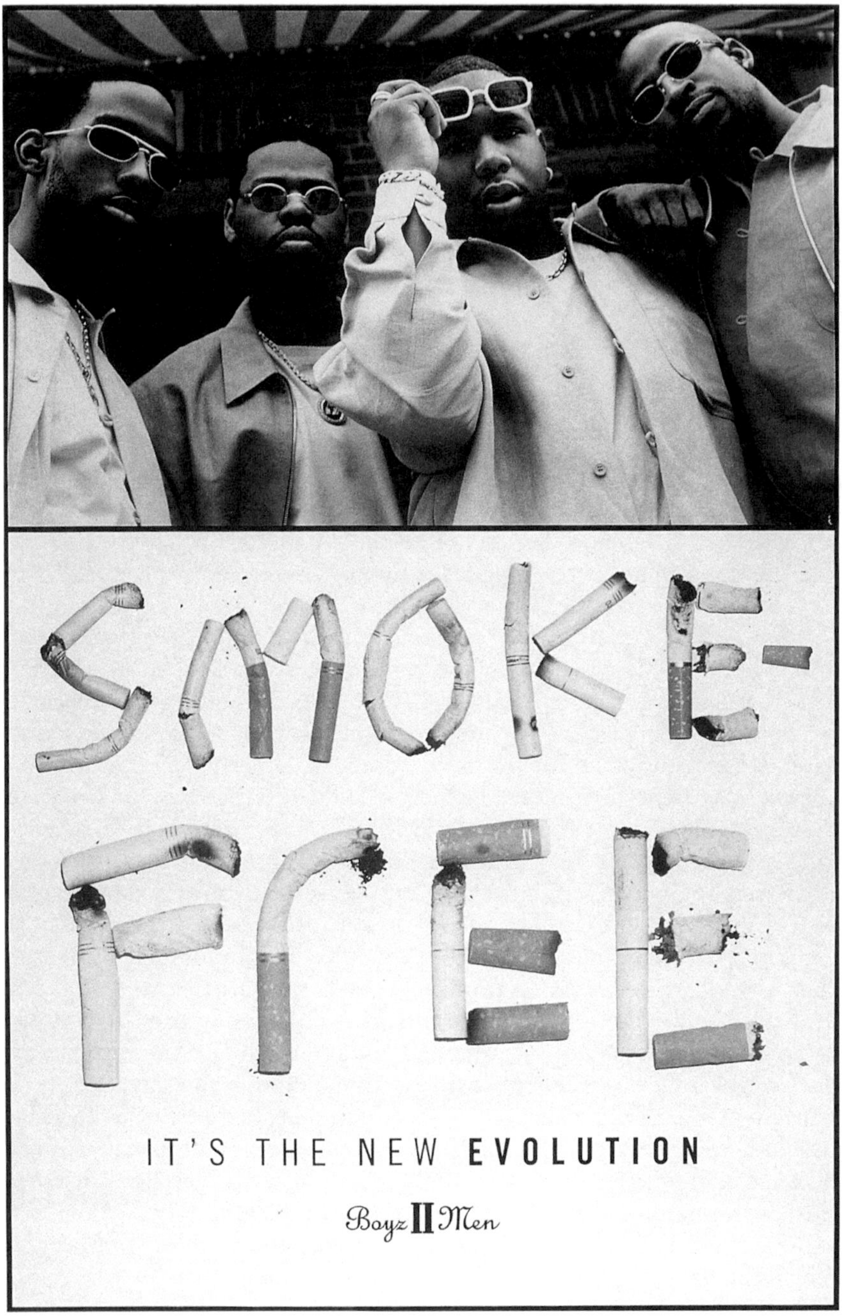

SOURCE: Centers for Disease Control and Prevention. Boys II Men.

Two programs that have emphasized local authority in program direction have achieved significant, community-wide effects on smoking cessation. One program addressed smoking among women in two counties in Vermont. By the third year of the program, local community boards had assumed the burden of responsibility for program planning and implementation. Relative to the counties used for comparison, the two counties achieved significantly greater levels of smoking cessation and lower smoking prevalences (Secker-Walker et al., 2000). A second program addressed smoking in three low-income, predominantly African-American neighborhoods in St. Louis, Missouri. Each neighborhood had its own wellness committee that helped coordinate a variety of peer-based and mass media activities to encourage nonsmoking. Declines in prevalence were significantly greater in St. Louis in comparison to untreated, comparable neighborhoods in Kansas City (Fisher et al., 1998).

A critical component of community-level programs is policy related to smoking. *Reducing Tobacco Use: A Report of the Surgeon General* (US DHHS, 2000b) identified several aspects of policy on smoking that are important, including bans on indoor smoking to reduce exposure to environmental tobacco smoke, policies that regulate the supply of tobacco and international trade in tobacco, policies that "ease economic diversification in tobacco-producing areas" (p. 359) to minimize economic dislocation from reduced tobacco sales, regulation of tobacco sales and promotion, especially to young people, and "substantial increases in the excise taxes on cigarettes [that] would have considerable impact on the prevalence of smoking and, in the long-term, reduce the adverse health effects caused by tobacco" (p. 359). As summarized in more detail in the section on smoking prevention, there is an emerging consensus that the use of tobacco control policies is an effective and efficient means of preventing smoking among youth.

Comprehensive statewide efforts that combine policy changes with prevention and cessation interventions have shown impressive results. Increased excise taxes and targeting of their proceeds to smoking prevention programs in California and Massachusetts have resulted in substantial statewide reductions in the prevalence of smoking (Biener et al., 2000; CDC, 1996; Pierce et al., 1998; Siegel et al., 2000). A combination of a broad campaign of public education in those states (including well-financed, creative, and hard-hitting advertisements and billboards countering tobacco marketing) with community-based coalitions, support services for cessation, smoking prevention programs aimed at youth, and multicultural approaches led to greater reductions in smoking than would have been brought about by increased sales taxes alone. Replication of the effort in Oregon identified a reduction in the per capita rate of tobacco consumption of 11.3 percent over the 2 years from 1996 to 1998, in contrast to nationwide reductions of only 1 percent per year (CDC, 1999a). Selected state initiatives in tobacco control are described in Box 4.2 (see Chapter 8, Box 8.4 regarding state provider training initiatives).

The United States has begun to realize some public health gains secondary to declines in adult smoking rates. A recent evaluation of nonsmoking campaigns in California found associations among (1) the imposition and then reduction of support of the program, (2) changes in smoking rates, and (3) changes in rates of death from heart disease (Fichtenberg and Glantz, 2000).

Cessation Programs to Reach Underserved and Minority Populations

Two key observations about channels for reaching disadvantaged minorities are that (1) they are relatively isolated from formal or mainstream channels of information and (2) they use informal sources of information and support (Dressler, 1991). Both of these observations lead to an emphasis on peer-based and community-based programs designed to enlist informal social networks to disseminate health messages and provide peer and informal support and encouragement for behavioral change (Fisher et al., 1992; Hatch and Derthick, 1992). Additionally, health promotion programs should reflect the emphasis on family found among members of African-American and other minority groups (Ness et al., 1997; Stolley and Fitzgibbon, 1997). Efforts at the promotion of smoking cessation among African Americans and other minorities have used churches, schools, lay health advisers, mass media, and community-based approaches.

Heart, Body and Soul was a smoking cessation program implemented through churches in the low-income, predominantly African-American neighborhoods of East Baltimore, Maryland (Voorhees et al., 1996). Churches were randomized either to a minimal self-help condition or to an intensive culturally specific intervention that included (1) pastoral sermons on smoking, (2) testimony of quitters during church services, (3) the use of trained volunteers as smoking cessation counselors, (4) spiritual audiotapes as part of individual and group support, (5) a day-by-day, guided quit booklet, and (6) baseline and follow-up health fairs with feedback on carbon monoxide levels as well as other risks for cardiovascular disease. In comparison to the minimal, self-help condition, these interventions in the churches resulted in observed but not statistically significant differences in quit rates as measured by self-reports and carbon monoxide levels. Statistically significant differences were found in the proportions who regressed, those who showed no change, and those who moved forward toward quitting or maintained abstinence.

As noted earlier, a program in predominately African-American neighborhoods in St. Louis (Fisher et al., 1998) emphasized the involvement of neighborhood residents, who helped direct the program through neighborhood wellness committees and who helped coordinate a variety of neigh-

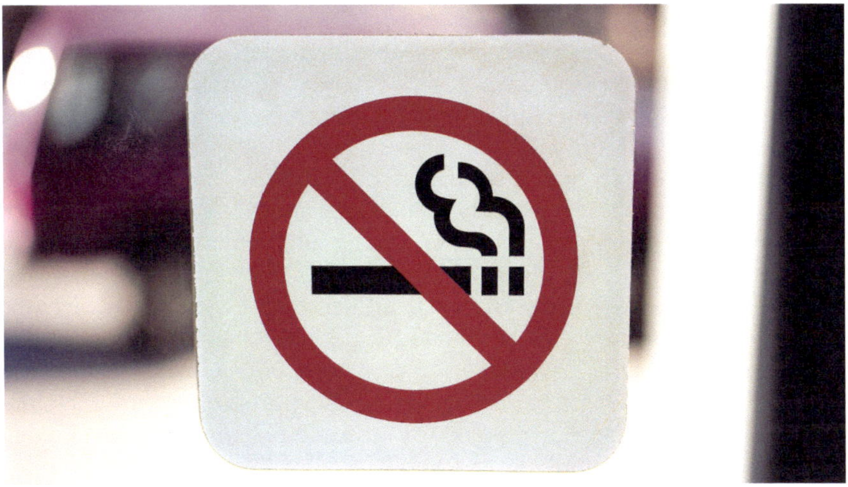

SOURCE: PhotoDisc, Inc.

borhood activities to encourage nonsmoking. Declines in the prevalence of smoking exceeded those in comparison neighborhoods.

PREVENTION OF TOBACCO USE

Because of the time course of exposure and disease incidence, reductions in cancer-related morbidity and mortality over the next two decades will result from smoking cessation rather than prevention of smoking initiation. Nevertheless, a critical public health goal is to achieve a generation of nonsmokers through widespread adoption of effective smoking prevention strategies. These strategies can range from behavioral and educational programs delivered directly to youth, to local, state, and federal tax policies that increase the cost of tobacco, to federal regulation of nicotine, the major addictive constituent of tobacco, as a drug. For more than 20 years, a state-of-the-art approach to the prevention of smoking among adolescents has developed that has emphasized programs that are implemented through key social channels (e.g., older peers) and that address social influences to smoke and social and personal skills for rebutting them. Reports of the positive impacts of these programs have been made throughout this period (Botvin et al., 1999; Perry et al., 1980). Such programs have been endorsed by several key reviews, including the 2000 Surgeon General's report *Reducing Tobacco Use* (US DHHS, 2000b). One study published subsequent to this review reported negative findings from a randomized trial of smoking prevention interventions implemented across grades 3 to 10. The intervention components stressed skills that helped students recognize and resist influences to smoke. Follow-up data were obtained through the 12th grade and the first 2 years past 12th grade (Peterson et al., 2000). The initial report finds no overall significant effect of the intervention on smoking prevalence in the 12th grade or 2 years later. In-depth analyses of the longitudinal results from that study have not yet been published. Still unanswered is whether the intervention had interim effects or whether such programs were more or less successful among subpopulations of children or schools (Cameron et al., 1999, 2001). Community-based approaches that encompass a broader array of social influences are likely needed to be effective (Peterson et al., 2001; Sussman et al., 2001). Such programs implemented on a statewide basis have shown success (see below).

Relatively little work has addressed family approaches to smoking prevention. This is somewhat remarkable, given the plethora of data linking parental and sibling smoking and family factors to the onset of smoking (Baumrind, 1991; Biglan et al., 1995; Chassin et al., 1996; Jessor et al., 1991). A recent study reported that a family-based approach succeeded in reducing the rate of smoking onset by 25 percent among non-Hispanic whites but not among other groups. This intervention included booklets mailed to families to help them prevent smoking among adolescents and follow-up telephone contacts by health educators (Bauman et al., 2001).

Evaluations of mass media and community-based approaches to the prevention of smoking have, as a group, achieved mixed results (Biglan et al., 2000; Sowden and Arblaster, 2000a,b).

Beyond school- and community-based educational programs, there is an emerging consensus that the implementation and enforcement of tobacco control policies are especially effective and efficient means of preventing smoking by youth (Altman et al., 1999; Farkas et al., 2000; Wakefield and Chaloupka, 2000). They can be less expensive to enact relative to preventive interventions, and they generally reach much larger populations of youth. Fueling such perspectives are findings such as those that show that nonsmoking teens who lived in towns in Massachusetts with local ordinances that restrict tobacco sales were significantly less likely (odds ratio = 0.60) to become smokers over a 4-year period than teens who lived in towns without such ordinances (Siegel et al., 1999). Another study of state tobacco control policies throughout the United States found evidence that policies can influence smoking initiation (Luke et al., 2000). States with the most extensive array of tobacco control policies had significantly lower youth smoking prevalence rates. They also tended to have lower percentages of teenagers who had smoked before age 13.

Statewide comprehensive campaigns to discourage smoking appear to be effective on a population basis (Institute of Medicine, 2000a; Warner, 2000). A review of studies from the United States and other countries (Willemsen and De Zwart, 1999) concluded that the best results are achieved through a combination of bans on tobacco advertising to youth, increased prices, restriction of sales to youth, mass media aimed at youth, and the intensification of school-based programs for youth. Reaching similar conclusions, another review (Lantz et al., 2000) emphasized implementation of programs in a manner that takes advantage of synergies among program components. Further supporting this approach, a recent review of the impacts of comprehensive state tobacco control programs in Arizona, California, Massachusetts, Oregon, and Florida found that the combination of increased taxes and comprehensive educational and promotional program elements reduced the level of tobacco consumption more than that expected from tax increases alone (Wakefield and Chaloupka, 2000).

PHYSICAL ACTIVITY INTERVENTIONS

For general health, it is recommended that every U.S. adult should accumulate 30 minutes or more of moderate-intensity physical activity on most—and preferably all—days of the week. Public health recommendations emphasize a lifestyle approach to increasing physical activity that includes common activities such as brisk walking, climbing stairs, doing housework and yard work, and engaging in recreational activities (US DHHS and Office of Disease Prevention and Health Promotion, 2000). In addition to the recommendation for general health, the recommendation for cardiorespiratory fitness includes 20 to 60 minutes of aerobic exercise of moderate to high intensity three or more time per week (Pate et al., 1995a). Although an association between cancer and physical activity is established, the exact exercise prescription for cancer prevention or treatment is not known. This section of the chapter summarizes evidence for interventions to promote adherence to national guidelines for physical activity and for physical activity interventions as part of multicomponent treatments for weight loss.

Distinctions between physical activity, exercise, and physical fitness are useful in understanding intervention research. Physical activity is "any bodily movement produced by the contraction of skeletal muscle that substantially increases energy expenditure." (US DHHS, 1996, p. 21). Exercise is considered a subset of physical activity that is "planned, structured, repetitive, and purposive in the sense that improvement or maintenance of one or more components of physical fitness is the objective." (US DHHS, 1996, p. 20). Physical fitness is "the ability to carry out daily tasks with vigor and alertness, without undue fatigue."(US DHHS, 1996, p. 20). The components of health-related fitness include cardiorespiratory endurance, muscular strength and endurance, flexibility, and body composition; the components of skill-related fitness include balance, agility, power, reaction time, speed, and coordination (US DHHS, 1996).

The way that physical activity is defined and measured varies widely. The studies described in this chapter have defined physical activity as vigor-

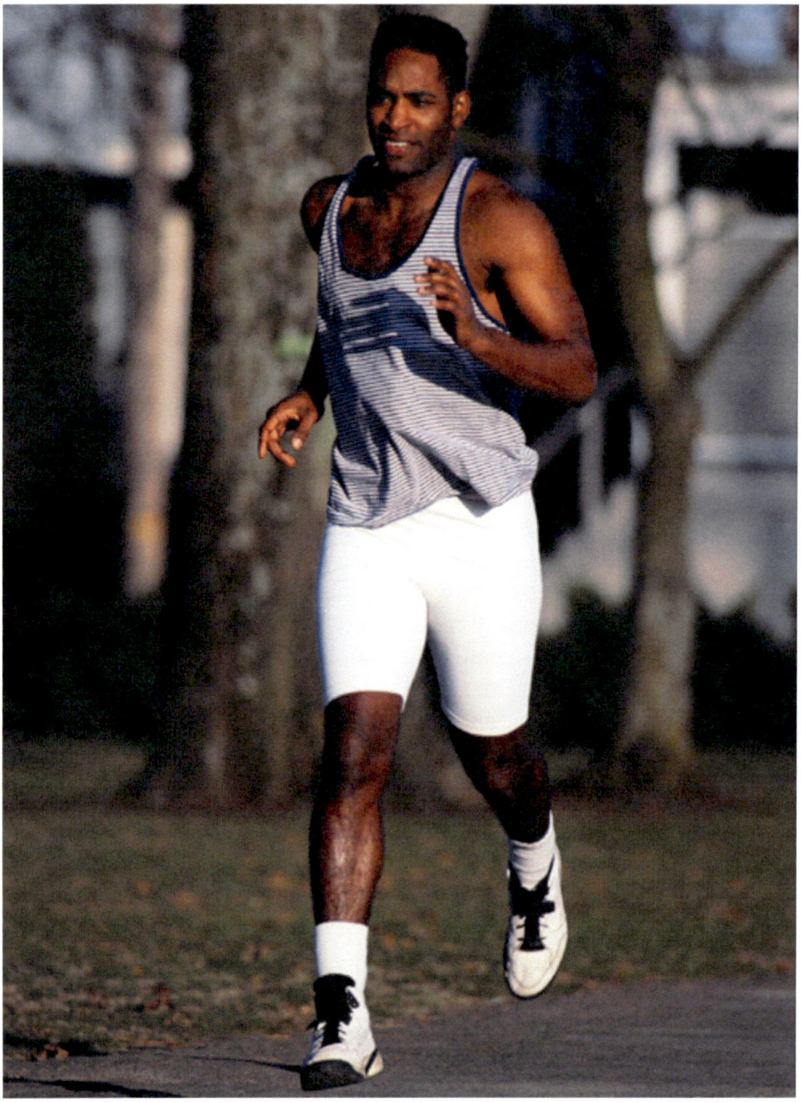

SOURCE: Corbis Corporation.

ous exercise, moderate physical activity, occupational physical activity, physical activity performed in school physical education classes, or lifestyle physical activity. Physical activity has been measured by a variety of means, including self-reports, physiological tests, observation, or technological monitoring. All these variations make comparisons of studies difficult and complicate efforts to summarize overall effects.

The Surgeon General's report on physical activity and health (US DHHS, 1996) concluded that physical activity has numerous beneficial physiological effects and that factors associated with success in promoting physical activity include the following:

1. Consistent influences on physical activity patterns among adults and young people include confidence in one's ability to engage in regular physical activity (e.g., self-efficacy), enjoyment of physical activity, support from others, positive beliefs concerning the benefits of physical activity, and lack of perceived barriers to being physically active.
2. For adults, some interventions have been successful in increasing physical activity in communities, worksites, and health care settings and at home.
3. Interventions targeting physical education in elementary school can substantially increase the amount of time students spend being physically active in physical education class (p. 8).

Interventions to Modify Physical Activity Levels and Patterns

Health Care Settings

Most studies of interventions to promote physical activity with individuals or groups of individuals have been implemented through health care settings. Patients report that they want information about physical activity from their physicians (Godin and Shephard, 1990), and several national initiatives recommend that all physicians and other health care providers advise and counsel their patients to be physically active (Simons-Morton et al., 1998). One of the goals outlined in *Healthy People 2010* is to increase the proportion of primary care providers who counsel their patients about physical activity from the 22 percent found in 1995 to 85 percent in 2010 (US DHHS and Office of Disease Prevention and Health Promotion, 2000). Because studies of the importance of increasing physical activity span several chronic diseases, provider counseling regarding physical activity is not typically disease-specific.

As defined in a recent review (Simons-Morton et al., 1998), physical activity interventions in health care settings fall into four categories:

1. advice or instruction such as a statement about increasing physical activity or the use of cognitive and informational approaches to increasing knowledge;
2. behavioral approaches such as feedback, reinforcement, goal setting, and staging;
3. provision of equipment; and
4. supervised training of groups or individuals.

Simons-Morton and colleagues (1998) reviewed 12 randomized controlled or quasi-experimental interventions conducted in primary care settings for general patients. All of the studies used moderate-intensity aerobic activity as the chief behavioral target. The behavioral theories underlying the interventions were described in six of the studies; of these, three reported significant effects, two reported short-term effects, and one reported long-term effects. Physicians delivered the majority of the physical activity interventions, with two delivered by nurses and two delivered by allied health care specialists. Of the seven randomized controlled studies, five reported significant increases in physical activity, but only two of these five reported significant long-term effects.

The review of Simons-Morton and colleagues (1998) also included studies of promotion of physical activity among patients with disease. Twenty-four studies of physical activity interventions in patients with cardiovascular disease were included. The majority of these studies included supervised exercise as the mode of intervention. Interventions were delivered in both inpatient and outpatient settings and by physicians, nurse counselors, and exercise specialists. Of the 24 studies, 13 reported significant changes in physical activity or cardiorespiratory fitness in the group that received the intervention compared with levels of fitness for the control group, or reported significant increases in physical activity or cardiorespiratory fitness before and after the intervention in the intervention group but no significant changes in the control group. Eleven studies had long-term interventions; eight of these had significant long-term effects, with some lasting as long as 4 and 5 years.

Education of providers and attention to how changes in clinic procedures can help providers encourage their patients to exercise appear to be useful. A combination of physician education, reimbursement for prevention counseling, and reminders to providers was followed by increases in the proportion of patients who started to exercise (Logsdon et al., 1989). Along similar lines, the Physician-Based Assessment and Counseling for Exercise program incorporated behavioral theory into individualized, brief counseling messages for patients. Evaluation of the program indicated that it improved health providers' knowledge about counseling for physical activity (Long et al., 1996) and led to greater improvements in the reported stage of readiness for physical activity, the reported amount of walking for exercise, and scores from an activity monitor (Calfas et al., 1996).

In addition to interventions by health care professionals, print materials and telephone-based interventions appear to be effective in promoting physical activity. A review of 21 studies of such interventions (Marcus et al., 1998d) found evidence that they have short-term impacts on physical activity, with prolonged interventions and those tailored to their audiences being more effective. Additionally, brief telephone contacts were valuable in maintaining adherence to physical activity programs (King et al., 1988, 1991, 1995a; Lombard et al., 1995; Schultz, 1993). Print materials can also be tailored to stage of readiness for exercise or readiness for motivation (Calfas et al., 1996; Cardinal and Sachs, 1996; Jarvis et al., 1997; Marcus et al., 1998d), but their impacts have not yet been documented.

Simons-Morton and colleagues (1998) identified the characteristics of successful physical activity interventions in health care settings. These included long-term interventions, multiple contacts, supervised exercise, provision of equipment, and the use of behavioral approaches.

Worksite Interventions

Many worksite-based health promotion programs include a physical activity or fitness component (Dishman et al., 1998). The mode and extent of physical activity or fitness promotion vary greatly by program. For example, some worksite-based programs offer very structured, supervised exercise or in-house exercise facilities, whereas others promote increased leisure-time physical activities, such as through physical activity contests or media programs. Among U.S. employees, access to wellness programs and fitness centers is highest among those employed by large establishments and among professional and technical employees (Table 4.3).

An early review (Shephard, 1996) reported that among 52 studies conducted in the United States and Canada, program participants showed small but favorable changes in body mass, skinfold thickness, aerobic power, muscle strength and flexibility, overall risk-taking behavior, blood pressure, serum cholesterol levels, and cigarette smoking. However, it was also noted that although participation in such programs can enhance health-related fitness, a population effect is limited by low participation rates. Also, the rates were often difficult to determine because of Hawthorne effects (individuals altering their behavior because they are being observed as part of a study), attrition rates, and poor definition of the intervention (Shephard, 1996).

Another recent review of worksite-based physical activity interventions (Dishman et al., 1998) found that the typical worksite-based intervention for increasing physical activity yielded small positive effects, but these were not significant. Interventions that use behavior modification or incentives were associated with medium positive effects.

One noteworthy program is the Live for Life program of Johnson & Johnson. This program consisted of a well-conducted, comprehensive, quasi-experimental study with a large study population. The Live for Life program reported a substantial increase in cardiorespiratory fitness, as assessed by clinical measures, in the intervention group versus the control group (Breslow et al., 1990).

TABLE 4.3 Access to Wellness Programs and Fitness Centers Among U.S. Full-Time Employees, by Type of Employer

Employer and Employee Group	Number of Full-Time Employees	Percentage of Employees with Access to: Wellness Program	Fitness Center
Small, Private Establishments (<100 employees), 1996			
All employees	39,816,173	8	4
Professional, technical	7,979,698	11	6
Clerical, sales	12,279,707	9	5
Blue collar, service	19,556,767	5	3
Medium and Large, Private Establishments (≥100 employees), 1997			
All employees	38,409,120	36	21
Professional, technical	10,659,842	44	31
Clerical, sales	9,168,433	36	19
Blue collar, services	18,580,845	32	16
State and Local Governments, 1998			
All employees	14,350,773	35	14
White-collar employees, except teachers	5,992,894	39	15
Teachers	3,816,292	31	7
Blue collar, service	4,541,587	33	20

SOURCES: U.S. Department of Labor, Bureau of Labor Statistics (1999a,b, 2000).

School-Based Programs

Because most children attend school, schools offer an exemplary setting for the promotion of physical activity to young people (US DHHS, 1996). Several interventions have been successful in increasing moderate-intensity physical activity during physical education classes (e.g., the CATCH study). Unfortunately, results from the School Health Policies and Program study revealed that although physical education is required by most states (94 percent), it is not required every year (Pate et al., 1995b). Additionally, observations of physical education classes report that insufficient time is spent engaging in physical activity (McKenzie et al., 1996).

Earlier interventions implemented in schools focused more on knowledge-based health education classes. Newer interventions include multiple components and address both the individual and the environment (US DHHS, 1996). These components include incentives to be more physically active, social support, and enhanced curricula in both health and physical education.

A recent review (Stone et al., 1998) synthesized information from 22 studies conducted in schools. Program components included physical education programs, classroom health curricula, and out-of-school physical activity. Analysis of the results of the studies concluded that improvements in knowledge and attitudes related to physical activity were generally found in the studies that measured these attributes, and variable increases in the amount of moderate-intensity physical activity were attained during physical education classes.

Seven of the studies (the CATCH study, the Oslo Youth study, the Australian School study, the Stanford Adolescent Heart Health study, Project Active Teens, ARTEC [Active Recreation Tertiary Education Campuses], and Project GRAD [Graduation Ready for Activity Daily]) found increases in the levels of out-of-school physical activity in the intervention group compared with those in the control group. Striking among these, the CATCH III follow-up study found that a significant difference in the amount of out-of-school physical activity still existed 3 years after the intervention. Most remarkable were the results of the Oslo Youth study. The initial results indicated that significantly more students in the intervention group than control students exercised at least twice a week. A follow-up conducted 12 years later indicated that 49 percent of the participants in the intervention group still reported that they exercise at least twice a week, whereas 40 percent of the participants in the reference group made such a report (Stone et al., 1998).

Other studies not included in the review of Stone and colleagues warrant discussion. Several smaller school-based studies target specific minority groups. The Jump into Action Program was geared toward low-income Hispanic children. This program demonstrated significant increases in exercise knowledge, self-efficacy, and frequency of exercise after the intervention compared with those before the intervention, but at a follow-up evaluation, most of the significant effect was lost (Holcomb et al., 1998). Davis and colleagues (1995b) described a significant difference in knowledge and self-reported levels of exercise in a school-based intervention geared toward Navajo and Pueblo youth. In study of Hispanic and African-American youth in middle school, students reported positive effects from an aerobic dance-based physical education intervention (Flores, 1995). Also, Hopper and colleagues (1992, 1996) conducted studies in rural schools that involved parents as well as grade-school-age children and reported significant increases in knowledge about exercise.

Two recent school-based studies promoted decreased amounts of television viewing as a component of their physical activity interventions (Gortmaker et al., 1999a; Robinson, 1999). Both studies were effective in reducing the amount of time spent watching television, and one (Robinson, 1999) reported favorably significant changes in BMIs and skinfold measurements as well. However, neither study measured whether the amount of physical activity increased as the amount of time watching television decreased.

Community-Based Programs

Comprehensive community-based approaches involve a complex series of physical activity-related interventions that cover multiple targets, channels of dissemination, and settings (King, 1991). These large-scale community-based programs often use multiple media channels and various health education techniques to address knowledge, attitudes, and beliefs about physical activity and normative physical activity behavior. The Stanford Five-City Study, the Minnesota Heart Health Project, and the Pawtucket Heart Health Project have all tested community-based approaches to promoting physical activity. In the Stanford Five-City Study, the only significant findings were from cross-sectional analyses indicating that the men in the treatment cities increased their daily energy expenditures and rates of participation in vigorous exercise. The women in the treatment cities increased their rates of moderate-intensity physical activity (Young et al. 1996). Six-year findings from the Minnesota Heart Health Project suggest that in the cities that received the intervention, the overall effects of the project in terms of behavioral changes related to greater levels of physical activity were modest (Luepker et al., 1994). In the Pawtucket Heart Health Project, there were no differences in self-reported knowledge of the benefits of physical activity, attempts to increase levels of participation in exercise, or prevalence of physical inactivity between Pawtucket (whose population received the intervention) and the comparison community (Eaton et al., 1999). Findings from those studies indicate that community-wide interventions for increased physical activity are feasible, acceptable to community residents, and potentially effective (King, 1991).

The heterogeneous groups that community-based programs seek to influence face diverse barriers to physical activity, and these barriers are special challenges to community-based programs. An analysis of the determinants of physical activity among U.S. women (King et al., 2000) found that the principal barrier for each racial or ethnic group of women varied. For example, white women cited a lack of time as the main barrier to physical activity, whereas African-American women reported a lack of a safe place to be physically active (King et al., 2000). Barriers can also be multilevel. In a report of a national cross-sectional study, Brownson and colleagues (2001) reported that personal barriers to physical activity included a lack of time, feeling too tired, and no motivation to exercise; in addition, they reported that there were environmental barriers to physical activity, such as neighborhood characteristics and heavy traffic. Tailoring interventions to accommodate these barriers is important but may be difficult in broad, community-based interventions.

An authoritative review of the effectiveness of interventions to increase physical activity has recently been released by the CDC (2001d). Its findings are consistent with those presented here.

Environmental and Policy Interventions

Environmental and policy interventions that can be used to increase levels of physical activity include the implementation of policies that result in improved access to facilities and programs or the provision of support for social environments that favor physical activity (Schmid et al., 1995). Examples include walking and bicycling trails, funding for public facilities, zoning and land use policies that facilitate participation in physical activities in neighborhoods, mall walking programs, building designs that encourage physical activity, policies and incentives that promote physical activity during the workday, and policies that require comprehensive school health programs (King et al., 1995b; Sallis et al., 1998).

Sallis and colleagues (1998) reviewed seven studies of environmental and policy interventions. An intervention that was as simple and low-cost as posting signs by stairs and escalators can substantially increase levels of physical activity (Andersen et al., 1998; Blamey et al., 1995; Brownell et al., 1980; Russell et al., 1999). More complex policy and environmental interventions have had varied results. Changes in policies and improvements in the physical environment designed to increase physical activity on a military base appeared to improve the fitness of military personnel (Linenger et al., 1991), although study design limitations hinder the ability to place confidence in these results. Policy and environmental changes made to increase the numbers of employees of a large plant in Finland who walk and bicycle to work resulted in only a 7 percent increase (Vuori et al., 1994). More promising results emerged from a quasi-experimental study of 14 publicly funded leisure centers that were opened in Northern Ireland (Roberts et al., 1989). These resulted in increased levels of participation in sports and physical activity among young adults as well as smaller improvements among those in other age groups.

Programs to Reach Underserved and Minority Populations

Several church-based programs that promote physical activity have been described in the literature, but they have not been fully evaluated (Hatch et al., 1986; Lasater et al., 1986). The Lose Weight and Win Program (Kumanyika and Charleston, 1992) demonstrated moderate success in reducing participants' blood pressure through exercise and dietary changes.

Several school-based programs have shown promise in improving rates of physical activity among minority youth. Davis and colleagues (1995b) described a significant difference in knowledge and self-reported rates of exercise in a school-based intervention geared toward Navajo and Pueblo youth. In a study with Hispanic and African-American youth in a middle school, students reported positive effects from an aerobic dance-based physical education intervention (Flores, 1995). Also, Hopper and colleagues

(1992, 1996) reported positive results of interventions in rural schools that involved parents as well as grade-school-age children.

Media-based approaches have the potential to reach minority populations in a way that may be less threatening and costly than meeting with a physician (Marcus et al., 1998d). Among the media campaigns that address minority populations, PROJECT WALK for sedentary minority women reported an increase in self-reported levels of walking (Chen et al., 1998). However, other mass media programs for physical activity have not been successful (Baranowski et al., 1990b; Nader et al., 1989).

Using a community approach, the Go Girls! Program targeted low-income, overweight, African-American adolescents (Resnicow et al., 2000). It achieved high levels of acceptance of and interest in physical activity, but it lacked a comparison group.

INTERVENTIONS TO ACHIEVE WEIGHT LOSS

Weight-loss treatments aim to modify eating habits and levels of physical activity. Decreasing energy intake, increasing energy expenditure, or a combination will result in decreases in body fat levels. To produce these changes, three main therapeutic elements are emphasized: dietary restriction, physical activity, and behavior modification. This section of the chapter synthesizes the treatment outcome literature for dietary restriction and behavioral programs.

Dietary Restriction

A caloric deficit of 3,500 calories (1 calorie = 4.2 joules) is needed to lose 0.5 kilogram (kg; 1 pound [lb]) of body fat. Thus, a reduction in caloric intake of 500 kilocalories per day (kcal/day) below requirements translates into a weight loss of about 0.5 kg (1 lb) per week; a reduction of 1,000 kcal/day translates into a weight loss of about 1 kg (2 lb) per week. Rather than trying to estimate current intakes and expenditures and then recommending a deficit of 500 to 1,000 kcal/day, it is typical to suggest a general range of calories and then to adjust the calorie level, as needed.

Low-Calorie Diets

The most common caloric regimen is the low-calorie diet (LCD). Typically, women are recommended a balanced deficit diet of 1,200 to 1,500 kcal/day and men are recommended a balanced deficit diet of 1,500 to 1,800 kcal/day. This regimen should produce a weight loss of 0.5 to 1 kg (1 to 2 lb) per week, which is the rate of weight loss typically recommended. Foods may be self-selected among conventional foods, recipes, and frozen entrees.

LCDs have been found to produce medically significant weight loss. For example, NHLBI reviewed 34 studies evaluating the effects of LCDs (National Heart, Lung and Blood Institute, 1998). In that review, the subjects in all 34 studies demonstrated significant weight loss, averaging 8 percent of initial body weight. The panel concluded that there was strong and consistent evidence that adherence to LCDs for 3 to 12 months produced medically significant weight loss in overweight and obese patients. The review also consistently showed that waist circumference decreased with the weight loss produced by LCDs. On the basis of these data, NHLBI recommended the LCD for the treatment of most overweight and obese persons.

Very-Low-Calorie Diets

Very-low-calorie diets (VLCDs) have traditionally been defined as diets consisting of energy intakes <800 kcal/day. As energy needs vary among individuals, investigators have recently suggested defining VLCDs in terms of the amount of caloric restriction induced by a given diet in a given individual. By using these criteria, a VLCD was defined as any diet providing ≤50 percent of an individual's predicted resting energy requirements (Wadden and Berkowitz, 2001).

VLCDs typically consist of liquid meal replacements (e.g., shakes) containing 100 percent of the recommended daily allowance of essential vitamins and minerals; these are consumed three to five times per day. No other foods are usually allowed. Since VLCDs can lead to dramatic shifts in fluid and electrolyte balances and may result in a significant loss of lean body mass, medical supervision is required.

VLCDs produce mean weight losses of about 20 kg (44 lb) in women and about 30 kg (66 lb) in men over 12 to 16 weeks. These reductions are two to three times greater than those produced by conventional diets of 1,200 to 1,500 kcal/day. The NHLBI review showed that VLCDs promoted weight loss of approximately 13 to 23 kg (29 to 51 lb) during the active phase of the VLCD intervention, whereas LCDs promoted weight loss of 9 to 13 kg (20 to 29 lb) (National Heart, Lung, and Blood Institute, 1998).

These favorable short-term results differ markedly from long-term outcomes. On average, patients treated by use of VLCDs regain 30 to 50 percent of their lost weight in the year following treatment and increasingly gain weight over time. In a 78-week trial, Wadden and colleagues (1989) compared a VLCD and an LCD. Weight loss was initially greater with the VLCD (12 kg [26 lb] versus 22 kg [49 lb]), but after 26 weeks the VLCD group began to regain weight, and by 52 weeks the weight loss was no longer different between the two groups.

These and other long-term data (National Task Force on the Prevention and Treatment of Obesity, 1993; Wing et al., 1994) have raised questions about the benefits of VLCDs and, in particular, of restricting caloric intake to less than 800 kcal/day. Although current VLCDs are generally safe when administered under appropriate medical supervision, they are usually limited to persons who have BMIs ≥30 kg/m^2 and who are resistant to less aggressive approaches with LCDs.

Portion-Controlled Diets

The effectiveness of VLCDs in promoting short-term weight loss likely lies in the form and manner of the VLCD rather than the goal of the VLCD (Foster et al., 1992). Portion-controlled diets capitalize on the advantages of both the LCD and VLCD approaches. Specifically, portion-controlled diets provide the same calories and macronutrients as a conventional LCD, but patients are encouraged to use portion-controlled servings. This can be in the form of drinks, bars, or prepackaged foods meant to replace a meal or snack. For example, patients could use a liquid formula at breakfast and lunch and a portion-controlled frozen dinner at night.

Recently, investigators reported that participants who consumed a liquid formula (i.e., Slimfast) for two meals per day lost more weight than those who consumed a conventional diet with an equivalent number of calories (Ditschuneit et al., 1999). In addition, continued use of meal replacements was related to the long-term maintenance of weight loss (Flechtner-Mors et al., 2000). Other studies in which the food was provided to participants in appropriate portion sizes (Jeffery et al., 1993b; McCarron et al., 1997; Metz et al., 2000) or in which detailed meal plans and grocery lists were distributed (Wing et al., 1996a) have also shown the benefits of structured eating plans relative to those of traditional LCDs. Taken together, these data suggest that portion-controlled diets enable individuals to lose weight effectively and provide healthy nutrition.

Macronutrient Composition

The macronutrient composition of the diet typically recommended for weight loss is based on the Food Guide Pyramid (U.S. Department of Agriculture, 1992). This represents a diet that is low in fat, high in carbohydrates and fiber, and that includes moderate amounts to no alcohol. This dietary composition capitalizes on the different caloric values of nutrients. Specifically, carbohydrates and protein have 4 calories per gram (cal/g), whereas alcohol has 7 cal/g and fat has 9 cal/g.

Because fat is the most calorically dense macronutrient, its consumption is likely to increase the risk of subsequent weight gain. Thus, reducing fat intake may help produce weight loss (Insull et al., 1990; Kendall et al., 1991). Randomized control trials evaluating the effects of low-fat diets report modest weight losses over the short term (4 kg [9 lb]) and long term (2 kg [4 lb]) (Jeffery et al., 1995; Schlundt et al., 1993). Similarly, NHLBI's review of the literature and a recent meta-analysis (Astrup et al., 2000) concluded that lower-fat diets promoted modest weight loss and also helped promote weight maintenance.

However, reducing the amount of dietary fat alone is not optimal for weight loss. Short- and long-term randomized control trials found that weight loss was significantly greater when low-fat diets were combined with caloric restriction than when caloric restriction alone or a low-fat diet alone was used (Pascale et al., 1995; Schlundt et al., 1993). NHLBI's review also found better weight loss and maintenance of weight loss when lower-fat diets were prescribed in combination with targeted caloric reduction (National Heart, Lung, and Blood Institute, 1998). These studies are supplemented by correlational data that also suggest the benefits of a reduced-fat diet. Greater decreases in the number of calories from dietary fat have been associated with greater short- and long-term weight losses (Harris et al., 1994; Jeffery et al., 1993b). In addition, several studies identified the consumption or the lack of consumption of specific high-fat foods (e.g., French fries and ice cream) as predictive of weight loss failure or success (Harris et al., 1994; Holden et al., 1992). Fast-food consumption or the lack thereof was also associated with weight loss failure or success (Holden et al., 1992). Thus, both the number of calories and the number of grams of fat in the diet should be monitored to achieve optimal weight loss. This is not surprising, given that many "low-fat" or "non-fat" food products compensate for the loss of fat (and calories) by increasing the amount of sugar (and calories) in the product.

Popular Diets

Diets with various energy levels and nutrient compositions have been used for weight loss. Many of the popular diets (e.g., the Atkins, Protein Power, Sugar Busters, and Zone diets) advocate reducing the amounts of specific nutrients or categories of food. These diets work for weight loss to the extent that they produce caloric deficits (Freedman et al., 2001). For example, individuals who are accustomed to a high-sugar diet but who adopt a sugar-free dietary plan may lose weight, at least in the short term, because they reduce their total intake of calories.

Most popular diets, however, have not been evaluated empirically; thus, their effects on weight loss and long-term health remain unclear. Popular diets may produce some short-term weight loss; however, there is no scientific basis for their long-term use. The available data indicate that individuals who are successful at maintaining their weight loss consume diets that are low in fat and high in carbohydrates (Klem et al., 1997). In addition, individuals derive the greatest health benefits from diets low in saturated fat and high in carbohydrates and fiber; these increase sensitivity to insulin and lower the risk for coronary heart disease.

In summary, LCD's consisting of 1,200 to 1,500 kcal/day can produce medically meaningful weight losses, averaging about 8 percent of initial body weight. Use of meal replacements and portion-controlled servings may help promote adherence to a diet and long-term weight maintenance. Diets that are low in fat and high in fiber and carbohydrates appear optimal for weight control and overall health.

Physical Activity Interventions to Promote Weight Loss and Maintenance

Many reviews and recommendations on the role of physical activity in the management of obesity have been published (Donnelly et al., 1991; Gleim, 1993; National Heart, Lung, and Blood Institute, 1998; Wing, 1999). Published research suggests that exercise alone (i.e., without adjunct dietary restriction) produces only modest weight loss. In the NHLBI review of the literature, 10 of 12 studies reported that exercise alone produced greater weight losses than no-exercise control conditions; however, the mean difference in weight loss was only 2.4 kg (5.3 lb) (National Heart, Lung, and Blood Institute, 1998). Therefore, the panel concluded that physical activity alone has only a modest effect or no effect on body weight. Similar findings have been reported in other reviews (Wing, 1999) and a meta-analysis of the literature (Garrow and Summerbell, 1995).

On the basis of these findings, the commonly held view is that exercise alone is not a very useful weight-loss strategy. However, the energy expenditures induced in the exercise-alone conditions of most of these studies were moderate, at best, and would not be considered enough to produce a substantial weight loss. Larger energy deficits (i.e., >3,500 kcal/week) do, in fact, promote weight loss (Bouchard et al., 1990; Sopko et al., 1985). Overall, when obese patients increase their levels of physical activity, a state of negative caloric balance is produced; at sufficiently high levels, this negative caloric balance can promote weight loss.

Induction of Weight Loss: Exercise Plus Dietary Restriction

Much research has also compared the effects of exercise, dietary restriction, and their combination in promoting weight loss. NHLBI's review reported that 12 of 15 studies showed greater weight loss in the group that used diet plus exercise than in the group that used diet alone (a 1.9-kg [4.2-lb] difference) (National Heart, Lung, and Blood Institute, 1998). In addition, the combination of diet plus physical activity improved cardiorespiratory fitness and produced modestly greater reductions in abdominal fat levels compared with those from dietary therapy alone. Wing's review

(1999), which included most of the same studies reviewed by NHLBI, noted that although the weight losses were greater in those who used exercise plus diet, only 2 of 13 studies showed statistically significant differences in weight loss between those in the group that used exercise plus diet and those in the group that used diet alone. Thus, although the combination of a reduced-calorie diet and increased physical activity produced greater weight loss, the effect was modest. However, given the modest increase in weight loss and the significantly greater improvements in cardiorespiratory health, the combination of a reduced-calorie diet and physical activity is the recommended treatment for obesity (National Heart, Lung, and Blood Institute, 1998).

Physical Activity and Maintenance of Weight Loss

Improving the rate of maintenance of weight loss remains a principal goal of obesity research. Empirical reviews of randomized control trials have reported that diet plus exercise generally increased long-term weight loss relative to that from diet alone, although the difference was often not statistically significant. Within these randomized control trials, those individuals who continue to perform the highest levels of activity achieve the best long-term results (Garrow and Summerbell, 1995; Jeffery et al., 1998; Pronk and Wing, 1994; Wing, 1999).

Correlational studies consistently show that the self-reported level of physical activity is a strong predictor of weight loss maintenance. In fact, exercise predicts weight loss maintenance significantly more than dietary adherence or use of other behavior modification techniques (Pronk and Wing, 1994; Wing, 1999). For example, Kayman and colleagues (1990) described the variables that differentiated weight maintainers (i.e., women who had successfully maintained their weight loss for at least 2 years), weight regainers (i.e., women who had previously lost 20 percent of their weight but had regained it), and normal-weight controls (i.e., women who had always been of average weight). One of the major factors that differentiated the three groups was adherence to exercise. Specifically, 75 percent of maintainers reported that they used exercise as part of their weight management strategy, whereas only 36 percent of weight regainers used exercise. In addition, 90 percent of maintainers and 82 percent of controls said that they had participated in exercise on a regular basis (i.e., >3 days/week for ≥30 minutes), whereas only 34 percent of regainers reported this behavior.

In a more recent example, the National Weight Control Registry described the weight-control behaviors of 784 men and women who had maintained an average weight loss of 30 kg (66 lb) for an average of 5.6 years (Klem et al., 1997). In that study, most participants reported extremely high levels of physical activity. Specifically, participants reported expending approximately 2,830 kcal/week, which is the equivalent of walking about 45 kilometers/week (28 miles/week) or more than 1 hour/day every day. Other correlational data have revealed similar findings (Pronk and Wing, 1994), further demonstrating the importance of physical activity in long-term weight control.

Given the low level of adherence to exercise by obese patients, identification of alternative ways to facilitate long-term adherence is paramount. One promising approach is to encourage engaging in multiple brief bouts of physical activity each day, that is, multiple 5- to 10-minute bouts of moderate-intensity activity throughout the day (Jakicic et al., 1995). Engaging in several short bouts rather than one long bout of physical activity may make it more convenient for patients to exercise. Jakicic and colleagues (1995) examined the effects of prescribing exercise in multiple short bouts (i.e., four bouts of 10 minutes each) versus one longer bout (i.e., 40 minutes). After 20 weeks, participants in the multiple-bout regimen had better rates of adherence to the exercise regimen and better initial weight loss. Both groups had similar improvements in fitness.

In a longer-term follow-up study, Jakicic and colleagues (1999) compared the effects of multiple short-bout exercise (10-min bouts), multiple short-bout exercise with home exercise equipment (i.e., a treadmill), and longer-bout exercise (40 minutes). After 18 months, the short- and long-bout exercise groups had similar weight losses and improvements in cardiorespiratory fitness, again suggesting the comparable benefits of short- and long-bout exercises. Interestingly, participants with the home exercise equipment maintained higher levels of exercise than participants in the short- and long-bout exercise groups; they also had significantly greater weight loss than participants in the short-bout exercise groups. As noted below, access to home exercise equipment may facilitate the maintenance of exercise, which can improve long-term weight loss.

Another approach to increasing physical activity is to promote lifestyle activity as an alternative or complement to programmed activity. Several studies have documented the benefits of increasing the amount of lifestyle activity (walking rather than driving, using stairs rather than escalators, and throwing away energy-saving devices such as television remote controls). For example, Andersen and colleagues (1999) found that both lifestyle activity and programmed exercise combined with a diet of 1,200 kcal/day produced weight losses of approximately 8.5 kg (19 lb) during a 16-week weight-loss program. A longer-term (2-year) study similarly reported that both lifestyle and structured exercise interventions produced significant and comparably beneficial changes in levels of physical activity, cardiorespiratory fitness, blood pressure, and the percentage of body fat (Dunn et al., 1999). Thus, the encouragement of lifestyle activity may be useful, particularly for patients who dislike programmed regimens.

Another approach is to have participants exercise at home rather than at a clinic or a health club. A number of studies have compared home-based and supervised exercise programs. For example, Perri and colleagues (1997) evaluated the effects of a supervised group exercise program versus those of a home-based exercise program. At 12 months, participants who had been randomly assigned to home-based exercise had better rates of adherence to exercise and greater weight losses. Similarly, King and colleagues (1991) found that participants were more adherent to exercises that they could complete at home than to those that had to be completed in supervised group settings. On the basis of these and other studies (Jakicic et al., 1999), home-based exercise appears to improve rates of adherence to exercise and may help in promoting long-term exercise adoption.

In summary, the combination of a reduced-calorie diet and increased physical activity is recommended since it produces the best maintenance of weight loss, the greatest increases in cardiorespiratory fitness, and the greatest decreases in abdominal fat levels. The accumulation of exercise through short bouts of exercise, lifestyle activity, and the use of exercise equipment in the home may help improve rates of adherence to physical activity regimens.

Behavioral Programs

A number of behavioral approaches have been incorporated into weight-control programs (Brownell, 1991; Wadden and Bell, 1990; Wing, 1996). Although little research examining the efficacies of specific components of behavior programs has been conducted, in general, a multimodal approach with numerous components works better than less-intensive behavior modification programs (National Heart, Lung, and Blood Institute, 1998).

Multicomponent behavioral programs integrate cognitive-behavioral skill training strategies with dietary restriction and physical activity. Typically, treatment consists of 16 to 20 weeks of group sessions, each lasting 60 to 90 minutes. Maintenance programs vary, but contact is typically decreased over time from weekly to biweekly sessions and then to monthly sessions. Each week, a group leader introduces a new weight-control skill that builds upon skills learned in previous sessions. To promote skill building and group cohesion, patients start and complete a program together, with no new participants added to the group. In addition to a weekly topic, session time is also spent reviewing homework, setting specific behavioral goals, and helping patients resolve barriers to their weight-loss efforts (Wadden, 1993). Sessions are structured by use of an agenda, and manuals may be provided (Brownell, 1991).

Short-Term Programs

Initial randomized control trials (conducted in the 1970s) showed that multicomponent treatment was consistently superior to comparison treatments, including treatments that included only psychoeducational and nutrition components. Weight losses averaged 3 to 4 kg (7 to 8 lb) in 8 weeks. Over time, both the duration and the content of treatment expanded. Specifically, the length of treatment doubled, from 8 to 10 weeks to 16 to 20 weeks. In addition, treatment began to emphasize caloric restriction and physical activity as key components for weight loss. As a result, weight losses nearly doubled (Brownell and Wadden, 1986). Today, treatment programs result in an average weight loss of 8.5 kg (18.7 lb) (9 percent of initial body weight), and attrition rates are generally low (<20 percent). Patients experience significant improvements in both cardiovascular and mental health (National Heart, Lung, and Blood Institute, 1998).

Long-Term Programs

The central problem with multicomponent treatment has been failure to promote the long-term maintenance of weight loss. In the year after treatment, patients typically regain about 30 to 35 percent of the weight that they initially lost. Weight regain generally increases with time. In 3 to 5 years after treatment, 50 percent or more of patients have returned to their baseline weight (Wadden et al., 1989).

Extending the length of treatment (i.e., to 52 or 78 weeks) can promote the maintenance of weight loss. On average, patients maintain their full end-of-treatment loss as long as they attend maintenance group sessions (Perri et al., 1988; Wadden et al., 1994; Wing et al., 1994). Unfortunately, attendance at these sessions declines over time, and after treatment ends, patients regain the weight that they lost (Perri et al., 1988; Wing et al., 1994).

A minority of individuals are able to maintain their weight by adhering to a low-calorie, low-fat diet and engaging in high levels of physical activity (Klem et al., 1997). Predicting who will succeed or fail treatment, however, has proven elusive. Personality traits, measures of psychopathology, the presence of binge eating, dietary restraint, and a history of weight cycling have all proved unreliable in predicting success. High levels of social support (Foreyt and Goodrick, 1991; Kayman et al., 1990) and greater initial body weight (Foreyt et al., 1982) are related to better short- and long-term weight-loss outcomes. In addition, the treatment variables of early weight loss (Wadden et al., 1998), consistent attendance at weight maintenance sessions (Guare et al., 1989; Jeffery et al., 1993b; Wadden et al., 1994), and adherence to self-monitoring (Jeffery et al., 1993b; McGuire et al., 1999) are also useful predictors.

In summary, multicomponent behavioral programs provide the skills and support needed to lose a medically significant amount of weight. A minority of individuals succeed at weight maintenance by adhering to a low-calorie, low-fat diet and maintaining a high level of physical activity. However, after treatment is terminated, most individuals regain weight. In some individuals who fail to achieve lasting weight loss by standard treatment, more aggressive treatments for obesity, including pharmacological or surgical treatments, may be considered.

Commercial Weight-Loss Programs

Very few empirical studies of commercial weight-loss programs have been conducted, although more people clearly receive their weight-loss counseling from such programs than from the research programs described above. Recently, Heshka and colleagues (2000) conducted an empirical study of the Weight Watchers program. That study showed that participants who were randomly assigned to receive self-help weight-loss materials lost 1.3 kg (2.9 LB) over 26 weeks, whereas those given free vouchers to attend a Weight Watchers meeting lost 3.9 kg (8.6 lb) (Heshka et al., 2000). The weight losses in the commercial program correlated significantly with attendance at the treatment meetings.

Maintenance of weight loss in former Weight Watchers participants who had reached their goal weight while in the program has also been studied (Lowe et al., 2001). Participants contacted 1 year after treatment had regained 31.5 percent of the weight that they had initially lost; after 2, 3, 4, and 5 years participants had regained 54, 60, 78, and 76 percent of the weight that they had initially lost, respectively. Even at 5 years, however, 43 percent of the participants maintained weight losses of >5 percent compared with their weight at the time of entry into Weight Watchers and 70 percent were below their weight at the time of entry into Weight Watchers.

The Trevose program is another self-help program with a different treatment approach (Latner et al., 2000). In this program, which is led by lay people, participants must regularly attend meetings and must achieve their weight loss goals to remain in the program. Given these contingencies, many who join the program do not remain in it long term; however, for a small group of participants the program appears to be quite effective.

Further study of commercial programs is clearly needed. For the present, it is recommended that overweight individuals who wish to use commercial programs select programs based on the following criteria: a good match between programmer and consumer, the soundness and safety of the program, and the short- and long-term outcomes of the program (Institute of Medicine, 1995b).

Mediated Approaches

Although programs that involve a face-to-face treatment approach appear to be the most effective for weight loss, many overweight individuals will not enroll in such programs. In an effort to increase the audience for weight-loss programs and to reduce the cost of such programs, several investigators have studied interventions delivered by phone (Hellerstedt and Jeffery, 1997; Wing et al., 1996b), mail (Jeffery et al., 1990; Leermarkers et al., 1998), television (Harvey-Berino, 1998; Meyers et al., 1996), or the Internet (Tate et al., 2001). In two studies that used telephone calls to remind people to self-monitor their intake, there were trends, but no significant differences, between those who received phone calls and those in a control condition who did not receive the calls (Hellerstedt and Jeffery, 1997; Leermarkers et al., 1998; Wing et al., 1996b). Leermarkers and colleagues (1998) compared a no-treatment control group with a home-based program delivered via mail and phone and a clinic-based program. Although participants in both the home-based and the clinic-based programs lost more weight than the controls, the weight losses achieved by both approaches were minimal, perhaps because the focus of the program was on weight gain prevention rather than on weight loss.

The presentation of treatment via television has appeared to be more effective. Using an interactive television technology in which patients could see and hear the therapist and other patients, Harvey-Berino (1998) achieved weight losses comparable to those achieved in a face-to-face program (7.6 versus 7.9 kg [16.8 versus 17.4 lb], respectively), over 12 weeks. A program delivered via cable television also produced weight losses comparable to those achieved in a clinic-based program over 8 weeks (Meyers et al., 1996).

Currently of interest is the use of the Internet and computer technology to deliver weight-control programs. Until recently, this approach focused mainly on the use of handheld computers to facilitate self-monitoring of eating and exercise behaviors and to provide feedback to participants (Taylor et al., 1991a; Winett et al., 1991). Recently, Tate and colleagues (2001) evaluated the effects of delivering a complete behavioral treatment program via the Internet and e-mail. Participants in the program delivered via the Internet received weekly lessons via e-mail and submitted their self-monitoring diaries to the therapist on a weekly basis. The therapist provided individualized feedback to the participants via e-mail. Weight losses in the group that received behavioral therapy via the Internet were significantly better than those in the control group that received weight-related information via a site on the World Wide Web (–4.1 versus –1.6 kg [–9.0 versus –3.5 lb]). This study raises the possibility that the Internet and e-mail can be useful in increasing the audience for weight-loss programs and helping these individuals achieve modest weight losses.

Pharmacological Treatments of Obesity

Obesity-related medications are recommended for use only by persons with BMIs of ≥ 30 kg/m^2 with no concomitant obesity-related risk factors or diseases (e.g., coronary heart disease or diabetes), or for patients with BMIs of ≥27 kg/m^2 in the presence of comorbid conditions (National Heart, Lung, and Blood Institute, 1998). In addition, medications should be used only as an adjunct to a comprehensive lifestyle modification program that includes diet, physical activity, and behavioral therapy (National Heart, Lung, and Blood Institute, 1998).

The history of pharmacotherapy for weight loss has been marked by several adverse experiences. In 1997, for example, fenfluramine and dexfenfluramine were withdrawn from the market because of their association with valvular heart disease (Weissman, 2001). Currently approved medications, however, appear to be generally safe and effective when used by appropriate persons under medical supervision.

The two medications currently approved for long-term use are sibutramine (Meridia, Abbott Laboratories) and orlistat (Xenical, Roche Pharmaceuticals). Sibutramine is a central nervous system agent that works by inhibiting the reuptake of norepinephrine and serotonin and that is associated with decreased food intake at meals. By contrast, orlistat is a gastric and pancreatic lipase inhibitor that works by blocking absorption of about one-third of the fat contained in a meal; the undigested fat is excreted in the stool.

Both medications in conjunction with dietary therapy promote weight losses of 5 to 13 kg (11 to 29 lb) of initial body weight, or approximately 3 to 9 kg (7 to 20 lb) more than those produced by placebo. Maximum weight losses are generally achieved by 6 months. Weight losses are generally well maintained, with only a minimal amount of regain for up to 2 years (Hauptman et al., 2000; Lean, 1997). Both medications appear to be useful in preventing weight regain after the use of other dietary approaches, such as a VLCD (Apfelbaum et al., 1999; Sjostrom et al., 1998). Unfortunately, few studies have compared the effect of monotherapy (i.e., medication or standard behavior modification treatment alone) versus that of combined treatment (medication plus standard behavior modification treatment). Thus, the benefits of adding medication to a comprehensive treatment program remain unclear. Nonetheless, current recommendations are that medication be used only in conjunction with a comprehensive behavioral treatment program.

Worksite-Based Interventions

Worksites are considered appealing locations for weight-loss interventions because they can reach large numbers of individuals, many of whom might not typically enroll in weight-loss programs, and these individuals can be treated cost-effectively. In addition, environmental changes can be made at the worksite to enhance treatment efficacy. Finally, worksite-based programs might be able to recover the cost of the programs through improved productivity and reduced health care costs (Hennrikus and Jeffery, 1996). The proportion of worksites offering weight-loss interventions gradually increased from 15 to 24 percent between 1985 and 1992.

Most worksite-based programs for weight control include an educational component, with information regarding diet, exercise, and behavior modification strategies presented as part of the program. Typically, this information is presented in small group meetings, held weekly for 8 to 16 weeks, which appear to parallel clinic-based programs. Some worksite-based programs also include financial incentives or prizes for attendance or weight loss. One special type of incentive system that is particularly appropriate in worksite settings is the use of team competitions (Brownell et al., 1984). These competitions may have weekly weigh-ins, posting of team progress, and other strategies to promote team cohesiveness and may provide financial awards, trophies, or T-shirts as prizes. With the exception of these team competitions, most worksite-based interventions have not really taken advantage of the worksite setting. A notable exception is one program that provided point-of-purchase information in the cafeteria, a special dieters lunch table, and nutrition information about vending machine choices (Summnex et al., 1986).

It is difficult to evaluate the effectiveness of worksite-based interventions because few randomized controlled trials have been conducted in the work setting. The median rate of employee participation among overweight employees averaged 39 percent across several studies that presented this information (Hennrikus and Jeffery, 1996). Although it thus appears that many will enter these programs, attrition rates have been high, especially in programs that do not involve group competitions or incentives. Weight losses appear to be modest. Jeffery and colleagues (1985) reported that participants in a worksite-based weight-loss program lost an average of 2.1 kg (4.6 lb) during the initial 3-month treatment, whereas those in the untreated control group gained 1.2 kg (2.7 lb). Few programs have included a maintenance component, but those that have suggest the benefits of continuing to see participants over time (Abrams and Follick, 1983). Long-term weight loss in worksite-based programs appears to be problematic, as is the case in other areas of weight control.

One of the largest worksite-based interventions was conducted by Jeffery and colleagues (1993a) between 1988 and 1990. Thirty-two worksites with a total of 20,000 employees were randomized to either an intervention or a control group. About 20 percent of all employees and 40 percent of the overweight employees enrolled in weight-loss classes that were offered at the worksite on four occasions over a 2-year period. The average weight loss of the program participants was 2 kg (4 lb) over 6 months. After 2 years, however, there were no differences in average BMI or change in BMI between individuals at the worksites that received the treatment and individuals at the control worksites.

In general, worksite-based programs have tended to merely provide clinical programs in a worksite setting. With the exception of team competitions, there has been very little effort to exploit the unique aspects of the worksite in developing these intervention programs.

Community-Based Interventions

Three large community-based intervention projects have sought to reduce smoking, high blood pressure, high cholesterol levels, and obesity. Weight reduction was viewed largely for its potential impact on blood pressure and cholesterol levels. In the Stanford Five-City Study (Taylor et al., 1991b), mass media, community organizations, and educational classes were used to increase knowledge and teach behavioral change skills related to changing diet and levels of physical activity. Both the treated and the control communities gained weight over the 6 years of the study. Although there was slightly less weight gain in the treated communities in cross-sectional analyses, no differences between the treated and the control communities were seen in a cohort analysis.

The Minnesota Heart Health Program (Jeffery, 1995) included interventions similar to those mentioned above for the Stanford Five-City Study but also included worksite-based programs, a home correspondence course, and interventions aimed at preventing weight gain. Again, the results were disappointing; there were substantial weight gains over the 7 years of the study in both the treatment and the control communities.

The Pawtucket Heart program (Carleton et al., 1995) also included both community-based and worksite-based programs; although there was less of an increase in BMI over 6 years in the treated community compared with that in the control community in the cross-sectional analysis, no differences were seen in the cohort analysis.

Thus, all three community-based programs had disappointing results for obesity. It is noteworthy that these community-based interventions were more effective for other risk factors. Perhaps the fact that all three studies occurred in the 1980s, when rates of obesity were increasing so dramatically, and the fact that none of these efforts focused on obesity alone may have limited their effectiveness.

Environmental Approaches to Treatment of Overweight

All of the approaches discussed above focus on providing the general population or the overweight population with education about healthy eating and physical activity and strategies to change their behaviors. An alternative approach is to focus on changing the environment. Over the past several decades there have been a large number of environmental changes that may be associated with the increasing rates of obesity. These include the increasing frequency of consumption of meals away from home, the explosion of fast-food restaurants, and the dramatic increases in portion sizes. Similarly, the increasing use of energy-saving devices, the large number of hours spent watching television and playing video games, and concerns about safety have led to decreases in amounts of physical activity.

To date, there have been few efforts to systematically evaluate the effect of modifying the environment on eating or exercise behavior and body weight. A number of studies have provided nutrition information to consumers in supermarkets, cafeterias, vending machines, and restaurants (Schmitz and Jeffery, 2002). Most of these have had mixed results. It may be difficult in settings such as grocery stores to provide nutrition information that can compete with the large amount of advertising and marketing that companies use to promote their products.

Rather than provide information or education, recent efforts have focused on changing the price or availability of healthy choices. Jeffery and colleagues (1994) found that increasing the numbers of fruits and salad items offered in worksite cafeterias and decreasing the costs of these items led to more purchases of these items; similar results were observed in a school cafeteria, but there was no postintervention maintenance of the effect (French et al., 1997b). Other investigators have studied the effects of changing prices and using promotional labels on vending machine choices (French et al., 1997a; Wadden and Berkowitz, 2001). Whereas the use of labels and signs had a small effect on purchases, price changes had quite dramatic effects: reducing the price of low-fat snacks by 10, 25, and 50 percent increased the levels of purchase of these items by 9, 39, and 93 percent, respectively. Interestingly, these manipulations had no significant effect on vending machine profits. The effectiveness of these environmental changes, in contrast to the limited effects of educational approaches, suggests that further research on these strategies should be conducted and that they should be tested in longer and larger research trials.

Many other environmental approaches have been suggested, but they have not been studied empirically. For example, taxes on high-fat foods, limiting food advertising during children's television programs, and building more bike paths have all been suggested, but they have not been empirically evaluated.

Programs to Reach Underserved and Minority Populations

African Americans often achieve less weight loss than whites in standard treatment programs (Kumanyika et al., 1991; Wing and Anglin, 1992; Yanovski et al., 1994). This may be due to physiological differences that impede weight loss in African Americans (Jakicic and Wing, 1998). Alternatively, current treatment programs may be less culturally relevant to African-American participants and other minority populations (Kumanyika,

2001). Intervention programs that are culturally adapted to the population—for example, programs that involve bilingual therapists, that discuss foods typically eaten by the participants or physical activities that are popular in the culture, that incorporate the family to a greater extent, and that involve relevant institutions such as the church—appear to be more effective (Cousins et al., 1992; Kumanyika, 2001; McNabb et al., 1993).

Overall, dietary interventions designed to be culturally relevant appear to be as effective as those designed for the general population. As with other programs for the general population, behavioral interventions for underserved groups are most effective when they are developed with input from the target population and are implemented within organizations respected and valued by the target community. Interventions that target change across multiple levels appear to be effective.

Treatment Approaches for Overweight Children

There has been a rapid rise in the prevalence of overweight among children and adolescents. Because overweight children and adolescents are at increased risk of becoming overweight adults and are likely to experience both negative psychological and physiological consequences of obesity, it is important to develop effective programs for these populations. Two general approaches have been used for childhood obesity: clinic-based interventions, which target overweight children or adolescents and their parents, and school-based interventions, which target an entire classroom of children.

Clinic-Based Programs

Epstein and colleagues (1990, 1994b, 1998) have conducted the most systematic research on clinic-based programs for children. Their program, which targets overweight children ages 6 to 12, has been effective in reducing the prevalence of overweight through 10 years of follow-up (Epstein et al., 1990, 1994b). At the 10-year follow-up, 34 percent of children who participated in these programs had lost 20 percent or more of their excess weight and 30 percent were no longer obese. The key components of this highly effective clinical intervention are discussed below.

Family-Based Intervention

Overweight children are likely to have overweight parents. Because the parents are responsible for most of the food purchases and food preparation and serve as important role models for their children, it is critical to involve the parents in the treatment program (Epstein et al., 1981). Epstein and colleagues (1980) showed that it was more effective to treat the child and the parents, targeting both for weight loss, than to focus only on the child or to have a nonspecific target. Typically, the child and parent attend separate group meetings, but they are seen together as a family to set specific behavior goals and rewards. Similarly, other research found that overweight adolescents treated with their mothers, but in separate groups, lost more weight than adolescents treated alone or in the same group as their mother (Brownell et al., 1983).

Multicomponent Program

Similar to the treatment of adults, Epstein and colleagues' effective treatment program for children involves diet, exercise, and behavior modification. Group meetings are typically held weekly for 8 to 12 weeks. These meetings present behavioral skills such as self-monitoring, stimulus control, contingency management, and praise. Several studies have shown that adding behavioral training to a standard diet program improves the results (Epstein et al., 1980; Israel et al., 1985).

Diet Epstein and colleagues used a "traffic-light" diet in which children are encouraged to increase their levels of consumption of green foods (unlimited foods), to eat yellow foods (foods with average nutritional value for their food group) in moderation, and to limit their intake of red foods (foods that provide less nutrient density per calorie) (Epstein et al., 1980, 1986; Valoski and Epstein, 1990). Studies that use this diet have shown significant decreases in rates of obesity among preadolescent children, with corresponding improvements in the nutrient composition of the diet and changes in food preference ratings (Valoski and Epstein, 1990). Other dieting approaches, including exchange-system diets and VLCDs (Figueroa-Colon et al., 1993), have also been used extensively in the treatment of overweight children. The success of these diets appears to depend on the context in which they are presented; no studies have compared different approaches with diet modification in overweight children.

Exercise

The combination of diet and exercise has been shown to be more effective in the treatment of childhood obesity than either diet or exercise alone (Epstein et al., 1998). This finding corroborates data obtained in studies with adults. Less structured, flexible lifestyle approaches to physical activity appear to be more effective than programmed aerobic activity, in which the child must set aside 40 minutes three times a week for structured exercise (Epstein et al., 1985). Moreover, a recent study showed that overweight children who were instructed to decrease the amount of time that they spend doing sedentary activities (watching television and playing video games) lost more weight and had improvements in fitness comparable to those for children who were instructed to increase the amount of time that they spend doing aerobic exercise or the combination (increase the amount of time that they spend doing aerobic activity plus decrease the amount of time that they spend doing sedentary activities) (Epstein et al., 1995).

School-Based Programs

Several school-based interventions have focused on modification of the diet and physical activity. Among the largest school-based interventions is the CATCH study, which was conducted in 56 elementary schools that received the intervention and 40 control elementary schools (Luepker et al., 1996). The intervention was aimed at children in grades 3 through 5 and included approaches to increasing activity, improving diet quality, and decreasing smoking. Although obesity was not a primary outcome, the fact that the intervention involved both diet and exercise makes the findings from the study relevant. The intervention included a classroom-based curriculum of diet and exercise, modification of the foods served in the school cafeteria, and increased amounts of moderate and vigorous levels of activity in physical education classes; in some schools there was also a family component to the intervention. After 3 years of intervention, positive changes were reported in the school environment (cafeteria foods had lower levels of total and saturated fats) and children spent more time participating in moderate and vigorous levels of activity during physical education classes; there were also positive changes in the children's self-reported eating behaviors and physical activity levels. However, the intervention had no effect on BMI or skinfold thickness.

Other school-based interventions with elementary school children have shown no effect on BMI. Donnelly and colleagues (1996) studied third to fifth graders in two school districts over a period of 2 years. The children in the schools that received the intervention received enhanced physical activity, grade-specific nutrition education, and a school lunch that consisted of foods with lower levels of fat and sodium. Although the children in the school that received the intervention showed improved behaviors in the school setting, their overall dietary intakes and physical activity levels remained unaffected. Similarly, there were no differences in BMIs.

Studies that use interventions that have focused more on decreasing sedentary activity have obtained better results. Planet Health (Gortmaker et al., 1999b) targeted sixth to eighth graders in Boston, Massachusetts, schools and focused on reducing the amount of television viewing to less than 2 hours/day as well as increasing the amount of moderate and vigorous levels of activity, decreasing the level of consumption of high-fat foods, and increasing the level of consumption of fruits and vegetables. These changes were encouraged in all aspects of the curriculum, with teachers given incentives to create lesson plans that increased the children's levels of activity or improved their diets. After 2 years, the intervention was found to be effective in reducing the prevalence of obesity among girls. Girls that received the intervention reported greater decreases in television viewing, the consumption of more servings of fruit and vegetables, and lower daily caloric intakes than control girls (but there were no differences in the levels of moderate or vigorous activity). There were no significant effects among the boys.

Decreasing the amount of television viewing was also shown to be effective in slowing the rate of weight gain in third and fourth graders (Robinson, 1999). In that study, children were taught to budget their television viewing time to 7 hours weekly. Both boys and girls in the intervention group had smaller increases in BMIs, waist circumferences, and triceps skinfold thickness over 6 months than children in the control group.

DIETARY INTERVENTIONS

There is general agreement that a healthful dietary pattern is one that emphasizes the consumption of vegetables, fruits, and grain products and that is low in fat, saturated fat, cholesterol, and sodium. According to nutritional guidelines specific to cancer risk reduction, individuals age 2 and older should (ACS, 1996; Willett, 1999):

1. Choose most foods from plant sources.
   a. Eat at least two servings of fruits daily.
   b. Eat at least three servings of vegetables daily, with at least one-third being dark green or orange vegetables.
   c. Eat other foods from plant sources, such as breads, cereals, grains, pasta, or beans several times each day.
2. Limit intake of high-fat foods, with total fat being no more than 30 percent of total caloric intake and saturated fat being no more than 10 percent of total caloric intake.
   a. Limit consumption of meats, especially high-fat meats.

These recommendations are consistent with those of the U.S. Department of Agriculture's Food Guide Pyramid (U.S. Department of Agriculture, 1992), the 2000 Dietary Guidelines for Americans (U.S. Department of Agriculture and US DHHS, 2000), and American Heart Association recommendations (Krauss et al., 2000).

Behavioral Interventions to Improve Eating Patterns

This section of the chapter reviews the effectiveness of behavioral interventions designed to improve fruit, vegetable, and fat intakes as defined by

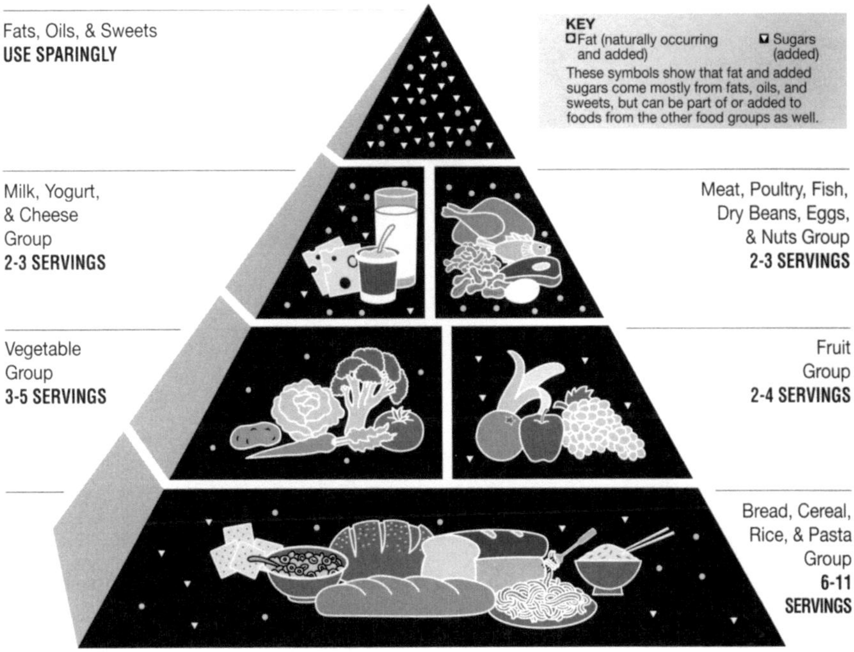

The food guide pyramid, U.S. Department of Agriculture.
SOURCE: http://www.nal.usda.gov:8001/py/pmap.htm.

current nutritional guidelines. A primary source for this review is the AHRQ *Evidence Report on the Efficacy of Interventions to Modify Dietary Behavior Related to Cancer Risk: Final Evidence Report* (hereafter referred to as the AHRQ Diet Report) (Agency for Healthcare Research and Quality, 2001a). Also reviewed are selected studies published from 1975 to 2000, a meta-analysis of studies of psychosocial factors and dietary change (Baranowski et al., 1999; Willett, 1995, 1999) and a NCI-sponsored review of the 5 A Day for Better Health Program (http://dccps.nci.nih.gov/5ad_1_intro.html).

Tables 4.4 and 4.5 summarize information from the AHRQ evidence report for fruits and vegetable (Table 4.4) and dietary fat (Table 4.5) intake. Interested readers are referred to the full report for an in-depth description of the study methods and rationale for data synthesis approaches. Results across 45 studies (12 for fruits and vegetables, 33 for dietary fat) are reported as median differences in percentage change in outcome. Thus, the numbers in the tables do not represent absolute changes in numbers of servings (fruits and vegetables) or percentage of energy from fat. For example, the median difference in percentage change in fruits and vegetables of +16.6 translates into an increase of approxi-

TABLE 4.4 Summary of AHRQ Analyses of the Efficacy of Interventions to Modify Dietary Behavior Related to Cancer Risk: Fruit and Vegetable Intake

Outcome	Number of Studies	Median (range)
Median differences between intervention and control groups in percentage change in fruit and vegetable intake		
Fruits and Vegetables (servings/day)	12	+16.6 (–3.7 to +60.9)
Fruits (servings/day)	9	+16.0 (0 to +73.4)
Vegetables (servings/day)	9	+5.7 (–17.2 to +153.2)
Median differences in percentage change in fruit and vegetable outcomes by intervention characteristics		
Social Support Component		
Yes	5	+17.3 (–3.7 to +18.6)
No	7	+15.9 (+6.9 to +60.9)
Interactions with Food		
Yes	7	+14.9 (–3.7 to +60.9)
No	6	+16.8 (+6.9 to +31.8)
Goal Setting		
Yes	5	+12.5 (–3.7 to +22.9)
No	7	+17.3 (+6.9 to +60.9)

SOURCE: AHRQ, 2001a.

mately 0.6 servings per day. The median difference for percent of energy from fat of –15.7 represents an estimated 7.3% reduction in percentage of calories from fat.

The majority of behavioral interventions to modify dietary patterns have been conducted within health care settings. The Diet Report reviewed 45 interventions conducted in health care settings, with most focused on persons at risk for chronic diseases (Agency for Healthcare Research and Quality, 2001a). The most frequently tested interventions used individualized counseling including self-monitoring, goal setting, and problem solving (Beresford et al., 1997; Chlebowski and Grosvenor, 1994; Simkin-Silverman et al., 1995), interactive recipe preparation (Boyd et al., 1996), or group sessions (Agurs-Collins et al., 1997; Coates et al., 1999; Lindholm et al., 1995; White et al., 1992). Two of the studies used computer or video components (Glasgow et al., 1996; Shannon et al., 1994). The intensities of the interventions ranged from 11 to 24 contacts, excluding the self-management or video interventions, in which contact was assumed to be ongoing. Follow-up contacts ranged from 3 months (Aubin et al., 1998) to 7 to 8 years (Boyd et al., 1996). Primarily on the basis of self-reported measures, these studies generally achieved positive results. All focused on fat consumption as the primary outcome of interest, whereas five also included

TABLE 4.5 Summary of AHRQ Analyses of the Efficacy of Interventions to Modify Dietary Behavior Related to Cancer Risk: Dietary Fat Intake (percentage of energy from fat)

Outcome	Number of Studies	Median (range)
Median differences in percentage change in dietary fat intake between intervention and control groups		
Total fat (% energy)	33	−15.7 (−76.4 to −1.0)
Total fat (grams/day)	7	−38.0 (−74.0 to −15.9)
Saturated fat (% energy)	16	−14.5 (−41.9 to +0.5)
Median differences in percentage change in total fat (% of energy) by population		
Risk Status		
General risk	12	−8.0 (−27.9 to −1.0)
High risk	20	−20.0 (−76.4 to −3.5)
Median differences in percentage change in total fat (% of energy) by intervention characteristics		
Social Support		
Yes	7	−26.7 (−76.4 to −3.5)
No	26	−10.4 (−44.2 to −1.0)
Interactions with food		
Yes	7	−11.0 (−26.7 to −3.2)
No	26	−17.8 (−76.4 to −1.0)
Goal Setting		
Yes	18	−18.9 (−44.2 to −2.7)
No	15	−11.0 (−76.4 to −1.0)

SOURCE: AHRQ, 2001a.

fruit and vegetable consumption. In general, studies in these health settings allowed retrieval of information on additional biochemical measures, including total cholesterol levels, and more intensive dietary measures (e.g., 3-day food records) that are not as frequently retrievable in other settings. These settings also allowed ongoing monitoring of at-risk groups.

A paper published subsequent to publication of the literature review in the AHRQ Diet Report extended these findings by showing both reduced levels of dietary fat intake and increased levels of fruit and vegetable consumption after an individualized intervention delivered by personalized mailings, standard dietary information, and personalized phone calls (Kristal et al., 2000a).

In summary, behavioral interventions tested in health care settings can have a significant impact on the dietary intakes of participants. These settings allow the targeting of participants at risk for disease, who may be more willing to engage in behavioral change, and offer an ideal environment for the monitoring of individuals.

Worksite Interventions

Worksites offer an environment in which effective behavioral changes can be promoted among large populations (Minkler and Wallerstein, 1997). Several studies used models of participatory research and included individuals from the worksite in the intervention development process. Although the levels of intensity of the interventions and the levels of participation in the interventions varied, those that were most successful used multiple strategies across multiple levels (the individual, the family, and the environmental levels).

According to the Diet Report's review of worksite studies (Agency for Healthcare Research and Quality, 2001a), fat intake was the primary outcome measured in three studies (Bauer et al., 1985; Sorensen et al., 1992; Strychar et al., 1998), fruit and vegetable consumption was the primary outcome measured in one study (Buller et al., 1999), and five studies addressed fat intake and fruit and vegetable consumption combined (Anderson and Dusenbury, 1999; Hanlon et al., 1995; Sorensen et al., 1992, 1996; Thompson et al., 1999; Tilley et al., 1999a). Interventions were delivered by a diverse group of professionals, including dietitians (n = 3 studies), doctors or medical staff (n = 2 studies), and peers or counselors (n = 2 studies). Family components were included in at least three studies (Bauer et al., 1985; Sorensen et al., 1992; Tilley et al., 1999a). Environmental changes such as increasing the availability of healthy food choices and labeling of foods were notable in two studies (Sorensen et al., 1992, 1996).

Multiple behavioral components were included in interventions addressing fat intake only. Four studies incorporated multiple theoretical perspectives into their intervention designs, including community organization and activation theories, social and adult learning theory, stages of change, social support, and the health belief model (Kristal et al., 2000b; Sorensen et al., 1992, 1996; Strychar et al., 1998). For example, the Treatwell study incorporated employee advisory boards to plan interventions that included organized screenings, courses, goal setting, and cafeteria modifications, in addition to a family component (Sorensen et al., 1992). The Working Well study included interactive activities and contests plus multiple environmental changes, such as altering food choices in vending machines, with significant effects on the levels of both fruit and vegetable consumption and fat intake (Sorensen et al., 1996).

The Next Step Trial targeted both fruit and vegetable consumption and fat intake for change. Strategies reflected various theoretical perspectives and included nutrition classes, individualized feedback on intakes, mailed self-help materials, and a family component to enhance home support for change (Kristal et al., 2000a; Tilley et al., 1999a). Measurements obtained from a food frequency questionnaire indicated at the 1-year follow-up that the intervention groups had significantly increased their levels of fruit and vegetable consumption and lowered their total level of fat intake. However, at the 2-year follow-up, there were no significant effects between groups for any of the dietary outcomes.

The Seattle 5 a Day Worksite Program randomized 28 worksites that had cafeterias and intervened in 14 sites with changes in the work environment and programs and activities targeting individual behavior change. Significant improvements in fruit and vegetable consumption were observed at the 2-year follow-up point (Beresford et al., 2001).

School-Based Interventions

Schools have been the setting for population-based interventions designed to lower the levels of fat intake and improve the levels of fruit and vegetable consumption of elementary and middle school children. As cited in the AHRQ Diet Report (Agency for Healthcare Research and Quality, 2001a), fruit and vegetable consumption was the focus of five school-based studies (Baranowski et al., 2000; Nicklas et al., 1998; Parcel et al., 1989; Resnicow et al., 1992), fat intake was the focus of four studies (Baxter et al., 1997; Harrell et al., 1996, 1998; Simons-Morton et al., 1991; Walter et al., 1988), and the combination of fruit and vegetable consumption and fat intake was the focus of three studies (Luepker et al., 1996; Perry et al., 1998a; Resnicow et al., 1992, 1998).

School-based interventions have generally focused on changing the dietary intakes of children in school settings in multiple ways, including through (1) one-to-one classroom instruction by teachers; (2) environmental change via modification of the foods served by the school cafeteria; and (3) family support through involvement in diet-related homework, activity packets, or group meetings (e.g., Gimme 5 [Baranowski et al., 2000], the Child and Adolescent Trial for Cardiovascular Health (CATCH) study [Luepker et al., 1996], 5 A Day Power Plus [Perry et al., 1998b]). For example, Parcel and colleagues (1989) included modeling, self-monitoring, and food demonstrations to enhance fruit and vegetable consumption, in addition to changes to the cafeteria environment. The Gimme 5 program attempted to improve fruit, juice, and vegetable consumption with changes to classroom curriculum and educational materials and programs for children and their parents (e.g., newsletters, videotapes, and point-of-purchase education) (Baranowski et al., 2000). Nicklas and colleagues (1998) included a media campaign with classroom, school lunch, and parental interventions. Finally, Perry and colleagues (1998b) collaborated with community food industries and the family and used other intervention components. In general, school-based behavioral interventions have yielded improvements in levels of fruit and vegetable consumption (Agency for Healthcare Research and Quality, 2001a). Studies such as the Cardiovascular Health in Children (CHIC) trial have also achieved significant reductions in total serum cholesterol levels (Harrell et al., 1998). Finally, the Child and Adolescent Trial for Cardiovascular Health (CATCH) has demonstrated that school-based interventions can influence the dietary behavior of a child by influencing the school lunch and physical education environments (Nader et al., 1999; Perry et al., 1998a; Stone et al., 1996).

In summary, schools are an important environment where dietary behaviors in youth can be addressed. Schools are where children spend a large amount of their time, offer a system for reaching students in a defined setting that allows environmental change, and can involve the family through extracurricular activities. School-based interventions across multiple levels of the ecological model can result in significant improvements in the levels of fruit and vegetable consumption by children and reductions in the levels of fat intake. The need to create innovative programs that encourage additional parental involvement and environmental changes at home continues to be important for future work.

Community-Based Interventions

The AHRQ Diet Report denotes 24 community-based studies that address dietary behavioral change at the community level (Agency for Healthcare Research and Quality, 2001a). Of these, 10 addressed fat intake as the primary outcome (Baranowski et al., 1990a; Domel et al., 1993, Campbell et al., 1999b; Cox et al., 1995; Jaycox et al., 1983; Nader et al., 1983, 1989; Simmons-Morton et al., 1998; Stern et al., 1976; Stolley and Fitzgibbon, 1997; Turnin et al., 1992), six addressed fruit and vegetable consumption (Campbell et al., 1999a; Cullen et al., 1997; Havas et al., 1998; Lutz et al., 1999; Marcus et al., 1998a,c), and nine addressed fruit and vegetable consumption and fat intake combined (Brug et al., 1996, 1998, 1999; Fitzgibbon et al. 1996; Hartman et al., 1997; Knutsen and Knutsen, 1991; Pierce et al., 1997; Rodgers et al., 1994; Tudor-Smith et al., 1998). The Stanford Three-City Study primarily defined communities by geographical location (Farquhar et al., 1984). More recently, studies have recruited participants from community-based organizations, such as Girl Scout troops (Cullen et al., 1997), clinics that sponsor participants in the Special Supplemental Food Program for Women, Infants, and Children (WIC) (Havas et al., 1998), cancer registries (Marcus et al., 1998b), churches (Campbell et al., 1999a), and participants recruited from health maintenance organizations (Lutz et al., 1999).

Several studies targeted outcomes related to changes in levels of fruit and vegetable consumption with individual change strategies (e.g., goal setting) and inclusion of family components (Baranowski et al., 1990a; Fitzgibbon et al., 1996; Jaycox et al., 1983; Knutsen and Knutsen, 1991; Nader et al., 1983, 1989; Stolley and Fitzgibbon, 1997). Peer or lay approaches have been used to deliver interventions in multiple studies (Cullen et al., 1997; Havas et al., 1998). For example, Havas and colleagues (1998) worked with WIC participants and trained peer educators to deliver education sessions and food demonstrations to enhance fruit and vegetable consumption. Discussion groups and mailings were also included, resulting in a significant increase in the levels of fruit and vegetable consumption by the intervention participants (0.56 versus 0.13 daily servings). Cullen and colleagues (1997) recruited Girl Scout troops and used nutrition classes, self-help materials, tasting sessions, and parental information sheets to encourage home support. This resulted in significant increases in levels of fruit and vegetable consumption. Other studies targeting changes in levels of fruit and vegetable consumption have reached the community through communication systems. Marcus and colleagues (1998c) delivered telephone messages based on participants' stage of change and offered follow-up mailings that resulted in improvements in the rates of adherence to the Five-a-Day program guidelines. Another intervention that included one call followed by two mailings to the home yielded significant improvements in the intervention group at the initial follow-up and at 4 weeks and 4 months of follow-up (Marcus et al., 1998a).

Interventions designed to decrease levels of fat intake have also used multiple components. The Stanford Three-City Community Study used variations of intensive instruction on diet and other cardiovascular risk factors and an extensive media campaign (Farquhar et al., 1984, 1990; Fortmann et al., 1990). Results showed significant decreases in the levels of saturated fat intake between the intervention and the control groups.

Several studies that have addressed fruit and vegetable consumption and fat intake combined have examined more intensive interventions, such as home visits with newsletters (Knutsen and Knutsen, 1991) and weekly classes or sessions (Fitzgibbon et al., 1996; Hartman et al., 1997), and minimal interventions such as computer-tailored letters (Brug et al., 1996, 1998, 1999) or telephone counseling (Pierce et al., 1997). Rodgers and colleagues (1994) altered supermarket environments to promote a significant positive dietary message. The North Karelia project used a range of interventions, from mass media educational campaigns to cooperation with agricultural and food merchandising groups, to improve the availability of healthy alternatives such as low-fat milk (Puska et al., 1985). The Minnesota Heart Health program and Project LEAN also used public-private partnerships to enhance the delivery of the dietary campaign message, further expanding on this collaborative concept (Heimendinger et al., 1996).

Community-based behavioral interventions have been effective in promoting dietary change. These programs have targeted change across multiple levels. In addition, they are more frequently delivered by nonprofessional, lay, or peer educators, ensuring ongoing resources and the development of a community capacity for ongoing dietary change.

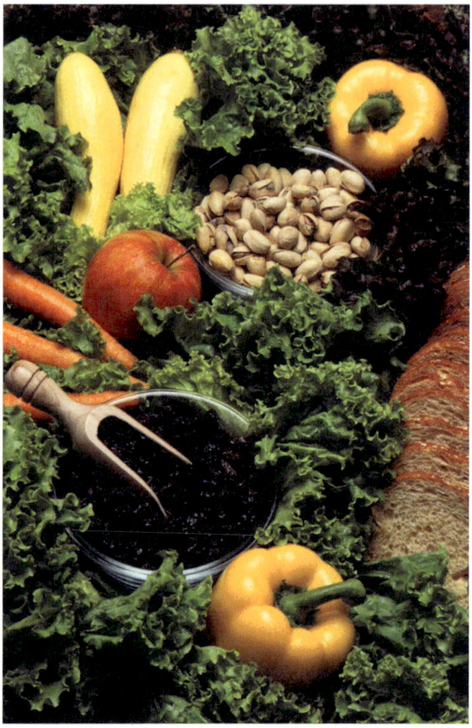

SOURCE: Agricultural Research Service, USDA. Photo by Scott Bauer.

Programs to Reach Underserved and Minority Populations

Among African Americans, diet may be an area of special vulnerability (World Cancer Research Fund and American Institute for Cancer Research, 1997). African Americans, particularly those living in rural communities, report poorer dietary intakes (Baranowski et al., 2000; Johnson et al., 1994; Lillie-Blanton et al., 1996; Schonfeld-Warden and Warden, 1997). Also, programs that promote healthy diets have not worked as well for African Americans as they have for other groups.

The availability of fruits and vegetables is a substantial predictor of intake (Hearn et al., 1998), and the availability of fruits and vegetables is lower in rural communities than in other areas. Additionally, the low levels of educational attainment and the limited literacy skills often found among individuals in minority and rural communities may result in limited exposure and receptivity to health messages designed for better-educated, urban groups (Kirby et al., 1995). This association is not limited to the United States and has also been reported in England (Margetts et al., 1998).

Community-based organizations have tested interventions in several population groups. Fitzgibbon and colleagues (1996) recruited Hispanic families from literacy training programs and offered a culturally specific curriculum over 12 weeks designed to improve both fat intake and fruit and vegetable consumption (Fitzgibbon et al., 1996). Stolley and Fitzgibbon (1997) recruited low-income mothers and daughters from a tutoring program to receive a low-fat, multicomponent intervention. Significant reductions in total fat intake were noted for both mothers and daughters. Auslander and colleagues (Auslander et al., 2000; Haire-Joshu et al., 1999) used a stage-based, personalized intervention implemented by peers and offered to overweight, low-income African-American women through a local neighborhood agency. The results showed significant benefits in terms of increased skills in the interpretation of food labels and improved knowledge of nutrition and the fat contents of foods.

Church-based approaches have also been effective in reaching ethnically diverse groups. A church program in Samoa used community-based organization approaches to program development and was successful in reducing waist circumference and eliminating weight gain in those at high risk for diabetes (Simmons-Morton et al., 1998).

A combination of church- and community-based approaches had promising effects on helping African-American participants consume a healthy diet (Campbell et al., 1999a). In each county randomized to the intervention, the pastors of local churches appointed a three- to seven-member Nutrition Action Team that was "responsible for organizing and implementing many of the program activities" (Campbell et al., 1999a, p. 1391). The intervention itself "used an ecological framework, targeting activities at the individual, social network, and community levels" (p. 1391). It included tailored bulletins and other print materials; group activities such as gardening, educational sessions, and personal recipe tasting; and the serving of more fruits and vegetables at church functions. To reinforce healthy eating habits, the program also included lay health advisers, pastor support, and community-based coalitions (these coalitions were located within each county and were composed of church members, representatives of local agencies, farmers, and grocers) and distributed materials through local grocers. Reflecting the strong community focus of the program, individual churches were also encouraged to implement their own activities, in addition to the planned intervention. These included "5-a-Day Sundays," gospelfests, and events for youth. The intervention lasted 20 months. It resulted in a significant difference (0.85 servings of fruits and vegetables per day) between the counties that received the intervention and the counties that received delayed treatment.

Members of minority and low-income groups can be reached effectively at worksites, and individuals who are members of important social networks at worksites can be used to influence the dietary behaviors of their co-workers. For example, Buller and colleagues (1999) encouraged the intake of five servings of fruits and vegetables per day via peers and managers at worksites with blue-collar workers. Informal social networks or cliques were used as a structure for the program. Workers from informal networks were trained to provide program interventions for their colleagues in those networks. The intervention included various print media and information sessions conducted by peer educators for large and small groups and included ethnically specific messages that encouraged the participants to increase their levels of fruit and vegetable consumption. In addition, the work environment was modified (through the use of cafeteria promotions). The intervention was found to have significant effects at 18 months (an increase of 0.77 servings) and 24 months (an increase of 0.41 servings) by use of dietary recall as the measurement method. However, use of food frequency methods showed a different effect at 18 months, but the effect remained significant (an increase of 0.46 servings); at 24 months there was no significant effect (an increase of 0.04 servings).

THE HEALTH CARE SYSTEM AND BEHAVIOR RISK REDUCTION

Health care organizations and settings and the providers who work in them have extraordinary opportunities to affect the health of a large percentage of people who are at risk for cancer. In 2000, 72 percent of U.S. adults reported going to a doctor's office or clinic to get care in the past year (Agency for Healthcare Research and Quality, 2001b), with this contact providing opportunities to offer counseling and other interventions. In addition to the high rate of contact, providers who are credible sources of health-related information frequently provide care on a regular basis in primary care settings. All types of clinicians—physicians, nurses, nurse practitioners, dentists, psychologists, pharmacists, health educators, dietitians, and many others—can effectively deliver prevention messages and prevention counseling (Fiore et al., 1996, US DHHS, 2000a).

Opportunities for the promotion and delivery of cancer prevention and control services can be found in a variety of locations where health care is delivered, including private physician office practices, integrated delivery systems or staff model health maintenance organizations (HMOs), and public health clinics. Health care providers in ambulatory health care settings have unique opportunities to promote the use of cancer prevention and early detection services; however, levels of access to such providers are not uniformly high. In 1998, the vast majority of individuals relied on doctors' offices and HMOs (70 percent) and on clinics or health centers (16 percent) for their routine and preventive care (1998 National Health Interview Survey, special tabulations by National Cancer Policy Board staff). A significant segment of the adult population (11 percent) reported that they did not have a usual source of routine care, which points to the limits of interventions aimed at health care professionals to improve access to cancer prevention and early detection services.

As summarized in the previous sections, there is evidence of the effectiveness of interventions for smoking cessation, physical activity, and dietary modification delivered in health care settings. Unfortunately, there has been little integration of these interventions into routine health care delivery. According to surveys with patients and providers, behavior risk factors are not routinely addressed.

With regard to tobacco use, only about one-half of patients who smoke report that they have received advice to quit (Doescher and Saver, 2000; Anda et al., 1987; CDC, 1993; Frank et al., 1991; Gilpin et al., 1993; Goldstein et al., 1997; Kottke et al., 1997; Pierce and Gilpin, 1994; Rogers et al., 1997; Thorndike et al., 1998) and far fewer report that they have received any smoking cessation assistance or follow-up (Goldstein et al., 1997; Rogers et al., 1997), as recommended by both the current clinical practice guidelines for tobacco treatment (US DHHS, 2000a) and the *Healthy People 2010* objective (US DHHS and Office of Disease Prevention and Health Promotion, 2000). The type of visit affects the rate of smoking intervention, with more interventions occurring during well visits than during acute care visits and with more interventions occurring for smokers with chronic tobacco-related illnesses than for smokers with non-tobacco-related illnesses (Jaen, 1997; Jaen et al., 1997, 1998; Sesney et al., 1997; Stange et al., 1994; Thorndike et al., 1998; Frame, 1995). The general infrequency of well visits and patients not being ready to stop smoking may help explain the less than desirable rates of smoking cessation interventions by physicians. Recent clinical practice guidelines call for intervening with all smokers at all visits, whether or not the visit is for an illness caused or complicated by tobacco use (US DHHS, 2000a). Despite evidence of the effectiveness of physician-delivered smoking interventions, physicians may view them as ineffective because of their clinical experience, in which only about 5 percent of patients advised to quit will do so in the course of a given year (Warner, 1998).

National data on the prevalence of provider provision of counseling to modify the diet as it relates to cancer prevention are lacking. *Healthy People 2010* Objective 19-17 is to increase to 75 percent the proportion of physician office visits made by patients with a diagnosis of cardiovascular disease, diabetes, or hyperlipidemia that include counseling or education related to diet and nutrition (US DHHS and Office of Disease Prevention and Health Promotion, 2000). Although this objective does not relate specifically to provider counseling for cancer prevention, it is the only *Healthy People 2010* objective that addresses provider counseling to modify the diet.

It is difficult to gauge the prevalence of diet modification counseling specific to cancer prevention or even general nutrition counseling (e.g., to decrease dietary fat intake, increase levels of consumption of fruits, vegetables, whole grains, and fiber, and limit red meat consumption) because available studies are based on provider practices in specific regions, organizations, or subpopulations and many of the studies suffer from low response rates. According to studies with acceptable response rates (above 60 percent) patients reporting that physicians offered dietary counseling ranged from 14 to 70 percent (Hunt et al., 1995; Kreuter et al., 1997; Taira et al., 1997). The rates of provision of diet modification counseling in selected studies that relied on physician self-report are somewhat higher, ranging from 66 to 79 percent (Glanz et al., 1995; Kushner, 1995; Ashford et al., 2000). On the basis of direct observation, the prevalence of counseling to modify the diet to reduce the risk of cancer ranged from 9 to 43 percent (Stange et al., 2000; Stange et al., 1998; Russell and Roter, 1993).

Roughly one-third (34 percent) of individuals who had visited a physician in the past year were counseled by the physician to begin or to continue any type of exercise or physical activity, according to estimates from the 1995 National Health Interview Survey (Wee et al., 1999). Estimates of the prevalence of physical activity counseling by providers range from 13 to 36 percent according to studies in which providers in health care settings were directly observed as they provided care (Podl et al., 1999; Russell and Roter, 1993; Stange et al., 1998; Stange et al., 2000). There is a tendency for primary care providers to discuss secondary prevention rather than focus on primary prevention (Wee et al., 1999). Although the goal is to have primary care physicians conduct primary prevention counseling, patients who have disease are more likely to be counseled about physical activity (Podl et al., 1999; Rosen et al., 1984; Wee et al., 1999), and the more risk factors a patient has, the more likely it is that the patient will be counseled (Kreuter et al., 1997). The lack of a standard protocol has been identified as a barrier to carrying out physical activity counseling (Gemson and Elinson, 1986; Orleans et al., 1985).

How a clinical practice is organized, its delivery capacity, and its manual and computerized administrative support systems can greatly affect a provider's ability to deliver preventive health care in general and address behavioral risk factors specifically. Medical chart prompts, checklists, and reminders improve the physician's ability to identify a patient's needs and behavioral risk factor counseling rates (Chang et al., 1995; Cohen et al., 1989; Cummings et al., 1989a,b; Fiore, 1991; Fiore et al., 1995; McIlvain et al., 1992; Ockene et al., 1996; Robinson et al., 1995; Solberg et al., 1990; Strecher et al., 1991). Smoking status designated as a vital sign on the chart increases the rate at which physicians ask their patients about smoking, discuss or advise cessation, and arrange a follow-up appointment or referral to a stop smoking program (Ahluwalia et al., 1999; Robinson et al., 1995). Most studies of the effects of computerized systems demonstrate that physicians who use such systems counsel their patients about changes in health behaviors at higher rates (McPhee et al., 1991; Ornstein et al., 1995). Computer-based reminder systems offer a quick and easy way to monitor patients (Frame and Werth, 1993), but such systems require considerable institutional commitment and resources.

Health risk appraisals (HRAs) provide individualized estimates of health risks and can be used as part of behavioral counseling in primary care settings. The evidence that HRAs improve rates of provider counseling is conflicting, with some showing improvements (Geiger et al., 1993; Gemson and Sloan, 1995) and some not noting such improved rates (Smith et al., 1985).

Periodic chart audits have been used as part of continuous quality improvement (CQI) initiatives as a way of assessing provider performance to provide feedback and improve compliance with clinical practice guidelines (Shortell et al., 1995). Trials of the effectiveness of CQI in improving prevention services have largely been negative (Solberg et al., 2000).

The need for multiple strategies is embodied in the U.S. Public Health Service clinical practice guideline for the treatment of tobacco use and dependence (US DHHS, 2000a). It emphasizes that, without supportive systems, policies, and environmental prompts, it is unlikely that the individual clinician will routinely assess and treat tobacco use. These guidelines include six strategies for systems-level interventions, modified here to encompass multiple behavioral risk factors:

1. implement a behavioral risk factor identification system in every clinic;
2. provide education, resources, and feedback to promote provider delivery of an intervention;
3. dedicate staff to provide treatment and include assessment of the delivery of this treatment in performance evaluations;
4. promote policies within the organization that support and provide behavior change treatment services;
5. include effective behavior change treatment as paid or covered services; and
6. reimburse clinicians and specialists for delivery of effective behavior change treatments and include these treatments in the defined duties of clinicians.

In addition to practice-specific factors, certain characteristics of the contemporary ambulatory care environment may not be conducive to preventive care practices (1998 National Ambulatory Medical Care Survey and 1998 National Hospital Ambulatory Medical Care Survey, special tabulations, NCPB staff):

- Prevention services are optimally provided in the context of routine health care visits or checkups, but such non-illness-related visits are relatively unusual, making up 17 percent of the estimated 717.6 million ambulatory care visits made by adults in 1998.

• Prevention services are more likely to be provided when patients see their primary care physician, but less than half (44 percent) of ambulatory care visits made by adults in 1998 were to a patient's primary care provider.

• Counseling about risk behaviors such as smoking cessation or describing the pros and cons of screening procedures can be time-consuming, yet most adult patients (63 percent) spend less than 15 minutes with the physician during their ambulatory care visits.

• During ambulatory care visits, adult patients generally spend time with physicians, but they also see other providers, although they see them less often. Patients see, for example, nurses, nurse practitioners, or physician's assistants, but these encounters occur during roughly only 20 percent of ambulatory care visits. These nonphysician providers can be important sources of counseling services, even though they are not frequently encountered.

One of the reasons most frequently cited by clinicians for not implementing prevention services is a real or perceived lack of time given the other demands of a primary care practice (Ashford et al., 2000; Battista and Mickalide, 1990; Burns et al., 2000; Cooper et al., 1998; Dunn et al., 2001; Jaen et al., 1994; Kottke et al., 1993; Kushner, 1995; Rafferty, 1998; Walsh et al., 1999). Responses to the patient's presenting complaints and concerns often take precedence (Burns et al., 2000; McBride et al., 1997; Stange et al., 1994). The total amount of time needed by the physician to deliver effective preventive services may not be prohibitive. Physicians can, for example, initiate a smoking cessation intervention, and this can be followed by provision of most of the intervention and follow-up by another clinician (e.g., a nurse, a nurse practitioner, or a physician's assistant). Physicians can deliver prevention services at high rates and still have a productive practice, as defined by relative value units, when formal systems for the delivery of prevention services are implemented (Kottke et al., 1993).

Systems of care may reduce institutional or organizational barriers to the use of prevention services with strategies that facilitate a usual source of care or a "regular doctor," the centralization of services, or the provision of an integrated structure (e.g., a centralized screening program [Thompson et al., 1995]), a requirement for minimal patient copayments for members, or reduction of clinicians' financial disincentives (Gordon et al., 1998; Weinick and Beauregard, 1997). Financial incentives, management strategies, the physical plant, and normative influences of colleagues can all interact to facilitate or hinder the provision of preventive services (Malin et al., 2000).

Organizational characteristics of HMOs might contribute to the relatively high rates of use of prevention services, for example, dedicated behavioral health programs, innovative use of personnel including nurse practitioners and health educators (Mullen and Zapka, 1982; Palitz et al., 1997), consumer expectation (Jordan et al., 1995; Trnka and Henderson, 1997), and systems of accountability (Box 4.3.). Although the model program described in Box 4.3. focuses on tobacco, its key elements are readily generalizable to other health behaviors. The most prominent effort to define and measure plan performance has been the National Committee for Quality Assurance's Health Plan Employer and Data Information Set (HEDIS®) (http://www.ncqa.org/programs/hedis/index.htm; Corrigan and Nielsen, 1993). This set of standardized performance measures helps purchasers and consumers reliably compare the performance of managed health care plans. In 2000, 273 organizations (health maintenance organizations, point-of-service plans, and other managed care plans) that collectively cover 63 million individuals voluntarily submitted performance data. In 2000, the median rate of advising smokers to quit reported by plans was 66 percent (National Committee for Quality Assurance, 2001). Expansion of measures to include obesity prevention and treatment and the promotion of physical activity could be considered.

A disincentive for providers to provide preventive services is a lack of, or inadequate, reimbursement. The Medicare program, for example, does not provide reimbursement for smoking cessation services. Other barriers to the provision of prevention services are more subtle. The benefits of effective prevention interventions may be viewed by physicians and health care systems as abstract because the costs in terms of time and finances are incurred up front, but the benefits may not be seen for years or decades (Ockene and Ockene, 1992).

SUMMARY AND CONCLUSIONS

Interventions to modify tobacco use, diet, and physical activity have substantial similarities in terms of their effectiveness. Separate educational, psychological, and behavioral models for interventions for each behavior are not needed. Rather, behavioral change efforts need to focus on common models that emphasize the skills needed for behavioral change, diverse and sustained interventions, and social and other forms of support for the maintenance of behavioral changes.

Two levels of intervention are generally found to be effective for all three preventive behaviors reviewed in this chapter. One level entails well-defined interventions delivered to individuals, such as counseling and prescription drugs for smoking cessation. The second level entails comprehensive, multicomponent, multichannel programs directed to large groups, for example, the statewide tobacco control programs that have emerged in the last decade. This finding is consistent with that of IOM's Committee on Health and Behavior: Research, Practice and Policy. They concluded that "health and

BOX 4.3 A Model Tobacco Control Program in an HMO

Group Health Cooperative (GHC) of Puget Sound is a large group model health maintenance organization established in 1947. The GHC program for smoking cessation targets interventions at three levels (Curry, 1998). On the practice setting level, interventions include self-help booklets, outreach telephone counseling, and group sessions. Several other interventions were prompted by the development and implementation of an evidence-based smoking cessation guideline. Training and ongoing consultation, patient questionnaires, education materials, chart stickers, vital sign stamps, patient flow sheets, and chart audit protocols are used.

Staffing for guideline implementation includes full-time employee support for physicians, health educators, and an implementation coordinator who works in the primary care clinics to assess staff readiness to implement the guideline, arrange appropriate education and training and follow-up for staff, facilitate ownership for the guideline, and encourage progress in tracking through the use of chart audits and feedback reports.

On the systems level, GHC tracks the percentage of audited charts with documentation of tobacco use status. GHC's benefits committee in 1992 approved a tobacco services benefit that went into effect in 1993. The benefit included access to the Free and Clear behavioral program with a 50 percent copayment and with nicotine replacement therapy fully covered for smokers who participate in the Free and Clear program (there is no coverage for nonparticipants). Implementation of this benefit resulted in a 10-fold increase in program attendance. GHC experimented with benefit design and learned that even with full coverage and the use of multiple strategies to enhance use of the benefit, the annual rate of use of the benefit among smokers was about 11 percent (Curry, 1998). The following strategies to increase the reach of their tobacco cessation services are being implemented:

- provision of full coverage for tobacco use cessation services (elimination of copayments),
- a streamlined referral and registration process for participants in the Free and Clear program,
- use of automated clinical information systems to track patient tobacco use and provider practices, and
- ensured adherence to the practice guideline in specialty care.

On the community and external environment levels, GHC has been involved in the formation of community coalitions, educational appearances on radio and television and in the print media, and community policy development (Thompson et al., 1995). Along with other health organizations, voluntary and state agencies, and tobacco control groups, GHC created the Washington Alliance for Tobacco and Children's Health to conduct lobbying and media advocacy. These actions led to plans for a tobacco trust account in Washington State with Tobacco Master Settlement Agreement funds (McAfee, 2000).

The GHC program has evolved over a period of about 15 years, demonstrating that development of multilevel programs takes considerable time, planning, and resources (Curry, 1998).

behavior are influenced by factors at multiple levels, including biological, psychological, and social. Interventions that involve only the person—for example, using self-control or willpower—are unlikely to change long-term behavior unless other factors, such as family relationships, work situation, or social norms, happen to be aligned to support a change" (IOM, 2001a).

A striking finding is the recurrent demonstration of the importance of interventions that combine several different channels of information or types of influence, are sustained, and address self-management or behavioral skills for the identification and attainment of personal goals and for the avoidance of temptations that would undermine those efforts.

A number of effective behavioral interventions exist, but no "magic bullet" or particular intervention is remarkably more effective than others. Additionally, different interventions may be effective in achieving similar goals. Thus, counseling as part of the delivery of primary heath care, mass media campaigns, and messages tailored to those not yet ready to change their behaviors may each be effective in reaching individuals and helping motivate change. Individual counseling, group programs, or self-help materials may each be effective in helping people plan their lifestyle changes and master behavioral self-management skills to avoid relapse. Follow-up from professionals, from trained volunteers, or through print or other media may help those who have changed their behavior maintain the healthy behavior.

To be successful, behavioral health interventions delivered in health care settings must overcome the principle barriers that confront providers and health care systems. The greatest barriers to providers' delivery of smoking cessation counseling are lack of education and training, limitations of time and practice setting systems, poor reimbursement levels, and a perceived lack of success with patients who smoke. For diet and physical activity, an additional critical barrier is the lack of clear guidelines regarding recommendations for cancer control.

The potential for combinations of effects and the importance of the use of multiple approaches underscore the need for the use of comprehensive approaches. There are many different effective interventions, and their aggregate effects may not be captured by the evaluation of each one in isolation. Comprehensive programs that combine different intervention methods and channels have appreciable effects on all key behaviors for the prevention of cancer (CDC, 1999a; Rimer, 1997). Within such comprehensive programs, no single intervention method or channel is necessary or sufficient, but several different sets of strategies and methods may achieve comparable results. What is important is the overall strategy of combining multiple methods and channels.

5

Potential of Screening to Reduce the Burden of Cancer[1]

A complementary strategy to preventing the occurrence of cancer (primary prevention) is early detection of cancer through screening (secondary prevention). The fundamental tenet of screening for cancer is that finding the disease before symptoms develop enables detection at a less advanced stage and that instituting treatment at that time leads ultimately to improved health outcomes. Although this syllogism seems intuitive and is widely assumed to be true by both health professionals and the lay public, its validity is unclear for many cancers.

The term *screening*, as used in this report, refers to the early detection of cancer or premalignant disease in persons without signs or symptoms suggestive of the target condition (the type of cancer that the test seeks to detect). Some investigators draw a distinction between screening and *case finding*, using the former term to describe population-based screening programs, such as those conducted at health fairs or shopping malls, and the latter term to refer to testing of patients in the clinical setting. This report refers to both forms of testing as screening because the evidence base is similar in both contexts. *Diagnostic testing*, which is not addressed in this report, refers to the evaluation of patients with signs or symptoms associated with cancer (e.g., a breast lump, blood in stool, fatigue, or weight loss), often by use of the same tests used for screening. *Surveillance*

[1]This chapter is a condensed version of a background paper prepared by Steven H. Woolf (www.iom.edu/ncpb).

refers to follow-up screening for new evidence of cancer in patients who have already been diagnosed with and treated for cancer or premalignant disease.

This chapter reviews the principles used for determination of the effectiveness of cancer screening and applies those principles in an examination of current scientific evidence regarding the benefits and harms of screening for four types of cancer (cancers of the colon and rectum, breast, prostate, and cervix). Chapter 6 examines strategies for optimization of the delivery of recommended cancer screening tests from the perspective of the health care system, providers, and, most importantly, the patient. Chapter 7 presents a case study that reviews the history and prospects for screening for lung cancer, illustrating the difficulties of adopting new technologies in the face of uncertain science.

PRINCIPLES FOR ASSESSMENT OF THE EFFECTIVENESS OF SCREENING FOR CANCER

The principal considerations in judging the effectiveness of cancer screening are (1) the burden of suffering, the frequency of cancer, and the severity of its health effects; (2) the accuracy and reliability of the screening test in detecting cancer and minimizing inaccurate test results; (3) the effectiveness of early detection, including the incremental benefit of detecting and treating cancer at an earlier stage; (4) the harms of screening, both from the testing process and from the incremental harms from evaluation and treatments that follow; and (5) costs. These considerations form the tradeoffs used to weigh the benefits and harms of screening. All of the preceding analytical steps are necessary to address the pivotal question of whether patients and populations experience better outcomes with screening than without it.

Burden of Suffering

The first consideration in assessing the effectiveness of cancer screening is the frequency with which cancer occurs in the population and its attendant health effects. The prevalence rate determines the pretest probability of disease or the average likelihood that a person in the screened population will have cancer. The lower this value is, the larger the number of tests that must be performed to detect one case of cancer (i.e., it will have lower *yield*) and, for statistical reasons discussed below, the greater the chances that a positive test result will be erroneous (a false-positive result).

Mortality rates and other measures of the probability of adverse health effects from cancer influence the absolute benefit of screening (see the discussion of *absolute benefit* versus *relative benefit* below). For example, if a screening test reduces the risk of dying from cancer by 20 percent (relative risk reduction), the number of lives saved by screening or the probability that a person undergoing screening will avert death (absolute benefit) depends directly on the baseline mortality rate in the screened population. If that rate is 30/100,000 per year, screening will save six lives per 100,000 screened. The same form of screening would save only one life in a lower-risk setting where the mortality rate is only 5/100,000. As detailed below, absolute risks influence the number of individuals who need to be screened to achieve a health benefit.

Most published rates for cancer morbidity and mortality are derived from patients with clinically detected disease (i.e., cancers that come to the attention of health care providers in the evaluation of abnormal symptoms or physical findings), but the types of cancers detected by screening also include those that were not destined to manifest clinical symptoms and that are therefore of uncertain clinical significance. Autopsy studies have demonstrated for decades that a large proportion of persons live their lives harboring occult cancers that cause little or no clinical symptoms because of their slow rate of growth or late onset. Screening often detects such lesions, but it is often difficult to determine at the time of diagnosis whether those cancers were destined to progress. This phenomenon of screening is known as *overdiagnosis* and is important because the degree to which cancers that are not destined to progress are represented among cancers detected by screening limits the net health benefits of screening.

Overdiagnosis figures prominently in debates about the benefits of screening for various cancers. A common criticism of screening for prostate cancer, for example, is that many of the cancers detected by screening are latent carcinomas that, due to that disease's slow growth characteristics, are unlikely to progress or cause clinical symptoms (Woolf, 1995). Screening mammography has led to increased detection of ductal carcinoma in situ (Feig, 2000; Winchester et al., 2000), the clinical significance of which is debated. Cervical cancer screening uncovers various forms of cervical atypia for which the need to treat and proper approach for follow-up are uncertain. Finally, new imaging technologies for lung cancer screening are finding small cancers and pulmonary nodules about which the natural history is uncertain (Frame, 2000).

Accuracies and Reliabilities of Screening Tests

The second consideration in judging the effectiveness of screening for cancer is whether the available test(s) can detect cancer at an early stage without producing large numbers of false-positive and false-negative results. Of greatest concern is the test's *accuracy*, the degree to which it measures the true value of the attribute it is testing, and its *reliability*, the consistency of the result when it is repeated. The principal parameters for measuring accuracy are sensitivity, specificity, and predictive value.

Sensitivity, Specificity, and Predictive Value

Sensitivity is the proportion of persons with cancer who correctly test positive, and *specificity* is the proportion of persons without cancer who correctly test negative (Box 5.1). Sensitivity and specificity are usually inversely related, so that tests with high sensitivities (i.e., those that miss few cases of cancer) tend to have low specificities (i.e., produce a higher proportion of false-positive results). If patients are put at substantial risk by receiving false-positive results, it may be worth compromising sensitivity—even though it means fewer cancers will be detected—in the interest of adopting a screening test or threshold with a higher specificity that generates fewer false-positive results.

Although the sensitivity and specificity of a cancer screening test are generally constant across populations and settings, this is not true for the *positive predictive value* (PPV), which is the probability that an abnormal

BOX 5.1 Definitions of Screening Test Performance

The performance of a screening test is often defined by three related measurements: sensitivity, specificity, and positive predictive value. The sensitivity (se) of a screening test is the proportion of people with the disease who test positive. Specificity (sp) is the proportion of people without the disease who test negative. The positive predictive value is the portion of individuals with a positive screening test who actually have the disease. If screened individuals are assigned a position in a 2 × 2 classification scheme based on their disease status and test result, values for the three measurements can be defined as follows:

	Actual Disease Status	
	+	–
Test Result	+ True Positive (TP)	False Positive (FP)
	– False Negative (FN)	True Negatives (TN)

Measurement: Question Answered:

Sensitivity (se) = $\frac{TP}{TP + FN}$ How often does the test correctly identify individuals with the disease?

Specificity (sp) = $\frac{TN}{TN + FP}$ How often does the test correctly identify individuals without the disease?

Positive predictive value = $\frac{TP}{TP + FP}$ Among individuals with an abnormal test, what proportion actually have the disease?

The positive predictive value is a function of sensitivity, specificity, and disease prevalence (P), with the following mathematical relationship:

$$ppv = \frac{(P)(se)}{\{(P)(se) + (1 - P)(1 - sp)\}}$$

result correctly indicates cancer (Box 5.1). The PPV depends on the pretest probability or likelihood that cancer is present at the time that the person is tested. For any cancer screening test, the PPV is lower (and the chances of false-positive results are higher) when there is a lower prevalence of cancer.

This important principle that underlies many concerns about cancer screening is best understood by example (Table 5.1). Suppose a test has a sensitivity and a specificity of 90 percent each. Clinicians would characteristically misinterpret these data to mean that a patient who has a positive result has a 90 percent likelihood of having cancer (i.e., PPV = 90 percent). In actuality the PPV is dependent on a third variable, the prevalence, or pretest probability, of cancer. Suppose the prevalence of cancer is 1 percent (1,000/100,000 population). This means that if 100,000 persons are screened, of whom 1,000 actually have cancer, then the 90 percent sensitivity means that 900 of these 1,000 will test positive, and the 90 percent specificity means that 89,100 of the 99,000 people without cancer will test negative. The chances that a positive test result is indicative of cancer (the PPV question asked above) would not be 90 percent, but 900/10,800, or 8 percent. The seeming accuracy conveyed by the "90 percent" figure for both sensitivity and specificity obscures the disturbing problem that the test would give false-positive information to 92 percent of those testing positive (11 people for every 1 person who truly had cancer). Because PPV correlates with prevalence, if the same test is administered in a community with a lower prevalence, the PPV would fall even further and the risk of producing false-positive results would climb higher (99 percent of those testing positive or 111 people for every 1 person who truly had cancer) (Table 5.1). The policy significance of these mathematics is that, regardless of the accuracy of a screening test, the administration of a test to populations or individuals with a low risk of cancer has

TABLE 5.1 Illustration of Influence of Prevalence on Positive Predictive Value

Prevalence = 1 percent, sensitivity = 90 percent, specificity = 90 percent

Test Result	No. with Disease Present	No. with Disease Absent	Total No.
Positive	900	9,900	10,800
Negative	100	89,100	89,200
Total	1,000	99,000	100,000

Prevalence = 0.1 percent, sensitivity = 90 percent, specificity = 90 percent

Test Result	No. with Disease Present	No. with Disease Absent	Total No.
Positive	90	9,990	10,080
Negative	10	89,910	89,920
Total	100	99,900	100,000

a potential to introduce major problems with false-positive results, leading to harms that can offset the benefits of screening.

Reliability

Reliability (or reproducibility) is the degree to which a screening test yields the same result when it is repeated under the same conditions. A laboratory assay for a serum tumor marker, for example, lacks reliability if it yields significantly different results when the test is repeated with a sample from the same tube of blood. Radiologists' interpretation of a screening chest radiograph can suffer from poor reliability due to either *interobserver variation* (differences between radiologists' interpretation of the same film) or *intraobserver variation* (different interpretations of the same film by one radiologist).

Effectiveness of Early Detection

A common mistake in determining whether screening for cancer is justified and a reason for premature enthusiasm for promoting screening tests is to limit consideration to the issues described above: burden of suffering and accuracy. Proponents argue that if the disease is serious and an accurate test is available, routine screening should be instituted. What this argument overlooks is the possibility that early detection of the disease may not improve outcomes either for the screened population as a whole or even for the individuals who will be found to have cancer.

Effectiveness of Treatment

The efforts and potential adverse effects of screening are not justified if an effective treatment is unavailable for persons found to have cancer. The tragedy of many cancers is that they progress inexorably, despite the use of the best available treatment regimens, because of the inability of these therapies to alter the natural history of the disease. Screening for such cancers serves only to identify the disease earlier in its course, not to improve the prognosis. This longer apparent survival time is not a benefit to the patient (and indeed may be a psychological and social cost) if that earlier diagnosis did not result in either less morbidity from treatment or longer life.

The benefits of early detection are muted for cancers that have a short preclinical period because the time window for early detection is short and the opportunity to affect outcomes is brief. Screening is also unlikely to confer benefits by detecting cancers that would have excellent outcomes under usual circumstances, when treatment is not initiated until patients present with symptoms. This concern underlies skepticism about the incremental benefit of screening for endometrial or testicular cancer, for example. Latent cancers detected by screening-induced overdiagnosis also may not benefit from early detection if the lesions were not destined to progress or affect the patient's health. Although little harm would have occurred if the cancer went undetected, the excellent outcomes of screening programs that predominantly detect such lesions are often cited as evidence of the benefits of screening. These principles are embodied in Whitmore's now-famous aphorism about prostate cancer: "Is cure possible for those for whom it is necessary, and is cure necessary for those in whom it is possible?" (Whitmore, 1988, pp. 7–11).

Incremental Benefit of Early Detection

Having an effective treatment is not enough. The logic behind screening rests on the argument that outcomes are improved by the early institution of treatment. If there is no incremental health benefit to early detection and patients fare just as well if their cancers are diagnosed after signs or symptoms appear, then there is not a good argument for screening. In this case, there are harms of screening, including adverse effects of screening on people without cancer, many of whom will experience anxiety and undergo workups for false-positive results, and the adverse effects of consumption of resources that would help patients more effectively if they were invested elsewhere.

The presumption that early detection improves outcomes is almost axiomatic in U.S. society. Epidemiological evidence would seem to support this belief. For almost all forms of cancer, 5-year survival rates are substantially lower for persons with advanced-stage disease (see Chapter 1). Such statistics are often mistakenly interpreted as evidence that patients are likely to live longer if their cancer is diagnosed early (see discussion of "lead time bias" below). Screening is consistently associated with the diagnosis of smaller and more localized tumors and with the familiar phenomenon of "stage shift," in which the proportion of cancers diagnosed at an earlier stage increases after screening is introduced. Also, observational studies demonstrate that patients whose cancers are diagnosed through screening often have better outcomes than those whose cancers are diagnosed otherwise. Many advocates of cancer screening find such evidence more than adequate to justify the intuitive notion that early detection is beneficial.

Whether such evidence is indeed adequate lies at the heart of many controversies about cancer screening. Critics of such evidence argue that such observations do not offer proof of benefit because the same patterns would be expected even if screening did not improve outcomes. For example, the fact that patients who participate in screening programs have better outcomes than those in other settings may be due to the fact that patients who participate in screening are more likely to have a college education, to be nonsmokers, and to have other healthier habits (Rimer et al., 1996b). Similarly, the fact that screening detects disease at an earlier stage and that patients diagnosed with localized disease have higher 5-year survival rates may reflect length and lead-time biases rather than true lengthening of life (Welch et al., 2000). The influence of these factors cannot be excluded unless outcomes are examined for a control group that is comparable in all respects other than exposure to screening, as has been done in trials of screening mammography.

Lead-Time Bias *Lead-time bias* refers to the overestimation of survival time simply due to a backward shift in the starting point for the measurement of survival as a result of early detection (Last, 1988). Patients diagnosed earlier can seem to live longer after diagnosis even if the time that they die does not change. For illustration, consider a man who is destined to develop symptoms from prostate cancer at age 65 and to die at age 70. His survival after diagnosis (5 years) can be doubled (10 years) if the cancer is detected through screening at age 60, even if he still dies from that same cancer at age 70. Because of lead-time bias, the fact that 5-year survival rates are higher for early-stage cancer than for advanced-stage cancer does not, by itself, prove that patients who are screened benefit from that screening and live longer; it may mean only that their disease is detected earlier. Similarly, the tendency of screening to detect smaller, localized tumors proves that cancers are being found at an earlier stage of their progression, not that the outcomes of that progression will necessarily be altered.

Length Bias *Length bias* refers to the tendency of screening to detect slowly growing lesions more readily than aggressive cancers. Rapidly progressive cancers, because they lead more hastily to death, are present in the screened population for a shorter period of time, thereby reducing their prevalence in the population and, thus, their odds of being detected when a screening test is administered. The consequence of length bias is that cancers detected by screening contain a higher proportion of slowly growing cancers than among cancers detected by symptoms. The favorable prognosis observed for cancers detected through screening may therefore imply a benefit from screening even when there is none.

Screening Interval and Duration Under conditions of uncertainty, in which the optimal frequency of screening has not been determined directly in clinical studies, there is a tendency to assume that a shorter interval is appropriate if the individual is at high risk of acquiring cancer. This assumption, which underlies the common advice that individuals in high-risk groups undergo more frequent screening, may be invalid because the proper determinants of the frequency of a screening test are the rate of progression of the disease and the sensitivity of the test. If these variables are held constant, increasing the frequency of testing offers little benefit, regardless of one's underlying risk of acquiring cancer (Frame and Frame, 1998).

Many controversies in cancer screening surround the question of when to stop. For most cancers, the absolute risk of dying from cancer increases with age, making elderly individuals the largest subset of people with cancer. On the other hand, the decreasing life expectancy and the greater likelihood of having other diseases that accompany advancing age tend to offset these benefits. One analysis, based on certain assumptions of efficacy, estimated that lifetime screening for breast cancer from age 50 until death results in a maximum potential life expectancy gain of 43 days, whereas the cessation of screening at age 75 or 80 would result in women giving up a maximum potential life expectancy gain of 9 or 5 days, respectively (Rich and Black, 2000). Rather than relying on such modeling data, which have their limitations, it would be preferable to examine direct evidence of the relative benefits of screening with advancing age, but most screening trials have limited enrollment to patients under the ages of 70, limiting access to definitive data. Because many older adults have excellent life expectancies and qualities of life, current thinking is shifting away from reliance on strict age cutoffs for screening and looking more closely at the life expectancy and health status of each individual to assess the potential benefits of screening.

Study Designs For the reasons outlined above, epidemiological studies reporting better outcomes for individuals with early-stage cancer tend not to persuade skeptics that early detection improves outcomes. Study designs fall in a hierarchy of persuasiveness (Box 5.2), in which uncontrolled epidemiological data and case series rank lowest in proving effectiveness.

Controlled observational studies compare outcomes among those who do or do not receive screening and bring investigators and clinicians one

BOX 5.2 Hierarchy of Effectiveness of Study Designs

Experimental trials
Randomized controlled trials
Nonrandomized controlled trials

Controlled observational studies
Cohort studies
Case-control studies
Cross-sectional comparisons
Historical (before-and-after) studies

Epidemiological studies without controls
Case reports, case series, descriptive analyses

step closer to having definitive evidence of the effectiveness of screening. *Historical studies* (before-and-after studies), such as a comparison of outcomes within a community before and after the introduction of a screening program, raise questions about the influence of temporal factors (e.g., improved treatment regimens) other than screening that occurred contemporaneously with the screening program. *Cross-sectional* comparisons, such as comparisons of outcomes for patients screened at a local institution with those for other patients in the community, also lack persuasiveness because of potential *confounding variables*: the characteristics of patients at these institutions may have an independent effect on the observed outcomes that are unrelated to screening.

In a *case-control study*, a retrospective review of medical records is undertaken to compare patients who died of cancer to a matched group of patients who did not die from cancer. If the patients who died from cancer were significantly less likely to have undergone screening, it is tempting to infer that the screening test was beneficial. The limitations of such studies include their retrospective design (e.g., medical records may not systematically capture relevant variables) and the difficulties of addressing confounding variables (persons who underwent screening may have other characteristics, such as healthier lifestyles, which may have contributed to the observed outcomes). Matching of the two groups by known confounding variables (e.g., age and risk factors) and the formulation of statistical adjustments in the odds ratios to control for such cofactors address some of these problems, but such studies cannot exclude the role of unknown or unmeasured confounding variables.

Prospective *cohort studies* overcome some of the limitations of retrospective analyses by establishing the variables of interest at the start of the study and collecting them systematically over time, often with long periods of follow-up, but the potential influence of confounding remains. Unless the decision to screen patients is made randomly, it is possible that screened and unscreened persons differ in characteristics other than screening that may account, at least in part, for the observed outcomes. It is this concern that accounts for the primacy of *randomized controlled trials* in demonstrating the effectiveness of screening (Jadad, 1998). The defining characteristic of such trials is that the assignment of patients to undergo screening is made randomly, creating comparison groups that are essentially the same in all respects other than exposure to screening. Unrecognized, as well as known, confounding variables are thereby distributed equally and should therefore not contribute to observed differences in outcomes.

Outcome Measures

The persuasiveness of evidence that screening does or does not improve outcomes depends in large part on which outcomes are considered. The outcomes that matter most are health outcomes, which in this report refer to outcomes that are perceptible to patients (e.g., pain, dysfunction, and death). Because of the lengthy follow-up periods and methodological challenges associated with the measurement of such outcomes, however, many studies infer effectiveness by measuring intermediate or surrogate outcomes. *Intermediate outcomes* are findings that are not health outcomes in themselves (e.g., histological features of a cancer) but that are thought to increase the risk of such outcomes. *Surrogate outcomes* are indicators that correlate with but that are not themselves health outcomes (e.g., length of hospital stay). One must be cautious, however, in relying on such indicators to infer effectiveness because screening can improve intermediate outcomes without necessarily improving health (Bucher et al., 1999; Gøtzsche et al., 1996).

The most definitive health outcome in terms of both importance to patients and relative ease of measurement is death, and thus, much of the focus in cancer screening is on evaluating whether death rates are lowered. As noted earlier, lead-time bias limits the utility of measuring survival after diagnosis, and thus, the conventional basis of comparison in screening trials is the proportion of persons in the intervention and control groups who die from cancer in a defined follow-up period.

The customary endpoint is the cancer-specific mortality rate and not mortality from all causes. In theory, a demonstrated reduction in all-cause mortality would be ideal, to ensure that death from cancer is not traded for death from another cause (such as fatal complications induced by screening or treatment). But because any specific cancer accounts for a relatively small proportion of all deaths in a population, the statistical power required to demonstrate an effect on all-cause mortality would require trials to have a sample size and duration that would render them unfeasible. Although most trials are therefore not powered to show an effect on all-cause mortality, their failure to do so is often mistakenly interpreted as evidence of a lack of benefit or, more erroneously, as evidence that screening somehow induces deaths from other causes.

Results can be statistically significant without having clinical or public health significance. Proponents of screening, in making their case, often emphasize the relative benefits rather than the absolute benefits of interventions. The *absolute benefit* of a 20 percent relative reduction in the risk of dying from cancer depends on the baseline probability of death. If that probability is 100/100,000 over some defined interval of time, the intervention reduces the risk of death to 80/100,000, an absolute difference of 20/100,000 or an absolute risk reduction of 0.02 percent, a far less impressive figure than the relative risk reduction of 20 percent. Although both figures are true, the absolute risk reduction has important policy implications, because it indicates that a large number of people must receive the intervention to save the life of one individual. The number of people who need to be treated to save one life is known as "the number-needed-to-treat" (NNT) which in this case is 100/0.02, or 5,000 people.

The NNT and its specific counterpart in screening, "the number-needed-to-screen" (NNS), have their limitations. They do not stipulate the health outcome prevented—two screening tests can have the same NNS, with, for example, one saving lives and the other one preventing fractures—nor do they address the harms and costs of interventions. In the context of screening, however, this measure can help place in context the size of the populations that do and do not benefit from early detection (Rembold, 1998). In the example presented above, most of the 5,000 people who must be screened to save one life will experience no personal benefits from screening but will be exposed to the inconvenience, discomfort, and potential harms of the screening experience. The difficult policy and ethical challenge in recommending that screening test would turn on deciding whether it is proper to expose that number of people to those particular harms to benefit one individual. Payers must decide whether it is worth the monetary costs (see below), but even without such considerations, for health reasons alone the NNS may sometimes be too large to make the argument that the population is better off with screening.

HARMS

Importance of Harms in Cancer Screening

The Hippocratic oath of *primum non nocere* (the first thing [is] to do no harm) establishes an ethical duty to ensure that medical interventions result in more good than harm. This duty is manifest throughout medicine but takes on special implications with regard to cancer screening (Ewart, 2000; Stewart-Brown and Farmer, 1997). Unlike patients who seek treatment for health complaints, persons undergoing cancer screening are, by definition, asymptomatic. With some exceptions (Rogers, 2000), most ethicists recognize a stronger moral imperative to avoid net harm in the case of preventive interventions and to ensure that what is offered is good for people.

Screening differs from conventional treatment interventions because in the latter case everyone exposed to a potential harm has a disorder, whereas the group exposed to potential harms from screening is the entire screened population, which is generally large (sometimes numbering in the millions) and predominantly free of disease. For every person found to have disease through screening, many more people in the screened population are exposed to potential harms. If the NNS for a screening test is 5,000, those who advocate screening must make the ethical argument that the large benefits to 1 individual justify the sum of the harms to which 4,999 people are exposed. Whether this holds up to moral scrutiny depends on the nature of the harms.

Test Procedure Although many screening test procedures are innocuous, involving little more than venipuncture, others (e.g., colonoscopy) are associated with various degrees of cost, discomfort, and potential complications (e.g., colonic perforation). Separate from the physical or psychological harms of the procedure are other difficulties such as the inconvenience of arranging testing, embarrassment in undergoing the procedure, and the unpleasantness of preparing for some procedures (e.g., bowel preparation for colonoscopy). The degree to which these matters are troublesome to patients is highly dependent on individual circumstances and personal values.

False-Positive and False-Negative Results The more common adverse effects of screening emanate from the information generated by testing. Positive or indeterminate test results plant the seed of anxiety, at least for some patients, and especially for serious diseases, and they usually require follow-up tests to determine whether the disease is present. In some cases the follow-up procedure is simple, such as a repeat blood test, but in other cases the patient is advised to undergo more invasive studies or procedures (e.g., biopsy) that may be associated with greater inconvenience, discomfort, or potential complications. Patients awaiting appointments for these confirmatory tests spend days or weeks, often in a state of worry and anxiety, not knowing whether they have a serious disease. The tally of harms against which the potential benefits of screening should be measured includes psychological morbidity and the accumulated potential physical risks associated with the cascade of tests and treatments triggered by screening. These harms are often borne by a sizable proportion of the screened population. For tests with a very low PPV, the net sum of the severity of harms experienced by persons without disease can outweigh the benefits to the small proportion of individuals with the disease.

For some individuals the harms do not end after the false-positive or false-negative error has been clarified. Patients who are ultimately told that their false-positive test results were erroneous may continue to believe that there is still something wrong. For example, as discussed later in this chapter, some studies of women who have received false-positive mammography results reveal continued anxiety on long-term follow-up, well after biopsies have shown no breast cancer.

These concerns, as well as ethical and legal ramifications, become more intense in the context of emerging technologies that screen for genetic susceptibility to cancer. Although such testing is currently considered primarily for families with a high likelihood of having uncommon familial cancer syndromes, technological advances raise the specter that screening of the population for genetic susceptibility to cancer will become more commonplace (Evans et al., 2001; Golub, 2001; Wilfond et al., 1997). The growing difficulty of keeping pace with the breathtaking advances in genetic technology makes it more likely that primary care physicians will provide misleading interpretations to patients undergoing genetic screening for cancer (Emery and Hayflick, 2001). The cascade of potential adverse consequences of genetic screening can reach beyond the patient to relatives and descendants.

Finally, normal results on screening are potentially harmful. False-negative results allow cancers to escape detection, but even true-negative results pose a potential risk. Patients may mistakenly assume that they are no longer in need of repeat screening at recommended intervals or that the clean bill of health makes it unnecessary to engage in other preventive behaviors or to seek clinical attention for abnormal signs or symptoms. Arguing against routine screening for lung cancer, Frame wrote: "A significant potential harm of screening is that smokers will interpret negative results of screening tests as assurance that they are disease free and will be less motivated to quit smoking" (Frame, 2000, p. 1982).

Harms of Treatment

The benefits of early detection of cancer must be weighed not only against the harms of screening but also against the harms of treatment. For some conditions it is possible for the adverse effects of treatment to offset the more modest benefits of screening. This is especially problematic when screening results in the overdiagnosis of latent cancers of uncertain clinical significance. Lesions that may pose little threat to patients' health are often treated, sometimes aggressively, with surgery, chemotherapy, radiotherapy, or other modalities that carry substantial risks of untoward side effects and complications.

A less obvious, but very real, harm of screening is the diversion of attention, time, and resources away from the primary prevention of cancer and other measures with greater health benefit to patients than screening. The American public has a particular fascination with technology (Smith, 2001) and is often more interested in getting a test for cancer than in adopting lifestyle measures that can prevent the very occurrence of cancer (e.g., the cessation of smoking or the consumption of a healthy diet). The limited time that individuals spend with clinicians is often consumed with testing, discussions of whether testing is necessary, and the interpretation of test results, leaving little time to talk about smoking cessation, dietary modification , or other primary prevention issues. This "opportunity cost" represents one of the most important arguments against the promotion of screening tests of unknown effectiveness, even if they are harmless and low-cost.

Costs

Expenditures for Screening

Those who are concerned about the costs of screening measure expenditures in different ways. The simplest measures are clinician and laboratory charges for screening. Charges are not the same as costs, however, especially if one considers the indirect costs of screening, such as the administrative overhead required to process the results or the patient's lost time from work. What counts as an expenditure also depends on one's perspective. The costs faced by a managed care organization or an employer differ from the copayments faced by the patient. A population-based perspective, which is recommended for economic analyses, considers all the costs faced by society, including time spent in treatment and time spent by unpaid caretakers (Gold et al., 1996).

The obvious criticism of considering only the up-front costs of screening is that it ignores the benefits, in both health and economic terms, of early detection. The pivotal economic question for most health services is not how much they cost but their *value* (the ratio of expenditures to benefits). An intervention with a low value, even if it is relatively cheap in terms of up-front costs, represents a poor use of resources, whereas a highly costly service may be an excellent value if it is highly effective. This argument makes perfect sense from a societal perspective but is often less compelling to insurance plans. Managed care organizations, for example, in which patients are unlikely to remain members for more than a few years, face the up-front costs of screening with little confidence that they will be the recipients of the downstream economic benefits.

Cost Analyses

The argument that screening pays for itself is often made on economic grounds, based on the contention that the up-front costs of screening are offset by the economic benefits of avoiding treatment for advanced-stage cancer. This argument is an example of *cost-benefit analysis*, in which the benefit is, by definition, measured in monetary units. This approach is not favored in economic analyses for both methodological and moral reasons. The methodological limitation stems from difficulties in quantifying the economic benefits of early detection and treatment. The moral difficulty is in assigning a monetary value to improved health or lengthened survival.

The more accepted approach is to compare health services on the basis of how much health benefit is purchased per dollar. A common measure is the *cost-effectiveness ratio*, in which the numerator is the monetary cost of the intervention and the denominator is the incremental health gain (e.g., years of life saved) with that expenditure. A screening test can be more or less cost-effective, depending on how it is used (Russell, 2000), and estimates can vary markedly depending on the methods used in the cost-effectiveness analysis. The greatest ambiguity surrounding cost-effectiveness analyses is the difficulty of which cutoff ratio constitutes a "good buy": how does one decide whether $50,000, $70,000, or $100,000 per year of life saved is a good value? As reviewed below, cancer screening escapes many of these quandaries because the cost-effectiveness ratios for recommended tests generally fall within widely accepted ranges of affordability, often below $20,000 per year of life saved.

The measurement of health benefits in terms of years of life saved does not capture the beneficial effects of screening on morbidity or quality of life, and thus, the ideal approach is to measure *cost-utility ratios*, in which health benefits are adjusted to reflect the relative importance of the outcome to patients. A common example of this ratio is the dollar cost of interventions per quality-adjusted life year (QALY), or disability-adjusted life year.

The validity of such comparisons—and the validity of economic calculations more generally—is highly dependent on the quality of the available cost estimates, which is often poor, and on the sophistication of the analytical methods. Standards for good cost-effectiveness analyses have been developed (Gold et al., 1996), but few published studies abide by these methods. Estimates of the cost-effectiveness of health services, cancer screening tests included, often vary widely because of differences in how the analyses were approached.

Trade-Offs and Shared Decision Making

Responsible decisions about whether cancer screening is appropriate require a methodical weighing of benefits and harms to determine whether the screened population gains more than it loses through screening. This judgment can be straightforward when the trade-offs are stark. Screening of all women for ovarian cancer, for example, is likely to result in unnecessary biopsies and laparotomies for a large proportion of women, few of whom will experience any proven benefit, making it clear that routine screening is inappropriate (National Institutes of Health, 1994). Cervical cancer screening illustrates a scale that tips the other way. The sizable benefits in terms of decreased mortality rates clearly offset the inconvenience of testing and the consequences of false-positive results, so that routine screening of the population has been widely accepted for decades and has been implemented around the world.

The more difficult controversies in cancer screening relate to what Kassirer and Pauker (1981) call "toss-ups," in which the balance between benefits and harms is less obvious, so which way the scales tip depends on subjective value judgments. Cancer screening tests often have both proponents and critics who, examining the same body of evidence, reach different conclusions about whether benefits outweigh harms. The facts (i.e., the data) are often less contentious than their interpretation. In some cases disagreements occur because reviewers set different thresholds for the quality of evidence that must be demonstrated to infer effectiveness. An element of subjectivity enters into assessments of science: the relative importance of various study design flaws, the validity of generalizing from one clinical context to another, and whether there have been enough studies with sufficient consistency.

However, the subjective value judgments that are perhaps most dominant in controversies about cancer screening do not concern the magnitude of benefits and harms but their relative importance. Differences in *utilities*, the relative importance that people assign to potential outcomes, explain why those examining the same data reach different conclusions about whether screening is appropriate. Proponents consider the benefits worth the harms, whereas skeptics take the opposing view. Guideline developers attempting to decide whether cancer screening is good or bad for a population inevitably apply their own value judgments (in effect, the average utility of the committee) in reaching a decision. Implicit in this act is the presumption that their value judgments are representative of the population to which their recommendations will be applied.

Studies have demonstrated that the relative importance that physicians assign to potential outcomes is often discordant with the relative importance assigned by their patients (Holmes et al., 1987), but even guideline panels composed of patients would have difficulty with "toss-up" screening controversies because of the degree to which preferences vary from person to person. If a hypothetical screening test with an NNS of 10,000 to prevent 1 death from cancer induces a non-fatal pulmonary embolus in 10 patients, people will differ regarding the appropriateness of screening, depending on the importance that they assign to these outcomes. Studies show that patients given the same facts about four colorectal cancer screening tests make different choices about which option is best (Leard et al., 1997; Pignone et al., 1999). When the best choice depends highly on personal preferences that vary substantially in the population, groups that issue uniform guidelines for or against screening expose a sizable proportion of the population to the wrong choice (Woolf, 1997a). Many who follow the guideline are screened (or not screened) in a manner that they would have deferred if given the opportunity to choose for themselves.

These considerations explain one of the most striking transitions in cancer screening guidelines in the last decade: for a growing number of screening tests, organizations are moving away from making uniform recommendations for or against screening and are instead encouraging clinicians to adopt shared decision making as part of an individualized, patient-centered approach to screening (Kassirer, 1994; Woolf, 1997a). This approach entails (1) giving patients information about potential benefits and harms, the probability of such outcomes, and the quality of evidence on which the estimates are based; (2) assisting them in considering their personal preferences and risk profile; and (3) helping them arrive at a choice that best suits their needs (Coulter, 1997; Frosch and Kaplan, 1999; Woolf, 1997a). The trend is toward giving patients the opportunity, if they so desire, to decide for themselves which choice is best.

A full discussion of the opposing arguments and logistical impediments to shared decision making is beyond the scope of this report and is addressed elsewhere (Barry, 1999; Elwyn et al., 1999; Frosch and Kaplan, 1999; Lang, 2000; Woolf, 2001). However, because consideration of patient preferences is embedded in many of the cancer screening guidelines discussed in this report, several fundamental challenges to the idea deserve mention. First, although most patients appreciate information about options, the degree to which they want to exert control over decisions is unclear (Deber et al., 1996; Strull et al., 1984). Many patients would rather have their physicians make such decisions and are overwhelmed both by the cognitive challenges of processing the facts and by the emotional toll of having made the wrong choice on a life-threatening matter.

For their part, physicians are unaccustomed to truly informed decision making, in one study doing so for only 9 percent of decisions (Braddock et al., 1999). Some physicians consider the sharing of decisions an abdication of their role as doctors and as a slight to their medical expertise. Others support the notion but in busy practices are too hurried to entertain the lengthy discussions that such decision making would require. In a recent survey, only 17 percent of internists reported that they would make their decision to order a prostate-specific antigen (PSA) test contingent on patient preferences (Dunn et al., 2001. The leading reasons for not discussing PSA testing were a lack of time (51 percent), the complexity of the topic (48 percent), and a language barrier between the physician and the patient (32 percent) (Dunn et al., 2001). Many physicians lack the knowledge, decision aids, or support staff to give patients the objective data that they need to make informed choices.

There are considerable difficulties in presenting risk information to patients (Bogardus et al., 1999) and uncertainties about how best to communicate probabilities (Goyder et al., 2000). In an intriguing study of 500 women, 96 percent of whom were high school graduates, 80 to 90 percent were unable to interpret simple probabilities (e.g., how many coin flips will come up heads?) or to understand relative or absolute risk reductions when they were applied to their perceived risk of breast cancer (Schwartz et al., 1997). How information is framed affects its interpretation: relative benefits are more impressive than absolute risk reductions, and percent gains are more attractive than percent losses. Visual displays to convey risks can help, but the optimal approach is unclear. A systematic review of 17 studies of aids for shared decision making concluded that they improved knowledge, reduced decisional conflict, and stimulated patients to engage in decision making without increasing their anxiety; but they had variable effects on decisions and no discernible effect on satisfaction (O'Connor et al., 1999).

The boundaries for shared decision making are indistinct (Woolf, 2001). It is unclear whether health systems and payers can afford to provide the choices that patients might prefer. Clearly, it is not the duty of clinicians and health systems to deliver services that patients might want but that are ineffective or medically contraindicated. What constitutes the dividing line between such services and the reasonable options from which patients have a right to choose must be delineated if the trend reflected in cancer screening guidelines continues its progression into other areas of medicine.

EFFECTIVENESS OF CANCER SCREENING

The remainder of this chapter focuses on four cancers for which there is a large body of evidence regarding the effectiveness of routine screening, including three cancers that are among the leading causes of cancer deaths in the United States: breast, colorectal, and prostate cancer. The review also examines cervical cancer, which claims fewer lives but for which important evidence and screening guidelines are available. Screening for lung cancer will be commented on in detail in Chapter 6, as this is a timely case study of the ongoing challenge of dealing with the uncertainties of screening efficacy as new screening technologies are developed.

Screening through routine self-examination, physician examination, or laboratory testing and imaging studies has been advocated for some of the cancers excluded from this report. Examples include cancers of the ovary, oral cavity, stomach, pancreas, bladder, endometrium, testis, and thyroid. For various reasons, however, few organizations recommend routine screening of the population for these conditions, and therefore, they are not reviewed here. Many guidelines do advocate screening for these cancers in individuals at especially high risk. For example, although no organization recommends routine screening of the population for ovarian cancer, a National Institutes of Health Consensus Conference did advocate screening of women at high risk for ovarian cancer due to their cancer family history (National Institutes of Health, 1994). Skin cancer screening is also excluded from this review. Although some organizations (e.g., American Cancer Society) recommend for the adult general population periodic examination of the skin by a physician, there is no direct evidence from either randomized trials or case-control studies that such screening reduces rates of morbidity or mortality from skin cancer (U.S. Preventive Services Task Force, 2001b). In a recent review, the Institute of Medicine (2000c) concluded that evidence was insufficient to support the adoption of a new program of clinical screening for skin cancer among asymptomatic Medicare beneficiaries.

The review presented in the remainder of this chapter focuses on the cancers detected and the screening options available in the United States. The findings may not be applicable in other countries, where there may be important differences in cancer prevalence, the availability and performance characteristics of screening tests, the values placed on benefits and harms, and the structures and resources of health care systems.

The evidence reviewed in this chapter was compiled from multiple sources, beginning with studies previously evaluated or currently under review by the U.S. Preventive Services Task Force (USPSTF) and other groups that have developed evidence-based cancer screening guidelines. It was supplemented by a manual search of recent literature on cancer screening and a computerized search of the National Library of Medicine's bibliographical MEDLINE database, conducted in February 2001, of relevant studies published since 1995, the closing year for the review of evidence for the second edition of the *Guide to Clinical Preventive Services*, the report of USPSTF (1996). Evidence published after that date is not included in the report.

Colorectal Cancer

The colorectal screening tests considered in the review in this part of the chapter are the fecal occult blood test (FOBT), flexible sigmoidoscopy, double-contrast barium enema, and colonoscopy. The review does not consider a variety of investigational technologies, such as computerized colography (virtual colonoscopy), and testing of feces for mutations in DNA (Traverso et al., 2002), which are less invasive than current screening options but which have not been sufficiently validated for routine use in the clinical setting.

Recent studies have shown an association between screening for colorectal cancer and a decreased incidence of the disease (Mandel et al., 2000), lending support to the notion that the removal of polyps, precipitated by screening, prevents colorectal cancer. For many years, the most compelling evidence was from the National Polyp Study, which demonstrated that the detection and removal of adenomatous polyps in patients with a prior history of such lesions could reduce the subsequent incidence of colorectal cancer by 76 to 90 percent (Winawer et al., 1993b). Such evidence lends support to the existence of an adenoma-carcinoma sequence: the hypothesis that colorectal cancer arises largely from adenomatous polyps. That said, an unknown proportion of colorectal cancers may arise de novo or from hyperplastic polyps (Bedenne et al., 1992). Concerns remain over flat lesions that are not discernible on colonoscopy and that may progress to cancer (Rembacken et al., 2000).

Certain patients are at increased risk for colorectal cancer, accounting for 30 to 35 percent of colorectal cancer cases (Winawer et al., 1997). Risk factors include a personal or family history of polyps or *prior* colorectal cancer and inflammatory bowel disease.

Fecal Occult Blood Testing

The test that has undergone the most extensive evaluation is the home FOBT, which in most studies consists of two samples from three consecutive specimens (six samples total) applied to guaiac-impregnated cards. The cards are mailed or delivered to the clinician's office or screening center, where a positive reaction indicates the possible presence of occult blood. The sensitivity of a single FOBT is limited and in some studies is as low as 40 percent (Ransohoff and Lang, 1997) because cancers and polyps may not bleed or may bleed intermittently and because blood is not fully distributed in the stool. The test is therefore typically repeated every 1 to 2 years to improve the likelihood of sampling blood and to thereby achieve greater "program" sensitivity. In screening trials, a program of FOBT every 1 to 2 years has been reported to detect 72 to 92 percent of colorectal cancers (Hardcastle et al., 1996; Kronborg et al., 1996; Mandel et al., 1993), with the higher values obtained by rehydration of the slides. Rehydration increases sensitivity at the expense of specificity, reducing the latter from approximately 98 percent (unrehydrated form) to 90 to 92 percent. FOBT is less sensitive for the detection of polyps than for the detection of cancers because polyps are less likely to bleed.

The chief limitation of FOBT is its limited specificity for the detection of colorectal neoplasms. False-positive results may occur if patients have ingested peroxidase-containing foods or gastric irritants (e.g., anti-inflammatory agents) or bleed from noncancerous sources anywhere in the gastrointestinal tract (e.g., gastritis or duodenal ulcers or hemorrhoids). The problems with specificity are reflected in the reported PPV of FOBT, which for unrehydrated slides is 5 to 18 percent for cancer and which for the combination of curable cancers or large adenomas is 20 to 40 percent (Ransohoff and Lang, 1997). In a trial with primarily rehydrated slides, the PPV was 2.2 percent (Mandel et al., 1993). Thus, a substantial majority of persons with abnormal FOBT results do not have neoplasms but must undergo further evaluation (typically colonoscopy) to rule out disease. In a 13-year trial of screening by FOBT, 38 percent of patients invited for annual screening underwent at least one colonoscopy (Mandel et al., 1993).

Office FOBT (testing of stool from the examination glove following a digital rectal examination) is thought to have lower sensitivity and specificity than home FOBT, but direct proof is limited. Studies have reported that the two tests have equivalent yields and PPVs (Bini et al., 1999; Eisner and Lewis, 1991), but because the profiles of the patient populations receiving each test may have been dissimilar, such findings provide a weak basis for contrasting the sensitivities and specificities of the tests.

Newer stool tests in development may increase the sensitivity and specificity of screening. These include immunochemical tests for blood and molecular biology-based analysis for neoplastic markers (e.g., testing for DNA markers of colorectal cancer present in the stool) (Ahlquist et al., 2000). One study of such a test for DNA reported sensitivities of 91 percent for cancer and 82 percent for adenomas (at least 1 centimeter [cm] in diameter) and a specificity of 93 percent (Ahlquist et al., 2000), though others have found less sensitivity for other mutations (Traverso et al., 2002).

Randomized controlled trials in Minnesota (Mandel et al., 1993, 1999, 2000), the United Kingdom (Hardcastle et al., 1996), and Denmark (Kronborg et al., 1996) have demonstrated that a program of annual or biennial screening by home FOBT reduces the rate of mortality from colorectal cancer by 15 to 33 percent (Table 5.2). This was achieved by referring patients with positive results on rehydrated FOBT slides for colonoscopy or barium enema. The Minnesota trial demonstrated that annual and biennial screening by FOBT reduced the mortality rates by 33 percent (Mandel et al., 1993) and 21 percent (Mandel et al., 1999), respectively. The European trials (in which screening was biennial, unrehydrated cards were used, and rates of colonoscopy were lower) reported lower reductions in the mortality rates (15 to 18 percent). Longer follow-up data from the Minnesota trial revealed that screening also reduced the incidence of colorectal cancer by 20 percent and 17 percent, respectively, for the annually and biennially screened groups (Mandel et al., 2000). This suggests that, in addition to secondary prevention (early detection of cancer), FOBT also achieves primary prevention (preventing the occurrence of cancer), presumably by leading those screened to colonoscopy, thus facilitating the detection (and removal) of premalignant polyps.

TABLE 5.2 Randomized Controlled Trials of Fecal Occult Blood Testing

Trial	Frequency of Testing	Duration (years)	Hydration	Colonoscopy Follow-Up (%)	Mortality Reduction (%)
Minnesota (Mandel et al., 1993, 1999, 2000)	Annual Biennial	10 18	Yes Yes	38 28	33 (17–49)[a] 21 (3–38)[a]
United Kingdom (Hardcastle et al., 1996)	Biennial	8	No	5	15 (2–26)
Denmark (Kronborg et al., 1996)	Biennial	10	No	5	18 (1–32)

[a]Screening also reduced incidence rates by 20 percent and 17 percent, respectively, for the annually and biennially screened groups (Mandel et al., 2000).

Flexible Sigmoidoscopy

Endoscopy (sigmoidoscopy or colonoscopy) has a high sensitivity for the detection of large adenomas and cancers, but only for the portion of the bowel that is directly visualized. The 60-cm flexible sigmoidoscope can reach as far as the descending colon in approximately 80 percent of examinations and is thus capable of reaching 40 to 60 percent of the colorectum (Winawer et al., 1997). Examiner skill, bowel preparation, and spasm influence the depth of insertion. Although the detection of distal lesions by sigmoidoscopy often prompts examinations by colonoscopy or barium enema that thereby can lead to the detection of proximal lesions beyond the reach of the sigmoidoscope, this approach fails to detect proximal lesions that are unaccompanied by distal disease. Colonoscopic studies suggest that 20 to 32 percent of advanced adenomas or cancers would go undetected if patients were screened only by sigmoidoscopy (Imperiale et al., 2000; Lieberman et al., 2000). Thus, even though sigmoidoscopy directly examines only the lower half of the colorectum, it can lead to the identification of advanced adenomas or cancers in 70 to 80 percent of people who have such lesions.

Although the specificity of sigmoidoscopy falls short of 100 percent because normal mucosa is occasionally mistaken as polyps, a more common form of "false-positive" result occurs even with tissue confirmation of an adenomatous polyp because most adenomas do not progress to cancer. Tubulovillous, villous, or large (greater than 1 cm in diameter) adenomas are an established premalignant precursor to colorectal cancer and their presence increases the risk of developing colorectal cancer (Atkin et al., 1992), but only some progress to cancer.

Randomized controlled trials of sigmoidoscopy screening with mortality as an endpoint are under way, and thus, prospective evidence that sigmoidoscopy has a benefit in terms of reducing the rate of mortality is lacking. The Prostate, Lung, Colorectal, and Ovarian trial sponsored by the National Cancer Institute has randomized more than 150,000 subjects to receive sigmoidoscopy screening or not, but the trial will not be completed until 2014 unless it is stopped early due to a large mortality benefit (Gohagan et al., 2000). Case-control studies have demonstrated, however, that patients who die of colorectal cancer are significantly less likely than matched controls to have undergone sigmoidoscopy (Muller and Sonnenberg, 1995; Newcomb et al., 1992; Selby et al., 1992). To address concerns that confounding variables might account for this observation, Selby and colleagues (1992) conducted an intriguing analysis in which they demonstrated that the benefit was observed only for lesions within 20 cm of the anus, a pattern consistent with an effect from sigmoidoscopy and unlikely to result from lifestyle or other confounders. The adjusted odds ratio for the detection of such lesions was 0.41 (95 percent CI, 0.25

to 0.69), suggesting a 59 percent reduction in the rate of mortality, whereas there was no benefit for the detection of more proximal colon cancers, beyond the reach of the scope (adjusted odds ratio 0.96) (Selby et al., 1992).

Several studies in California report an association between a lower incidence of distal colorectal cancers and increased rates of screening by sigmoidoscopy (Cress et al., 2000; Inciardi et al., 2000). It is unclear whether these temporal trends can be attributed to sigmoidoscopy or other confounding variables, such as dietary or environmental changes.

The combination of FOBT and sigmoidoscopy is often recommended to enhance effectiveness, but evidence of its incremental benefit is limited. A nonrandomized trial found that adding FOBT to rigid sigmoidoscopy detected more colorectal cancers on initial screening, but the mortality rate was not significantly lowered (Winawer et al., 1993a). Other trials have examined the incremental benefit of adding flexible sigmoidoscopy to FOBT and have found that the amount of previously unrecognized disease identified was significantly increased compared to FOBT alone (Berry et al., 1997; Rasmussen et al., 1999).

Barium Enema

Data regarding the accuracy of barium enema for the detection of polyps and colon cancer in asymptomatic screened populations are limited. Studies that were poorly designed to assess test accuracy report sensitivities of 70 to 90 percent for the detection of polyps larger than 1 cm and 55 to 85 percent for the detection of colorectal cancer and specificities of 90 to 95 percent and 99 percent, respectively (Winawer et al., 1997). One study reported that double-contrast barium enema has a sensitivity of 85 percent for the detection of colorectal cancer (Rex et al., 1997b). In one study, patients undergoing surveillance for previously diagnosed adenomatous polyps underwent double-contrast barium enema followed by colonoscopy in which the endoscopist was unaware of the results of the barium enema. (The endoscopist was later given the results if a neoplasm was seen so that the involved segment could be reexamined.) Compared with colonoscopy, barium enema detected only 48 percent of the polyps larger than 1 cm and had an estimated specificity of 85 percent (Winawer et al., 2000). No trial has studied the effect of barium enema screening on the incidence of or rate of mortality from colorectal cancer.

Colonoscopy

Colonoscopy serves as the reference standard for most studies, and thus, its sensitivity and specificity are difficult to determine. Back-to-back colonoscopic examinations report a sensitivity of 90 percent for the detection of polyps larger than 1 cm (Rex et al., 1997a). Specificity for the correct tissue diagnosis by biopsy approaches 100 percent. As noted earlier, however, a large proportion of polyps, although correctly identified by colonoscopy, do not progress to clinically significant disease.

A trial to test the effect of colonoscopy screening on mortality rates is under consideration. Given the evidence from sigmoidoscopy screening reviewed above, one can postulate that the effect of colonoscopy screening on mortality would be of equal or, more likely, of greater magnitude, but direct evidence is lacking. One of the previously mentioned case-control studies of sigmoidoscopy, which also included colonoscopic examinations, reported that the odds ratio for reduced colon cancer mortality was 0.47 (95 percent CI, 0.37 to 0.58) for patients who underwent colonoscopy (Muller and Sonnenberg, 1995), but this subgroup analysis is of limited persuasiveness in proving a benefit in terms of a reduction in the rate of mortality.

Colonoscopy screening is routinely advocated for patients with a family history of familial polyposis syndrome and hereditary nonpolyposis colorectal cancer or for patients with inflammatory bowel disease. Controlled observational studies suggest that such screening improves survival from familial polyposis syndrome, a hereditary syndrome associated with an extremely high risk of colorectal cancer (Heiskanen et al., 2000). A randomized trial to confirm the benefits of this practice is unlikely for ethical reasons.

Harms

Performing the FOBT is not harmful, but the results can be distressing. Patients screened for colorectal cancer were distressed by an invitation letter, a positive test result, and delay in the process of screening (e.g., a wait of 10 days to colonoscopy) but later reported that it was worthwhile to have had the test (Mant et al., 1990). The more important consequence is the large proportion of patients who must undergo colonoscopy because of false-positive FOBT results. Aside from the risks of bleeding and perforation outlined below, patients experience the discomfort, embarrassment, and inconvenience associated with bowel preparation and the examination itself, and the anxiety and other negative consequences of awaiting the evaluation of positive results.

A British screening trial of sigmoidoscopy screening reported that bleeding and moderate to severe pain were reported by 3 and 14 percent of patients, respectively (Atkin et al., 1998). Bowel perforation is estimated to occur in 1 to 2 sigmoidoscopy examinations for every 10,000 performed (Winawer et al., 1997). An audit of 49,501 sigmoidoscopies performed over 10 years at the Mayo Clinic in Scottsdale, Arizona, reported perforations in 1 in 25,000 examinations (Anderson et al., 2000).

Bowel perforation is more common with colonoscopy than with sigmoidoscopy, although the exact incidence is uncertain and varies depending on whether the procedure is diagnostic or therapeutic. It has been estimated that 1 in 1,000 patients experience perforation, 3 in 1,000 have major hemorrhage, and 1 to 3 in 10,000 die from the procedure (Winawer et al., 1997). A British trial reported a colonoscopy complication rate of 1 in 200, and most of these complications required surgical intervention (Robinson et al., 1999). An audit of 10,486 colonoscopies performed over 10 years at the Mayo Clinic in Scottsdale, Arizona, reported perforations and colonoscopy-related deaths in approximately 1 in 500 and 1 in 5,000 examinations, respectively (Anderson et al., 2000). Perforations are estimated to occur in 1 in 25,000 barium enema examinations, and death occurs in 1 in 55,000 examinations (Winawer et al., 1997).

Uncertainties About Periodicity

Direct evidence about the optimal frequency of screening exists only for FOBT, for which annual and biennial screening intervals were prospectively evaluated in the trials discussed earlier. Although sigmoidoscopy screening was once recommended every 3 years and more recently every 5 years, such guidelines are based on expert opinion and not outcomes data. Indirect evidence from case-control studies of sigmoidoscopy suggests that an interval of at least 6 years (Muller and Sonnenberg, 1995) or even 9 to 10 years (Selby et al., 1992) may have an equivalent benefit. Colonoscopy screening is recommended every 10 years not on the basis of direct evidence but on the basis of inferences about the time it takes for the evolution from normal mucosa to invasive carcinoma (approximately 10 years). A 5-year interval for barium enema screening is advocated because of concerns that its lower sensitivity makes it more likely that extant lesions would escape detection in the interim (Smith et al., 2001).

Cost-Effectiveness Studies

A series of recent analyses (Frazier et al., 2000; Khandker et al., 2000; Sonnenberg et al., 2000; Theuer et al., 2001) have confirmed the findings of earlier reports (Eddy, 1990a; Wagner et al., 1996; Winawer et al., 1997) that screening for colorectal cancer has acceptable cost-effectiveness ratios. Calculations of the cost-effectiveness of screening for colorectal cancer are highly sensitive to certain assumptions, such as the time assumed to evolve from polyps to cancer and the performance characteristics of tests. Thus, individual reports often reach different conclusions about which test or which combination of tests is most cost-effective. The options that tend to dominate most analyses are the combination of annual FOBT and flexible sigmoidoscopy every 5 years or colonoscopy alone every 10 years. Cost-effectiveness ratios also vary to some extent by racial and ethnic group (Theuer et al., 2001). Nonetheless, in most reports every option, including colonoscopy, costs less than $20,000 per quality-adjusted life year (QALY).

Subjective Value Judgments

Although there is universal agreement that screening for colorectal cancer beginning at age 50 is worthwhile, the controversy over which test is best is heavily influenced by subjective value judgments. The current trend is to promote colonoscopy as the "preferred" test, a message promoted by celebrities and the news media (Gorman, 2000) and a formal position recently adopted by one gastrointestinal specialty society (Rex et al., 2000). Advocacy for colonoscopy is fueled by its superior accuracy over other screening tests. Accepting the alternative of sigmoidoscopy was said in one editorial to be the equivalent of performing mammography on one breast (Podolsky, 2000). The counterargument is that sigmoidoscopy screening can detect 80 percent of people who have significant neoplasms and that the incremental benefit of colonoscopy may be offset by its added harms, costs, and lack of availability.

In actuality, which screening test is best from an individual's perspective depends on subjective judgments regarding multiple variables: the relative importance that one assigns to scientific certainty, accuracy, benefit, safety, acceptability, costs, and feasibility (Woolf, 2000a). One value judgment concerns whether the absolute benefit of screening is large enough, which some question (Budenholzer, 1998). Although the relative reduction in mortality rates in FOBT trials was large (15 to 33 percent), the absolute benefit of screening is limited by the low prevalence of clinically significant disease in the screened population. The prevalence of advanced neoplasia (cancer, adenoma, or villous histology) in screened populations is only 6 percent (Imperiale et al., 2000; Lieberman et al., 2000), and cancers account for a relatively small proportion of these lesions. By one calculation, 1,374 patients must undergo screening by FOBT for 5 years to prevent 1 death from colorectal cancer (Rembold, 1998).

Research has shown that patients' preferences, given the same factual information, vary considerably. For example, Leard and colleagues (1997) gave 100 patients a 10-minute, scripted oral presentation about the benefits and risks of the four screening tests for colorectal cancer. When the patients were asked which test they would prefer on the basis of the information that they had just heard, 38 chose colonoscopy, 31 chose FOBT, 14 selected barium enema, and 13 chose sigmoidoscopy (Leard et al., 1997). Another study found that preferences for FOBT and sigmoidoscopy changed with more information. When patients received general descriptions of colon cancer and the two tests, their order of preference was FOBT alone (45 percent), both tests (38 percent), and sigmoidoscopy alone (13 percent).

When they next learned about test accuracy, more patients preferred both tests (47 percent) and fewer wanted FOBT alone (36 percent). When they were then told about out-of-pocket costs, preferences for FOBT alone rose to 53 percent and requests for both tests fell to 31 percent (Pignone et al., 1999).

With an appreciation of this heterogeneity in patient preferences, shared decision making was recommended in a guideline produced in 1997 by a consortium led by the American Gastroenterological Association and endorsed by the American Cancer Society and a dozen other organizations. Beginning with a generic statement that screening was recommended for average-risk persons beginning at age 50, it offered five options for screening regimens and encouraged physicians to individualize the choice: "Decisions about which test or tests to use should take into account the patient's preferences, the patient's age, any existing comorbidity, and local resources and expertise. The panel considers planning of colorectal cancer screening an ideal opportunity for clinicians to share the decision making process with their patients as well as for exercising their own clinical judgment" (Winawer et al., 1997, p. 603).

Subsequent guidelines, including a recent update from the American Cancer Society (Smith et al., 2001), continue to advocate this shared decision-making approach to increase the likelihood that patients will be screened in a manner that suits their preferences. Preliminary evidence suggests that such engagement gives patients the knowledge they need to make informed choices. A randomized trial that compared the effect of giving elderly patients an informational intervention that simulated one of two informed consent presentations (with one emphasizing absolute risk and the other emphasizing relative risk) versus the effect of a brief scripted message about screening options showed that they created no differences in interest in screening—63 percent of patients in both groups intended to be screened. The informational intervention group demonstrated a more accurate understanding of the PPV, but those receiving the absolute risk information rated efficacy lower than did those who received relative risk information; controls rated efficacy highest (Wolf and Schorling, 2000).

Current Guidelines

Most organizations are in agreement that all Americans age 50 and older should be periodically screened for colorectal cancer and should be allowed to choose from options that include FOBT, flexible sigmoidoscopy, colonoscopy, or double-contrast barium enema (see Box 5.3 for guidelines published since 1996). Most organizations offer additional guidelines on the screening of adults at increased risk for colorectal cancer. For example, the American Cancer Society recommends colonoscopy screening beginning at age 40 (or 10 years before the age of occurrence of colorectal cancer

BOX 5.3 Recommendations for Colorectal Cancer Screening in Average-Risk Persons

Organization	Recommendations
U.S. Preventive Services Task Force, 2002 (http://www.preventiveservices.ahrq.gov)	Screening for colorectal cancer is strongly recommended for men and women 50 years of age or older. Several screening methods are effective in reducing mortality from colorectal cancer. There is good evidence that periodic fecal occult blood testing (FOBT) reduces mortality from colorectal cancer and fair evidence that sigmoidoscopy alone or in combination with FOBT reduces mortality. There is no direct evidence that screening colonoscopy is effective in reducing colorectal cancer mortality; efficacy of colonoscopy is supported by other evidence (e.g., its integral role in trials of FOBT, extrapolation from sigmoidoscopy studies). Double-contrast barium enema offers an alternative means of whole-bowel examination, but it is less sensitive than colonoscopy, and there is no direct evidence that it is effective in reducing mortality rates. There are insufficient data to determine which strategy is best in terms of the balance of benefits and potential harms or cost-effectiveness, but colorectal cancer screening is likely to be cost-effective regardless of the strategy chosen.
American Cancer Society (Smith et al., 2001)	Adults at average risk should begin colorectal cancer screening by age 50. The screening options are (1) FOBT annually, (2) flexible sigmoidoscopy every 5 years, (3) annual FOBT plus flexible sigmoidoscopy every 5 years, (4) double-contrast barium enema every 5 years, or (5) colonoscopy every 10 years. The digital rectal examination is not recommended as a stand-alone screening test for colorectal cancer.
American College of Gastroenterology (Rex et al., 2000)	The preferred screening strategy is colonoscopy every 10 years. An alternative strategy is an annual FOBT plus flexible sigmoidoscopy every 5 years.
American College of Obstetricians and Gynecologists, 2000	Beginning at age 50, the recommendation is for a yearly FOBT plus flexible sigmoidoscopy every 5 years, colonoscopy every 10 years, or double-contrast barium enema every 5 to 10 years, with a digital rectal examination performed at the time of each screening sigmoidoscopy, colonoscopy, or double-contrast barium enema.
American Academy of Family Physicians, 2000	Adults age 50 and older should be screened for colorectal cancer by FOBT (annually), sigmoidoscopy, colonoscopy, or barium enema.

BOX 5.3 *(continued)*

American Society of Colon and Rectal Surgery (Simmang et al., 1999)	Beginning at age 50, low- or average-risk persons should have an annual digital rectal examination and FOBT and should have a flexible sigmoidoscopy every 5 years. If the patient has a family history of colorectal cancer, colonoscopy or barium enema is recommended every 10 years if the relative is not a first-degree relative. A family history of colorectal cancer involving first-degree relatives is not classified as average risk, and the guideline recommends more intensive screening.
American Gastroenterological Association (Winawer et al., 1997)[a]	Screening for colorectal cancer and adenomatous polyps should be offered to all men and women without risk factors beginning at age 50. Offer FOBT each year, flexible sigmoidoscopy every 5 years, both annual FOBT and sigmoidoscopy every 5 years, double-contrast barium enema every 5 to 10 years, or colonoscopy every 10 years.

[a]Panel originally established by the Agency for Health Care Policy and Research (now the Agency for Healthcare Research and Quality). The recommendations were endorsed by a consortium that included the American Cancer Society, American College of Gastroenterology, American Gastroenterological Association, American Society of Colon and Rectal Surgeons, and other groups.

or adenomatous polyps in the youngest affected person in the family) for persons with a first-degree relative who has or who has had colorectal cancer or adenomatous polyps before age 60 or for persons with two or more first-degree relatives who have or who have had colorectal cancer or adenomatous polyps at any age (Smith et al., 2001; Winawer et al., 1997). Most groups recommend early colonoscopy screening (by puberty or age 21) in persons with a family history of familial adenomatous polyps or hereditary nonpolyposis colon cancer and colonoscopy screening of persons with inflammatory bowel disease within 8 years of the onset of pancolitis. Guidelines for surveillance of persons with previously diagnosed polyps or colorectal cancer have also been disseminated but fall outside the scope of this review.

Breast Cancer

The screening tests reviewed here include clinical breast examination, mammography, screening for mutations in *BRCA1* and *BRCA2* (mutations of breast cancer-associated tumor suppressor genes), and breast self-examination. Ultrasound and newer technologies that offer promise in improving the accuracy of breast cancer screening (e.g., full-field digital mammograms, magnetic resonance imaging, and filmless imaging) are not reviewed because their performance characteristics and incremental benefits over existing screening modalities require further evaluation before they are suitable for routine clinical use (Lewin et al., 2001; Orel, 2000). They are likely to offer important advances in the screening of high-risk groups, such as women suspected of carrying breast cancer susceptibility genes (Brown et al., 2000; Kuhl et al., 2000; Tilanus-Linthorst et al., 2000). The review also does not examine computer-based algorithms and other measures used to improve the accuracy of mammographic interpretations (Boccignone et al., 2000; Floyd et al., 2000).

The incidence of ductal carcinoma in situ (DCIS) (and of mastectomies) has increased in association with more widespread screening mammography (Ernster et al., 1996). DCIS now represents 12 to 20 percent of all newly diagnosed breast cancers (Feig, 2000; Winchester et al., 2000). In one community case series, DCIS accounted for 41 percent of cancers detected by screening in women ages 40 to 49 (Linver and Paster, 1997). The American Cancer Society estimated that 46,400 cases of carcinoma in situ breast cancer were diagnosed in 2001, and of these, approximately 88 percent were DCIS (Greenlee et al., 2001). A spectrum of controversy surrounds DCIS, ranging from those who are convinced that DCIS is potentially fatal to those who consider it a false-positive finding. There is no direct evidence from controlled trials that women benefit from the early detection and treatment of DCIS (Ernster et al., 1996). Observational data suggest that it is a major risk factor for the development of invasive carcinoma and for death from breast cancer (Ernster et al., 2000), but a large proportion of DCIS cases remain indolent (Page et al., 1995; Winchester et al., 2000). Among women diagnosed with DCIS, the 10-year death rate from breast cancer is 3.4 percent (Ernster et al., 2000). Diagnostic criteria for DCIS are imprecise, producing inconsistencies in the differentiation of low-grade DCIS from ductal hyperplasia. Whether small nonpalpable foci of DCIS require treatment and the proper treatment modalities are also debated (Morrow and Schnitt, 2000).

Clinical Breast Examination

An analysis based on pooled data from controlled trials and case-control studies calculated that the sensitivity and specificity of the clinical breast examination were 54 and 94 percent, respectively. Clinical breast examination was estimated to detect 3 to 45 percent of breast cancers that screening mammography missed (Barton et al., 1999). A sensitivity of 59 percent and a specificity of 93 percent were recently reported in an evaluation of 752,000 clinical breast examinations (Bobo et al., 2000). The sensitivity of the clinical examination appears to be higher in younger women, although it is less likely than mammography to detect small lesions. In a Canadian trial, lesions at least 20 millimeters (mm) accounted for 56 percent of cancers detected in women screened only by physical examination, whereas they accounted for 21 percent of cancers detected in women screened only by mammography (Miller et al., 2000). False-positive results are common, however. The PPV of the clinical breast examination ranges from 4 to 50 percent (Barton et al., 1999), reflecting differences in prevalence rates, technique, and case definitions. In one study, the cumulative risk of a false-positive finding over 10 years of screening by clinical breast examination was 22 percent (Elmore et al., 1998).

There is limited evidence about the effect on mortality of routine clinical breast examination in isolation. Trials have evaluated it in combination with mammography and have reported significant reductions in rates of mortality (Alexander et al., 1999; Shapiro, 1988), but the contribution of the clinical breast examination to outcomes is uncertain because similar effects were observed in trials that evaluated mammography alone.

Mammography

Because several clinical trials combined screening mammography with clinical breast examination, the performance characteristics of mammography in isolation are uncertain. The sensitivity, specificity, and PPV reported by trials that examined mammography alone are 68 to 88, 95 to 98, and 4 to 22 percent, respectively (Fletcher et al., 1993). Another review that used modified definitions of sensitivity and specificity reported sensitivity and specificity ranges of 83 to 95 and 94 to 99 percent, respectively (Mushlin et al., 1998). The sensitivity of mammography is somewhat lower (e.g., 72 percent) in some community practice audits (Poplack et al., 2000). Higher and lower sensitivities have been reported in individual trials depending on case definitions, the length of follow-up, and the number of views and interpreters. A retrospective review found discernible cancers in 5 to 50 percent of older films obtained before incidence cancers were diagnosed, depending on the methods and number of radiologists involved (Moberg et al., 2000).

Estimates of the specificity of mammography vary widely (82 to 99 percent in one review), as do the reported PPVs (4 to 22 percent) (Fletcher et al., 1993). The Canadian Breast Cancer Screening Initiative reported a PPV of 7 to 8 percent in population-based screening across seven provinces (Paquette et al., 2000). As these values indicate, most abnormal screening mammograms are falsely positive. In one study, among 2,400 women screened over 10 years (median of four mammograms per woman), 24 percent had at least one false-positive mammogram; the estimated cumulative risks of a false-positive result and the need to have a biopsy increased to 49 and 19 percent, respectively, after 10 mammograms (Elmore et al.,

1998). There are also considerable inter- and intraobserver variations among radiologists in the interpretation of mammograms (Kerlikowske et al., 1998).

The sensitivity of screening mammography appears to be lower for women under age 50 than for older women, approximately 14 to 20 percent lower in most screening trials (Fletcher et al., 1993; Kerlikowske et al., 1996, 2000). This is likely due to differences in breast density, the more rapid growth of cancers in younger women, or both. Sensitivity also appears to be lower with longer intervals between examinations. In one study, the sensitivity of the first mammogram for registry-confirmed breast cancer was 99 percent with 7 months of follow-up, but sensitivities were 93 and 86 percent with 13 and 25 months of follow-up, respectively (Kerlikowske et al., 1996).

As with any screening test, the PPV of screening mammography depends on the prevalence (pretest probability) of breast cancer. The PPV of the first screening mammogram is between 5 and 38 percent (Kerlikowske et al., 1993) and is generally higher with increasing age or a positive family history (Kerlikowske et al., 2000). In a Canadian trial, the rates of false positivity for the combination of screening mammography and clinical breast examination were 7 to 10 percent for women ages 40 to 49 and 5 to 8 percent for women ages 50 to 59 (Miller et al., 1992a,b). In an American analysis of claims data, for every 1,000 women aged 65 to 69 who underwent mammography, 85 had follow-up testing in the subsequent 8 months (23 had biopsies); the PPVs of mammograms requiring further testing were 8 percent for women aged 65 to 69 and 14 percent for older women (Welch and Fisher, 1998). An audit of 36,850 screening mammography examinations of women with a mean age of 59 reported that 5 percent of the examinations were abnormal, and approximately 25 percent of these led to a biopsy. The PPV of an abnormal mammogram was approximately 10 percent (Dee and Sickles, 2001). A modeling analysis predicted that the cumulative probability of experiencing a false-positive result over nine mammograms in women ages 40 to 69 was 43 percent, but it ranged widely, depending on the combination of risk factors for false-positive results (Christiansen et al., 2000). These included young age, the number of breast biopsies, family history of breast cancer, estrogen use, time between screenings, no comparison with previous mammograms, and the radiologist's tendency to label mammograms as abnormal.

Effectiveness of Early Detection

Although the effectiveness of early detection of breast cancer has been examined in observational (e.g., case-control) studies, eight randomized controlled trials of screening mammography provide more compelling evidence and are less subject to bias from confounding variables and other methodological factors. This review therefore focuses on the trials.

The eight trials include studies from Scotland (Alexander et al., 1999), Canada (Miller et al., 1992a,b, 2000), and the United States (Shapiro, 1988) and four trials from Sweden: Malmö (Andersson and Janzon, 1997), Kopparberg and Östergotland (the Swedish Two-County Trial) (Tabàr et al., 1999, 2000), Stockholm (Frisell and Lidbrink, 1997), and Gothenburg (Nyström et al., 1993) (Table 5.3). The studies, conducted from 1963 to 1990, varied in certain important respects: the age of the women at entry ranged between 39 and 74 years; individual, cluster, and combined methods of randomization were used; the mammograms included one or two views; and clinical breast examination was not part of the intervention in most trials. The subjects underwent between two and six rounds of screening at intervals that ranged from 12 to 33 months, and follow-up in the most recent reports varied between 11 and 20 years.

Despite these differences, the results of the trials are relatively consistent. Most reported that screening mammography reduced the risk of death from breast cancer, with relative risk reductions ranging from 3 to 32 percent. The relative risk reduction achieved statistical significance in only a few trials, but the combined data from all trials show a highly significant reduced risk. The pooled relative risk ratio reported in one meta-analysis (across all age groups) was 0.79 (a 21 percent reduction in the risk of dying from breast cancer) (Kerlikowske et al., 1995), and the pooled relative risk ratio in a more recent meta-analysis based on longer follow-up data was

TABLE 5.3 Results of the Randomized Clinical Trials of Screening Mammography

Trial	Entry Years	Age at Entry (years)	Number of Women	Median Follow-Up By 2002 (years)	RR for Death from Breast Cancer (95% CI)
Mammography alone					
Stockholm	1981–85	40–64	60,261	13.8	0.91 (0.65–1.27)
Gothenburg	1982–88	39–59	49,533	12.8	0.76 (0.56–1.04)
Malmö	1976–86	45–70	42,283	17.1	0.82 (0.67–1.00)
Swedish Two-County	1977–85	40–74	133,065	17.0	0.68 (0.59–0.80)
Mammography plus CBE					
Canada NBSS I	1980–87	40–49	50,430	13.0	0.97 (0.74–1.27)
Canada NBSS II[a]	1980–87	50–59	39,405	13.0	1.02 (0.78–1.33)
HIP	1963–69	40–64	60,496	16.0	0.79
Edinburgh	1978–85	45–64	54,643	13.0	0.79 (0.60–1.02)

[a]Compared mammography + clinical breast exam to clinical breast exam alone, RR = Relative Risk (A value less than one indicates fewer breast cancer deaths among screened women), CI = Confidence Interval.
Adapted from: Humphrey et al., 2002.

0.84 (95 percent CI, 0.77–0.91) (Humphrey et al., 2002). The narrow 95 percent CI around this estimate denotes the high level of statistical certainty about the magnitude of benefit.

That said, the designs of these trials were imperfect and have been criticized (Berry, 1998; Gøtzsche and Olsen, 2000). A recent analysis by Danish investigators, published as a Cochrane Collaboration report (Olsen and Gøtzsche, 2001), drew attention to poor documentation of concealment of allocation, imbalances in the baseline characteristics, inconsistent data on the number of subjects, and inadequate accounting for loss to follow-up and breast cancer ascertainment.[2] In contrast to the positive findings in other trials, the combined evidence from the two trials that the investigators considered "adequately randomized" (Canada, Malmo) showed no effect on breast cancer mortality (pooled relative risk, 1.04; 95 percent CI, 0.84 to 1.27). The investigators concluded that screening mammography is unjustified, generating a flurry of broadcast and print media reports in early 2002 questioning the merits of mammography and prompting an announcement by the National Cancer Institute PDQ advisory panel expressing reservations about the evidence (Kolata, 2001a,b; Kolata, 2002a; Circling the Mammography Wagons, 2002; Henderson, 2002; Kolata and Moss, 2002; Ernster, 2002; Excerpts from Speech, 2002; Kolata, 2002b).

There has not been uniform acceptance of the conclusions of Olsen and Gøtzsche within the scientific community. Most of the design flaws of concern to the Danish authors have been discussed in the literature, and by the investigators themselves, for many years. Their review therefore did less to "discover" these problems than to give them public airing. The disagreement is less about whether the trials have flaws but whether such imperfections are grounds, as the Danish authors contend, for invalidating the results. Not all analysts and review groups agree that the design flaws are fatal (Duffy and Tabar, 2000; Cates and Senn, 2000; Law et al., 2000; Moss et al., 2000; Nyström, 2000; Hayes et al., 2000; de Koning, 2000; Duffy et al., 2001; Wald, 2000; Smith et al., 2002; Miller, 2001; Lee and Zuckerman, 2001; Senn, 2001; Duffy et al., 2001; Duffy et al., 2002; Nyström et al., 2002; Gelmon and Olivotto, 2002; Humphrey et al., 2002).

Those who are willing to accept the trial data advance a variety of arguments. They note that some design imperfections, such as the imbalance between groups that occurs with cluster randomization, were fully expected at the outset and are a necessary compromise in conducting population-based

[2]Although this chapter is based on a review of evidence available in February 2001, this review was published in October 2001 as a follow-up to a January 2000 article. It is given special attention here because of the questions it has stimulated about the effectiveness of mammography.

screening trials. Other flaws that seem unacceptable by today's standards, such as failure to conceal allocation or lack of blinding, received less attention in prior decades when these trials were designed. Rather than rejecting trials in a formulaic fashion because of the presence of such flaws, groups such as the U.S. Preventive Services Task Force examine whether the biases potentially introduced by these design flaws were of sufficient magnitude, duration, and direction to account for the observed mortality reductions. They concluded that the mortality patterns are more likely attributable to a real effect from mammography than to an artifact from improper study designs (US Preventive Services Task Force, 2002; Humphrey et al., 2002). Others disagree with the very premises that underlie the Danish critique, noting the lack of empirical evidence demonstrating that the types of design flaws of concern to the Danes are more likely to produce invalid data. Others question the appropriateness of using all-cause mortality to judge the merits of a cancer screening test, or the analytical methods used in their meta-analysis (Cates and Senn, 2000; Duffy and Tabàr, 2000; Hayes et al., 2000; Law et al., 2000; Moss et al., 2000; Nyström, 2000; Woolf, 2000b).

Prior to this recent controversy, debates within the scientific community about mammography have historically centered less on whether mammography is effective than on questions about the magnitude of benefit and the proper starting and stopping ages and interval for screening. Controversies about magnitude relate to uncertainties about the relative risk reduction associated with screening (values vary somewhat from one meta-analysis to another) and how this uncertainty impacts estimations of absolute benefit. Even with a relative risk reduction of 20–25 percent, large numbers of women (perhaps 1,000) must be screened to prevent a single death from breast cancer, raising a legitimate question about whether the benefit is of sufficient magnitude to outweigh potential harms (see below).

Since the 1980s there has been controversy regarding the effectiveness of screening mammography for women under age 50. The results for women who were age 40 to 49 at entry into the trials tend to be smaller in magnitude and less statistically significant than results for women ages 50 and older, possibly because the trials were not designed with sufficient statistical power (sample size, length of follow-up) to detect a difference in outcome for this age group. At the frequency with which mammography was conducted in the trials, the mortality benefits that do occur for women ages 40 to 49 appear to be delayed. A clear separation in survival curves suggesting a mortality benefit did not become apparent in most studies until after 8 to 10 years of follow-up, whereas benefits were observed within 4 to 5 years of screening in women ages 50 to 69.

Because of the modest reduction in absolute benefit observed when women ages 40 to 49 were screened, it has been uncertain whether the lower mortality rates observed in this age group are statistically significant or due to chance. For many years, no trial had reported reductions in mortality that were statistically significant for women ages 40 to 49 at the time of screening. Early meta-analyses for this age group also failed to demonstrate statistical significance. The pooled relative risk ratios reported by Kerlikowske and colleagues (1995) and Smart and colleagues (1995) were 0.92 (95 percent CI, 0.75 to 1.13) and 0.84 (95 percent CI, 0.69 to 1.02), respectively, suggesting no significant benefit. A 1993 overview of the data from the Swedish trials for women ages 40 to 49 reported a pooled relative risk ratio of 0.90 (95 percent CI, 0.65 to 1.24) (Nyström et al., 1993). The ratio was 0.91 (95 percent CI, 0.72 to 1.15) when the results were updated through 1997 (Jonsson et al., 2000). A meta-analysis by an Australian team, limited to seven trials, yielded a pooled relative risk ratio of 0.95 (95 percent CI, 0.77 to 1.18) (Glasziou et al., 1995).

In recent years, however, extended follow-up of women who were ages 40 to 49 when they were recruited into the trials and at the start of screening has revealed a delayed separation in survival curves that approaches or achieves statistical significance. This trend was first reported at a 1996 conference in Falun, Sweden (Swedish Cancer Society and the Swedish National Board of Health and Welfare, 1996). In 1997, updates from the Gothenburg and Malmö trials revealed for the first time a statistically significant reduction in the mortality rate for women in this age group. The relative risk ratios were 0.56 (95 percent CI, 0.32 to 0.98) (Bjurstam et al., 1997) and 0.64 (95 percent CI, 0.45 to 0.89) (Andersson and Janzon, 1997), respectively. A meta-analysis incorporating the new data with the results from other clinical trials concluded that the pooled relative risk ratio for women ages 40 to 49 was 0.82 (95 percent CI, 0.71 to 0.95) (Hendrick et al., 1997). Other meta-analyses suggested slightly more modest benefits that bordered on statistical significance, yielding values of 0.84 (95 percent CI, 0.71 to 1.01) (Kerlikowske, 1997), 0.85 (95 percent CI, 0.71 to 1.01) (Glasziou and Irwig, 1997), and 0.85 (95 percent CI, 0.73 to 0.99) (Humphrey et al., 2002). An updated 1997 meta-analysis of the Swedish trials yielded a relative risk of 0.77 (95 percent CI, 0.59 to 1.01) (Larsson et al., 1997).

The estimates presented above rely on subgroup analysis of the cohort aged 40 to 49. The only trial designed specifically to evaluate screening for women ages 40 to 49 was the Canadian National Breast Screening Study. That randomized trial, which assessed the effectiveness of the combination of annual mammography, physical breast examination, and teaching of breast self-examination, initially reported a relative risk ratio of 1.36 (95 percent CI, 0.84 to 2.21) (Miller et al., 1992a), which some interpreted as evidence that screening was harmful. The ratio reported at the latest follow-up was 1.06 (95 percent CI, 0.80 to 1.40) (Miller et al., 2002), supporting an interpretation of no effect.

The design and conduct of the Canadian trial have been criticized. Questions have been raised about the randomization methods, prompted by differences in the baseline characteristics of the study arms (Boyd, 1997; Burhenne and Burhenne, 1993; Tarone, 1995). However, independent investigations have disclosed no evidence that the randomization process was flawed or subverted (Bailar and MacMahon, 1997; Cohen et al., 1996). Critics have also asserted that the physical examination that preceded mammography may have confounded its effects, that the mammographic technique used by some centers was outdated or of poor quality, that the trial lacked statistical power, and that the trial included excess numbers of individuals with advanced disease (Burhenne and Burhenne, 1993; Kopans et al., 1994). Moreover, because patients in the control arm received clinical breast examination (rather than the "usual care" that control arms in other trials received) many have suggested that the trial was less likely to show a benefit, or at least tested a different question than did other mammography screening trials. To provide further evidence, additional trials of screening in this age group are under way or are being considered in Europe and the United States (Forrest and Alexander, 1995; Moss, 1999).

Whether the existing evidence is sufficient to justify routine screening mammography for women ages 40 to 49 has long been a matter of debate (Smith, 2000). Beyond concerns about statistical significance, some question the absolute benefit of screening, given the low prevalence of breast cancer in premenopausal women. Analyses suggest that 1,500 to 2,500 women aged 40 to 49 would require screening mammography for 10 to 15 years to avert 1 death from breast cancer (Berry, 1998; Salzmann et al., 1997). In light of the 8- to 10-year delay in observing a significant separation in survival curves for women who are aged 40 to 49 at the start of screening, some speculate that the benefit does not occur until after age 50 and could be retained if screening was deferred until that age. In the Health Insurance Plan (HIP) trial, for example, all of the decrease in mortality observed among women who began screening at age 45 to 49 occurred among those whose breast cancer was detected at ages 50 to 54 (Shapiro et al., 1982).

For their part, proponents of screening at age 40 to 49 argue that the modest benefit observed in clinical trials is due to limitations in study design. The trials were not designed to test the effectiveness of screening in this age group, recruiting instead a large proportion of older women, and the studies lacked adequate sample sizes and adequate durations of follow-up to detect a difference in this subgroup. They note that the trials used outdated methods (e.g., single views) and screened women too infrequently (e.g., every 2 years) to detect rapidly growing tumors (Feig, 1996). They also emphasize that the age of 50 years is an arbitrary cutoff point that has little biological significance; younger women with certain risk factors face the same absolute risk of breast cancer and may benefit as much from mammography as older women with fewer risk factors (Gail and Rimer,

1998). Indeed, the pooled relative risk reductions in the various meta-analyses reported above suggest that screening mammography reduces mortality by an average of 15–21 percent for women in all age groups, with reductions being smaller on average for younger women (e.g., ages 40 to 49) than for those age 50 and older.

Most of the evidence from screening trials suggests that the effectiveness of mammography is equivalent whether it is performed annually or every 2 years. However, a body of natural history and modeling evidence suggests that an annual interval may be more effective (Boer et al., 1999; Michaelson et al., 1999; Ren and Peer, 2000), especially among women ages 40 to 49. Breast cancer appears to have a shorter mean sojourn time in premenopausal women (Moskowitz, 1986; Tabàr et al., 1995). A greater ratio of interval cancers (cancers that arise between screenings) to total cancers among women ages 40 to 49 may account for the diminished effectiveness of mammography observed in clinical trials, most of which screened women every 18 to 24 months. (Only the American and Canadian trials screened women ages 40 to 49 annually.) The limited number of women of this age in the trials gave the trials inadequate power to conclude whether the difference in relative risk reduction between annual and less frequent screening is statistically significant. Indirect evidence suggests that annual screening might significantly lower the rate of mortality from breast cancer (Feig, 1995) without increasing the frequency with which women are recalled for follow-up imaging studies (Hunt et al., 1999).

Women Age 70 and Older Data from studies that have evaluated the effectiveness of screening of older women for breast cancer are lacking because most trials enrolled women younger than age 69. The Swedish Two-County Trial, in which women up to age 74 were enrolled for screening, reported a 32 percent reduction in the rate of mortality from breast cancer (95 percent CI, 0.51 to 0.89) for women aged 70 to 74 at the time of randomization (Chen et al., 1995). Modeling studies also support the screening of women over age 65 (Mandelblatt et al., 1992), but beyond age 69 the relative improvement in detecting metastatic cancer may be lower (Smith-Bindman et al., 2000) and the incremental benefit in terms of reduced mortality may be modest (Kerlikowske et al., 1999). Others have argued that the evaluation of incremental benefit should give greater consideration to differences in life expectancy, comorbidities, effects on treatment, and value preferences (Mandelblatt et al., 2000). It is generally held that continued screening is unwarranted in elderly women who have significant morbidities, poor functional status, low bone mineral density (an indicator of low estrogen levels), or an unwillingness to accept the potential harm of screening (Parnes et al., 2001).

Testing for BRCA1 and BRCA2 Mutations

Cloning of the *BRCA1* and *BRCA2* genes has made it possible to identify individuals who carry the mutations for breast cancer susceptibility in the *BRCA1* and *BRCA2* genes. In one British study, carriers of mutations in the *BRCA1* and *BRCA2* genes accounted for 2 percent of breast cancer cases diagnosed before the age of 55 in population-based screening (Anglian Breast Cancer Study Group, 2000). Advances in genetic technology may soon enable testing for other disturbances in molecular pathways to identify women susceptible to breast cancers unrelated to the early-onset familial form (Golub, 2001).

The potential benefits of early identification of genetic susceptibility to breast cancer include the opportunity for earlier or more frequent screening, antiestrogen therapy, prophylactic surgery, and lifestyle modifications (Goodwin, 2000). Because these mutations are also associated with an increased risk of ovarian cancer, the opportunity to consider prophylactic oopherectomy is another potential benefit. There is some evidence that testing influences women's choices. In a Canadian survey of women who tested positive for mutations in the *BRCA1* or *BRCA2* genes, 58 percent indicated that their screening practices had changed, 28 percent had undergone prophylactic mastectomy, and nearly two-thirds were considering prophylactic mastectomy or oopherectomy (Metcalfe et al., 2000). In a Dutch study, 51 percent opted for prophylactic mastectomy (Meijers-Heijboer et al., 2000).

Breast Self-Examination

There is limited evidence regarding the accuracy of breast self-examination. The upper limit of its sensitivity has been estimated at 12 to 25 percent (Fletcher et al., 1993), making it considerably less sensitive than either clinical breast examination or mammography. Its specificity is unknown, but Chinese women instructed in breast self-examination in a large randomized trial (see below) identified 331 cases of breast cancer but also had 1,457 false-positive findings, whereas the control group (which received education about low back pain) found 322 cancers and had 623 false-positive results (Thomas et al., 1997).

There remains little direct evidence that breast self-examination improves the outcomes from breast cancer. A nonrandomized study in the United Kingdom found that two centers at which women were invited to education sessions on breast self-examination had combined mortality rates that were similar to those at control centers, but one of the two centers did have significantly lower death rates (Lancet, 1999).

A randomized trial in Russia sponsored by the World Health Organization is evaluating the effectiveness of the training of small groups in breast self-examination combined with reinforcement techniques. Over 10 years there has been no significant difference in mortality rates, although the intervention group has had more physician visits, referrals, and breast biopsies (Semiglazov et al., 1999). Methodological limitations raise doubts about the ability of this trial to rule out a benefit associated with the intervention. A randomized trial in Shanghai, China, involved 267,040 textile workers in which the intervention group received instruction in breast self-examination and reinforcement interventions. No reduction in mortality was observed at the 5-year follow-up (Thomas et al., 1997).

Harms

The potential harms of screening mammography relate primarily to false-negative and false-positive results (which some define as including detection of cancer of unknown clinical significance such as DCIS). The latter can be especially significant because of the emotional (e.g., anxiety) and physical (e.g., biopsy) implications. Approximately 8 to 12 percent of women who undergo screening mammography must be reevaluated because of abnormal results, which typically entails repeat and more intensive imaging studies (Carney et al., 2000; Paquette et al., 2000; Poplack et al., 2000).

A growing literature has analyzed the psychological impact of this experience. Not surprisingly, women who have had abnormal mammogram results are substantially more worried about getting breast cancer than women who have not had such results (Lipkus et al., 2000a). Although the psychological impact of false-positive results requires further study (Lerman and Rimer, 1995), surveys suggest that after receiving a false-positive result women experience increased anxiety at both short-term and long-term follow-ups and experience added stress when they undergo biopsy (Gilbert et al., 1998; Gram et al., 1990; Lerman et al., 1991b; Lowe et al., 1999; Olsson et al., 1999). In one survey, 41 to 47 percent of women with suspicious mammograms expressed anxiety and worry about breast cancer (Lerman et al., 1991b). In a British study, psychological effects were reported for at least 5 months by 44 to 61 percent of women (Brett et al., 1998). About half of the women with normal mammograms said that the results reduced their fears, but concerns about breast cancer persisted for 28 percent.

These feelings do not appear to dampen interest in future screening. Among American women, having had a false-positive mammogram does not diminish interest in subsequent screening and may even heighten interest (Burman et al., 1999; Pisano et al., 1998b). In one study, women who had had an abnormal mammogram within the 2 years before the interview were more likely to be on schedule for mammography than women who had never had an abnormal mammogram (Lipkus et al., 2000a). Similarly, although moderate to extreme discomfort from mammography was reported by 52 percent of American women, it was not associated with disinterest in future testing (Dullum et al., 2000). A Dutch study reported that 73 percent of women found mammography mildly to severely painful, but only 3 percent indicated that the pain would deter them from future screening (Keemers-Gels et al., 2000).

It has been estimated that for every 1,000 mammographic examinations, between 3 and 42 biopsies are performed to investigate abnormal results (Fletcher et al., 1993). Recall examinations, often with special views, can reduce the need for unnecessary biopsies (Sickles, 2000b). A more recent audit of 36,850 consecutive screening mammographies reported that 1.4 percent of women were biopsied; these women represented approximately 25 percent of all those with abnormal mammograms (Dee and Sickles, 2001). In recent community studies, 22 to 38 percent of biopsy specimens were positive for cancer (Dee and Sickles, 2001; Poplack et al., 2000). At the biopsy rate in the Canadian trial, women have a 10 to 20 percent chance of undergoing biopsy at some time during 5 years of screening by annual mammography and clinical breast examination (Fletcher et al., 1993). The probability of undergoing a biopsy for a false-positive result depends on breast cancer risk factors. The false-positive rate may be higher among younger women and is dependent on other risk factors. In the Stockholm trial, 41 to 56 percent of the costs related to false-positive results occurred in women who were under age 50 when screening began (Frisell and Lidbrink, 1997). In an American study, women ages 40 to 49 having their first mammogram underwent twice as many diagnostic tests per cancer detected compared with the number for women ages 50 to 59 (43.9 versus 21.9 diagnostic tests) (Kerlikowske et al., 1993).

There is no direct evidence that ionizing radiation from mammography causes breast cancer. Given a mean dose to the breast of 0.1 rad during mammography, modeling based on data from studies of higher levels of radiation exposure suggests that 100,000 women screened annually from ages 50 to 75 would lose 12.9 years from radiogenic cancers but would gain 12,623 years from an assumed 20 percent reduction in the rate of mortality from breast cancer (Feig and Ehrlich, 1990). The benefit-risk ratio was narrower in a Swedish model (Mattsson et al., 2000). Other models have estimated that mammography would detect 114 to 815 cancers for every case of cancer that it might induce (Beemsterboer et al., 1998; Law, 1993).

Testing for mutations in the *BRCA1* or *BRCA2* genes introduces complex psychological, medical, social, and legal consequences if women are informed that they are carriers (Fasouliotis and Schenker, 2000; Koenig et al., 1998). A study of a kindred tested for a *BRCA1* mutation reported higher levels of psychological distress (Croyle et al., 1997), but such experiences are not uniform. A prospective study of families that underwent testing for *BRCA* mutations revealed that individuals found to be noncarriers of a mutation reported fewer depressive symptoms and functional impairment and that mutation carriers did not exhibit increased levels of depression; 1 month later, 17 percent of carriers intended to have mastectomies (Lerman et al., 1996). Those who declined the test and who had high baseline levels of cancer-related stress had higher rates of depression at 1 and 6 months of follow-up (Lerman et al., 1998). At 1 year only 3 percent of unaffected carriers of a mutation in the *BRCA1* or *BRCA2* genes had undergone prophylactic mastectomy. Although their mammography rates were higher than those for noncarriers, analysis revealed that this was because noncarriers decreased their rate of adherence to screening (Lerman et al., 2000). Another study reported that women who underwent prophylactic mastectomy had lower levels of psychological morbidity than those who decided not to have prophylactic mastectomy (Hatcher et al., 2001).

The potential harms of genetic screening reach beyond the patient being tested. When women in one survey were asked whether it was appropriate to share genetic test results with family members, 100 percent were supportive if the only option was prophylactic mastectomy, 97 percent were supportive if it was a preventable disease, and 85 percent were supportive if it was a nonpreventable disease (Lehmann et al., 2000). Even if the individual was opposed to sharing the results with family members, 16 to 22 percent of respondents said the physician should seek out and inform the family members against the patient's wishes. A survey of adults in one study revealed that one-fourth would permit testing of children (under age 18) (Hamann et al., 2000). Under such a policy, minors (who are not in a position to choose otherwise) would be preempted from living their lives without knowing their genetic susceptibility, a choice they might make as adults. The ripple effects of genetic testing for mutations in the *BRCA1* and *BRCA2* genes pose formidable challenges to the physician attempting to offer patients informed consent before undergoing such testing (Miesfeldt et al., 2000).

Cost-Effectiveness

A review of economic evaluations of breast cancer screening published through 1997 found that estimates ranged widely. Estimates of the cost per case of cancer detected ranged from $5,226 to $58,331 (Brown et al., 1999). Studies suggest that the cost-effectiveness of screening mammography is within customarily accepted ranges: approximately $16,100 to 21,400 per year of life saved (Leivo et al., 1999; Rosenquist and Lindfors, 1998; Salzmann et al., 1997). Studies in other countries estimate the cost at $3,750 (U.S. dollars) per year of life saved (Wan et al., 2001).

Compared with beginning screening at age 50, however, the incremental cost-effectiveness of beginning screening at age 40 appears to be high, perhaps as much as $105,000 per year of life saved (Salzmann et al., 1997).

The incremental costs of performing mammography annually rather than biennially may also be substantial, especially for older women (Boer et al., 1999). The incremental cost-effectiveness of continuing screening mammography beyond age 69 for women with increased bone mineral density was estimated to be $66,773 per year of life saved (Kerlikowske et al., 1999).

Given certain assumptions, a modeling study estimated that the cost-effectiveness of screening Ashkenazi Jewish women for *BRCA1* and *BRCA2* mutations ranged from $20,717 to $72,780 per year of life saved, depending on which surgical options were selected by carriers, but testing followed only by surveillance was not cost-effective ($134,273 per year of life saved) (Grann et al., 1999).

Subjective Value Judgments

The longstanding controversy about whether mammography screening should begin at age 40 underscores the important role of subjective value judgments in the crafting of screening guidelines. For some time the argument centered on statistical significance because no individual trial or meta-analysis could exclude the possibility that lower mortality rates in that age group were due to chance. The extended follow-up data now available has convinced most analysts that mammography reduces breast cancer mortality in women ages 40 to 49 as well. The *relative* risk reduction is probably slightly less than that observed in women age 50 and older, but not markedly so. The more important distinction between these age groups is the difference in *absolute* benefit. The probability of acquiring breast cancer is much lower for premenopausal women, so that even an equivalent relative risk reduction in both age groups would mean that a much larger number of women would need to be screened to prevent a breast cancer death—that is, the NNS would be higher—than is the case for older women.

Unless one is a payer concerned about costs, a higher NNS is, by itself, an inadequate argument against screening. It is the trade-off between benefits and harms that makes a higher NNS a concern. Weighing that trade-off is made more complicated for younger women because of their higher probability of receiving false-positive results. The precise nature of that trade-off is unclear; estimates of the NNS and the risk of harms for women ages 40 to 49 vary, depending on the data and methods used for the calculation and the risk profile of the woman involved. Several analyses suggest that the NNS to prevent a breast cancer death over 10 years is 1,500 to 2,500, and the risk of follow-up biopsy or surgery during that decade is 8 to 20 percent (Harris and Leininger, 1995; Kerlikowske, 1997; National Institutes of Health, 1997).

Whether this trade-off is worthwhile has no objective answer and is clearly dependent on personal values. Some women, perhaps the majority (Schwartz et al., 2000), would say that the benefits outweigh the risks. Some women might feel otherwise. A consensus panel convened in 1997 by the National Institutes of Health, faced with this evidence, concluded that it was inappropriate to issue a uniform recommendation for all women ages 40 to 49. Instead, it recognized the diversity of women's views and recommended that the choice be individualized for each woman on the basis of "how she perceives and weighs each potential risk and benefit, the values the woman places on each, and how she deals with uncertainty" (National Institutes of Health, 1997, p. 1015). The recommendation ignited a firestorm of controversy, beginning at the conference and followed by harsh criticism in the lay press, a unanimous resolution by the U.S. Senate denouncing the statement, congressional pressure on the National Cancer Institute to take a firm position in favor of screening, and hearings on Capitol Hill. The pressure ultimately culminated in the issuance of guidelines by the National Cancer Institute in favor of screening women beginning at age 40 and an immediate announcement at the White House of expanded Medicare coverage for such screening (Begley, 1997; Taubes, 1997).

Debates of similar intensity erupted more recently in response to the critique of the mammography trials by Gøtzsche and Olsen. Fueled by the prominent attention it received from the news media, organizations and agencies were compelled to take public positions on the importance they assigned to design flaws in trials, stances that ultimately reflected subjective value judgments rather than hard facts. Following the announcement that the Physician's Data Query (PDQ) panel of the National Cancer Institute was also concerned about the design flaws, a dozen professional and cancer advocacy organizations published a full-page advertisement in the *New York Times* to reassure women that guidelines in favor of mammography screening were still in effect, and the National Cancer Institute reaffirmed its 1997 guideline in favor of screening (http://newscenter.cancer.gov/pressreleases/mammstatement31jan02.html). A subsequent editorial in the same newspaper accused the groups of "circling the wagons" and urged an independent review of the evidence by an impartial body (Circling the Mammography Wagons, 2002). When the Secretary of Health and Human Services announced the results of just such a review (the U.S. Preventive Services Task Force completed its 3-year update of its recommendations shortly thereafter), skeptics questioned whether the conclusions had been influenced by politics.

Much has been written in the medical literature about what occurred at the 1997 National Institutes of Health consensus conference (Ernster, 1997; Fletcher, 1997; Kassirer, 1997; Pauker and Kassirer, 1997; Ransohoff and Harris, 1997; Woolf and Lawrence, 1997) and much more will probably be written about the more recent controversy. Concerns that swirl around both incidents include the intrusion of politics into science, the loss of comity by the belligerents in the debate, and the difficult circumstances in which the consensus panel in 1997 and the U.S. Preventive Services Task Force in 2002 were placed. The intensity of the acrimony was amplified by the strong emotions surrounding breast cancer and the powerful agendas of interest groups. Analyses of the disparate perspectives of these parties and the larger policy implications of this controversy are covered elsewhere (Woolf and Dickey, 1999). What underlies these debates are ultimately differences in value judgments. The pivotal decision points for setting policy—e.g., whether design flaws are fatal, the NNS is too high, or benefits outweigh harms—are in many ways matters of opinion.

In the context of this report, it is also worth noting why the 1997 consensus panel's recommendation for shared decision making—a position scientifically justified for the reasons outlined above and consistent with the patient-centered theme appearing in screening guidelines for other cancers issued at the same time by other groups—met with such misfortune. The answer is complex and reflects in part the challenges of satisfying the public desire for clear, explicit guidelines when scientific uncertainty precludes such statements. Some of the resistance stemmed from fundamental discomforts with the entire notion of shared decision making and the tension between "paternalists" and "pluralists" in defining which choice is best (Woolf and Lawrence, 1997).

However, it is also conceivable that nuances in the wording of the recommendation, prepared hurriedly under pressure from the National Institutes of Health to produce a statement within 1 day of hearing the evidence, influenced its reception. A close examination of the recommendation (italics added) reveals the degree to which the language implied that the decision was the patient's rather than a shared decision as the panel intended: "*Each woman should decide for herself* whether to undergo mammography. . . . *Her decision* may be based . . ." (National Institutes of Health, 1997, p. 1015). This wording may have fueled the adverse press coverage, which accused the panel of abdicating its authority and leaving to women the responsibility for a decision that experts could not make.

If the locus of control over decisions is viewed as a continuum, with physician paternalism on one extreme and patients making independent decisions on the other, it is important for guidelines that advocate shared decision making to use precise language that occupies the middle ground. Research indicates that only a small minority of patients, characterized by a high degree of self-empowerment and autonomy, are comfortable at the far extreme and that most patients who want to share decisions prefer a partnership role. The success with which the language used in recent prostate cancer screening guidelines has clarified this role is discussed in the next section of this chapter.

Increasingly evident in the years since the consensus conference is that the risk of breast cancer is not a dichotomous variable in which the need for subjective value judgments exists only before age 50. The artificial demarcation of the age 40 to 49 cohort is an artifact of the recruitment ages in the mammography trials. In reality there is a continuum of risk with advancing age; the probability of benefit increases and the probability of false-positive results decreases as women grow older, and there is nothing distinctive at age 50, other than approximating the age of menopause, that disrupts this pattern (Smith, 2000). Whatever the age, the magnitude of benefit that outweighs the risk is a subjective judgment that varies from woman to woman. If the appropriateness of screening mammography in a 48-year-old women depends on how she weighs the NNS against the risk of a false-positive result, the same is true of a 52-year-old woman; it is only the ratios, and not the need for value judgments, that change with time. As Smith advocated, rather than continuing to focus on women ages 40 to 49 as a distinct cohort, "an alternative and more productive view is that women of all ages need to be fully informed about the benefits and limitations of breast cancer screening" (Smith, 2000, p. 331). This should include elderly individuals, whom studies indicate are significantly less likely to be offered active involvement in decision making about mammography (Burack et al., 2000a).

The presumption in considering personal preferences is that a substantial proportion of women will defer screening because of concerns about false-positive results. The first studies to examine this subject are challenging that premise, suggesting that women are not terribly troubled by the downsides of screening (Cockburn et al., 1999; Schwartz et al., 2000). It is unclear whether these data reflect true preferences, patient overestimation of risk for breast cancer (Lipkus et al., 2000a), the challenges of understanding the meaning of relative and absolute risk reductions (Schwartz et al., 1997), or an artifact of the ways in which questions are framed (Peticolas, 2000). In one survey (Schwartz et al., 2000), women expressed a high degree of tolerance of a 20 percent risk of false-positive results, with 63 percent of women indicating that 500 or more false-positive results per life saved was a reasonable trade-off. Fully 37 percent were willing to tolerate a rate of 10,000 or more false-positive results per life saved. Only 8 percent viewed mammography as potentially harmful, and 62 percent indicated that they did not want to consider false-positive results when deciding about screening.

The challenge of shared decision making lies in ensuring that preferences are expressed on the basis of an accurate understanding of the facts. Software tools have been developed for use in the physician-patient discussion to help women quantify their personal risk of developing breast cancer (Gail and Rimer, 1998). Materials in both English and Spanish are being developed for this purpose (Lawrence et al., 2000). However, the difficulties of presenting probabilistic information in a narrative, numerical, or graphic format will need to be overcome to help women make choices that are grounded in accurate perceptions of likely outcomes.

In response to the renewed controversy surrounding mammography, the National Cancer Institute has formed a Breast Screening Working Group to promote timely examination of issues related to breast screening and to track research progress in these areas (P. Greenwald, Director, Division of Cancer Prevention, personal communication to Roger Herdman, National Cancer Policy Board, March 21, 2002). A subcommittee on mammography and communication issues will focus on approaches to evidence synthesis and communicating the implications of evolving evidence to the public. Other subcommittees will focus on the basic biology of early breast cancers, and new technologies and molecular methods to advance early detection.

Box 5.4 summarizes selected recommendations for breast cancer screening from major organizations.

BOX 5.4 Recommendations for Screening for Breast Cancer

Organization	Recommendations
U.S. Preventive Services Task Force, 2002 (http://www.ahcpr.gov/clinic/3rduspstf/breastcancer/)	The USPSTF recommends screening mammography, with or without clinical breast examination, every 1–2 years for women aged 40 and older. The precise age at which benefits from screening mammography justify the potential harms is a subjective judgment and should take into account patient preferences. The recommendation for women to begin routine screening in their 40s is strengthened by family history of breast cancer having been diagnosed before menopause. The precise age at which to discontinue screening is uncertain. There is insufficient evidence to recommend for or against clinical breast exams or teaching or performing breast self-examination.
American Cancer Society (Smith et al., 2001)	Women should conduct a breast self-examination monthly beginning at age 20, should have a clinical breast examination every 3 years at ages 20 to 39 and annually starting at age 40, and should have annual mammography starting at age 40.
American Academy of Family Physicians, 2000	The standard recommendation is to offer mammography and clinical breast examination every 1 to 2 years for women ages 50 to 69. The guideline is to

continued on next page

	counsel women ages 40 to 49 regarding potential risks and benefits of mammography and clinical breast examination.
American Geriatrics Society Clinical Practice Committee, 2000	Physicians should strongly consider recommending annual or at least biennial mammography until age 75 and biennially or at least every 3 years thereafter, with no upper age limit for women with an estimated life expectancy of 4 or more years. It is recommended that clinical breast examination be performed annually. For women with the manual dexterity or a willing partner to perform (breast self-examination), instruction with annual refreshers during clinical breast examination is recommended. The recommended interval for breast self-examination is monthly.
American College of Obstetricians and Gynecologists, 2000	Low-risk women should have a routine mammography every 1 to 2 years beginning at age 40 and annually beginning at age 50. This supplements annual clinical breast examinations.
American College of Radiology (Feig et al., 1998)	Asymptomatic women age 40 or older should have an annual screening mammography, monthly breast self-examination, and an annual clinical breast examination. Screening mammography before age 40 may benefit women who are at high risk for breast cancer.
National Institutes of Health, 1997	At present, the available data do not warrant a single recommendation for mammography for all women in their 40s. Each woman should decide for herself whether to undergo mammography. Her decision may be based not only on an objective analysis of the scientific evidence and consideration of her individual medical history but also on how she perceives and weighs each potential risk and benefit, the values that the woman places on each, and how she deals with uncertainty.
American College of Preventive Medicine (Ferrini et al., 1996)	There is inadequate evidence for or against screening mammography of women under age 50. Women between ages 50 and 69 should have an annual or biennial, high-quality, two-view mammography. Women ages 70 or older should continue undergoing screening mammography, provided their health status permits breast cancer treatment.
American Society of Clinical Oncology, 1996	Genetic testing for cancer susceptibility should be offered only when (1) the person has a strong family history of cancer (e.g., families with well-defined hereditary syndromes) or very early age of onset of disease, (2) the test can be adequately interpreted, and (3) the results will influence the medical management of the patient or family member.

Prostate Cancer

This part of the chapter on prostate cancer screening examines digital rectal examination and PSA (prostate-specific antigen) testing as screening tests for prostate cancer. Investigational tests of potential usefulness for screening (e.g., testing for the human glandular kallikrein 2 protein) are not discussed (Partin et al., 1999).

Digital Rectal Examination

The digital rectal examination lacks sensitivity for the detection of small tumors (McNeal et al., 1986). By definition, stage A tumors are nonpalpable. The digital rectal examination has a PPV of 15 to 30 percent and a sensitivity of approximately 60 percent. There is little evidence that digital rectal examinations reduce the rate of mortality from prostate cancer. One observational study of digital rectal examination found evidence of benefit (Jacobsen et al., 1998), but several others have reported no effect (Friedman et al., 1991; Gerber et al., 1996; Jacobsen et al., 1998; Richert-Boe et al., 1998) and all have been the target of methodological criticisms (Weiss et al., 1999).

Prostate-Specific Antigen Testing

A PSA concentration greater than 4 nanograms per deciliter (ng/dl) has a sensitivity of up to 80 to 85 percent in detecting prostate cancer (Catalona et al., 1994; Jacobsen et al., 1996). Analyses of archived blood samples suggest that PSA level elevations (and low free PSA ratios [see below]) precede the development of prostate cancer by as much as 13 years before diagnosis (Gann et al., 1995; Parkes et al., 1995; Tibblin et al., 1995; Tornblom et al., 1999). PSA testing appears to be significantly more sensitive for the detection of aggressive prostate cancers than for the detection of nonaggressive (small, well-differentiated) prostate cancers.

PSA testing has limited specificity, producing false-positive results in the presence of benign prostate disease. About 25 to 46 percent of men with benign prostatic hypertrophy have elevated PSA levels (Oesterling, 1991; Sershon et al., 1994). Biological variability and differences among PSA assays can also affect accuracy (Wu, 1994). PSA levels fluctuate by as much as 20 to 30 percent for physiological reasons (Komatsu et al., 1996; Stamey et al., 1995). The specificity of PSA testing is age-related. On the basis of population data from one region in the United States, the specificities of PSA testing are 98, 87, and 81 percent for men ages 50 to 59, 60 to 69, and 70 to 79, respectively (Jacobsen et al., 1996).

In asymptomatic men, the PPV of a PSA level above 4 ng/dl is 28 to 35 percent (Bretton, 1994; Catalona et al., 1991, 1994; Cooner et al., 1990);

that is, roughly two of three men with elevated levels of PSA do not have prostate cancer. The reported PPV when the digital rectal examination is negative is 20 percent (Andriole and Catalona, 1993). It is unclear whether these data can be extrapolated to healthy men screened in clinical practice. Most of the participants in those studies were either patients seen at urology clinics or volunteers recruited from the community through advertising. Such volunteers may not be representative of men in the general population (Demark-Wahnefried et al., 1993). In one PSA screening study, 53 percent of the volunteers had symptoms of prostatism (Catalona et al., 1994).

Recent interest has focused on the incremental benefit of lowering the cutoff for abnormal PSA levels to below 4.0 ng/ml, especially in men with a suspicious digital rectal examination. The increased sensitivity of this change is accompanied by a decreased specificity. In one study of this approach, the PPVs were 5, 14, and 30 percent depending on whether the PSA level was 0.0 to 1.0, 1.1 to 2.5, or 2.6 to 4.0 ng/ml, respectively (Carvalhal et al., 1999a). In another study the PPV of a digital rectal examination and transrectal ultrasound for men with PSA levels below 4.0 ng/ml was 9.7 percent. It was estimated that only 37 percent of prostate cancers were diagnosed by using a cutoff PSA level of 2 to 4 ng/ml (Schroder et al., 2000).

There is little direct evidence regarding the optimal periodicity for performing PSA tests. A cohort study suggested that few curable cancers would be missed in men with PSA levels less than 2.0 ng/ml if screening occurred every 2 years (Carter et al., 1997). Modeling studies suggest that biennial screening is most cost-effective and may reduce the need for biopsies (Etzioni et al., 1999a; Ross et al., 2000).

Other Strategies to Improve PSA Specificity Most research on PSA screening has focused on improving specificity to reduce the probability of false-positive results and unnecessary biopsies. Several approaches have been used. PSA density is the concentration of circulating PSA divided by the gland volume as measured by ultrasound (Bazinet et al., 1994). This measure accounts for the relationship between PSA and prostatic enlargement apart from cancer. A value greater than 0.15 ng/ml^2 may be predictive of cancer (Benson et al., 1992). PSA velocity is the rate of change in PSA levels over time. An increase of at least 0.75 ng/ml within 1 year has a reported specificity of 90 percent in differentiating cancer from benign disease (Carter et al., 1992). PSA cutoff levels can also be defined for specific age and race categories, as PSA levels generally increase with age and are higher in certain racial or ethnic groups (Kalish and McKinlay, 1999; Morgan et al., 1996; Oesterling et al., 1993). Tables that stratify normal PSA levels by the age or the race or ethnicity of the patient have been created. Finally, free PSA is the ratio of the amount of free PSA to the amount of PSA bound to α_1-antichymotrypsin and other moieties (Catalona et al., 1998). A low free PSA ratio (e.g., <25 percent) is more common with prostate cancer than with benign prostatic hypertrophy. Free PSA has garnered much interest in recent years. A cutoff of 15 percent has been reported to be most discriminatory in predicting favorable outcomes (Southwick et al., 1999). Some recommend the use of this ratio for men with total PSA levels of 2.51 to 4 ng/ml to optimize cancer detection and minimize unnecessary biopsies (Catalona et al., 1999b). Assays for the specific moieties to which PSA binds offer promise in further reducing the rates of false-positive results. However, no single approach has yet been proved to be more accurate than the others (Hayek et al., 1999; Wald et al., 2000), although the age-specific PSA level tends to be less sensitive than either free PSA or PSA density (Catalona et al., 2000).

Many cancers detected by testing for PSA (true positives) lack clinical significance. Autopsy studies suggest that 30 percent of men over age 50 have histological evidence of latent prostate cancers that are unlikely to produce symptoms or affect survival (Scardino, 1989; Woolf, 1995). Because of the indolent behavior of most prostate tumors, men are more likely to die of other causes (e.g., coronary artery disease or stroke) before their prostate cancers progress to clinical significance or metastasize. There are methodological challenges to ascertaining the true cause of death of men with prostate cancer (Albertsen, 2000), but one analysis of elderly American decedents known to have prostate cancer reported that 61 percent died of other causes (Newschaffer et al., 2000). Other investigators have reported similar findings (Satariano et al., 1998). Whether screening leads to the overdiagnosis of such cases is controversial. One study estimated that overdiagnosis increased the number of cases by 51 and 93 percent for men screened at ages 60 and 65, respectively (Zappa et al., 1998).

A subset of tumors detected by PSA testing do progress and are fatal. Certain histopathological features provide important clues regarding the likelihood of progression; observational studies and modeling data suggest that advanced tumor grade, stage, and volume increase the probability of progression and metastasis (Chodak et al., 1994; Epstein et al., 1993; Stamey et al., 1999). Gleason scoring is a system used by pathologists to grade cell differentiation of prostate cancers. Patients with Gleason scores of 2 to 4 (well-differentiated cancer) face a 4 to 7 percent probability of dying from prostate cancer within 15 years when treated conservatively, but the mortality rate is 60 to 87 percent when the Gleason scores are 8 to 10 (poorly differentiated cancer) (Albertsen et al., 1998).

The high prevalence of unfavorable histopathological features in tumors detected by PSA testing suggests that PSA-detected cancers might be more clinically important than latent cancers detected on autopsy. Pathological staging of cancers detected through PSA screening and radical prostatectomy reveals extension beyond the prostate capsule, poorly differentiated cells, large gland volumes, and metastases in 31 to 41 percent of PSA-detected patients (Catalona et al., 1993; Epstein et al., 1994a; Humphrey et al., 1996; Mettlin et al., 1994; Smith and Catalona, 1994). Other retrospective studies also report high prevalences of large tumor volumes, extracapsular extension, and positive surgical margins in cancers detected through PSA screening (Scaletscky et al., 1994; Stormont et al., 1993).

Effectiveness of Early Detection

Few studies to date have used randomized controlled designs to test whether screening for prostate cancer reduces rates of morbidity or mortality. One randomized controlled trial of screening has reported preliminary results: Canadian men offered screening were reported to have a 67 percent reduction in the rate of mortality from prostate cancer (Labrie et al., 1999). Critics have expressed concern about the design of the study: men were not randomized to screening but, rather, to receiving a letter of invitation for screening, introducing a potential imbalance in volunteer bias. Substantial crossover occurred between groups, and the investigators did not perform an intention-to-treat analysis. The latter, applied to the available data, suggests no significant reduction in mortality rates (Ruffin, 1999). Other randomized controlled trials of screening are under way in Europe (Schroder et al., 1995) and the United States (Gohagan et al., 2000). The results of these trials will not be available for at least several years, however, leaving only indirect evidence with which to evaluate effectiveness.

Indirect evidence that early detection improves outcome is also limited. Men with localized tumors at diagnosis appear to live longer and have higher 5-year survival rates than those with more advanced disease. Five-year survival rates are 98 to 100 percent for patients diagnosed with localized disease but are only 30 to 32 percent for those diagnosed with distant metastases (Greenlee et al., 2001). Men who undergo PSA screening are more likely to have early-stage tumors at diagnosis (stage shift) (Catalona et al., 1993; Mettlin et al., 1998; Rietbergen et al., 1999). Ongoing screening programs in countries and regions where PSA screening is prevalent report that the proportion of cancers that are clinically or pathologically advanced has been steadily decreasing over time (Farkas et al., 1998; Labrie et al., 1996; Smith et al., 1996a; Spapen et al., 2000). Many have not been persuaded by this evidence, however, because of concerns about lead-time and length biases.

Recent attention has focused on evidence that prostate cancer mortality rates began declining in the United States (Tarone et al., 2000) and Canada (Meyer et al., 1999; Skarsgard and Tonita, 2000) within several years of the introduction of PSA screening. The same pattern has been observed in Olmsted County, Minnesota, where PSA screening has been longstanding (Roberts et al., 1999). Preliminary reports from a province of Austria,

Tyrol, indicate a 42 percent decrease in mortality 5 years after the introduction of PSA screening, although death rates remained unchanged throughout the rest of Austria (Bartsch et al., 2001). Epidemiologists indicate that some (Hankey et al., 1999), but not all (Etzioni et al., 1999b), of this decline may be attributable to PSA screening. A decline so suddenly after the introduction of screening would be unexpected for a cancer known for its long latency. Other potential contributors to these trends (e.g., misclassification of deaths and improved treatment) therefore cannot be excluded (Feuer et al., 1999).

Efficacy of treatment for prostate cancer. The principal treatment options for localized prostate cancer include radical prostatectomy, external beam or interstitial radiation therapy, hormonal treatment, cryosurgical ablation, brachytherapy, and no treatment (expectant management or "watchful waiting"). New and investigational treatments, such as gene therapy, are not reviewed here.

For men with localized prostate cancer, the stage of disease for which screening is intended, there are no results from controlled trials to indicate that any treatment improves survival over watchful waiting. Studies that suggest otherwise tend to be uncontrolled case series (Bagshaw et al., 1994; Catalona and Smith, 1998; Gerber et al., 1996; Hanks et al., 1994, 1995; Lerner et al., 1995; Shipley et al., 1999; Tefilli et al., 1999; Zincke et al., 1994), which suffer from a host of methodological problems. These include the lack of internal control groups (to which another treatment or no treatment was offered), the selection of subjects on clinical grounds that introduce a favorable selection bias, failure to control for confounding, and defining "cure" and progression on the basis of surrogate measures (e.g., PSA levels) rather than hard clinical endpoints. Biochemical failure is an unreliable surrogate for survival (Chodak, 1998; Jhaveri et al., 1999).

Aside from these problems, the survival rates reported from those studies differ little from the expected rates after adjustment for stage and grade of disease. A number of randomized trials have compared the relative benefits of one treatment regimen over another, and to the extent that some have shown benefit, it could be argued that treatment is effective; but most trials rely on intermediate and surrogate outcomes. Some studies do report improved survival with specific treatments (Adolfsson et al., 1993), but the differences typically lack clinical and statistical significance because of confounding variables and wide confidence intervals.

A randomized controlled trial of the effectiveness of treatment was conducted in the United States in the 1970s (Graversen et al., 1990) and found no difference in 15-year survival rates between radical prostatectomy and watchful waiting, but the sample size may have been too small to observe an effect. Larger randomized controlled trials comparing radical prostatectomy with expectant management are under way in Scandinavia

(Johansson, 1994) and the United States (Wilt and Brawer, 1994), but the results will not be available for some years.

Conservative treatment. Enthusiasm about the efficacy of treatment has been dampened by evidence that long-term survival for localized prostate cancer may be good even without treatment. In a widely cited study, Johansson et al. (1997) monitored a population-based cohort of 223 men with prostate cancer who were initially untreated. After a mean follow-up period of 12.5 years, 10 percent had died of prostate cancer and 56 percent had died of other causes (Johansson, 1994). Although regional extension occurred in more than one-third of the patients and metastases occurred in 17 percent, the 15-year disease-specific survival rate was 81 percent (Johansson et al., 1997). By comparison, 10-year survival rates after radical prostatectomy in the United States are 75 to 97 percent for patients with well-differentiated and moderately differentiated cancers and 60 to 86 percent for patients with poorly differentiated disease (Krongrad et al., 1997).

Critics of the Swedish study worry that survival rates were high because of the large proportion of older men with small, well-differentiated tumors (Walsh and Brooks, 1997). Other studies, however, have also reported high 10-year survival rates (74 to 96 percent) in untreated men with palpable but clinically localized prostate cancer (Adolfsson et al., 1994, 1999; Warner and Whitmore, 1994). A retrospective 16-year cohort study of American patients ages 65 to 75 who underwent conservative treatment for localized prostate cancer (either no treatment or hormonal treatment) found that life expectancy was unchanged from that of the general population if the tumor was low grade (Albertsen et al., 1995). However, survival was reduced by 4 to 5 years if the tumor was moderate grade and 6 to 8 years if it was high grade.

Other studies have reported more pessimistic outcomes from conservative therapy. A retrospective study in Sweden reported a disease-specific mortality rate of 50 to 100 percent for patients with conservatively treated localized tumors, but the denominator included only men who had died of prostate cancer (Aus, 1994). The same denominator problem affects other studies reporting high mortality rates with conservative treatment (Borre et al., 1997). A prospective Canadian study reported that 60 percent of men (median age, 75 years) placed in a watchful waiting program had clinical progression (McLaren et al., 1998). A study of Danish men with prostate cancer who survived for at least 10 years reported that it was the direct cause of death in 43 percent of the men (Brasso et al., 1999).

Researchers have attempted to model the natural history of untreated prostate cancer by pooling the results of the studies mentioned above, but the assumptions used in the models are controversial. On the basis of the results of six studies, one model concluded that conservative management (delayed hormone therapy but no surgical or radiation therapy) was associated with 10-year disease-specific survival rates of 87 percent for men with well-differentiated or moderately differentiated tumors and 34 percent for men with poorly differentiated tumors (Chodak et al., 1994). For patients alive after 10 years, the probabilities of having metastatic disease were 19, 42, and 74 percent for those with well-, moderately, and poorly differentiated cancers, respectively. Critics of the analysis disagree with the study's probability estimates (Catalona, 1994; Scardino et al., 1994).

An older review using pooled data from 144 articles estimated that the annual risks of metastasis and death from untreated prostate cancer were low (1.7 and 0.9 percent, respectively) (Wasson et al., 1993). That study has been criticized for including a large proportion of patients with well-differentiated tumors and those receiving early androgen deprivation therapy (Walsh, 1993). A different review calculated higher annual rates of metastasis and death (2.5 and 1.7 percent, respectively), but that analysis was limited to studies of patients with palpable, localized cancers and excluded cancers found incidentally at prostatectomy (Adolfsson, 1993).

Harms

Screening all men age 50 and older in the United States (35 million persons) would expose a large population to potential harms. Both false-positive and false-negative results commonly occur with PSA screening. On the basis of the reported PPV of 20 to 35 percent (see above), two to four men with abnormal results on routine PSA screening will not have cancer for every man who does. These individuals must generally return for one or more repeat PSA measurements and rectal examinations or more invasive testing (e.g., ultrasound and fine-needle biopsy) to rule out cancer. If PSA levels are suspicious, one or more biopsies may be required. In one recent study, approximately 75 percent of the men who underwent biopsy did not have cancer (Naughton et al., 2000a). As with breast cancer, the psychological morbidity that may occur while the patient awaits the possibility of having cancer may be significant, but fewer studies have been performed on this topic.

Biopsy itself carries its own morbidity. In a large American screening program, needle biopsy was performed for 18 percent of patients screened by digital rectal examination and PSA testing (Catalona et al., 1994). Discomfort from the biopsy procedure is reported by half of men. Patients recall more pain 2 and 4 weeks after the procedure than immediately after the biopsy (Naughton et al., 2000b). The standard sextant (6-core) biopsy procedure allows cancers to escape detection, prompting recent interest in obtaining 12 cores, which appears to increase the incidence of hematochezia and hematospermia but which has no incremental adverse effect on quality of life (Naughton et al., 2000b, 2001). Other potential harms include local infection (0.3 to 5 percent of patients), sepsis (0.6 percent of patients), and significant bleeding (0.1 percent of patients) (Aus et al., 1993; Cooner et al., 1990; Desmond et al., 1993; Hammerer and Huland, 1994). One study reported that bacteremia occurred in 16 percent of patients and that 12 percent of patients described dysuria 1 day after the procedure (Lindert et al., 2000).

Published rates of mortality from radical prostatectomy are 0.2 to 2 percent, with lower rates reported at specialized centers or for patients under age 65 (Andriole et al., 1994; Catalona and Avioli, 1987; Kramer et al., 1993; Lu-Yao et al., 1993; Mark, 1994; Murphy et al., 1994; Optenberg et al., 1995; Wasson et al., 1993; Wilt et al., 1999; Zincke et al., 1994). The potential iatrogenic complications of treatment for prostate cancer are substantial. Chief among these are impotence and incontinence, but several other adverse effects are possible. Surgical complications have been reduced to some extent by using bilateral nerve-sparing techniques and by limiting the operation to younger and healthier men; at experienced centers, recovery of erections occurs in 68 percent of preoperatively potent men (with bilateral nerve-sparing surgery), and 92 percent of men regain continence (Catalona et al., 1999a). One such center, at the Washington University School of Medicine, evaluated men at least 1 year after starting treatment and reported that urinary control was a problem for 9 percent. Sexual function was a moderate or major problem for 58 percent of those treated by prostatectomy, 48 percent treated by radiotherapy, 64 percent treated by hormonal therapy, 45 percent treated by cryoablation, and 30 percent treated by observation (Smith et al., 2000). Overall dissatisfaction with treatment, primarily because of urinary dysfunction and bothersome symptoms, was reported by 11 to 21 percent of patients who underwent prostatectomy, 14 percent of those treated with radiotherapy, and 8 percent of those treated by observation (Carvalhal et al., 1999b).

Such outcomes in experienced hands are not always reproducible in normal community practice (Talcott et al., 1997). In a study of 1,291 men, 56 to 66 percent of men who were potent before radical prostatectomy complained of impotence at least 18 months later, and 8 percent were incontinent (Stanford et al., 2000). Other surveys report high complication rates (Shrader-Bogen et al., 1997). An audit of procedures performed from 1986 to 1996 at veterans' hospitals revealed major cardiopulmonary, vascular, and colorectal injury complications in 1.7, 0.2, and 1.8 percent of men, respectively (Wilt et al., 1999). Complication rates are lower in healthier and younger patients (Zincke et al., 1994).

The reported incidences of acute and chronic gastrointestinal complications and genitourinary complications from radiotherapy are 55 to 76 and 11 to 12 percent, respectively (Leibel et al., 1994). Sexual dysfunction is common, with approximately 40 percent of persons who were potent before diagnosis being impotent 24 months later (Hamilton et al., 2001). Comparisons across studies to contrast the relative safety of radical prostatectomy and radiation therapy are generally unreliable because of differences in study design, patient populations, and outcome measures. Patients tend to report more bowel dysfunction with radiation therapy and more sexual dysfunction with radical prostatectomy (Shrader-Bogen et al., 1997). At a median follow-up of 14 years, patients who undergo radiotherapy report worse bladder, bowel, and erectile functions than are reported for men without prostate cancer (Johnstone et al., 2000). A recent study reported that almost 2 years after treatment, men receiving radical prostatectomy were more likely than men receiving radiotherapy to be incontinent and impotent. Radiotherapy produced greater declines in bowel function (Potosky et al., 2000).

Cost-Effectiveness

The widespread performance of PSA testing is costly. A 1995 Canadian study reported screening of all eligible men in Canada would have cost $317 million (Canadian dollars) (Krahn et al., 1999). An older U.S. article claimed 1 year of PSA screening could cost the United States $28 billion (Kramer et al., 1993).

Several cost-effectiveness analyses have been published. One estimated that digital rectal examination and PSA screening at ages 50 to 69 would cost $12,491 to $18,769 per year of life saved (Coley et al., 1997). An analysis from the Medicare perspective by the Office of Technology Assessment of the U.S. Congress estimated that, given favorable assumptions, a one-time digital rectal examination-PSA screening would cost from $14,200 per year of life saved at age 65 to $51,290 per year of life saved at age 75, although the report emphasized that the estimates were highly sensitive to arguable assumptions (U.S. Congress, 1995). Similarly, other analyses have conjectured that screening for prostate cancer would have favorable cost-effectiveness ratios given certain assumptions about benefits and performance characteristics (Benoit and Naslund, 1997; Littrup, 1997). A screening program in Sweden estimated that screening costs about $14,900 per patient (U.S. dollars, 158,000 SEK) (Holmberg et al., 1998). Claims of cost-effectiveness are dubious if the denominator, the magnitude of benefit from screening, is uncertain and if assumptions used in the model are debatable.

Modeling Studies to Weigh Trade-Offs

In contrast to many of the other forms of cancer screening reviewed in this report, investigators studying prostate cancer screening have attempted to use modeling techniques to quantify the influence of subjective value judgments on the weighing of benefits and harms. The models take account of potential harms by adjusting for patient utilities. Older analyses found that screening achieves minor improvements in absolute survival (Love et al., 1985; Thompson et al., 1987), but more recent analyses that adjust for utilities have concluded that screening produces, at best, a modest gain, measured in days to weeks, or a net loss in QALYs (Cantor et al., 1995; Coley et al., 1997; Krahn et al., 1994; Mold et al., 1992). According to those studies, the harmful effects of screening and treatment on quality of life undercut the potential gains in life expectancy, but the assumptions used in the models have been challenged (Miles et al., 1995).

Some modeling studies have compared the relative impacts of different testing protocols. One examined the benefits of conducting screenings less frequently, estimating for a hypothetical population of 1,000 men that annual PSA testing beginning at age 50 would require 10,500 PSA tests, prevent 3.2 deaths, and require 600 biopsies, whereas a policy of PSA testing at ages 40 and 45 years followed by biennial testing beginning at age 50 would require 7,500 PSA tests, prevent 3.3 deaths, and require 450 biopsies (Ross et al., 2000).

Other decision analyses have focused on treatment. An analysis for men aged 60 to 75 concluded that treatment increases quality-adjusted survival by less than 1 year (in most cases, by less than 0.2 QALY) compared with observation (Fleming et al., 1993). For men over age 70 and younger men with well-differentiated disease, treatment appeared to be more harmful than watchful waiting. Critics of the analysis questioned the probabilities for certain components of the model and the inclusion of a relatively older population of men with low-volume and low-grade tumors (Beck et al., 1994; Walsh, 1993). The investigators emphasize that the data were adjusted for age and tumor grade. Other studies also concluded that radical prostatectomy and radiation therapy produce a net decrease in quality of life, even after adjusting for prevalence rates for sexual and urinary dysfunction (Litwin et al., 1995). Although some patients are willing to risk these complications of treatment, others do not believe that the risks are justified. In one study, 26 percent of patients (mean age, 66 years) indicated a preference for expectant management over surgery, even if the latter would extend life by 10 years (Mazur and Merz, 1996).

Subjective Value Judgments

Given the lack of direct evidence about the benefits of early detection, the uncertainty about complication rates, and the indefinite implications of modeling studies, the ultimate judgment of whether benefits outweigh harms remains subjective (Woolf and Rothemich, 1999). Physicians who weigh the trade-offs are affected by personal beliefs about the intuitive benefits of early detection, clinical training and experience, practice norms, patients' expectations, insurance coverage, and medicolegal concerns. Many clinicians feel compelled to screen patients for prostate cancer to protect themselves against litigation and damages should patients later develop prostate cancer.

However, what is best for the individual patient depends on personal preferences, subjective values, and individual risks (Woolf, 1997a,b). A man's fears, lifestyle plans, and priorities dictate whether the balance of benefits and harms is favorable. These issues received little attention in the early 1990s, when PSA screening guidelines first emerged, and organizations assumed polar positions on whether men should receive the test. Groups on one extreme recommended that all men uniformly undergo screening (American College of Radiology, 1991; American Urological Association, 1992; Mettlin et al., 1993), and opposing groups argued against routine screening (U.S. Preventive Services Task Force, 1989). Most guidelines now take account of the importance of patient preferences (Box 5.5). The move toward a policy of shared decision making has subdued the heated controversy that once characterized guidelines on this topic and is giving way to an emerging consensus around a patient-centered approach. The shift in policy began to occur in 1997 when the American College of Physicians, a group previously associated with its resistance to prostate cancer screening, recommended that the physician "describe the potential benefits and known harms of [prostate] screening . . ., listen to the patient's concerns, and then *individualize the decision to screen*" (American College of Physicians, 1997, p. 482) (italics added). In 1998, the American Academy of Family Physicians adopted a similar policy (American Academy of Family Physicians, 1998), advising that physicians "counsel [men] regarding the known risks and uncertain benefits of screening for prostate cancer" (American Academy of Family Physicians, 2000, p. 14). In 2000, the American Urological Association, once the staunchest advocate of routine screening, stated that "early detection of prostate cancer should be *offered*" and emphasized in its 2000 practice policy that "the decision to use PSA for the early detection of prostate cancer should be individualized. Patients should be informed of the known risks and the potential benefits" (American Urological Association, 2000, p. 271). The 2001 guidelines of the American Cancer Society state that "the PSA test and the digital rectal examination should be *offered*. . . . Information should be provided to patients about benefits and limitations of testing. Specifically, prior to testing, men should have an opportunity to learn about the benefits and limitations of testing for early prostate cancer detection and treatment" (Smith et al., 2001, pp. 42–43).

Referring to the controversy surrounding the National Institutes of Health consensus conference statement on breast cancer screening, the absence of a similar phenomenon for prostate cancer screening and the likely role that language has played in the acceptability of the prostate cancer screening policy are worth noting. The organizations' consistent advice that physicians "offer" choices to patients conveys a sense of partnership and

BOX 5.5 Recommendations for Screening for Prostate Cancer

Organization	Recommendations
American Cancer Society (Smith et al., 2001), pp., 42–43	The PSA test and the digital rectal examination should be offered annually beginning at age 50 to men who have a life expectancy of at least 10 years. Men at high risk should begin testing at age 45. Information should be provided to patients about the benefits and limitations of testing. Specifically, before testing, men should have an opportunity to learn about the benefits and limitations of testing for early prostate cancer detection and treatment. High-risk men (men of sub-Saharan African descent or with a first-degree relative with a diagnosis of prostate cancer at a young age) should begin testing for early prostate cancer detection at age 45. The digital rectal examination should be included whenever appropriate.
American Urological Association, 2000, p. 271	Early detection of prostate cancer should be offered to asymptomatic men age 50 or older with an estimated life expectancy of more than 10 years. It is reasonable to offer testing at an earlier age to men with defined risk factors, including men with a first-degree relative who has prostate cancer and African-American men.
American Academy of Family Physicians, 2000	As a guideline, for men ages 50 to 65, counsel them regarding the known risks and uncertain benefits of screening for prostate cancer.

places the locus of control at a more moderate position in the continuum of control than did the National Institutes of Health consensus conference's reference to the "woman's decision" about mammography.

Guidelines that individuals use to make decisions about their personal choices about prostate cancer screening differ in important respects from the guidelines that governments and policy makers for health plans must use to make decisions for populations of individuals (Woolf, 1997b; Woolf and Rothemich, 1999). Which way the scales tip for a population depends on the average utilities of men as a whole. Although some men favor screening, modeling studies that incorporate the full distribution of men's utilities, cited above, suggest that screening decreases QALYs. Population policy also requires consideration of resources: whether it is appropriate to invest in screening, especially for an intervention of uncertain effectiveness and safety, if it comes at the expense of other services.

Policy positions opposing routine screening of the population for prostate cancer have therefore been issued in the United States by the U.S. Preventive Services Task Force (1996) and the Office of Technology Assess-

American College of Preventive Medicine (Ferrini and Woolf, 1998), p. 84	The American College of Preventive Medicine recommends against routine population screening by digital rectal examination and for PSA. Men age 50 and older with a life expectancy of greater than 10 years should be given information about the potential benefits and harms of screening and the limits of current evidence and should be allowed to make their own choice about screening, in consultation with their physician, on the basis of personal preferences.
American College of Physicians, 1997, p. 482	Rather than screening all men for prostate cancer as a matter of routine, physicians should describe the potential benefits and known harms of screening, diagnosis, and treatment; listen to the patient's concerns; and then individualize the decision to screen.
U.S. Preventive Services Task Force, 1996, p. 129[a]	Routine screening for prostate cancer by digital rectal examination, evaluation for serum tumor markers (e.g., PSA), or transrectal ultrasound is not recommended. Patients who request screening should be given objective information about the potential benefits and harms of early detection and treatment. If screening is to be performed, the best-evaluated approach is to screen by digital rectal examination and for PSA and to limit screening to men with a life expectancy of greater than 10 years.

[a]The USPSTF guidelines on prostate cancer screening are being updated.

ment (U.S. Congress, 1995), as well as in Canada (Canadian Task Force on the Periodic Health Examination, 1994), the United Kingdom (Morris, 1997), Sweden (Swedish Council on Technology Assessment in Health Care, 1996), and Australia (Australian Health Technology Advisory Committee, 1996). For reasons that are too extensive to outline in this report, such positions are not inconsistent with the clinical recommendations presented above that each man should decide for himself whether to be screened (Woolf, 1997b).

A factor that influences the balance of benefits and harms at the societal level is the cascade effect of screening on stimulating inappropriate procedures. For example, the dramatic escalation in PSA screening in the United States in the early 1990s was accompanied by a striking increase in the performance of radical prostatectomies (Lu-Yao and Greenberg, 1994; Wilt et al., 1999). Many of these operations, especially the large number performed on men over age 75, may not have been indicated. A similar phenomenon is becoming apparent in other countries, such as the Netherlands (Spapen et al., 2000) and Australia (Ansari et al., 1998).

Cervical Cancer

This section of the chapter reviews the Pap (Papanicolaou) smear and adjunctive technologies that can be used to improve the accuracy of detection of cervical cancer. Alternative screening strategies, such as testing for human papillomavirus (HPV), testing for molecular biomarkers (e.g., fluorescent immunochemical labeling) (Patterson et al., 2001), and cervicography, are not reviewed.

Pap Smear

A fundamental difficulty in the evaluation of screening tests for cervical cancer is the lack of reliability of the reference standard: cytological and histological interpretation of cervical specimens. Even among expert pathologists, interobserver variations in interpreting atypical squamous cells of undetermined significance and low-grade squamous intraepithelial lesions are substantial (Stoler and Schiffman, 2001).

A principal limitation of the Pap smear is its poor sensitivity. A recent meta-analysis calculated that the sensitivity and specificity of the Pap smear were 51 percent (95 percent CI, 37 to 66 percent) and 98 percent (95 percent CI, 97 to 99 percent), respectively (Agency for Health Care Policy and Research, 1999). False-negative results are due to both sampling errors (in obtaining the sample from the cervix and in cell collection and cell preparation techniques) and interpretation errors, with the latter accounting for about one-third of false-negative results. Efforts to improve sensitivity have included the introduction of the cytobrush, broom brushes, and plastic spatulas to gain better access to the squamocolumnar junction and endocervix. Other measures have been programmatic, such as federal legislation mandating manual reexamination of a portion of negative slides under the Clinical Laboratory Improvement Amendments.

Adjunctive Technologies

New technologies have been introduced in recent years to improve the sensitivity and specificity of screening. These include thin-layer cytology (ThinPrep), computerized rescreening neural network technology (Papnet), and algorithm-based computer rescreening (AutoPap). Although these innovations offer the promise of improving the sensitivity and specificity of screening, a systematic review by the Agency for Health Care Policy and Research concluded that existing data for making comparisons were inadequate to reach conclusions about their incremental impacts on health outcomes (Agency for Health Care Policy and Research, 1999). Coupling Pap smears with screening for HPV infection has also been advocated, but testing for HPV plays a larger role (including the evaluation of cervical atypia) that is beyond the scope of this review.

Following introduction of the Pap smear by Papanicolaou in the 1930s, experience has revealed a consistent association between the routine use of cervical smears for cytological examination and lower rates of mortality from cervical cancer. Virtually all evidence of a benefit in terms of a lower rate of mortality is observational rather than from experimental trials. The consistency of the evidence is impressive, however, with evidence coming from studies conducted over time, ecological studies, cross-national comparisons, and case-control studies. A body of literature suggesting a 20 to 60 percent relative reduction in mortality rates has been reviewed by the U.S. Preventive Services Task Force (1996).

Harms

There are no direct harms from cervical cancer screening aside from the inconvenience, discomfort, and embarrassment that may accompany the examination procedure. The principal harms relate to the consequences of false-positive and false-negative results. As with other screening tests, psychological harms are a potential concern. In one study, 3 months after a positive Pap smear result, women were significantly more worried about cancer and had greater impairments in mood, daily activities, interest in sexual activity, and sleep patterns (Lerman et al., 1991a). Other studies have also reported an association between a positive Pap smear result and adverse emotional reactions, fears of cancer, decreased sexual function, social dysfunction, and feelings of unattractiveness (Khanna and Phillips, 2001). False-positive results also incur the inconvenience of follow-up reexaminations and colposcopic procedures. False-negative results introduce the risk of failing to detect interval dysplasia and cancer and underlie concerns about the need for frequent screening.

Periodicity of Screening

Although many physicians recommend an annual interval for Pap smears, there is little evidence to suggest that it confers greater benefit than screening every 2 or 3 years. A collaborative study of screening programs in eight countries, published in 1986 by the International Agency for Research on Cancer, shed considerable light on the incremental benefit of frequent screening. The analysis clarified the limited difference in the protection afforded by screening every year compared with that afforded by screening every 3 years. Relative to no screening at all, the protection afforded by screening was many-fold greater than no screening, across a wide range of screening intervals. Relative to no screening at all, screening at intervals less than one year offered about 15-fold protection, at intervals between 1–2 years about 12-fold protection, and at intervals of 2–3 years about 8-fold protection (IARC Working Group on Evaluation of Cervical Cancer Screening Programmes, 1986).

More recent insights have been gained from a large prospective cohort study of 128,805 women at community-based clinics throughout the United States who were screened for cervical cancer within 3 years of normal smears (Sawaya et al., 2000a). It documented that the yield of screening is relatively low (for high-grade squamous intraepithelial lesions or lesions suggestive of squamous cell carcinoma, the incidence per 10,000 women was 66 for women under age 30, 22 for women ages 30 to 49, 15 for women ages 50 to 64, and 10 for women ages 65 and older). Moreover, the incidence rate did not differ significantly on the basis of the frequency of screening: 25/10,000 for screening at 9 to 12 months, 29/10,000 for screening at 13 to 24 months, and 33/10,000 for screening at 25 to 36 months. In previously screened postmenopausal women, in whom the incidence of new cytological abnormalities was low, the PPV of an abnormal smear was zero 1 year after a normal smear and 0.9 percent within 2 years. On the basis of this evidence, the investigators concluded that cervical smears should not be performed for postmenopausal women within 2 years of normal cytological results (Sawaya et al., 2000b).

Cost-Effectiveness

A variety of studies document that cervical cancer screening has acceptable cost-effectiveness ratios compared with those for no screening (Agency for Health Care Policy and Research, 1999). In one analysis, the cost-effectiveness ratios for screening every 1 or 3 years were $7,345 and $2,254 per year of life saved, respectively, and cost savings seemed likely if screening was targeted to women who have not had regular screenings (Fahs et al., 1992). Several analyses have cast doubt on the incremental cost-effectiveness of computerized rescreening versus conventional cytological evaluation (Meerding et al., 2001; Troni et al., 2000). The imprecision of the available data makes it inappropriate to draw conclusions about the relative cost-effectiveness of these modalities (Agency for Health Care Policy and Research, 1999), but the ratios tend to be more favorable if screening is less frequent. For example, in one analysis, annual use of the AutoPap cytology smear was estimated to cost $166,000 per year of life saved, whereas use of AutoPap every 4 years cost $7,777 per year of life saved (Brown and Garber, 1999). Some have cautioned that the resources expended to pay for these adjunctive technologies could compromise the delivery of cervical cancer screening to high-risk groups (Sawaya and Grimes, 1999).

Box 5.6 summarizes the cervical cancer screening recommendations of selected organizations.

BOX 5.6 Recommendations for Screening for Cervical Cancer

Organization	Recommendations
American Cancer Society (Smith et al., 2001), p. 40	All women who are or who have been sexually active or who have reached age 18 should have an annual Pap test and pelvic examination. After a woman has had three or more consecutive satisfactory normal annual examinations, the Pap test may be performed less frequently at the discretion of the physician.
American College of Obstetricians and Gynecologists, 2000	Women should have a pelvic examination and Pap smear every year beginning at age 18 or earlier if she is sexually active. If the patient is at low risk, testing may be continued periodically at the discretion of the physician and the patient after three consecutive normal tests.
American Academy of Family Physicians, 2000	The standard is to offer a Pap smear at least every 3 years.
U.S. Preventive Services Task Force, 1996, p. 112	Regular Pap tests are recommended for all women who are or who have been sexually active and who have a cervix. Testing should begin at the age when the woman first engages in sexual intercourse. Adolescents whose sexual history is thought to be unreliable should be presumed to be sexually active at age 18. There is little evidence that annual screening achieves better outcomes than screening every 3 years. Pap tests should be performed at least every 3 years. There is insufficient evidence to recommend for or against an upper age limit for Pap testing, but recommendations can be made on other grounds to discontinue regular testing after age 65 in women who have had regular previous screening in which the smears have been consistently normal. There is insufficient evidence to recommend for or against routine cervicography or colposcopy screening for cervical cancer in asymptomatic women, nor is there evidence to support routine screening for HPV infection. Recommendations against such screening can be made on other grounds, including poor specificity and costs.
American College of Preventive Medicine (Hawkes et al., 1996	Screening for cervical cancer by regular Pap tests should be performed for all women who are or who have been sexually active and should be instituted after a woman first engages in sexual intercourse. If the sexual history is unknown or is considered unreliable, screening should begin at age 18. At least two initial screening tests should be performed 1 year apart. For women who have had at least two normal annual smears, the screening interval may then be lengthened at the discretion of the patient and physician after considering the presence of risk factors, but it should not exceed 3 years. Screening may be discontinued at age 65 if the following criteria are met: the woman has been regularly screened, has had two satisfactory smears, and has had no abnormal smears within the previous 9 years.

SUMMARY AND CONCLUSIONS

The intuitive notion that early detection saves lives is supported by scientific evidence for some cancers. As detailed in this chapter, studies demonstrate that screening for colorectal, breast, and cervical cancer significantly lowers cancer mortality rates. For other cancers, however, the evidence is less direct. Although screening increases the likelihood that cancer will be diagnosed at an early stage, when survival rates are generally higher than those for individuals with advanced-stage disease, these findings do not necessarily prove that screening improves outcomes because of potential statistical artifacts (e.g., length and lead-time biases). Doubts about the value of screening grow even stronger when the available treatment options appear to be of limited efficacy and are unable to alter the natural progression of the disease.

Given the alarming death toll from cancer, many would argue that the mere possibility of benefit from screening offers sufficient grounds for moving forward, even in the absence of scientific certainty. However, screening can itself be harmful. A substantial proportion of a population that is screened for cancer can receive false-positive or false-negative results (depending on the accuracy of the test), and this misinformation can set off a cascade of adverse physical and emotional health consequences. Even for those in whom cancer is accurately diagnosed, the incremental benefit of early detection may be outweighed by the side effects and complications of treatment.

The monetary costs of screening, which can be substantial, may be offset by the savings achieved through early detection, but quantifying the health gains achieved per dollar invested in screening requires evidence that screening produces health gains. Determining whether resources spent on screening are wise investments are concerns not only of insurance companies and other third-party payers but also of society at large. This is an era in which escalating health care costs and the mounting pressures on service delivery are stretching the capacities of the U.S. health care system to the point of compromising quality (Institute of Medicine, 2001c) and threatening patient safety (Institute of Medicine, 2000e). Under such conditions it is reasonable to examine whether resources spent on screening tests of uncertain benefit would save more lives and achieve greater health gains if they were invested in health care services for which effectiveness is more certain.

Health care organizations, government agencies, advocacy organizations, and expert panels have struggled for decades with these issues in deciding what constitutes prudent policy and guidelines for cancer screening. Groups that develop such guidelines approach these issues from different perspectives—depending on their audiences, methods of developing guidelines, and the importance that they place on supporting scientific evidence (Woolf and George, 2000; Woolf et al., 1996)—and have reached different conclusions about who should be screened, how often, and by which tests (see Boxes 5.3 to 5.6).

Despite these inconsistencies, however, a core consensus has emerged about the appropriateness of certain types of cancer screening. There is essentially universal agreement across organizations that all adults age 50 and older should be screened for colorectal cancer, that all women should receive mammograms every 1 to 2 years beginning at least by age 50 (some say age 40), and that all sexually active women with a cervix should be screened regularly for cervical cancer. Of course, controversies about cancer screening persist, the details of which receive some attention in this report and are dissected in detail elsewhere (U.S. Preventive Services Task Force, 1996). The debate over whether men should routinely receive the PSA test symbolizes such controversies. A case study describing efforts to screen individuals for lung cancer, first using chest radiography and more recently using low-dose spiral computed tomography (CT), is presented in Chapter 7 to illustrate the dilemma of adoption of a new screening technology in the face of uncertain science.

From a public health perspective, the disturbing paradox is that the cancer screening tests for which there is a core consensus are not being administered to a large proportion of the Americans for whom they are recommended. Upward trends in the proportion of Americans receiving recommended cancer screening tests are heartening, but disparities in screening by socioeconomic status are substantial, many individuals are tested too late to obtain the full benefits of early detection, they are tested incorrectly, or their results receive inadequate follow-up. Chapter 6 examines the size of this gap and reviews evidence regarding potential strategies to improve the delivery of cancer screening services.

6

Improving Participation in Cancer Screening Programs[1]

Screening programs can effectively reduce the burden of cancer if they ensure that people get the tests that they need and that tests are performed accurately, are not conducted too often, and are followed up in a timely and appropriate manner. The principal challenges to optimizing the delivery of effective cancer screening services and reducing inappropriate testing lie in changing the behaviors of (1) systems of care, to make cancer screening services available to eligible populations; (2) health care providers, to perform cancer screening as recommended, on time, and with skill when they encounter patients eligible for screening; and (3) individuals, to obtain recommended screening tests and pursue follow-up tests. This chapter describes the major challenges to delivering cancer screening and reviews the literature to identify interventions that are successful in improving rates of participation in screening. Although there is a fairly extensive literature on barriers to access to screening, less is known about ways to optimize the delivery of screening to ensure quality and cost-effective testing. Resources can be wasted and harm can be done if screening is delivered badly, and more research is needed to assess ways to ensure quality in screening programs.

---

[1]This chapter is based on a background paper prepared by Steven H. Woolf. Additional references were drawn from two other background papers commissioned for this report, the first by Edwin B. Fisher, Ross C. Brownson, Amy A. Eyler, Debra L. Haire-Joshu, and Mario Schootman, and the second by Judith Ockene, Jane Zapka, Lori Pbert, Suzanne Brodney, and Stephenie Lemon (www.iom.edu/ncpb).

CHALLENGES FOR SYSTEMS OF CARE

One fundamental barrier to cancer screening imposed by the structure of the U.S. health care system is that a large proportion of the eligible population lacks access to health care. The policy issues surrounding the amelioration of the current situation in which some 39 million Americans (14 percent of the population) lack some type of health insurance are beyond the scope of this report, but the situation clearly constitutes a fundamental obstacle to optimizing the potential of cancer screening in the United States (http://www.census.gov/Press-Release/www/2001/cb01-162.html).

Even among persons with health insurance, the private payers and governmental programs that finance health care services face economic barriers to offering coverage for cancer screening. For payers and employer benefits managers, monetary costs pose an impediment to offering coverage for cancer screening, as they do for many other health care services, although the literature suggests that their cost-effectiveness ratios generally fall within affordable ranges. Managed care plans, whose members often remain enrolled for an average of just a few years, may be reluctant to extend coverage to screening tests with high up-front costs. Public insurance programs, such as Medicare and Medicaid, face similar concerns and statutory restrictions against covering prevention services, although the latter have been less of a concern in recent years. Between 1965 and 1990, the U.S. Congress introduced 453 bills proposing coverage for prevention services under Medicare, but the first prevention service was not covered until 1980 (Schauffler, 1993).

Developments in recent years have shifted payer policy toward more extensive coverage for cancer screening tests, making insurance coverage less of an impediment to screening than it was as recently as one decade ago. In addition, the competitive marketplace of private health insurance and the public's interest in obtaining preventive care have made coverage of cancer screening a potent marketing tool, with coverage of cancer screening heavily promoted by the managed care industry, thereby providing an infrastructure for the delivery of cancer screening services. In fact, at least some studies suggest that patients who belong to health maintenance organizations are more likely to receive cancer screening tests than those covered by indemnity plans (Phillips et al., 2000; Gordon et al., 1998; Hsia et al., 2000).

Data from the Health Plan Employer Data and Information Set (HEDIS) reported to the National Committee for Quality Assurance reflect the successes of this infrastructure in the delivery of cancer screening at 273 organizations (health maintenance organizations, point-of-service plans, and other managed care plans) that collectively cover 63 million Americans. In 2000 these organizations reported that 76 percent of their female members aged 52 to 69 had received a mammogram within the past 2 years and that 80 percent of women aged 21 to 64 had received at least one Pap test during the past 3 years (National Committee for Quality Assurance, 2001).

Coverage of prevention services has expanded under Medicaid and Medicare, with the latter now covering annual mammography beginning at age 40, Pap smears and pelvic examinations, prostate cancer screening (annual digital rectal examination and prostate-specific antigen [PSA] testing), and screening for colorectal cancer (annual fecal occult blood testing [FOBT] and flexible sigmoidoscopy every 4 years). This coverage has important policy implications for Medicare, whose 39 million beneficiaries make it the largest health insurance plan in the United States. Its coverage of colorectal cancer screening was recently expanded to include colonoscopy every 10 years, with barium enema covered as a substitute for either sigmoidoscopy or colonoscopy (see Chapter 9 for further discussion of the screening services covered by Medicare and Medicaid).

The coverage policies of the Medicare program appear to influence screening rates. When coverage for biennial mammography was offered beginning in 1991, it was followed by increased mammography use, at least among women with access to a usual source for primary care (Kelaher and Stellman, 2000). Similar influences are noted through initiatives at the state level. As of 2000, 43 states and the District of Columbia mandated coverage of cancer screening, even though the provisions of the mandates were not always in compliance with evidence-based guidelines (Rathore et al., 2000). Federal legislation establishing a national program for breast and cervical cancer screening services has had some salutary effects on screening rates (Lillquist, 2001).

Legislative and regulatory efforts by government and professional organizations have also focused on enhancing the quality with which screening tests are delivered to ensure that they are performed well and interpreted accurately and to ensure that patients receive appropriate follow-up. For example, the Mammography Quality Standards Act of 1992 (PL 102-539) seeks to improve the performance standards of mammographic facilities (Monsees, 2000). In 1999, the act was amended to require that mammographers send a written summary of findings directly to patients in terms easily understood by laypersons. The American College of Radiology maintains detailed standards for the performance of screening mammography (American College of Radiology, 2000) and has established the National Mammography Database, an effort to improve the quality of mammography through a reporting system for breast imaging facilities, regions, and states (www.acr.org/departments/stand_accred/nmd-intro.html).

Local and regional factors influence successes and failures in the delivery of cancer screening. For example, a major concern about making colonoscopy the preferred screening test for colorectal cancer is that some communities and regions lack an adequate supply of gastroenterologists to absorb the volume; therefore, unqualified examiners may offer screening services and thereby increase the risk of complications. Communities struggling with the stresses of poverty, poor housing, inadequate jobs, domestic stresses, and crime have residents with urgent priorities that compete with cancer screening. The absence of public transportation, of social service agencies to support disadvantaged and non-English-speaking individuals, and of community health centers, free clinics, and public health departments impose added barriers to access to cancer screening. In attempting to correct the problem, communities face a variety of barriers, including state and local budget constraints and political dynamics.

Finally, the systems of care that deliver cancer screening within the community—primary care offices, clinics, emergency departments, urgent care centers, integrated health care delivery systems, hospitals, and institutions that provide long-term care—encounter a variety of operational barriers in delivering effective health care services that are too broad to review here. The systems that clinicians need to deliver effective cancer screening (see below) depend on supportive management structures; efficient patient-flow procedures; and information systems that support reminder systems, documentation of screening, timely follow-up and referrals, and coordinated communication with providers and institutions across the community. Some providers have succeeded in establishing such systems. Approximately 50 percent of capitated medical groups and independent practice associations in California mail patients reminders for mammography and Pap testing (Malin et al., 2000). The financial, organizational, and technological barriers that health systems face in making such reconfigurations are formidable and are the subject of a recent report by the Institute of Medicine (2001c).

CHALLENGES FOR INDIVIDUALS

Whether an individual is a physician or a patient, improvements in cancer screening practices (and most other changes in behavior) require a series of steps well known to psychologists. The four steps include knowledge, attitudes, ability, and reinforcement (Woolf, 2000a). The relevance of this framework is illustrated by considering how they result in changes in the behaviors of clinicians and patients.

Challenges for Clinicians

Knowledge

Clinicians do not promote or perform screening tests without the basic prerequisite of knowing that such screening is recommended and appropriate. Many studies have shown that simply disseminating a guideline is, for a variety of reasons, an inadequate means to change practice behavior (Bero et al., 1998; Davis et al., 1992). For one, physicians may not see the guideline or retain its recommendations. Studies confirm that physicians tend to have limited familiarity with published practice guidelines, especially recent ones. A 1995 survey found that baseline mammograms, a practice no longer recommended, were still being ordered for women ages 30 to 39 (Reifel et al., 1998).

Physicians' knowledge of practice guidelines tends to be uneven across organizations. The American Cancer Society guidelines on cancer screening, which were first issued in 1980 (ACS, 1980a), tend to be the most well known by physicians and the general public (Hamblin and Connor, 1998). When primary care physicians in Colorado were surveyed about the influence of guidelines on their screening practices for prostate cancer, 89 percent rated the American Cancer Society guidelines as moderately or highly influential, whereas fewer than one-third rated the guidelines of the U.S. Preventive Services Task Force as moderately or highly influential (Moran et al., 2000). A clear understanding of what is recommended is made more difficult by inconsistencies between the recommendations of different organizations and controversies over whether scientific evidence supports the practice.

Attitudes

Even if physicians are knowledgeable about recommendations, they may not agree that the proposed policy represents good care, is supported by valid evidence, meets accepted norms for their specialty or among local opinion leaders, or is applicable to their practice. Studies of family physicians in Ohio demonstrated disagreement with a substantial proportion of recommendations against cancer screening issued by the U.S. Preventive Services Task Force (Stange et al., 1992; Zyzanski et al., 1994). Finally, physicians may agree that it is appropriate for patients to obtain certain screening tests but disagree that it is their role to provide the service.

Ability

Clinicians who agree that screening is appropriate may be unable to offer testing and follow-up for a variety of operational reasons. These include lack of time, skills, personnel, equipment, adequate reimbursement, information systems, freedom from bureaucratic obstacles and medicolegal liability, and patient cooperation (see below). As noted earlier, the practice systems in which clinicians care for patients must be configured in an efficient design to facilitate the recognition of when patients are in need of screening (e.g., through the use of prompts or flow sheets); ease in administering tests or expediting referrals for testing elsewhere; and tracking systems to ensure receipt, interpretation, reporting, and appropriate follow-up of test results. An integrated, multifaceted approach to the reconfiguration of clinical operations and personnel duties is often necessary to make this happen. Studies have shown that such changes can improve cancer screening rates, although some randomized trials have shown modest incremental benefit (Dietrich et al., 1994b, 1998; Solberg et al., 1998).

Reinforcement

Even when providers are able to deliver screening tests well, reminder systems and feedback are important to identify when the need for rescreening has arisen. Tracking systems are necessary to indicate when the results of screening tests have not returned and to ensure that prompt and appropriate action is taken for patients with abnormal results. In an era when patients change providers and relocate geographically on a frequent basis, providers have limited ability to determine retrospectively from medical records when screening was last performed, and patients' memories are an imprecise substitute.

Measures to address these behaviors are not uniformly effective. The Cochrane Collaboration, an international effort to systematically review randomized clinical trials of health care, analyzed 18 systematic reviews of methods for the dissemination and implementation of evidence in practice. Although some interventions were consistently effective (e.g., educational outreach, reminders, multifaceted interventions, and interactive education), others were rarely or never effective (e.g., educational materials and didactic teaching) or were inconsistently effective (e.g., audits, feedback, local opinion leaders, local adaptation, and patient-mediated interventions) (Bero et al., 1998). Similarly, a review of 58 studies of strategies for the improvement of preventive care found that most were effective in some studies but not others (Hulscher et al., 1999).

A review of 187 studies by the RAND Corporation on behalf of the Health Care Financing Administration (now the Centers for Medicare and Medicaid Services) evaluated interventions that can be used to increase the rates of delivery of mammography, Pap smears, and FOBT (HCFA, 2001). Organizational changes and financial incentives most consistently produced the largest improvements in screening services. Examples of successful organizational changes include the use of a prevention team that includes standing orders for mammography by nurses (i.e., nurses may routinely refer eligible patients for mammograms), the use of nurses to distribute kits and instruct patients in the completion of FOBT, and the use of a health educator to contact patients via telephone to offer counseling or to assist in the scheduling of an appointment for cervical cancer screening. Patient reminders were somewhat less effective than organizational changes or financial incentives. Patient reminders that are personalized or signed by the provider appear to be modestly more effective than generic reminders. Provider education is moderately effective at increasing cancer screening, but patient education and provider feedback were least effective. Multiple interventions were more effective than single measures. Computer-assisted provider reminders are more cost-effective than patient reminders in the few studies that have addressed the issue.

What these reviews indicate is that there is no "magic bullet" that can be used to improve rates of cancer screening. A more rational strategy is to take a diagnostic approach, to identify which barriers account for the unsatisfactory screening practices, and to tailor strategies accordingly (Grol, 1997; Woolf, 2000b). Depending on which barrier(s) is(are) pertinent, a menu of options for improvement of the quality of interventions is available.

Challenges for Patients

Patients face the same four-part spectrum of challenges faced by clinicians (knowledge-attitudes-ability-reinforcement), although patients face these challenges from a different perspective.

Knowledge

The first impediment that patients face in pursuing cancer screening is inadequate knowledge of a variety of issues related to cancer: simple awareness of the existence of the cancer, knowledge of the fact that they face a risk of acquiring cancer, the cancer-associated morbidity and mortality, the availability of screening tests that can reduce these risks, and recommendations regarding when and how often they should be screened. People are unlikely to consider, let alone pursue or obtain, screening without this information. Not surprisingly, people with limited education and limited exposure to health information are less likely to have this knowledge. Knowledge about breast and cervical cancer among Hispanic women, for example, is related to age, education, income, language preference, and recent screening history (Ramirez et al., 2000a).

Inaccurate knowledge can influence screening behavior, leading to overutilization and underutilization of cancer screening. As noted earlier, research has documented that many patients have inaccurate perceptions about the magnitude of their risk from cancer (Clarke et al., 2000) and the likely benefits that they will obtain from screening.

Attitudes

Even if people have the facts about cancer screening right, they may lack motivation to obtain screening for a variety of attitudinal reasons.

Personal and cultural beliefs may influence attitudes about the importance of cancer, the acceptability of the tests that they must undergo, and the mores of trying to alter the natural history of disease rather than allowing nature to take its course (Mandelblatt et al., 1999; Paskett et al., 1997; Bowen et al., 1997; Tortolero-Luna et al., 1995). Fears of cancer and fears of knowing whether it is present also influence the motivation to get tested. Finally, attitudes about cancer prevention exist in the context of the competing priorities patients face in their daily lives. Concerns related to one's livelihood, income, family, or safety are often too substantial to make cancer screening a priority.

These attitudinal factors vary across ethnic and cultural traditions. Hispanic or Latino population groups are often treated as a monolithic entity on this (and many other) topics without consideration of heterogeneous cultural diversities. For example, Mexican Americans and Puerto Ricans may have more negative or fatalistic views about breast and cervical cancer than Cubans or Central Americans do (Ramirez et al., 2000a). Understanding of these cultural contexts and, more importantly, the involvement of individuals from within the particular culture who are sensitive to these concerns help craft interventions that are effective in shifting attitudes. For example, one randomized controlled trial found that the intervention that was effective in improving rates of screening for breast and cervical cancer among Latinas was organization of educational group sessions led by *consejeras*, lay Latino community volunteers (Navarro et al., 1998). Other research suggests that lay health advisers are effective among low-income women (Margolis et al., 1998; Skinner et al., 2000). Self-reported Pap smear utilization rates doubled in 6 months when lay health advisers assisted American Indian women (Dignan et al., 1996).

Ability

Even if people are knowledgeable about cancer and want to be screened, they may not be able to. A fundamental impediment is a lack of access to screening services. People who lack health insurance are less likely to receive cancer screening tests (Breen et al., 2001; Gordon et al., 1998; Hsia et al., 2000; Potosky et al., 1998), and this applies to a large proportion of U.S. citizens. In 1997, 22 percent of adults ages 18 to 44 and 12 percent of adults ages 45 to 64, respectively, were uninsured; among individuals under age 65 classified as poor or near poor, 34 and 36 percent, respectively, were uninsured. The proportion of older persons (age 65 and older) who are uninsured, however, is 1 percent because of Medicare coverage (National Center for Health Statistics, 2000). As noted earlier, people with health insurance typically find that most cancer screening tests are covered under their plans, although there are notable exceptions and an increasing requirement for copayments, a factor known to reduce the rate of adherence to screening tests

(Solanki et al., 2000; Solanki and Schauffler, 1999; Partnership for Prevention, 1997). Studies from the early 1990s suggested that individuals with Medicaid coverage were screened at lower rates than those with private insurance (Makuc et al., 1994); however, more recent studies suggest comparable screening rates for the two groups (Potosky et al., 1998).

A related but separate part of access to health care is having a provider, in particular, a regular source of primary care. Adults who receive regular care from a family physician are more likely to receive mammography and Pap smears (McIsaac et al., 2001). Low-income individuals and families are less likely to enjoy this degree of access. In 1997, 9 to 16 percent of adults reported that they needed to see a doctor but could not because of the cost, irrespective of insurance status (CDC, 2000a). Even among individuals with a health problem, however, 12 percent had no physician contact within the past year (the rates were 21 and 12 percent for poor or near-poor men and women, respectively) (National Center for Health Statistics, 1998).

Patients with insurance and access to providers face other barriers that impede their ability to be screened. Work, school, or family responsibilities may make the tasks of scheduling and traveling to appointments, undergoing tests, and arranging and attending follow-up procedures too time-consuming or inconvenient. Women who report that they must take time off from work to see a physician are less likely to be screened (Lantz et al., 1995). Inconvenience of appointments, long waits for appointments, and scheduling difficulties may also discourage screening and follow-up (Glasgow et al., 2000; Marcus and Crane, 1998; McCarthy et al., 1996). On-site technology, such as a mammography unit (Potter et al., 1996) or a sigmoidoscope (Schroy et al., 1999), and extended and convenient hours (Potter et al., 1996) can increase screening use in primary care settings.

Physical limitations, such as those imposed by frail health in elderly individuals, may interfere with the ability to perform or undergo screening tests (e.g., handling of stool for FOBT or suitability for colonoscopy). Illiteracy, cognitive deficits, or language barriers may make it difficult to understand or follow instructions from medical staff. Patients referred to specialists to obtain screening tests or follow-up procedures may be unable to understand or navigate the increasingly onerous administrative tasks of dealing with health plans to obtain referrals to the recommended provider or facility, scheduling appointments, and being adequately prepared on arrival.

Reinforcement

Finally, even if patients are willing and able to be screened, remembering that screening is due or remembering to perform self-examination is often difficult simply because of forgetfulness. This is especially problematic for screening tests with long recommended intervals between testing. Patients who are advised to return for sigmoidoscopy in 5 years or colonoscopy in 10 years may have difficulty remembering when the test must be done and relating to new providers which test they underwent previously.

Intermingling of Challenges

The disentangling of health systems, providers, and patients as separate sources of challenges to screening is a somewhat artificial construct given their complex interrelationships. The example of the barriers to optimizing colorectal cancer screening, seen from the provider's perspective, illustrates the intermingling of the three groups (Box 6.1).

CLOSER EXAMINATION OF SPECIFIC CANCER SCREENING TESTS

Using the four-part model of behavioral change (knowledge-attitudes-ability-reinforcement) as an organizational framework for understanding the patient's perspective on reasons for inadequate screening, this section reviews in greater detail the evidence regarding the factors associated with cancer screening and the effectiveness of interventions that can enhance the appropriateness of screening practices. Evidence is examined for screening for cancer of the colon-rectum, breast, prostate, and cervix. (Lung and skin cancer are not considered in this discussion because of the lack of an organized interest in promoting screening for lung cancer and the lack of current evidence regarding efforts to improve skin cancer screening. The history of attempts to screen for lung cancer is described in Chapter 7). Evidence regarding predictors of cancer screening is understandably derived largely from observational studies, but, where possible, evidence regarding the effectiveness of interventions to improve screening rates emphasizes evidence from randomized controlled trials. The review considers the evidence available as of February 2001 but not more recently published evidence.

Colorectal Cancer Screening

Size of the Gap

Many of the lives claimed each year by colorectal cancer are attributable to the small proportion of the population that undergoes screening. As of 1999, approximately 60 percent of U.S. adults age 50 and older reported that they had never been screened for colorectal cancer (by FOBT, sigmoidoscopy, or colonoscopy). Others had been screened, but not recently. Only 19 percent had undergone home FOBT within the past year, 32 percent had undergone sigmoidoscopy or colonoscopy within the past 5 years, and 44 percent had received at least one of the tests within the preceding 5 years (CDC, Behavioral Risk Factor Surveillance System, 2000; CDC, 2001c).

BOX 6.1 Challenges to Providers in Improving Rates of Screening for Colorectal Cancer

Knowledge

Many physicians are unaware of the evidence that screening for colon cancer reduces the rate of mortality from that disease. Until recent trials demonstrated otherwise, the conventional wisdom was that colorectal cancer screening had no proven benefit. Furthermore, clinicians may not know current protocols for screening. Many assume that guaiac testing in the office, performed with the glove used in a rectal examination, constitutes FOBT screening (the procedure that lowered the rates of mortality in clinical trials was the collection of six specimens, two specimens from three consecutive stools, at home). Physicians know little about the effects of rehydrating FOBT cards (which results in a better sensitivity but a decreased specificity, increasing the probability of obtaining false-positive results and the need for workups). They do not know which types of polyps are premalignant and, having detected them by endoscopy or barium enema, the sizes of polyps that require biopsy.

Attitudes

Clinicians can know the facts but remain uneager. For many years, colorectal cancer screening was the focus of conflicting guidelines and controversy. Not until 1996 did the U.S. Preventive Services Task Force abandon the position that there was insufficient evidence to make a recommendation. That this group—and most others—now enthusiastically recommends colorectal cancer screening is not well known. The ambiguity and the dismal compliance rates of patients are fresh in mind, and many clinicians give priority to other prevention services (e.g., counseling against tobacco use and control of blood pressure, and lipid levels). Some physicians who know the data are not impressed by the magnitude of benefit; by one calculation, 1,374 patients must undergo screening by FOBT for 5 years to prevent one death from colorectal cancer.

Ability

Even enthusiastic physicians cannot screen patients if they lack time, patient cooperation, office help, ease of referral to gastroenterologists, and insurance coverage. They cannot perform endoscopy skillfully without training and without conducting a large volume of procedures. Changes in the practice environment, for example, implementing an office system to generate reminders for screening and follow-up, can enhance practice.

Reinforcement

Screening cannot occur if clinicians do not remember when patients are due for screening or forget to act on abnormal results.

The probability of having done FOBT at home was 18.2 percent for whites, 20.3 percent for African Americans, 14.2 percent for Hispanics, and 12.3 percent for American Indians (CDC, Behavioral Risk Factor Surveillance System, 2000). The probability of having had a flexible sigmoidoscopy or colonoscopic examination within the past 5 years was 30.4 percent for whites, 28.2 percent for African Americans, 22.4 percent for Hispanics, and 27.6 percent for American Indians (CDC, Behavioral Risk Factor Surveillance System, 2000).

An additional problem beyond access to screening is the quality of testing. Patients with positive FOBT results often receive incomplete follow-up investigation (Shields et al., 2001).

Predictors of Screening

Knowledge A likely reason for the failure of many Americans to obtain screening for colorectal cancer is unfamiliarity with the disease (Newman, 2001). In contrast to breast cancer, most people have never heard of colorectal cancer. Although breast cancer claims 11,000 fewer lives each year, it is perceived as a more deadly threat to health. Many women misperceive colorectal cancer as a man's disease (Burke et al., 2000). Most women know about breast and cervical cancer screening, and an increasing number of men know about screening for prostate cancer, but both women and men are generally unaware that all adults should be screened for colorectal cancer beginning at age 50. Some evidence suggests that physicians are not providing patients with the information that they need to facilitate screening. Individuals not screened by sigmoidoscopy report that their physician did not recommend it (Beeker et al., 2000; Vernon, 1995; Weitzman et al., 2001). A recent study of Massachusetts residents found that only 34 percent of people aged 50 to 64 and 43 percent of people aged 65 and older reported that a physician had ever recommended sigmoidoscopy (Erban et al., 2001). Among a sample of family physicians in Washington state, 30 percent of age-appropriate patients had received recommendations for screening sigmoidoscopy within the previous 5 years (Montano et al., 2000). In another study, only 58 percent of older women in a large health maintenance organization reported that they had been encouraged by their physician to receive screening for colorectal cancer, but this factor was strongly related to screening participation (Mandelson et al., 2000).

Attitudes Among people who are aware of colorectal cancer and the recommendation to be screened, attitudes about the disease, the anatomic part of the body involved, and the nature of the tests pose barriers to screening. Some find distasteful or inconvenient the notion of handling stool specimens for FOBT at home (Myers et al., 1991). The inconvenience of having to avoid certain foods in the days preceding the test may dissuade patients from completing the test (Robinson et al., 1994). Others anticipate discomfort and embarrassment from screening by endoscopy or barium enema or the bowel preparation procedure that precedes those tests. Their attitudes may be amplified if their prior screening examinations were unpleasant.

As with other screening tests, however, patients' attitudes are more likely to shift in favor of screening if a physician recommends the test. If a physician recommends the test, approximately 50 to 70 percent of patients complete the FOBT and 25 to 50 percent undergo sigmoidoscopy (Vernon, 1997).

Ability Patients who want to be screened for colorectal cancer may be unable to do so. They may lack insurance coverage or access to care. In certain communities and regions of the country, gastroenterologists who can perform screening colonoscopic examinations, radiology facilities where high-quality double-contrast barium enemas can be performed, or openings on schedules for timely appointments may not be available to patients. Patients may be unable to understand, perform, or tolerate bowel preparation procedures. Reading and language barriers can make instructions useless. Older patients with poor vision or manual dexterity may have difficulty collecting stool specimens for FOBT.

Reinforcement For patients who want to undergo annual FOBT, few may remember when 1 year has passed. Even fewer remember, 5 years hence, that it is time for another sigmoidoscopy. Reminders from the physician who performed the test help little if the patient has moved out of the area or, as occurs frequently in the current environment of managed care, has acquired a new physician.

Interventions to Enhance Colorectal Cancer Screening

Knowledge Interventions In recent years, considerable effort has gone into heightening public awareness of colorectal cancer. Much of this has been accomplished by celebrities, a noteworthy example being Katie Couric, a television personality, who has spearheaded an effort to promote screening for colorectal cancer (Gorman, 2000; Newman, 2001). A live television broadcast of her colonoscopy screening examination was associated with a subsequent increase in requests for screenings and referrals to gastroenterologists.

In 1997 the CDC and the American Cancer Society established the National Colorectal Cancer Roundtable, a coalition of medical professional, consumer advocacy, and volunteer organizations committed to raising awareness about colorectal cancer. The U.S. Congress designated March of each year the National Colorectal Cancer Awareness Month. The annual program Screen for Life, A National Colorectal Cancer Action Campaign, is a collaboration among the CDC, the National Cancer Institute, and the Centers for Medicare and Medicaid Services (formerly the Health Care Financing Administration) and promotes the distribution of television and radio public service announcements, brochures, posters, and fact sheets for the public and providers (http://www.cdc.gov/cancer/colorctl/calltoaction).

Attitude Interventions The review of the literature for this chapter found little current evidence of whether the efforts described above have been effective in shifting attitudes about the acceptability of screening tests for colorectal cancer.

Ability Interventions It is difficult for the large proportion of the U.S. population that lacks health insurance or access to health care providers to obtain colorectal cancer screening. Interventions to correct this formidable defect in the U.S. health care system are beyond the scope of this review. For insured populations, however, major steps have been taken to expand coverage for colorectal cancer screening. Most private health plans offer coverage for screening by FOBT and flexible sigmoidoscopy, a growing number offer coverage for colonoscopy, and congressional legislation may mandate such coverage. As already noted, the Medicare program began offering coverage for colorectal cancer screening tests in 1998 and now includes coverage for colonoscopy.

The review of the literature for this chapter found little current published evidence of organized efforts to address the potential shortage of physicians available to screen the millions of Americans for whom it is recommended by current guidelines. Low reimbursement rates for screening work against efforts to expand the workforce for this task (Lewis and Asch, 1999). Studies have demonstrated that nurses can be trained to perform sigmoidoscopy and even colonoscopy and thereby expand the number of health professionals available to perform screening (see Chapter 8).

The lack of a requirement for dietary restrictions before home FOBT was shown in one randomized trial to improve adherence rates (Robinson et al., 1994). The present review otherwise found few published studies about efforts to enhance the patient's ability to schedule, prepare, and undergo colorectal cancer screening tests, although manufacturers, public health departments, and community health centers have undertaken efforts with these aims, with a particular focus on patients with limited education and limited English-language proficiency.

Reinforcement Interventions Some work has gone into developing reminder systems to alert physicians and patients when screening for colorectal cancer is due. Computerized reminder systems have been shown to improve compliance with screening by FOBT (Litzelman et al., 1993). In a review of the effectiveness of interventions aimed at increasing rates of screening by FOBT, Vernon (1997) showed that studies that deliver minimal or relatively impersonal interventions were generally not effective (King et al., 1992; Myers et al., 1991, 1994). In general, the rate of adherence was lowest when persons were asked to pick up a test kit or to mail in a reply card to receive a kit (Lallemand et al., 1984; Nichols et al., 1986). More intensive interventions appeared to be more effective (Vernon, 1997), such as combining reminder telephone calls with self-help screening booklets (Myers et al., 1991).

As discussed below with regard to breast cancer screening, the ability of physicians' offices and clinics to establish reminder systems and institute appropriate follow-up for colorectal cancer screening appears to be facilitated by the adoption of comprehensive office system changes (e.g., through the use of office chart reminders, patient health maintenance cards, on-site training and start-up assistance visits, continuing education seminars, and quality assurance feedback). Such programs have proved effective in increasing the rates of performance of FOBT (Manfredi et al., 1998). In one randomized trial, the intervention consisted of an 11-minute video about colon cancer screening, the selection of a color-coded educational brochure reflecting degree of interest in screening, and a marker of the same color attached to the chart. The numbers of requisitions for FOBT and flexible sigmoidoscopy and the rates of completion of these tests increased significantly under this program (Pignone et al., 2000).

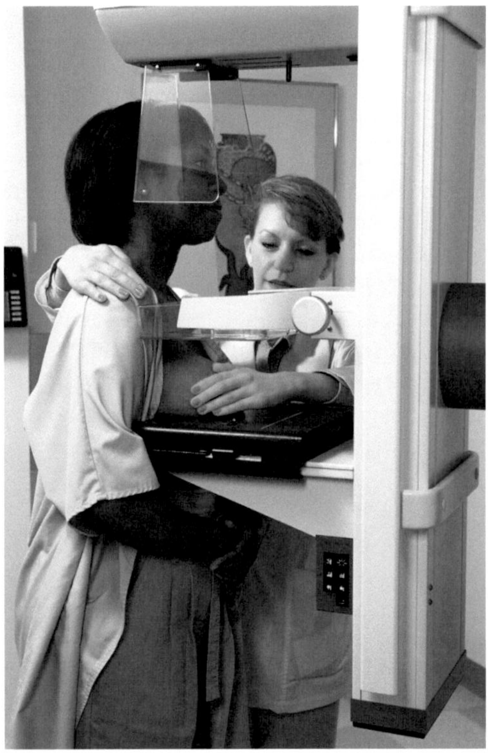

SOURCE: PhotoDisc, Inc.

Breast Cancer Screening

Size of the Gap

In contrast to colorectal cancer screening, a relatively large proportion of women have availed themselves of screening mammography. Approximately 64 percent of women age 50 and older report that they have had a mammogram in the past year (CDC, Behavioral Risk Factor Surveillance System, 2000), and 74 percent report that they have had one within the past 2 years (CDC, 2000a). Approximately 57 percent of women in this age group have also reported that they have had a clinical breast examination in the past year (CDC, Behavioral Risk Factor Surveillance System, 2000), and 66 percent have reported that they have had both a mammogram and a clinical breast examination within the past 2 years (CDC, 2000a). Fully 59 percent of women age 40 and older reported that they have had a mammogram within the preceding year (CDC, Behavioral Risk Factor Surveillance System, 2000). In fact, breast imaging accounts for 10 percent of all examinations performed by radiologists (Sickles, 2000a).

These numbers, however, leave a substantial proportion of women who have not been screened recently and a disturbing minority of women who have never been screened, a more common occurrence among poor women. Whereas 72 percent of women age 50 and older with family incomes at or above the poverty level have had a mammogram in the past 2 years, the same is true for only 53 percent of women of the same age who have family incomes below the poverty level. (National Center for Health Statistics, 2000). Among women age 40 and older, the probability of having had a mammogram within the past 2 years was 73 percent for women with at least some college education but 55 percent for those with less than a high school education (National Center for Health Statistics, 2000). Screening rates are lower in urban inner-city America (Ekeh et al., 2000; Taylor et al., 1998). In community-based screening in Albuquerque, New Mexico, only 50 percent of women aged 50 to 74 were screened each year in the study period from 1994 to 1997 (Gilliland et al., 2000).

There are important racial and ethnic disparities in breast cancer screening rates, but in contrast to other areas of health care, African Americans do not appear to be disadvantaged in terms of screening for breast cancer. After controlling for income, African-American women are just as likely (if not more so) to have had a recent mammogram as white women. The probability of having had a mammogram within the past 2 years is 73.7 percent for whites, 76.1 percent for African Americans, and 63.5 percent for Hispanics (CDC, Behavioral Risk Factor Surveillance System, 2000). In fact, among poor women, African-American women were about 60 percent more likely than white women to have had a recent mammogram (National Center for Health Statistics, 1998). Also, in contrast to other areas of health care, African-American women do not appear to be more likely to receive substandard mammographic services (Jones et al., 2001).

Other minority groups, particularly Hispanic and Asian women, are more likely to receive substandard screening. In one study in Albuquerque, New Mexico, only 20 percent of Hispanic women ages 50 to 74 had received routine annual mammograms (Gilliland et al., 2000). Breast cancer screening rates are significantly reduced among Asian Americans and Pacific Islanders (Kagawa-Singer and Pourat, 2000). Only 47 percent of Korean Americans have had a mammogram in the past 2 years (Juon et al., 2000). Among Cambodian Americans, approximately 40 percent are up to date on their clinical breast and mammography examinations (Tu et al., 2000). Screening rates are also low among American Indians. A 1995 audit of diabetes care at Indian Health Service centers found that at some centers as few as 35 percent of women had ever had a mammogram, and at one center only 28 percent had received a clinical breast examination in the past year (Giroux et al., 2000).

Access to mammography is also affected by age, with older women less likely to have kept up to date with screening mammography. An audit of 110,000 mammograms in New Hampshire confirmed that the rate of screening was higher for younger women (40 to 48 percent for those ages 44 to 64) than for older women (34 to 39 percent for those ages 65 to 84) (Carney et al., 2000). Overuse and exposure to unnecessary false-positive results are potential risks for elderly women. A chart review of women age 75 and older in a skilled nursing facility revealed that an average of 1.9 mammograms were performed per patient, with 45 percent producing abnormal results requiring investigation (Kerins et al., 2000).

Gaps exist not only in breast cancer screening rates but also in what happens next if the findings are abnormal. In one health maintenance organization, in 34 percent of patients, follow-up for an abnormal mass or a suspicious calcification detected on mammography was not completed within 1 month, and it was delayed beyond 2 months in an additional 35 percent of patients (Burack et al., 2000b). Another analysis estimated that 14 percent of patients with abnormal findings on breast cancer screening received inadequate follow-up (Schootman et al., 2000). In a setting where most physicians advise annual mammograms, the median time to subsequent screening was 18 months (Ulcickas Yood et al., 1999).

Predictors

Knowledge Studies of women who receive inadequate screening mammographies reveal women's misperceptions of their perceived and actual risks of breast cancer (Clemow et al., 2000). There are misconceptions that mammography is unnecessary unless a mass is palpable. In one study of low-income African-American women, those who lacked breast symptoms were more likely to miss appointments (Crump et al., 2000).

Misperceptions about whether one is supposed to have a mammogram is an obvious and proven correlate of whether screening occurs (MacDowell et al., 2000), and confusion on this topic is more prevalent in certain groups. Older women (i.e., those over age 65), for example, are more likely to express doubts about whether they need to have a mammogram (King et al., 1993a; Taplin and Montano, 1993). Only 53 percent of women attending an urban emergency department knew the correct age to begin screening mammography or the recommended frequency of breast self-examination, and knowledge tended to be poorer among African Americans, Asians, and Hispanics (Takakuwa et al., 2000). In a telephone survey of Hispanic women, accurate knowledge of the screening guidelines ranged from 58 percent for Mexican Americans to 72 percent for Cubans (Ramirez et al., 2000a). A study of urban Chinese-American women age 60 and older revealed that a low level of perceived need affected whether they had had a mammogram in the past year (Tang et al., 2000).

Knowledge in the form of misperceptions also contributes to overdemand for screening mammographies that may not be recommended. Although experts debate whether mammography has significant benefit for women ages 40 to 49 (see Chapter 5), a survey of American women (Woloshin et al., 2000) revealed that 83 percent believed that it did. In fact, 38 percent believed that benefit was proven for women younger than 40 years. Most women suggested that women should begin screening mammography before age 40, whereas only 5 percent believed that it should not begin until age 50. When asked why mammography was controversial, the lead answer (49 percent of respondents) was cost.

Whether a woman acquires accurate knowledge about breast cancer screening is obviously affected by language barriers, an important problem in certain ethnic minority groups. For example, proficiency with the English language is a correlate of recent mammography among Korean-American women (Juon et al., 2000).

Attitudes Personal emotions and values and beliefs about breast cancer and mammography affect the motivation to be screened (King et al., 1995b). An important attitude through which women filter their knowledge of breast cancer screening is fear, including both worry about breast cancer and fear of learning that one has breast cancer (Clemow et al., 2000). Women's attitudes are influenced by the experiences of family and friends who have had breast cancer (King et al., 1995b).

Women may be reticent to be screened because of fatalistic beliefs. This is especially true for older, African-American, and less educated women (Mayo et al., 2001). In one study, older women (ages 65 to 74) who had never had a mammogram expressed anxieties about the consequences, stating that having a mammogram means "looking for trouble" and that it "makes me nervous" (King et al., 1993a). Other considerations that dampen attitudes about screening include fear of embarrassment (Crump et al., 2000) or discomfort and being in poor health (Taplin et al., 1994). External influences also affect attitudes about screening. A woman is less likely to have a mammography if a family member or friend discourages it or if her social network lacks someone with whom to discuss health concerns (Pearlman et al., 1997).

An important external influence on women's attitudes about mammography, both in general and in ethnic and racial groups, is the advice of their health care provider to have the test (Gnanadesigan et al., 2000; Halabi et al., 2000; Juon et al., 2000; MacDowell et al., 2000; Pearlman et al., 1997; Simon et al., 1998; Tang et al., 2000). Such advice may come irregularly, however. Most physicians regularly recommend screening mammography for asymptomatic women ages 50 and older, with estimates ranging from 53 to 81 percent of physicians in recent studies (Lane et al., 2000; May et al., 1999; O'Malley et al., 2001). Uninsured and underinsured women are, however, less likely to receive a recommendation from their doctors to be screened (Lane et al., 2000; May et al., 1999). Studies have not consistently linked age, income, or race or ethnicity to the likelihood of a physician recommendation (Lane et al., 2000; O'Malley et al., 2001; Solberg et al., 1997a). With respect to physician characteristics, asymptomatic women seeing female physicians or younger physicians (i.e., physicians age <40) report receipt of mammography recommendations most often (Lane et al., 2000; Levy et al., 1992).

Having the clinical encounters that provide the opportunity to get screening advice depends on access to health care and health insurance, barriers (O'Malley et al., 2001) discussed below under "Ability," but the propensity of clinicians to give the advice appears to be influenced by some of the patient's other socioeconomic conditions, independent of access. Women age 65 and older are less likely to receive a physician recommendation with increasing age and decreased income and education (Lane et al., 2000). Rural women in a study conducted in North Carolina were significantly less likely to be advised to have a mammogram if they were older, less educated, or had a lower family income (O'Malley et al., 2001).

Women may also be influenced by the type of provider who gives the advice. One study found that low-income African-American women were less likely to miss their appointment if they were referred by a physician's assistant or a nurse practitioner than if they were referred by a physician (Crump et al., 2000).

Aside from what they hear from their personal physician, women's attitudes are affected by the messages conveyed in practice guidelines and the controversies that they engender. One survey conducted following the controversial 1997 NIH Consensus Development Conference on breast cancer screening for women ages 40 to 49 found 28 percent confused about the schedule on which women should have mammograms. Confusion was a significant predictor of being off schedule (Rimer et al., 1999). Studies of women who have had a mammogram but who have not returned for timely repeat screening find that they are more likely to be confused about screening guidelines and to express ambivalence than those who have kept current with their screening mammographies (Halabi et al., 2000). A survey of American women revealed that 95 percent were aware of the debate over screening mammography guidelines. Half reported being upset by the public disagreement among experts, and only 24 percent said the discussion had improved their understanding (Woloshin et al., 2000). Another survey of women conducted in western Washington state suggests that conflicting recommendations do not necessarily depress use of mammography. More important than controversy surrounding guidelines was physician recommendation and women's self-reported likeliness to follow physician advice (Taplin et al, 1997b).

Values about the importance of breast cancer screening vary by race and ethnicity, but it is difficult to disentangle the extent to which these relate to socioeconomic variables. This interrelationship illustrates the overlaps between knowledge, attitudes, ability, and reinforcement as determinants of cancer screening. For example, researchers have used "willingness to pay" for mammography as an indicator of the relative importance that women assign to screening. One study of low-income, ethnically diverse women found that this willingness, which varied by ethnic group, was statistically associated with elements that this report classifies under *knowledge* (perceived risk of cancer or the knowledge that one needs a mammogram even after a clinical breast examination) and elements related to *ability* (household income) (Wagner et al., 2000).

Attitudes that are unmistakably cultural and ethnic also influence interest in breast cancer screening. Acculturation and the proportion of a woman's life spent in the United States are important factors among some immigrant and ethnic populations, such as Korean women (Juon et al., 2000). A study of urban Chinese-American women age 60 and older revealed that acculturation and issues surrounding modesty affected ever having had a screening mammography or a clinical breast examination, and the lack of a physician recommendation affected having it in the past year. Cambodian women, even those with Asian-American physicians, are less likely to be screened if the physician is a man (Tu et al., 2000). Within Hispanic populations, attitudes differ among ethnoregional subgroups (Ramirez et al., 2000b).

Ability Access to health care and insurance coverage are closely correlated with whether women obtain screening mammography. As noted earlier with regard to HEDIS indicators, health maintenance organizations report that large proportions of their female enrollees have received regular screening mammographies. By 1992, 75 percent of women who had been members of the Kaiser Permanente, Northwest Region, health maintenance organization for at least 2 years had undergone a screening mammography (Glass et al., 1996).

The potential for confounding variables in this association is strong, given the linkages between income and private insurance and the tendency of such women to have greater knowledge about breast cancer screening (Takakuwa et al., 2000). Many of the seemingly cultural differences in obtaining screening mammography are functions of poverty and educational status (Facione and Katapodi, 2000). Nonetheless, even after multivariate logistic regression analysis for other preventive health behaviors, education, and socioeconomic status, access to health care and insurance coverage remain independent predictors of screening (Qureshi et al., 2000). Along with low income, they tend to have a disproportionate role as barriers to breast cancer screening among Asian Americans and Pacific Islanders (Coughlin and Uhler, 2000; Kagawa-Singer and Pourat, 2000; Tang et al., 2000).

In an era when screening mammography is increasingly covered by health insurance, it is important to recognize that insurance status is not the only factor limiting the ability of women who want mammograms to obtain them. Other barriers include not knowing the name of their primary care physician (Simon et al., 1998), difficulty with access (King et al., 1995b), and geographic distance from the provider (Hyndman et al., 2000; Taplin et al., 1994).

Reinforcement As with other cancer screening tests, the maintenance of schedules for breast cancer screening is influenced by forgetfulness (Crump et al., 2000). For similar reasons, women forget to perform breast self-examination (Tang et al., 2000).

Interventions to Enhance Breast Cancer Screening

By far, the most extensive research on interventions that improve the effectiveness of cancer screening is in the area of promoting mammography and clinical breast examinations. A 1999 meta-analysis attempted to summarize this evidence by reviewing 43 studies of 63 interventions. It concluded that behavioral interventions increased the rate of breast cancer screening by 13.2 percent (95 percent confidence interval [CI], 4.7 to 21.2 percent). Cognitive interventions that used generic education strategies had little impact, but those that used theory-based education (e.g., health belief model) increased rates of screening by 23.6 percent (95 percent CI, 16.4 to 30.1 percent). Sociological interventions also increased screening rates (Yabroff and Mandelblatt, 1999).

This literature is examined in more detail below by using the four-part knowledge-attitude-ability-reinforcement model as an organizational framework. The interventions are reviewed in terms of their effectiveness in improving screening rates, focusing primarily on evidence from randomized controlled trials. The incremental benefit of these interventions in improving rates of screening mammography is often marginal in comparison with their costs, yielding various estimates of their cost-effectiveness (Lantz et al., 1996; Saywell et al., 1999; Wagner, 1998). These monetary factors must be considered by health care systems in determining whether the costs per additional mammogram are worth the benefit, but such considerations are not the focus of this review.

Knowledge Interventions Some efforts to promote breast cancer screening rely on dissemination of information about the disease and the importance of screening. Much of this comes through press reports, television and radio broadcasts, articles about breast cancer in women's magazines, and advertisements. Research by the Annenberg School of Communication has documented the influence of media coverage, independent of physician's advice, on women's decisions to have mammograms, especially women without regular access to or contact with a physician (Yanovitzky and Blitz, 2000). One study in Washington state has confirmed the expected correlation between community newspaper advertisements and mammography use (Urban et al., 1995). Others have concluded that messages in the media can heighten awareness and increase behavioral intention but are unlikely to assert their influence beyond awareness of breast cancer screening (Rimer, 1997).

Attitude Interventions The sources of information and promotional messages have important influences on attitudes, and considerable research and programmatic activity have gone into the effort to deliver messages through venues and individuals who have greater credibility with women. Much of this work has targeted the populations that are least adequately screened, including inner-city low-income women, rural women, and women in certain ethnic and minority groups.

Interventions aimed at reminding physicians and health care systems to advise women about the need for screening mammography, an important motivator that shapes women's attitudes about the importance of screening, also serve as reminder systems when screening is overdue and are therefore reviewed below under "Reinforcement Interventions." Other studies have engaged other health care professionals in the community in this role. For example, a before-and-after study reported that a program that was conducted by pharmacists and that incorporated risk assessment software and education and training about breast self-examination, clinical breast examination, and mammography was associated with a substantial increase in the rate of adherence to guidelines (Giles et al., 2001).

Some interventions focus on enlisting the aid of individuals familiar to women. A randomized trial sponsored by the American Cancer Society demonstrated that screening mammography rates increased among women who received a telephone call from a friend offering encouragement to have a mammogram (Calle et al., 1994). Other strategies focus on empowering women to become involved in screening choices. In one study, older women in an urban setting were more likely to have current mammograms because they took an active role and had recurrent participation in screening (Gnanadesigan et al., 2000).

Other interventions tend to be multifaceted and highly coordinated group or community-based efforts that often rely on volunteers and community outreach. Rural communities have used volunteers for individual counseling or community activities (Andersen et al., 2000). In Minneapolis, Minnesota, a randomized trial targeting low-income women in public housing high-rise buildings found that screening rates increased for women living in buildings where health professionals spoke about screening and where community volunteers held small group discussions and the women had an opportunity to request assistance with obtaining mammograms or mammogram reminders (Slater et al., 1998). In Hawaii, Kokua Groups, which provide culturally tailored education to native Hawaiian women in a group setting, have observed some improvements in screening activities (Gotay et al., 2000).

Researchers have worked toward understanding how to more effectively shift attitudes about breast cancer screening by crafting messages with an understanding of different ethnic, racial, and cultural traditions. Research suggests, for example, that African-American women's intentions to get mammograms following receipt of such messages are influenced by both the message's arguments and the degree of favorable "peripheral cues" (Kirby et al., 1998). A randomized trial involving inner-city Spanish-speaking Hispanic women found success with a culturally sensitive, linguistically appropriate computerized education program with an interactive soap opera format, the viewers of which demonstrated increased knowledge and altered beliefs about breast cancer compared with controls (Jibaja et al., 2000).

Ability Interventions The same interventions that would eliminate a lack of access to health care and inadequate health insurance as barriers to breast cancer screening are those that would solve these problems for the U.S. health care system in general and are beyond the scope of this review. It is the case that some women—because they misunderstand their insurance coverage status, their covered benefits, or the affordability of obtaining screening without insurance—are under the misconception that these barriers make them unable to be screened. Simply mailing a notice to Medicare beneficiaries indicating that mammography was subsidized under the program was associated with increased rates of utilization (Fox et al., 2001).

Other problems that affect the ability to be screened, such as ease of access and geographical proximity to mammography services, have been eased in some communities by offering screening at nontraditional sites such as workplaces and churches, operating mobile mammography vans, and establishing geographically dispersed imaging facilities (see Box 6.2). The more organized health care systems and managed care plans have developed systems that streamline the process of obtaining referrals and arranging mammography to remove operational impediments that frustrate, delay, or sabotage the efforts of women who want to obtain a mammogram (Taplin et al., 1997a).

Reinforcement Interventions Although some women who know they are due for screening proactively visit their physician or radiology facility to obtain a breast examination and mammogram, it is important that women who are unaware of this need receive timely reminders so that their screening is not delayed. One strategy is for physicians or mammography facilities to mail reminder letters or postcards to patients when their mammogram is due. Studies of the effectiveness of this intervention

BOX 6.2 Cancer Screening at Worksites and Places of Worship

Worksites

Relatively few worksites provide cancer screening services, but screening at worksites represents an opportunity to increase access to screening. As of 1995 an estimated 7 percent of worksites offered cancer screening; and of these, 59 percent offered breast cancer screening, 25 percent offered colorectal screening, and 17 percent offered cervical cancer screening (CDC, 1997b). Occupational health nurses often manage the screening programs, and key organizational factors associated with success in at least some worksites include the endorsement of upper management and the employee's immediate supervisor (Caplan and Coughlin, 1998). Most worksites that offer breast cancer screening use mobile mammography units (Caplan and Coughlin, 1998; Dershaw et al., 1992; Kessler et al., 1991), which appear to be cost-effective (Schrammel et al., 1998). Few studies, however, have assessed the effectiveness of cancer screening programs at worksites (Hart et al., 1998; Lee, 1983, 1991; Marcus and Crane, 1998; Tilley et al., 1999b; Vernon, 1997), but some evidence suggests that workplace settings could offer a complementary location for the delivery of screening services.

Places of Worship

Although places of worship are often noted to be key channels for reaching African Americans and Hispanic groups (e.g., Davis et al., 1994; Fisher et al., 1992; Ransdell, 1995), few studies that have evaluated interventions aimed at improving cancer screening at places of worship are available. Results from some church-based efforts appear to be promising (Bailey et al., 2000; Marcus and Crane, 1998), whereas the results of other efforts have been disappointing (Mitchell-Beren et al., 1989).

have yielded mixed results. Some randomized trials and community studies report a significant improvement in the rate at which women return for mammography (King et al., 1994; Mayer et al., 2000; Urban et al., 1995). A randomized trial in a Philadelphia health maintenance organization found that a birthday card reminder was more effective than a personalized letter from the medical director accompanied by materials promoting mammography (Davis et al., 1997b). A 1998 meta-analysis of 16 articles concluded that women who received reminders were 50 percent more likely to get a mammogram and that tailored letters were more effective than generic reminders (Wagner, 1998). Women with family histories of breast cancer are more likely to obtain mammograms if reminders are tailored to emphasize that history and the consequent increased importance of testing (Curry, 1993).

Other studies have reported more pessimistic results. Randomized trials have reported no benefit when a radiology department (Bodiya et al., 1999) or a health maintenance organization serving urban, predominantly African-American women (Burack et al., 1996) sent reminder letters. A subsequent article from the same research team noted that although 48 percent of the recipients of the reminder letter completed a mammogram within the following year and 72 percent remembered that they had received it, only 5 percent responded to its recommendations (Simon et al., 1998). Having the letter come from the primary care physician rather than the program director had no incremental benefit in one randomized trial, but sending a subsequent reminder postcard doubled screening mammography rates (Taplin et al., 1994).

Some work has focused on the incremental benefit of following reminder letters with telephone contacts that offer reminders or encouragement to obtain a mammogram. These calls are generally made to women who are overdue for a mammogram, have not responded to previous reminders, are older, or are in low-income groups. The results are generally positive; but the magnitude of benefit varies depending on the content of the conversation, motivational techniques, the stage of readiness to change of the women, the number of repeat calls, whether the opportunity to schedule a screening appointment is included, and whether past mammography experiences are discussed (Bodiya et al., 1999; Crane et al., 2000; Davis et al., 1997a; Janz et al., 1997; King et al., 1994, 1995b; Lantz et al., 1995; Ludman et al., 1999; Taplin et al., 2000).

Telephone calls may be more effective than mailed reminders, at least in some trials (Lipkus et al., 2000b). Calls placed by church-based volunteers delivering culturally specific information about mammograms and where to obtain them at low cost appear to attract women who were previously not adherent to screening recommendations (Duan et al., 2000). One randomized trial found that calls by trained counselors focusing on barriers to screening were no more effective than annual mailed reminders but did produce some modest benefit in the subset of women who had previously undergone mammography (Costanza et al., 2000). Another trial found no difference between a simple reminder telephone call and a motivational call addressing barriers (Taplin et al., 2000). Calls placed by medical assistants from a primary care office appear to be more effective than those placed by physicians and are considerably more cost-effective (Mohler, 1995).

It is important that women who do not receive reminders by mail or telephone or who forget to act on them be reminded to get an examination or mammogram when they visit their primary care physician for other reasons and that they receive assistance in expediting the process. For this to occur efficiently, practices and providers must have in place systems that identify women who are overdue for screening and that remind or prompt providers to notify women who are overdue for screening. In addition, it is important to have in place a streamlined process for obtaining examinations and mammograms that removes impediments that account for failures or delays in screening.

A number of randomized trials have examined different strategies for reconfiguring office and clinic operations and modifying manual or computerized information systems to provide these services in a comprehensive and efficient format. The components of such interventions have included various combinations of on-site training and start-up assistance, patient-administered computer reminder software in the waiting room, office chart reminders (notices placed in the medical record), computerized reminder systems, physician and office staff training to enhance counseling skills, patient health maintenance cards, continuing education seminars, and quality assurance feedback.

These trials have generally reported promising results from such efforts, including improved rates of clinical breast examinations (Manfredi et al., 1998; Williams et al., 1998) and mammograms (Burack and Gimotty, 1997; Litzelman et al., 1993; Williams et al., 1998), although successes were not uniform across practices (Burack et al., 1996). One trial reported an increase in the mention of mammography but not of mammography rates among women who have been the targets of such efforts (Kinsinger et al., 1998). Another trial found the effort no more effective than mailing annual reminders to patients, although it did offer modest incremental benefit among women who had previously had a mammogram (Costanza et al., 2000). One study found that screening rates improved by coupling mammography with completion of a clinical breast examination or a Pap smear (Cummings et al., 2000).

Some interventions focus on easing the difficulties that women face in obtaining referrals to mammographic facilities and arranging their appointments. The barriers are modest (e.g., the inconvenience) for many women but are overwhelming for women who are elderly, have limited education, or have language barriers or other difficulties that make it difficult to navigate the health care system. One strategy to reduce the inconvenience is to arrange same-day mammography services for women who are advised to have a mammogram. Such programs have improved screening rates in urban academic general medicine practices (Dolan et al., 1999). A British study suggests that fixed appointments are more effective than inviting women to telephone to make their own arrangements (Stead et al., 1998).

More intensive assistance (case management) in obtaining mammograms has been evaluated in settings where obtaining mammograms is especially difficult. For example, a primary care referral project operating within an urban emergency department improved screening rates by offering older minority women a brief motivational interview and a mammography referral and scheduling a next-day, no-cost appointment (Bernstein et al., 2000). A randomized trial reported a tripling of mammography rates among inner-city women by offering case management by culturally sensitive community health educators (Weber and Reilly, 1997). Case management at senior citizens' housing facilities encouraged mammography through the distribution of a Medicare mammography benefit flier, community education, and arrangements for mammography appointments and transportation, but primarily among women who were already predisposed to having the test. The investigators suggested that individual targeted interventions may be needed for women who have not had or who do not wish to have a mammogram (King et al., 1998).

Multiple interventions directed at patients, physicians, the health care system, and the community may provide the best approach to improving rates of screening for breast cancer (Rimer, 1997). In one review, 33 percent of studies that used single interventions and 85 percent of multicomponent trials were associated with increased rates of screening (Rimer, 1994). Diverse strategies, such as patient and community education, enabling legislation, and efficacious screening technology, can play independent yet synergistic roles (Zapka, 1994; Montano et al., 1997). According to one meta-analysis, all types of provider-targeted strategies to increase use of mammography were found to be effective, but those targeting both patients and providers were not significantly better at increasing screening than those targeting providers alone (Mandelblatt and Yabroff, 1999). The behavior involved in obtaining mammograms is complex, and it is usually not sufficient to solely target women. Without a physician recommendation, the behavior might not be enabled. Without access-enhancing and cost-reducing strategies, even a physician recommendation might not be enough (Rimer, 1994).

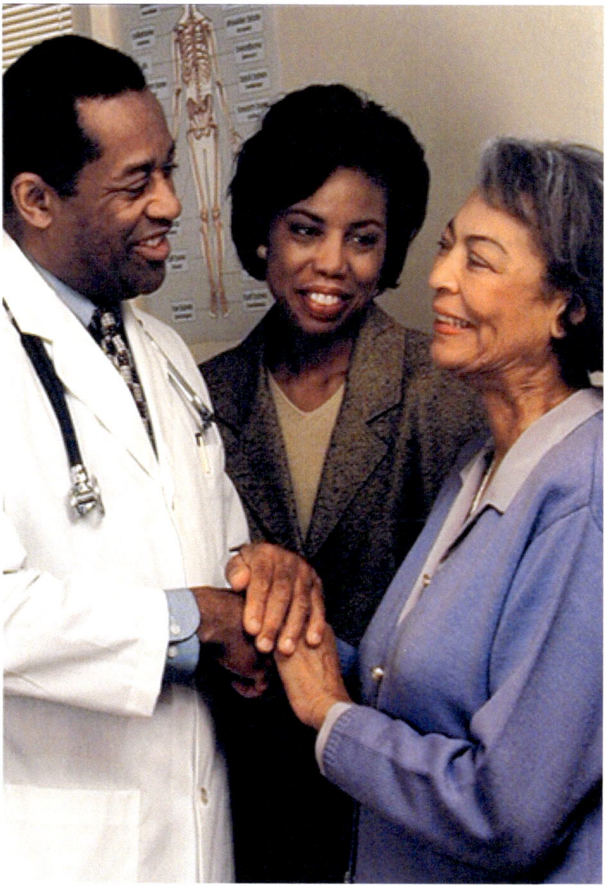

SOURCE: Centers for Disease Control and Prevention.

Prostate Cancer Screening

Awareness of prostate cancer in the United States has increased significantly in association with public education campaigns, media attention, and advocacy spearheaded by celebrities and prominent national figures. Screening for prostate cancer by testing for PSA is increasingly common in the United States. According to one survey, 87 percent of family physicians and 98 percent of urologists reported using the test for screening (McKnight et al., 1996). Studies conducted by the New York State Department of Health suggest that 60 to 64 percent of men age 50 and older have heard of the PSA test and have had it done (Smith et al., 2001). A 1997 survey in Texas revealed that 37 percent of men age 40 or older had received the PSA test (CDC, 2000b).

Given the controversy surrounding the appropriateness of PSA screening, it is unclear whether failure to be screened is properly viewed as a "gap" in care or carries the same public health significance as gaps in receiving tests with proven benefits in terms of reducing rates of mortality (e.g., colorectal, breast, and cervical cancer screening).

In fact, recent data support concerns about excessive PSA screening in the United States. Men for whom most professional organizations do not recommend PSA screening are receiving this test. Examples of such categories include men older than age 75, asymptomatic men with a life expectancy of less than 10 years, asymptomatic men with no risk factors who are younger than age 50, and men with risk factors before age 40. Studies report that 17 to 21 percent of PSA tests are ordered for such men (McNaughton Collins et al., 2000; Poteat et al., 2000). Although some of this testing probably represents a response to high patient demands or efforts by physicians to minimize medicolegal liability, to some extent it represents physicians' misconceptions about appropriate indications. In one survey, 16 percent of urologists and 43 percent of radiation oncologists recommended routine PSA testing in men with a life expectancy of less than 10 years (Fowler et al., 2000). This tendency is not limited to specialists. In one survey, 65 percent of primary care physicians reported "almost always" ordering a PSA test for men aged 70 to 74; 53 percent reported doing so for men aged 80 and older (Barry et al., 1996).

Even for men for whom current guidelines consider screening appropriate (for a description of current guidelines, see Box 5.4 in Chapter 5), what is advised is shared decision making rather than routine testing. Yet patients often undergo PSA screening without receiving any information about the consequences and sometimes without even being told that they received the test. In one study, more than 50 percent of men who had undergone PSA screening 2 weeks earlier said that they had not heard of the test and were unaware that they had received it (Diefenbach et al., 1996). As long ago as 1995, when PSA screening was less entrenched, 55 percent of primary care physicians reported ordering the PSA test "often" or "always" as part of the periodic health examination (Austin et al., 1997). In a study discussed in Chapter 5, a recent survey of internists found that only 17 percent consider patient preferences before ordering a PSA test (Dunn et al., 2001).

Randomized trials involving videotapes and pamphlet aids on the decision to undergo PSA screening have consistently demonstrated their effectiveness in improving patients' knowledge about the test (Flood et al., 1996; Schapira and VanRuiswyk, 2000; Volk et al., 1999). In most cases the intervention resulted in a statistically significant reduction in the rates of PSA testing (Flood et al., 1996; Schapira and VanRuiswyk, 2000; Volk et al., 1999; Wilkins et al., 1999), on average reducing interest in undergoing PSA screening by 65 percent (Volk and Spann, 2000).

Cervical Cancer Screening

Size of the Gap

The proven efficacy of cervical cancer screening and its remarkable success in reducing the disease to being an uncommon cause of cancer death in the United States have focused attention on screening failures as the primary cause of continued deaths from this disease. It has been estimated that 60 percent of cases of cervical cancer are associated with absent or deficient screening (Sawaya and Grimes, 1999). As of 1999, 88 percent of women ages 18 to 44 and 81 percent of women ages 45 or older have received a Pap smear within the past 3 years (CDC, Behavioral Risk Factor Surveillance System, 2000). The fact that more than 80 percent of women have had a Pap smear within the past 3 years is encouraging, but considerable progress needs to be made to achieve the goal set forth in *Healthy People 2010* (US DHHS and Office of Disease Prevention and Health Promotion, 2000), that is, for 90 percent of all women ages 18 and over to have had a Pap smear screen within the past 3 years.

The proportions of women who have had a Pap smear within the previous 3 years decline with age: among women ages 55 to 64, 65 to 74, and 75 and older, the median proportions across states are 83, 77, and 58 percent, respectively (CDC, 1999c). Other analyses show that higher income levels and higher levels of educational attainment are associated with an increased likelihood that eligible women have had a Pap test within the past 3 years (Blackman et al., 1999).

The probability of having had a Pap test within the past 3 years is 85 percent for whites, 91 percent for African Americans, 81 percent for Hispanics, and 95 percent for American Indians (CDC, Behavioral Risk Factor Surveillance System, 2000). Cervical cancer screening rates are significantly reduced among Asian Americans and Pacific Islanders (Kagawa-Singer and Pourat, 2000). For the period from 1994 to 1997, approximately 74 percent of women in these groups who were age 18 or older (and who had not undergone a hysterectomy) had received a Pap smear within the past 3 years (Coughlin and Uhler, 2000). Only 50 percent of Korean-American women have had a Pap smear in the past 2 years (Juon et al., 2000). American Indian women are more likely than others to report never having had a Pap test and to have a higher proportion of abnormal results (Benar et al., 2001). In a study of American Indians with diabetes, some Indian Health Service centers reported that as few as 26 percent of women had received a Pap smear test in the last year (Giroux et al., 2000).

Follow-up for an abnormal screening test result is an extremely important step in the cancer control process, yet many women fail to receive timely or any resolution of an abnormal screening test result. In one study, rates of nonresolution varied considerably across settings and populations, ranging between 7 and 49 percent (Yabroff et al., 2000). Factors associated with incomplete or delayed follow-up included younger patient age, financial barriers, lower education and income levels, non-white race, and certain psychosocial characteristics.

Predictors of Screening

Knowledge Most American women are familiar with cervical cancer screening and consider the Pap smear and pelvic examination a standard component of the well-woman examination. It is less likely that they have an accurate understanding of screening guidelines, in particular, the lack of necessity for annual or more frequent screening. The level of knowledge about cervical cancer screening is lower among certain socioeconomic and ethnic groups. A telephone survey of Hispanic women demonstrated that the proportions of individuals who had knowledge of guidelines ranged from 41 percent for Puerto Ricans to 56 percent for Cubans (Ramirez et al., 2000a). Follow-up for an abnormal Pap smear is associated with a memory of being informed of the test results (McKee et al., 1999) and understanding the purpose of colposcopy (Lerman et al., 1992).

Attitudes Several studies have demonstrated that poor adherence to cervical cancer screening is associated with attitudinal factors, such as fear of cancer and treatment (Khanna and Phillips, 2001; Lerman et al., 1992), but some have suggested that poor adherence is not associated with such factors (McKee et al., 1999). In Hispanic and Latino cultures, especially among Mexican Americans, Central Americans, and Cubans, social integration networks have a significant influence on cervical cancer screening rates (Suarez et al., 2000).

Ability As with the other screening tests evaluated in this chapter, insurance coverage, access to care, time, money, and transportation are important determinants of Pap smear use and adequate follow-up (Lerman et al., 1992). A lack of insurance, a low level of income, and a lack of a usual source of health care appear to play disproportionate roles as barriers to cervical cancer screening among Asian Americans and Pacific Islanders (Coughlin and Uhler, 2000; Kagawa-Singer and Pourat, 2000).

Reinforcement Many women have difficulty remembering how much time has elapsed since their last Pap smear and become overdue for screening. A lack of follow-up for abnormal smears has been linked to forgetting the appointment (Lerman et al., 1992).

Interventions to Enhance Cervical Cancer Screening

The review conducted for this chapter found little current evidence regarding the effectiveness of interventions to influence the knowledge or attitudes of women about cervical cancer screening or their ability to obtain the tests. Studies have examined reinforcement interventions. Randomized trials have not found physician or patient reminders to be particularly effective in improving cervical cancer screening rates (Buehler and Parsons, 1997; Burack et al., 1998; Ward and Proude, 1999), but the statistical powers of some studies may have been limited. A meta-analysis of randomized controlled trials assessing the value of patient letter reminders concluded that they increase the rate of cervical cancer screening, but are less effective among lower socioeconomic groups (Tseng et al, 2001). At least one randomized trial indicated that the combination of a physician reminder letter and a telephone contact increased the rate of Pap smear testing (Lantz et al., 1995). Another randomized trial involving low-income minority women who had received an abnormal Pap smear result reported higher rates of follow-up from telephone calls about the need for follow-up colposcopy (Miller et al., 1997).

Comprehensive office system changes such as those described above for breast cancer screening have proved effective in increasing Pap smear testing rates (Manfredi et al., 1998). One randomized trial reported higher Pap smear testing rates among Vietnamese women by use of such a program that also included Vietnamese-language educational materials, newsletters, and oncology data-query programs (Nguyen et al., 2000).

Some evidence suggests that lay health advisers can effectively promote cervical cancer screening (Dignan et al., 1996; Marcus and Crane, 1998). The use of such outreach staff may be enhanced when their work is coordinated with existing resources in the community, such as residents of low-income housing, and door-to-door recruitment (Davis et al., 1994; Dignan et al., 1996; Dunn and Sprunt, 1955; Evans et al., 1980; Hulka, 1966, 1967). The use of outreach clinics or mobile examination rooms also appears to increase rates of screening (Satariano et al., 1982; White et al., 1990). Educational campaigns to promote these clinics are required to ensure increases in rates of screening (Hirst et al., 1990; Holland et al., 1993).

PRIORITIZING CANCER SCREENING

Limited resources, both personal and economic, make it necessary for providers, health care systems, payers, and patients to set priorities in cancer screening. Ideally, this would be determined by knowing which approaches to cancer screening are most likely to improve health. From the patient's perspective, it would be useful to know whether one screening test may reduce the risk of premature death more substantially than another. Policy makers would benefit from knowing whether more gain in health is purchased by intensifying delivery of a particular screening test (e.g., introducing more frequent or more accurate testing or expanding coverage of screening to populations with limited access) or by directing resources to other screening maneuvers.

Given the larger goal of preventing premature death from cancer, consideration might also be given to the relative benefits of focusing on primary prevention over screening. Resources directed at smoking cessation and the consumption of a healthy diet might offer greater incremental benefits than the intensification of screening campaigns. The even larger aim of preventing premature morbidity and mortality might be achieved by directing resources to the prevention of coronary artery disease, stroke, or diabetes rather than optimizing the delivery of cancer screening tests. Studies indicate that as many disability-adjusted life years are claimed by road traffic collisions as by lung cancer (Michaud et al., 2001). Directing public resources toward effective injury prevention strategies might ultimately save more lives.

The modeling tools needed to make definitive comparisons of the relative health benefits of preventive maneuvers are not fully developed, offering patients, providers, and policy makers limited data with which to set priorities. Progress in this area has been inhibited by the paucity of firm data and methodological difficulties in arriving at valid projections. Even the crude modeling efforts undertaken thus far, however, hint at the relative importance of competing priorities in terms of preventive maneuvers. By one analysis, for example, closing the gap in the proportion of Americans who receive annual FOBT and screening mammography would prevent 9,632 and 4,475 deaths per year, respectively, whereas eliminating cigarette smoking would prevent 328,044 deaths (Woolf, 1999). By application of the same model to a hypothetical 45-year-old woman who smokes, the probability that stopping smoking would prevent her death before age 75 is 10.9 percent, whereas the probability that mammography every 1 to 2 years would do so would be 0.5 percent.

A modeling effort undertaken by the Partnership for Prevention in collaboration with the CDC and the Health Care Financing Administration (now called the Centers for Medicare and Medicaid Services) compared prevention services on the basis of preventable burden, the burden of disease that could be reduced if the service was delivered to 100 percent of the target population. The numbers of quality-adjusted life years (QALYs) that could be added by optimizing screening according to this model were 357,554 for cervical cancer, 293,092 for colorectal cancer, and 268,780 for breast cancer. By comparison, screening for high cholesterol levels would add 585,000 QALYs (Coffield et al., 2001).

The broadest approach to priority setting would take account of the other determinants of health, such as income disparities and inadequate education. Given the documented disadvantage that certain populations face in overcoming the burden of cancer and other chronic diseases, it is conceivable that efforts directed at improving access to health care and correcting social impediments to self-care and productivity (e.g., improving education and job security) might accomplish more in reducing rates of morbidity and mortality than investing further in refining screening technologies.

SUMMARY AND CONCLUSIONS

The possible benefit of cancer screening in the United States falls far short of its potential, costing health and lives. The lost opportunities take several forms: a substantial proportion of eligible persons are never screened or are screened too infrequently to achieve early detection, those who are screened may not be screened well, and the follow-up steps for abnormal results are often inadequate.

Inadequate screening occurs more commonly among certain segments of the population. Age, socioeconomic status, race or ethnicity, education, and health status account for marked disparities in the access of Americans to cancer screening tests. Older women, for example, are less likely than younger women to be screened for breast and cervical cancer (Mandelblatt and Yabroff, 2000). Women who do not receive breast cancer screening are also less likely to undergo cervical cancer screening (Cummings et al., 2000; Glasgow et al., 2000). Screening is also less common among low-income households and those with limited education or limited or no health insurance.

Members of certain ethnic and racial groups are significantly more likely to develop cancer and suffer higher mortality rates than whites. The reasons for this are not entirely clear but are certainly multifactorial. One important contributor may be the disproportionate difficulties that these individuals face in obtaining cancer screening. For virtually every cancer reviewed in this report, certain ethnic and racial minorities are less likely to be screened, making early detection less likely.

The complex interrelationships among the demographic variables mentioned above—income, education, and race and ethnicity—make it difficult to know the extent to which the reasons for inadequate screening are racial or ethnic status itself rather than the socioeconomic characteristics with which racial or ethnic status is often associated. An extensive body of social epidemiological research has examined this issue (Berkman and Kawachi, 2000), and data support the concern that race and ethnicity influence cancer screening even after adjustment for these cofactors (Smith, 1998; Institute of Medicine, 1999b).

Underuse of cancer screening is not the only problem in the United States. Overuse of screening tests (the widespread performance of screening tests that are not recommended or the performance of testing too frequently) potentially exposes patients to net harm and consumes resources needed for more effective health care, including cancer screening services for high-risk groups. Examples of overuse include the use of routine chest radiographs to screen for lung cancer or the rising use of whole-body computed tomography scanning to screen for various cancers and other health conditions (Smith, 2001) (see Chapter 7). Excessive levels of resource consumption and rates of false-positive test results are also amplified when screening is performed too frequently, such as when Pap smears are performed every 6 months.

To enhance the use of effective screening tests, multilevel approaches are recommended. Optimization of the delivery of effective cancer screening services and reductions in the numbers of inappropriate tests that are performed lie in changing the behaviors of the following:

- systems of care, to make cancer screening services available to eligible populations;
- health care providers, to perform cancer screening as recommended, on time, and with skill when they encounter patients eligible for screening; and
- individuals, to obtain recommended screening tests and to pursue follow-up.

Elimination of financial and access barriers to screening improves screening rates, for example, through the use of health insurance coverage, reduced cost sharing, and the availability of free screening at public clinics. In addition, certain organizational innovations are tied to improved rates of screening, such as the implementation of office systems to prompt health care providers to recommend screening, facilitate referrals, and remind patients and providers of the need for rescreening. Other opportunities to improve screening rates, particularly among underserved populations, include the use of nurses to provide outreach and education, case management, and facilitation. Increased opportunities for the provision of screening in health care settings (e.g., screening in emergency departments and screening during acute care visits) and the encouragement and provision of screening in nontraditional settings such as worksites and places of worship also hold some promise, although evidence of their effectiveness is limited.

Evidence suggests that multistrategy interventions are more effective than any one intervention alone (Sin and Leger, 1999). Examples include programs that integrate case management by culturally sensitive community health educators and the print or other media to communicate the benefits of mammography, general education of the community regarding screening, and the handling of logistic barriers by arranging appointments for mammography and transportation to those appointments (King et al., 1998; Weber and Reilly, 1997). Systematic and integrated approaches such as these offer great promise in the effort to optimize the quality and timeliness of cancer screening available to Americans.

7

Adopting New Technology in the Face of Uncertain Science: The Case of Screening for Lung Cancer[1]

Lung cancer, an uncommon type of cancer at the start of the 20th century, is the leading cause of cancer death in the United States at the start of the 21st. Surpassing deaths from breast, colon, and prostate cancer combined, there were an estimated 155,000 deaths from lung cancer in 2002 (ACS, 2002a). The prognosis after diagnosis is dismal. Five-year sur-vival rates remain less than 15 percent, changing little over the past 30 years (Travis et al., 1995). While lung cancer is mostly preventable through avoidance of tobacco products, smokers, health care providers, and scientists have unsuccessfully tried other preventive approaches, such as screening for early disease with chest radiographs and sputum cytology (secondary prevention).

Finding cancer earlier by screening seems intuitively appealing. Successful early detection of cervical cancer with Pap testing, breast cancer with mammography, and colon cancer through finding and removing polyps has lowered mortality from these cancers, thus providing impetus to search for early detection methods for other cancers. Unfortunately, the value of screening for other cancers, such as prostate-specific antigen (PSA) testing for prostate cancer, is less clear and has become more contentious (see also Chapter 5). Some cancers may be more amenable to early detection methods than others. For lung cancer, the prominent failures of chest radiographic and sputum cytology screening to lower disease mortality have led most organizations to recommend against screening for it.

[1]This chapter is based on a background paper prepared by Parthiv J. Mahadevia, Farin Kamangar, and Jonathan M. Samet (www.iom.edu/ncpb).

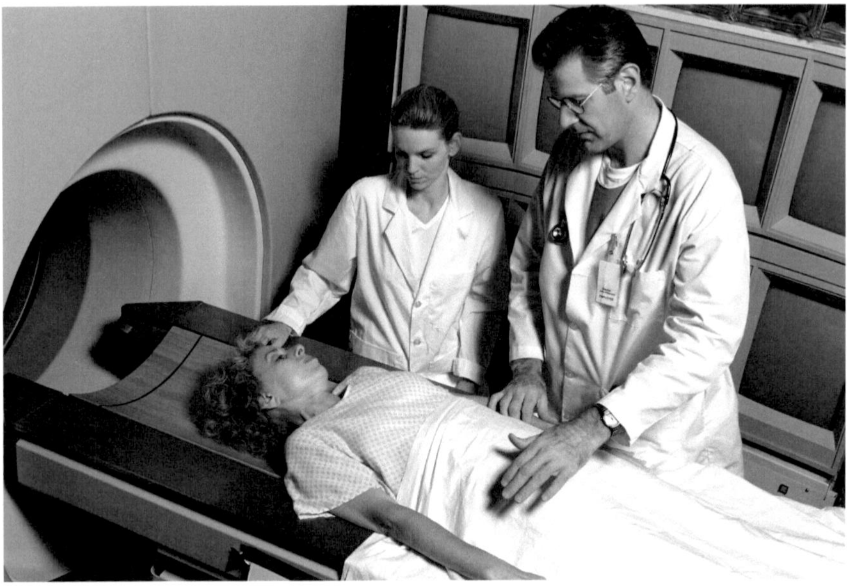

SOURCE: Corbis Corporation.

Recently a "high-tech" medical imaging device called spiral or helical computed tomography (CT) scan has renewed hope for finding an early detection method that can reduce mortality from lung cancer (Brice, 2000). Promising preliminary studies report that spiral CT scans can detect lung cancers at a smaller size than can chest radiographs (Henschke et al., 1999; Henschke et al., 2001; Sobue et al., 2002; Sone et al., 2001; Swensen et al., 2002). However, the clinical significance of these findings is unclear since long-term outcome data are unavailable. Randomized controlled trials evaluating spiral CT screening for lung cancer have only recently begun and conclusive efficacy data could be 5 to 10 years away.

Despite the lack of clear benefit, direct-to-consumer marketing of spiral CT screening is being offered by entrepreneurial radiology practices (Lee and Brennan, 2002). Early dissemination of an unproven screening test raises many concerns and questions. Concerns include false-positive and false-negative tests, harms from subsequent invasive procedures or treatments, and sizable costs to consumers, payers, and society. Decision makers have many questions. Should consumers get these scans? How should health care providers counsel high-risk individuals interested in this technology? Should managed care organizations and other third-party payers cover the costs of screening? What experimental or observational study designs provide the best data in the most efficient manner?

The case study presented in this chapter evaluates this high-technology screening test through a review of past and current scientific evidence. Clinical studies of lung cancer screening techniques have close to a 50-year history. Using a historical perspective, we review the lessons learned from past attempts to assist individuals, clinicians and policy makers in making decisions on the use of lung cancer screening technology despite the uncertainty of its effectiveness.

SCREENING FOR LUNG CANCER BY CHEST RADIOGRAPHY AND SPUTUM CYTOLOGY

In the early 1950s several researchers noted that "X-ray surveying" of the population detected lung cancers in asymptomatic individuals (Lilienfeld, 1966), raising the possibility that screening for lung cancer by chest radiography might detect cancers at earlier stages, when there might be hope of operative resection and cure. At that time there was already lengthy experience with mass screening for tuberculosis with a similar goal: identification of cases at a stage when intervention was most likely to be effective. Screening for tuberculosis was a major public health activity, and screening clinics with mobile radiographic facilities were successfully used for this purpose. It seemed reasonable to extend these same approaches to an emerging epidemic of another fatal pulmonary disease.

Four prospective cohort studies of lung cancer screening were started in the 1950s to determine if screening by chest radiography could improve lung cancer survival rates: the Veterans Administration-American Cancer Society (VA) Study (Lilienfeld, 1966), the Philadelphia Neoplasm Research Project Study (Weiss et al., 1982), the South London Lung Cancer Study (Nash et al., 1968), and the Tokyo Metropolitan Government Study (Hayata et al., 1982). Those studies used survival data to evaluate effectiveness and found 5-year survival rates that ranged from 8 to 20 percent (Table 7.1), not a meaningful improvement from the historical lung cancer survival rate. Survival rates among patients who had undergone surgical resection were 12 to 44 percent, higher than the overall survival rate. Unfortunately, the four studies did not incorporate control groups, and any improvement in survival from screening could not be assessed.

Two other nonrandomized studies, the North London Lung Cancer study (Brett, 1969) and the Erfurt County, Germany, study (Wilde, 1989), evaluated screening by chest radiography and did have control groups (Table 7.1). Both studies included an intervention group that received chest radiographs every 6 months and a control group that had either no screening or less frequent screening than the intervention group. In both studies, the 5-year survival rate was higher among the intervention group than the control group (15 versus 6 percent in the North London Lung Cancer study and 14 versus 8 percent in the Erfurt County study). However, lung cancer

TABLE 7.1 Summary of Nonrandomized Prospective Trials of Lung Cancer Screening (1950s to 1970s)

Study	Veterans Administration American Cancer Society Study, 1958–1961 (Lilienfeld, 1966)	Philadelphia Neoplasm Research Project, 1951–1965 (Weiss et al., 1982)
Design	Uncontrolled prospective study	Uncontrolled prospective study
Population and Number Screened[a]	14,607 males ages 45 and older	6,136 males ages 45 and older
Screening Interval and Method	6-month chest radiographs and sputum cytology	6-month chest radiographs
Incidence Rate (per 1,000 person-years)	0.52 percent[b]	2.3 percent
Number of Cancers Found	73 cases	121 cases
Overall 5-Year Survival Rate	17 percent[c]	8 percent
Percentage of Cancers Resected	36 percent	27 percent
5-Year Survival Among Those Who Had Resection	12 percent	18 percent
Lung Cancer Mortality Rate (per 1,000 person-years)	0.7 percent[b]	47 percent
Number of Cancers Found Between Screenings	5 cases	NR[d]
Comments	High attrition rate; VA domiciliary sample	Volunteer sampling; high attrition rate

[a]Numbers are incidence screened.
[b]Reported as a proportion (percent) of all patients only rather than as a rate.
[c]Reported as the 32-month survival rate.
[d]NR = not reported.
[e]Reported as 4-year survival rate.

Tokyo Metropolitan Government study (Hayata et al., 1982)	South London Lung Cancer Study, 1959–1963 (Nash et al., 1968)	North London Cancer Study, 1959, (Brett, 1969)	Erfurt County Study, 1953–1979 (Wilde, 1989)
Uncontrolled prospective study 1,871,374 radiographs	Uncontrolled prospective study 67,400 males ages 45 and older	Controlled prospective study Screened group, 29,733; control group, 25,311 males ages 40 and older	Controlled prospective study Screened group, 41,532; control group, 102,348 males
Annual chest radiographs	6-month chest radiographs	6-month chest radiographs	Screened group, 6-month chest radiographs; control group, 18-month chest radiographs
10.3 cases/100,000 radiographs	1.4 percent	Screened group, 1.1 cases; control group, 1.0 case	Screened group, 0.9 percent; control group, 0.65 percent
193 cases	147 cases	Screened group, 101 cases; control group, 77 cases	Screened group, 374 cases; control group, 667 cases
20.6 percent	27 percent[e]	Screened group, 15 percent; control group, 6 percent	Screened group, 14 percent; control group, 8 percent
56 percent	56 percent	Screened group, 44 percent; control group, 29 percent	Screened group, 28 percent; control group, 19 percent
43.6 percent	47 percent[e]	Screened group, 32 percent control group, 23 percent	Screened group vs. control group, 52 vs. 27 percent; 10-year: 39 percent vs. 19 percent
NR	NR	Screened group, 0.7 percent; control group, 0.8 percent	Screened group, 0.8 percent; control group, 0.6 percent
67 cases	87 cases (estimated)	36 cases	Screened group, 199 cases; control group, 485 cases
No mention of attrition or compliance	High attrition rate	High attrition rate	County-specific study

mortality rates were the same in both the intervention and the control groups. The discrepancy between the improved survival rate and the unchanged mortality rate was later explained by the previously mentioned biases that often affect screening data (see also Chapter 5).

These early studies were nonrandomized intervention studies that might be called "demonstration projects" today. Although the clinical trial was an established method for the evaluation of therapeutic interventions at the time, it had not yet been applied to the evaluation of screening. The landmark randomized controlled screening trial—the Health Insurance Plan of New York, which studied breast cancer—was not started until the mid-1960s (Shapiro, 1997).

Although most of the early lung cancer screening studies used chest radiography as the principal screening test, the VA study also evaluated sputum samples as another method for the detection of cancer. Oscar Auerbach (Auerbach, 1969), a pathologist, showed that a spectrum of histologic abnormalities could be found in the respiratory epithelia of smokers, ranging from normal cells to frank malignancy. Geno Saccomanno and colleagues (Saccomanno et al., 1974), who developed the techniques needed for the preparation of specimens of respiratory cells for cytological examination, showed that this spectrum of abnormalities was mirrored in exfoliated cells from the lung. These observational studies provided a rationale for screening for lung cancer by cytological examination of sputum (sputum cytology), which was considered a screening technique complementary to chest radiography. Radiography was presumed to be better at finding radiographically visible peripheral cancers, which originate in the small airways and alveoli (air sacs) of the lung, whereas sputum cytology would find centrally located and hence radiographically invisible cancers arising from the larger airways of the lung, the bronchi. The VA study estimated that the addition of sputum cytology increased the rate of detection of lung cancer by 50 percent compared with that by the use of chest radiography alone.

On retrospective assessment, these early lung cancer-screening studies had serious flaws, including a failure to have a control group and to randomize the participants to screened and nonscreened groups. Consequently, the results may have been affected by the time-related biases that arise in screening studies. Their results were also limited by attrition of the study populations, poor compliance with the screening regimen, difficulties with sputum collection, and high rates of mortality from surgery.

For screening to be effective, most enrollees should be compliant with the screening regimen. In the VA study, roughly 30 percent of the initial enrollees failed to return for a second chest radiograph. By the third year, only 685 of the initial 14,607 enrollees received their recommended chest radiographs. The Philadelphia Neoplasm Research Project study noted that noncompliant individuals had a 76 percent higher rate of lung cancer than participants who complied. If dropouts are more likely to have the disease, the effectiveness of any screening program may seem to be lower, as the individuals at greatest risk are less likely to receive the intervention.

The quality of screening by sputum cytology in these studies was not optimal. International standards for cytological classification were not yet developed, and there was a high degree of variability in interpretation of abnormalities that fell between the normal and the malignant states (Fullmer, 1970). The significance of finding "atypical" cells was unclear. In 1970, Fullmer noted that priority areas for the enhancement of sputum cytology as a screening method included further refinements in the sample collection technique, education of the technicians who performed the cytological examination, reductions in costs, and establishment of international standards. A positive sputum cytology result requires follow-up by another test to localize the cancer. The VA study had difficulty finding the lung cancer when the sputum cytology result was considered positive but the chest radiography result was negative. The poor localization of cancer made surgical resection less effective, if not impossible. Finally, postoperative death rates were high, approaching 30 percent in the Philadelphia Neoplasm Research Project study.

Randomized Controlled Trials of Chest Radiographic and Sputum Cytology Screening

Building on the earlier studies, the NCI sponsored three randomized controlled trials of lung cancer screening in the 1970s: the Johns Hopkins Lung Project (the Hopkins study) (Tockman, 1986), the Memorial Sloan Kettering Lung Project (the Memorial study) (Melamed et al., 1984), and the Mayo Lung Project (the Mayo study) (Fontana et al., 1986). A fourth randomized controlled trial was performed in the Czech Republic (Kubik and Haerting, 1990). The studies addressed the key design deficiencies of the earlier studies: assignment to screening was by randomization, and careful conduct of the studies addressed issues of compliance and attrition (Berlin et al., 1984). Technological advancements such as CT and flexible fiberoptic bronchoscopy improved the ability to localize the cancer in persons positive by screening. In addition, surgical techniques had improved, and the postoperative mortality rate had declined since the earlier studies.

The individuals in the intervention arms of all three NCI studies underwent both chest radiography and sputum cytology every 4 months. The individuals in the control arms of the Hopkins and Memorial studies also underwent chest radiography annually. The Mayo study had a different control arm; enrollees were given advice only at the time of enrollment to have chest radiography and sputum cytology performed annually. In the Czech study, which lasted 3 years, the intervention group underwent chest radiography and sputum cytology every 6 months, whereas the control group had both tests at the beginning and at the end of the study.

TABLE 7.2 First Screening (Prevalence) Results from NCI-Sponsored Randomized Controlled Trials of Lung Cancer Screening Using Chest Radiographs and Sputum Cytology

Study	Johns Hopkins Lung Project, 1973–1978 (Tockman, 1986)	Memorial Sloan Kettering Lung Project, 1974–1978 (Melamed et al., 1984)
Population and Numbers Screened	10,387 male volunteers, ages 45+ with median 28.5 pack-year history of smoking	10,040 male volunteers, ages 45+ with median 31.2 pack-year history of smoking
Screening Intervention (number of subjects in each group)	I (5,226): CXR and SC C (5,161): CXR	I (4,968): CXR and SC C (5,072): CXR
Prevalence Rate (per 1,000 persons)	Overall: 7.6 I: 7.5 C: 7.8	Overall: 5.3 I: 6.0 C: 4.5
Number of Cancers Detected	I: 39 C: 40	I: 30 C: 23
5-Year Survival Rate in Study Group(s)	I: 59 percent C: 35 percent	I: 47 percent C: 31 percent
Number of Stage 1 Cancers Detected	I: 26 C: 16	I: 14 C: 8
5-Year Survival Rate for All Stage 1 Disease[b]	90 percent	85 percent
Percentage of All Cancers Resected	I: 69 percent C: 42 percent	I: 60 percent C: 48 percent
Cancers Detected by Sputum Cytology Alone	11	9
Number of Second Primary Lung Cancers	8	6
Comments	2 postoperative deaths	2 postoperative deaths; 16 surgeries for non-malignant lesions

NOTE: Results are reported separately for groups receiving the intervention (I) and those that were controls (C). CXR = chest radiography; SC = sputum cytology.

[a]The NCI intervention group includes all of the Mayo study subjects and the intervention groups in the Hopkins and Memorial studies. These are then compared with the control groups in the Hopkins and Memorial studies.

Mayo Lung Project, 1971–1976 (Fontana et al., 1986)	NCI composite results of the above three trials[a] (Berlin et al., 1984)	Czech study (Kubik and Haerting, 1990)
10,933 male volunteers, ages 45+ with median 20 pack-year history of smoking	31,360 males	6,364 males ages 40–64 with 32-year smoking history
All enrollees received CXR and Sputum Cytology	I (21,127): CXR and SC C (10,233): the control cases in the Hopkins and Memorial studies	All enrollees received CXR and Sputum cytology
Overall: 8.3	Overall: 7.1 I: 7.6 C: 6.2	Overall: 3.0
Overall: 91	I: 160 C: 63	Overall: 19
Overall: 40 percent	Hopkins/Memorial I: 55 percent; Mayo group: 40 percent; Hopkins/Memorial C: 35 percent Overall: 45 percent	Overall: 26 percent
Overall: 41	Overall: 105 I: 81 C: 24	Overall: 5
70 percent	80 percent	NR
54 percent	I: 76 percent C: NR[c]	33 percent
17	37	NR
7	21	NR
3 postoperative deaths; 28 surgeries for non-malignant lesions		

[b]These survival rates reflect those that were resected, not all stage I disease.
[c]NR = not reported.

TABLE 7.3 Incidence Screening Results from Randomized Controlled Trials of Lung Cancer Screening Using Chest Radiographs and Sputum Cytology

Study	Johns Hopkins Lung Project, 1973–1978 (Tockman, 1986)
Population and Numbers Screened	10,387 male volunteers ages 45+ with median 28.5 pack year history of smoking
Screening Intervention (numbers in each group	I (5,226): CXR and SC C (5,161): CXR
Incidence rate (per 1,000 person-years)	I: 4.6[b] C: 4.9[b]
Number of Cancers Detected	I: 155 C: 162
5-Year Survival in Study Groups	I: 20 percent[c] C: 20 percent[c]
Number of Early vs. Advanced Cancers Found[a]	I: early vs. advanced 83 and 111 C: early vs. advanced 93 and 109
Percentage of All Cancers Resected	I: 47 percent[c] C: 44 percent[c]
5-Year Survival for Cancers That Were Resected	NR[d]
Mortality Rate (1,000 person-years)	I: 3.4 C: 3.8
Number of Cancers Found Between Screenings or Due to Symptoms	193 total
Additional Number of Cancers Found by SC	22

NOTE: Results are reported separately for groups receiving intervention (I) and those that were controls (C). CXR = chest radiography; SC = sputum cytology.
[a]Early cancers are those staged as 0, 1, or 2, and late cancers are those staged as 3 or 4.
[b]These results are based on interim results; the final results did not report these statistics.
[c]Eight-year survival.
[d]NR = not reported.
[e]These results are for stage 1 cancers only.

Memorial Sloan Kettering Lung Project, 1974–1982 (Melamed et al., 1984)	Mayo Lung Project, 1971–1976 (Fontana et al., 1986)	Czech study (Kubik and Haerting, 1990)
10,040 male volunteers ages 45+ with median 31.2 pack-year history of smoking	10,933 male volunteers ages 45+ with median 20 pack-year history of smoking	6,364 males ages 40–64 with 32-year smoking history
I (5,072): CYR and SC C (4,968): CXR	I (4,618): CXR and SC C (4,593): annual advice to get CXR	I (3,171): CXR and SC every 6 months for 3 years C (3,174): CXR and SC 3 years apart
I: 3.7 C: 3.8	I: 5.5 C: 4.3	I: 6.0 C: 4.5
I: 114 C: 121	I: 206 C: 160	I: 108 C: 82
I: 36 percent C: 33 percent	I: 33 percent C: 15 percent	I: 18 percent C: 18 percent
I: early vs. advanced, 54 and 85 C: early vs. advanced, 68 and 86	I: early vs. advanced, 99 and 107 C: early vs. advanced, 51 and 109	I: early vs. advanced, 55 and 53 C: early vs. advanced, 36 and 46
I: 51 percent C: 53 percent	I: 46 percent C: 32 percent	I: 23 percent C: 23 percent
80 percent[e]	50 percent	26 percent
I: 2.7 C: 2.7	I: 3.2 C: 3.0	I: 3.6 C: 2.6
I: 44 C: 56	I: 116 C: 160	I: 47 C: 44
18	18	2

The Hopkins and Memorial studies thus evaluated the contribution of sputum cytology to early detection, whereas the Mayo and the Czech studies were designed to assess the combined effects of sputum cytology and chest radiography.

Results were reported for the first screening interval, also called the prevalence screening interval, separately from subsequent or incidence screening intervals (see Table 7.2 versus Table 7.3). This distinction was appropriate since prevalence data measure the burden of disease in the population as the study starts. Prevalence information indicates the potential benefit of one-time or short-term screening, but prevalence gives no insights into the effect of screening for new cases or for reductions in the rate of mortality from the disease. Length-time bias typically introduces apparent screening effectiveness into the prevalence screening results (Melamed et al., 1984). The effectiveness of screening tests is best measured by determining whether those individuals who were negative after the first screening benefit from ongoing screening. When this initially negative population is screened repeatedly, any subsequent new cancers are thought to be more representative cases of the disease in terms of the growth characteristics of the disease. This subsequent screening, or incidence screening, provides the needed estimate of the value of long-term screening.

Prevalence data from these randomized controlled studies showed 3 to 8 cancers per 1,000 persons screened (Table 7.2). The Hopkins and Memorial studies randomized their study populations from the start of the study. The combined 5-year survival rates for both studies were 55 percent for the screened groups and 35 percent for the control groups. The Czech and Mayo studies, which did not separate the groups into screened and control groups at the first screening, had overall survival rates of 26 and 40 percent, respectively. Composite results for all three NCI-sponsored trials show that 51 percent (81 of 160) of the lung cancer cases among the intervention group were stage I, whereas 38 percent (24 of 63) of the lung cancer cases in the control group were stage I. The 5-year survival rates among all individuals with stage I cancers ranged from 70 to 90 percent. Forty-two to 76 percent of the cancers were surgically resected. Chest radiography was more sensitive than sputum cytology for the detection of peripheral cancers. The addition of sputum cytology as a screening technique was considered complementary to chest radiography because 37 cancers were detected by sputum cytology alone. Nearly all cancers detected by cytology were centrally located squamous cell carcinomas. Persons with these cancers had the best survival rates compared with the survival rates for the persons in the other groups, suggesting that these cancers tend to have slower growth rates.

NCI concluded that the preliminary data were encouraging. The composite 5-year survival rate was 45 percent, much higher than the historical survival rate. The NCI investigators wrote optimistically, "It is probable that some of the patients who had lung cancer detected by screening and successfully resected, and are alive and free of cancer today, would have died of their cancers had they not been screened. . . . Chest radiographs were the most sensitive method for detecting lung cancer" and sputum cytology for squamous cell cancers (Berlin et al., 1984). They cautioned that the high 5-year survival rate was artificially elevated because of the effects of lead-time bias, length bias, and overdiagnosis bias. Mortality rates from subsequent incidence data would determine whether screening was effective.

Incidence data from the randomized controlled trials showed annual new cancer rates of 4.3 to 6.0 per 1,000 persons. The Hopkins and Memorial studies found similar numbers of cancers in each group (intervention group versus control group in the Hopkins study, 155 versus 162; intervention group versus control group in the Memorial study, 114 versus 121) (Table 7.3). The Mayo and Czech studies found more cancers among the intervention group than the control group (206 versus 160 in the Mayo study and 108 versus 82 in the Czech study).

As mentioned earlier, an effective screening test should result in the detection of a greater proportion of early-stage cancers and a lower proportion of late-stage cancers (a stage shift). Among all three of the NCI studies, the total numbers of early cancers detected were 240 in the intervention groups and 212 in the control groups; that is, 28 more early-stage cancers were found in the intervention groups. Unfortunately, the gain in the numbers of cases of early-stage cancer was not offset by a decrease in the number of cases of advanced, late-stage cancer: 303 in the intervention groups and 304 in the control groups. Thus, a stage shift did not take place and the increased number of cases of early-stage cancer suggests possible overdiagnosis bias (Eddy, 1990b). The large number of interval cases—that is, cases not detected by screening but diagnosed between scheduled visits—is further evidence of the ineffectiveness of the screening interventions. Either the prior screening missed the tumors or the tumors represent new, aggressively growing tumors not amenable to screening.

The survival and mortality rate data were disappointing. Of the four randomized controlled studies, only the Mayo study had a favorable 5-year survival advantage for participants in the intervention group: 33 percent for the intervention group compared with 15 percent for the control group. These data need to be interpreted with consideration of potential biases, as described above. The other studies showed no survival advantage for screened participants, and all four studies showed no meaningful reduction in the rate of mortality from lung cancer as a result of screening. In the Mayo and Czech studies, the mortality rates were actually worse for those receiving the screening intervention.

Other studies that have evaluated screening for lung cancer by chest radiography include three case-control studies and a historical cohort study

(Ebeling and Nischan, 1987; Hillerdal, 1996; Okamoto et al., 1999; Sobue et al., 1992b). The case-control study of Okamoto and colleagues (Okamoto et al., 1999) was the only one to find a statistically significant beneficial effect of screening. The other three studies did not show significant benefits for screening. The case-control studies are subject to many biases inherent to retrospective data collection, in addition to the time-related biases that can affect interpretation of any data on screening. Selection of an appropriate control group is often difficult, and information obtained from records and interviews may be flawed.

Lessons Learned from Lung Cancer Screening Studies

Why was screening with chest radiographs and sputum cytology unsuccessful? Trial investigators and epidemiologists have offered several explanations. In her analysis of the lung cancer screening studies, Hulka (1986) offered two scenarios that could have explained the lack of mortality reduction in these trials. First, the duration of the preclinical phase of lung cancer may be short, implying that most of these malignancies are too aggressive to benefit from early detection. Secondly, sputum cytology and chest radiography may not have had the accuracy needed for early detection and subsequent mortality reduction.

With regard to the preclinical phase, the rate of mortality from a fatal disease can be reduced by screening only if the preclinical phase is sufficiently long and early detection leads to more effective interventions. For clinically diagnosed lung cancer, which is invariably fatal unless it is treated, the duration of the preclinical phase is not well characterized. Walter and colleagues (Walter et al., 1992) estimated the preclinical phase from the data from the Czech study, offering an estimate of 7 to 8 months (95 percent confidence interval, 6 months to a year), which is shorter than that for other cancers. They recommended that, at a minimum, biannual screening would be needed to detect the majority of cancers during the preclinical phase. Flehinger and colleagues (Flehinger et al., 1993), using data from the Mayo study, estimated that the mean duration of early-stage disease is 4 years. The rate of detection of disease at the early stage was low (less than 25 percent) (Flehinger et al., 1993). An analysis of the data from the Hopkins and Memorial studies by some of the same investigators found similar results (Flehinger and Kimmel, 1987). The actual duration of the average preclinical phase of lung cancer remains unclear.

Was the choice of diagnostic tests an issue? Inadequate sensitivity[2] of the tests was found in the studies. The VA study reported the sensitivities of

---

[2] See Chapter 5 for the definitions of screening parameters such as sensitivity, specificity, and predictive value.

chest radiography and sputum cytology to be 42 and 33 percent, respectively. The Hopkins study and a study conducted in Osaka, Japan (Sobue et al., 1991), estimated the sensitivities of chest radiography to be 50 and 57 percent, respectively. The corresponding estimates for the sensitivity of sputum cytology were 25 and 31 percent. All three trials estimated the combined sensitivities for both screening modalities: 63 percent in the VA study, 67 percent in the Hopkins study, and 72 percent in the Osaka study. A systematic review of the sputum cytology literature, including studies done as early as 1935, found a wide range of test sensitivities, 22 to 98 percent, with the average being 64 percent (Bocking et al., 1992). Tockman (2000) reviewed the accuracy of chest radiography and sputum cytology for all cancers diagnosed in the NCI randomized trials. Both tests together detected 49 percent of all cancers, and sputum cytology alone detected 11 percent. The specificities of chest radiography or sputum cytology, or both, were generally high, about 95 percent.

The inaccuracy of chest radiography for lung cancer detection has also been shown by studies evaluating its rate of false-negative results. False-negative results represent the proportion of cancers present but missed by the screening test. Chest radiographs are known to detect cancers as small as 6 millimeters (mm) in diameter if the cancers happen to lie in the intercostal spaces (the clear area between the ribs). However, radiologists often miss cancers smaller than 10 mm on a chest film. In a study of missed lung cancers, the average size of the tumors was 16 mm and the largest tumor was 34 mm (Austin et al., 1992). In the Mayo study, only 1 of 50 peripheral cancers detected by screening was less than 10 mm. Seventeen measured between 10 and 20 mm, and 19 were between 20 and 30 mm (Sanderson and Fontana, 1982).

Other potential problems with these studies have been described. Using the Mayo study as an example, the study's investigators gave insightful comments regarding the contamination of study groups, a lack of stage shift, and possible overdiagnosis (Fontana et al., 1991). They noted that the control group had high rates of screening by chest radiography during the last 2 years of the screening phase. At the time it was common practice to screen for lung cancer, and contamination of the control group could not be avoided. Nearly 75 percent of control subjects underwent radiography. In addition, the intervention group complied with the 4-month regimen of sputum cytology and chest radiography only 75 percent of the time, thereby reducing the possibility of observing the full impact of the screening. Even under conditions of no contamination, the statistical power of the Mayo study was limited (statistical power refers to the likelihood that a study will find a particular effect if the effect exists). Small reductions in the rate of mortality from lung cancer (reductions on the order of 10 to 20 percent) could easily have been dismissed as not statistically significant (Flehinger et al., 1993).

Excess cases were diagnosed among the screened groups, suggesting the possibility of overdiagnosis. If both groups were appropriately randomized, the risk for lung cancer would be equivalent, and similar numbers of cancer cases should be detected in each group. Yet, at the end of 10 years of follow-up, the intervention group had 46 more cases of disease than the control group. It is possible that some in the control group, who were less closely monitored than the screened group, died from other causes before a diagnosis of lung cancer could be made (Type II Pseudodisease); therefore, the 46 cases could have been overdiagnosed. Fontana et al. (1991) noted that the death rate from all causes was high among this population. "Predictably, the great majority of deaths were attributable to ischemic heart disease (which alone accounted for 50 percent of all deaths)" (p. 1160).

Strauss and colleagues (Strauss et al., 1995) argue that overdiagnosis bias is an unlikely problem in lung cancer, given the aggressive course of lung cancer and the rarity of undiagnosed lung cancers found in autopsy studies. The rate of survival among patients with stage I cancers who refused surgery is dismal, suggesting that practically all lung cancers are lethal if left untreated (Sobue et al., 1992a). Others contend that the natural history of early-stage cancers is unknown and that overdiagnosis bias is possible, even though it is difficult to document (Black, 2000).

Mortality from surgery and unnecessary therapy took place in the trials. Seven deaths were reported after the 122 surgeries. The Mayo and Memorial studies reported that 40 surgeries were performed for conditions that mimicked lung cancer. Common diagnoses among these cases included hamartomas, healed infarcts, granulomatous lung diseases such as tuberculosis, and rare tumors such as mesothelioma and thymoma. One man with a benign condition died from a myocardial infarction after surgery. Given the persistent risks of thoracic surgery, the harm that may result from false-positive diagnoses cannot be dismissed.

In general, survivors of a first lung cancer are at higher risk for the development of another lung cancer and may need more frequent screening. Among the studies evaluated here, second primary lung cancers occurred in 21 (17 percent) of the 122 lung cancer patients who had surgical resections (Berlin et al., 1984; Fontana et al., 1972; Frost et al., 1984; Melamed et al., 1984). Other lessons from these studies include the difficulty of motivating smokers to participate in regular screening, the need for close follow-up since the requirements for additional workups are high, and the costs attendant to such care.

Screening Recommendations from Medical Organizations

The American Cancer Society, which had recommended the annual screening of "heavy cigarette smokers" and workers exposed to asbestos by chest radiography, dropped this recommendation in 1980 (Eddy, 1980a).

Eddy wrote, "The Society has changed its policy and does not recommend any tests for the early detection of cancer of the lung, but urges a focus on primary prevention: helping smokers to stop (or switch to low tar and nicotine cigarettes), and keeping nonsmokers from starting. People with signs and symptoms of lung cancer should consult their physicians" (p. 205). The rationale for the policy change was that screening techniques must reduce morbidity and mortality from the disease, which these trials clearly did not establish. Furthermore, harm from screening due to false-positive workups and iatrogenic complications with corresponding costs would make such screening unattractive. The NCI trials were done at respected academic medical centers with well-trained health care professionals. If widespread mass screening were incorporated, the rates of workups because of false-positive results and subsequent harm would rise, given the inexperience and wide variability in the quality of care. A lack of experienced cytologists to read the sputum smears was cited as an example of the limitations of the infrastructure available for the implementation of widespread mass screening.

The American Cancer Society's position paper did leave the door open for change: "Although at present there is insufficient evidence that screening is effective in reducing lung cancer mortality, there is no proof that it is not effective. As stated before, every case is different, and it may be that even knowing the lack of evidence of benefit and the potential risks, some individuals may choose to have early detection examinations. The Society's recommendations are not meant to discourage this" (Eddy, 1980a, p. 206).

A U.S. Preventive Services Task Force (1990) position paper stated, "screening asymptomatic persons for lung cancer with routine chest radiographs or sputum cytology is not recommended" (p. 1763). They noted "accuracy of the chest radiograph is limited by the capabilities of the technology and by variation in interpretation among radiologists" (p. 1763). "Furthermore, the yield of screening chest radiography to detect cancer is low, largely because of the low prevalence of lung cancer in the general population and even among asymptomatic smokers" (p. 1763) and the low yield due to the uncommon nature of the disease. The NCI prevalence data indicate that only 0.39 percent of the screened population had lung cancer. Sputum cytology was a less effective technique since chest radiography detected the majority of cancers. The paper concluded that $1.5 billion would be spent if mass screening for high-risk groups was advocated and that there would be significant harm from follow-up testing. It concluded, "Primary prevention may be more effective . . . cigarette smoking is responsible for more than 90 percent of lung cancers and should therefore be the principal focus of clinical efforts to help prevent this disease" (U.S. Preventive Task Force, 1990, p. 1765).

The NCI, the Food and Drug Administration, the American College of

Radiology, the Royal College of Radiologists, the World Health Organization, and the Canadian Task Force on Periodic Health Examinations reached the same conclusions. All strongly endorsed smoking cessation as the principal method of prevention.

A NEW MEDICAL IMAGING SCREENING TEST: THE SPIRAL CT SCAN

As a lung cancer screening test, chest radiography lacked the sensitivity to find early-stage cancers. When a cancer is seen on a radiograph it is now common clinical practice to obtain a CT scan to evaluate the lesion. The conventional CT scan is more precise in measuring the size of the lesion, the shape of the lesion, the number of microcalcifications contained in or around the lesion, and enlargement of lymph nodes (for spread of malignancy). CT scans are more sensitive than chest radiographs in finding small cancers hiding around blood vessels and old scars (Sone et al., 2000). If CT scans are superior imaging tests, why could they not be used to screen for lung cancer?

Conventional CT scanning emits higher dose of ionizing radiation than chest radiographs. Chest radiographic radiation exposure ranges from 13 to 20 millirads (mrads). Conventional CT scans can emit 1,400 mrads of exposure, or 70 times the dose of a single chest radiograph (Naidich et al., 1990). The average radiation dose from natural sources, which comes primarily from indoor radon, is estimated to be 300 mrads per person per year (Black, 1999b). Widespread mass screening with this level of ionizing radiation could cause harm in many individuals and could even increase the incidence of lung cancer (Eddy, 1980a). Furthermore, conventional CT scans are time-consuming for radiologists to read, are costly to produce, and produce more false-positive results than chest radiographs.

Spiral CT scanning has some advantages over conventional CT scanning for screening purposes. First, spiral CT scans emit less radiation, estimated around 260 mrads, than conventional CTs, prompting the description "low-dose" CT. Several studies have investigated spiral CT scanners that emit yet lower radiation (Anderson et al., 1991; Diederich et al., 1999; Kanazawa et al., 1998; Nitta et al., 1998; Nitta et al., 1999), so-called ultra-low-dose CT scanners. The radiation doses from these machines are lower and the diagnostic accuracy is reportedly not compromised. Secondly, by scanning in a spiral fashion, spiral CT scans are fast and scanning can be completed in a single breath hold of 15 to 30 seconds. Finally, out-of-pocket charges to the consumer for a spiral CT screen are approximately $300 (Brice, 2000), which is less than for a conventional CT scan but more than for a chest radiograph. Similar to conventional CT scanning, radiologist time for interpretation and false-positive test results remains a problem with spiral CT scanning as a screening test.

Four nonrandomized, uncontrolled studies have reported spiral CT screening data for both prevalence and incidence screening (Tables 7.4 and 7.5). Two studies, the Early Lung Cancer Action Project, or ELCAP, study (Henschke et al., 1999; Henschke et al., 2001), and a Mayo Clinic study (Swensen et al., 2002) were performed in the United States while the other two, the Anti-Lung Cancer Action, or ALCA study, (Kaneko et al., 1996; Sobue et al., 2002) and a Shinshu University study (Sone et al., 2001; Sone et al., 1998) were conducted in Japan.

All studies initially compared lung cancer detection rates using spiral CT scanning to chest radiographs. Three of the studies, ELCAP, the Mayo Clinic and Shinshu University, performed annual spiral CT screening, and the ALCA study recommended screening biannually. Participants who had abnormal scans, defined as having an indeterminate lung nodule, were asked to return for surveillance with conventional CT scans on a periodic basis. For example, the ELCAP trial recommended those with indeterminate nodules to have 3-, 6-, 12-, and 24-month conventional CT scans. If nodule growth was detected, then surveillance was stopped and a definitive invasive diagnostic procedure was performed. This nodule triaging process aimed to limit the number of unnecessary invasive tests and any harm performed for those without lung cancer.

The demographic composition of the participants varied widely across the studies. The United States studies had combinations of current and former smokers, with the ELCAP trial enrolling the highest-risk population, older individuals (mean age 66 years) with a heavy smoking history (median 44 pack-year). The Japanese studies included never smokers, which are at low risk for lung cancer. Also, many participants in one study, ALCA, had undergone screening with chest radiographs in prior years, making this a more prescreened population than in the other three trials.

While all of the studies used spiral CT scan technology, the radiological parameters of the spiral CT scans were slightly different for each trial. Notably, the Mayo Clinic study used newer spiral CT scan technology, a multi-detector scanner with thinner slice thickness (5 mm in the Mayo Clinic study vs. 10 mm in the other studies), which significantly improves the resolution and detection capability of the spiral CT scan.

During the prevalence screening, spiral CT scans detected 30 lung cancers among 1,000 participants in the ELCAP study for a cancer detection rate of 30 per 1,000 screenings. The cancer detection rate at the Mayo Clinic study was 13.8 per 1,000 screenings. For the Japanese studies the spiral CT cancer detection rate was lower, 8.1 per 1,000 screenings for ALCA and 4.0 per 1,000 screenings for Shinshu University. ELCAP, which enrolled a high-risk population, had the highest lung cancer detection rate. The Shinshu University study, which enrolled the largest numbers of never smokers, had the lowest lung cancer detection rate. Nonetheless, every

TABLE 7.4 Spiral CT Lung Cancer Screening Trials: Prevalence Data

	Baseline Screening Data				
Trial	Henschke et al. (1999)	Swensen et al. (2002)	Sone et al. (1998)	Kaneko Sobue et al. (1996)	Weighted Average
Study location	United States		Japan		
Study design	Prospective uncontrolled cohort study	Prospective uncontrolled cohort study	Prospective uncontrolled cohort study	Prospective uncontrolled cohort study	
Study years	1993–98	1999	1996–98	1993–98	
Recommended screening interval	1 year	1 year	1 year	6 months	
Participant demographics	54% male, 44 pack-year, Mean age 66	52% male, 61% CS, 39% FS, Mean age 59	54% male, 46% ES, 54% NS, Med. age 64	88% male, 62% CS, 25% FS, 14% NS, Mean age 59	
Spiral CT scan parameters (all protocols used 120–140 kVp and between 40–50 mA)	Single detector 10 mm ST	Multi-detector 5 mm ST	Single detector 10 mm ST	Single detector 10 mm ST	

Participants screened	1,000	1,520	5,483	1,611	9,614
Number of screening tests performed	1,000	1,520	5,483	1,611	9,614
New indeterminate lung nodules detected	233	782	676	192	1,883
Rate of new indeterminate nodules per screening, %	23	51	12	12	20
Benign biopsies or surgeries (harm)	3	4	7	8	22
Clinical Stage Distribution					
IA NSCLC	22	13	21	10	66
IB NSCLC	1	1	2	1	5
IIA NSCLC	1	4			5
IIB NSCLC					0
IIIA NSCLC	2	2		2	6
IIIB NSCLC	1			1	2
IV NSCLC	1				1
Unclassified NSCLC	2				2
SCLC		2			2
Total lung cancers	30	22	23	14	89

NS = Never smoker, ES = Ever smoker, FS = Former smoker, CS = Current smoker.
CT = Computerized Tomography, NSCLC = Non-small-cell lung cancer, SCLC = Small-cell lung cancer.
ST = slice thickness, kVp = kilovolt peak, mA = milliangstroms.

TABLE 7.5 Spiral CT Lung Cancer Screening Trials: Incidence Data

	Annual Repeat Screening				
Trial	Henschke et al. (2001)	Swensen et al. (2002)	Sone et al. (1998)	Sobue et al., (2002)	Weighted Average
Study location	United States		Japan		
Study design	Prospective uncontrolled cohort study	Prospective uncontrolled cohort study	Prospective uncontrolled cohort study	Prospective uncontrolled cohort study	
Study years	1993–98	1999	1996–98	1993–98	
Recommended screening interval	1-year	1-year	1-year	6-months	
Participant demographics	54% male, 44 pack-year, Mean age 67	52% male, 61% CS, 39% FS, Mean age 60	54% male, 46% ES, 54% NS, Med. Age 65+	88% male, 62% CS, 25% FS, 14% NS, Mean age 60	
Spiral CT scan parameters (all protocols used 120–140 kVp and between 40–50 mA)	Single detector 10 mm ST	Multi-detector 5 mm ST	Single detector 10 mm ST	Single detector 10 mm ST	
Participants screened	841	1,464	8,303	1,180	11,788
Number of screening tests performed	1,184	1,464	8,303	7,891	18,842

New indeterminate lung nodules detected	35	191	518	770	1,514
Rate of new indeterminate nodules per screening, %	3	13	6	10	8
Benign biopsies or surgeries (harm)	1	3	9	27	40
Clinical Stage Distribution					
IA NSCLC	5		32	18	55
IB NSCLC					0
IIA NSCLC	1	1	1	1	4
IIB NSCLC		1	1		2
IIIA NSCLC	1		1	1	3
IIIB NSCLC			1	1	2
IV NSCLC			1	1	2
Unclassified NSCLC					0
SCLC	2	1			3
Total number of lung cancers	9	3	37	22	71
Spiral CT Test Performance					
Sensitivity, %	78	67	92	86	87
Specificity, %	98	87	94	90	92
Rate of lung cancers detected per 1,000 screenings	5.9	1.4	4.1	2.4	3.3
Rate of benign biopsies/surgeries per 1,000 screening	0.8	2.0	1.1	3.4	2.1

NS = Never smoker, ES = Ever smoker, FS = Former smoker, CS = Current smoker.
CT = Computerized Tomography, NSCLC = Non-small-cell lung cancer, SCLC = Small-cell lung cancer.
ST = slice thickness, kVp = kilovolt peak, mA = milliangstroms.

study reported that chest radiographs detected fewer lung cancers than spiral CT scans. All together, 89 lung cancers were found during prevalence screening, of which 3 were missed by spiral CT scans.

The lung cancers detected by spiral CT scans were mostly localized clinical stages. Of the 89 lung cancers found, 66 were clinical stage IA non-small-cell lung cancers (NSCLC), 5 stage IB NSCLC, 5 stage IIA NSCLC, 6 stage IIIA NSCLC, 2 stage IIIB NSCLC, 1 stage IVA NSCLC, 2 NSCLC and were classified as being in the right and left main stem bronchus and 2 were small-cell lung cancers. Viewed another way, 82 percent of all NSCLC found in these studies were at clinically localized stages (stage IA and IB).

For the incidence screening years, the ELCAP study once again found the highest lung cancer detection rate, 5.9 cancers per 1,000 screenings compared to 1.4 per 1,000 screenings at the Mayo clinic, 4.1 per 1,000 screenings at Shinshu University, and 2.4 per 1,000 screenings at ALCA. Out of 68 NSCLC, 55 or 81 percent were localized stage IA or IB. Furthermore, the average size of these localized staged cancers was small, usually less than 14 mm in diameter (Sone et al., 2001).

Negative findings such as the frequency of indeterminate lung nodules and harms were also reported. During the Mayo Clinic's prevalence screening, 782 out of 1,520 participants (51 percent) had indeterminate lung nodules that required further periodic surveillance with one or more conventional CT scans. Out of these 782 individuals only 22 had lung cancer; that is, more than 97 percent of those with indeterminate lung nodules were believed to be not cancerous (false positives). The average rate of new indeterminate lung nodules across all studies was 196 per 1,000 screenings (19.6 percent) for the prevalence screenings. This rate decreased but remained sizable, 80 per 1,000 screenings, during incidence screenings.

Harms from screening include invasive diagnostic testing or treatment for individuals without disease (false positives). During the prevalence screening years, 22 participants underwent an invasive test or surgery for a benign lesion. For incident screenings, 40 participants had invasive procedures resulting in a benign diagnosis. The ratio of individuals potentially benefiting from screening to those potentially harmed can be obtained by comparing the rate of lung cancers detected by spiral CT screening to the rate of benign diagnoses from unnecessary invasive procedures. Screening with spiral CT scans found 3.3 lung cancers per 1,000 screenings and 2.1 benign diagnoses per 1,000 screenings (unnecessary testing). Therefore, for every 3 lung cancers successfully found (potential benefit), almost 2 individuals received unnecessary testing and potential morbidity and mortality. In the spiral CT trials, there were no reported deaths among the disease-free individuals who underwent unnecessary testing.

As with past chest radigraphic screening trials, non-compliance with helical CT screening is a major problem. Sizable numbers of participants did not followup for incident screenings in some of these spiral CT screening trials. For example, in the Shinshu University study, 1,035 of 5,460 participants without identifiable cancer, 19 percent of all eligible participants, did not return for their second year screening. In contrast, the Mayo Clinic Study reported a low non-compliance rate of only 3 percent per year, suggesting that low rates of non-compliance are achievable.

One study, ALCA, has reported 5-year survival estimates. Among lung cancers found with prevalence screening, the 5-year survival was 76.2 percent and among those found on incidence screening, the 5-year survival was lower, 64.9 percent. The authors acknowledged that these estimates could be influenced by length, lead-time, and overdiagnosis biases. The lower survival among lung cancer participants detected during incidence screenings suggests the presence of length bias among the prevalent screening cancers.

Implications of Lung Cancer Screening with Spiral CT Scans

The results from these uncontrolled trials are promising and leave little doubt that spiral CT is more sensitive in detecting lung cancers than chest radiographs. However, while encouraging, they do not provide conclusive evidence for long-term efficacy. Even had they provided long-term outcome data, a full understanding of the clinical significance of the results would not have been gained as these trials, like the demonstration projects of the 1950s, all lack a control group. Simply finding smaller-sized cancers does not mean mortality is lowered. In one study, among localized stage cancers, smaller tumor size was not associated with better outcomes, demonstrating that some biologically aggressive forms of lung cancer may metastasize early, even when they are 1–5 mm in size (Patz et al., 2000b).

Elevated survival rates also do not prove efficacy. Survival rates are affected by selection, lead-time, length and over-diagnosis bias (see Chapter 5 for definitions), hence inferences about screening efficacy made from these data alone become speculative. Cancers with longer latency periods or with the potential for length bias are likely to be over-sampled in the early screening years, and inflated survival estimates may result, as shown in the ALCA results. Overdiagnosis bias is also a concern, since very small cancers have been found and the natural course of disease in individuals with tumors of this size is not known. Could some of these cancers grow very slowly, fail to progress, or perhaps regress? Excluding the possibility of overdiagnosis bias will be difficult, as the identification of a lung cancer mandates curative therapy and observation without therapy would not be considered ethical. Estimates of overdiagnosis bias may best be gained after the fact through autopsy screening (Black, 2000). Despite the many weaknesses of the CT studies, they have spurred interest and investments into randomized controlled trials of spiral CT screening.

Concerns such as physical and psychological harms from screening have been raised in the spiral CT screening studies. A case of a 73-year-old woman, Mrs. S., who decided to undergo lung cancer screening with spiral CT, illustrates the downside of screening. As described in the *New York Times*, Mrs. S.'s spiral CT scan showed a collapsed lung, presumably due to an obstructing lung cancer. However, after open lung surgery, surgical pathology showed no evidence of lung cancer. Her doctor writes, "While this news is welcome, Mrs. S.'s surgery and a rocky postoperative course had drained her both physically and emotionally. When she returned home, it took her several months to recover. She is still paying her hospital bills" (Lerner, 2002, p. D6). This individual did not benefit from screening and her case describes the possibility of unintended consequences of spiral CT screening.

Psychological harms can affect many individuals in these trials. Uncertainty as to the diagnosis of an indeterminate lung nodule can cause much anxiety, as the affected individuals may have had to wait months to years before learning that their nodules were not growing and hence not of concern. More than half of all participants in the Mayo Clinic Study had indeterminate nodules. This study, which used the most updated screening technology, found a higher rate of lung nodules than in other studies. Trials of spiral CT face the difficult challenge of appropriately triaging these very common nodules and counseling participants. Wardle and Pope (1992) pointed out that psychological costs from early detection are worrisome, and Reich argued that so far lung cancer "screening does no good and may do much harm" (1995, p. 557).

Edward Golub (1999) wrote, "It is not overdramatic to say that the entire nature of the future life of a patient can depend on the results of. . .[these] tests, what the person can and cannot do, how much time the person has to do it in, what the person's self-perception is, and how others think of and behave toward the person" (p. 13). The implications for otherwise healthy participants of screening tests are even more striking since they are at risk of being "transformed" from wellness into sickness. Another potential harm of screening would occur if smokers receiving a negative screening test decided that they did not need to quit smoking.

These spiral CT studies have been performed at referral centers with highly motivated staff, investigators, and participants. If widespread mass screening by spiral CT were adopted today, could their results be replicated elsewhere? It is possible that they could, but the costs of developing the infrastructure required to deliver top-quality care would be substantial. Standards for the detection and measurement of lesions by spiral CT scanning need to be established. Costs for the training of personnel and investments to purchase scanning instruments are required. Furthermore, capacity would also be needed to carry out diagnostic workups and follow-up.

Given the potential harms, logistical hurdles to minimize harm and costs, and, most importantly, the lack of evidence of efficacy, judgment on using spiral CT as a lung cancer screening test should be reserved until evidence from well-designed clinical trials can be evaluated.

Sputum Cytology as an Adjunctive Screening Test

While spiral CT scans are superior to chest radiographs for detecting lung cancer, CT could still miss cancers hiding in endobronchial locations. Sputum cytology is considered a good adjunctive screening test since it frequently detects endobronchial cancers, which are usually squamous cell carcinomas. The randomized controlled trials that were started in the 1970s showed that of the four major histologic types of lung cancer, the best prognosis was for squamous cell carcinoma. Squamous cell cancers represented 25 percent of all cancers found, and the 5-year survival rate for those with squamous cell cancers detected by cytology only was 85 to 90 percent (Berlin et al., 1984). Another cohort study that monitored lung cancer patients with radiographically occult malignancies identified by sputum cytology reported 5-year survival rates of 74 percent (Bechtel et al., 2000). Kennedy and colleagues (2000) pointed out that the number of deaths caused by squamous cell carcinoma of the lung is similar to the number caused by breast or colon cancer, for both of which screening is recommended. Thus, if squamous cell carcinoma is the slowest growing of the lung cancers and therefore the most likely to be detected early, screening for this particular type of lung cancer by sputum cytology may be warranted (Kennedy et al., 2000).

Advances in the screening of sputum samples hold promise, as do new bronchoscopic methods for examination of the lung. Researchers have identified precancerous and early cancerous states in sputum by identification of certain abnormal genes in sputum cells and improved localization of early cancers through fluorescent bronchoscopy, which consists of the identification of malignant cells by bronchoscopic examination under fluorescent light (Lam et al., 1998; Palmisano et al., 2000; Tockman, 2000). For example, Palmisano and colleagues (2000) found that certain cancer-fighting genes in the sputum cells of smokers had an abnormality called hypermethylation. On examination of sputum specimens several years before cancer developed, they found that hypermethylation antedated lung cancer in each of 21 persons who eventually developed lung cancer. They reported that "aberrant methylation . . . can be detected in DNA from sputum in 100 percent of patients with squamous cell lung carcinoma up to 3 years before clinical diagnosis" (Palmisano et al., 2000, p. 5954). This specific molecular abnormality is only one of many that appear to be promising as targets for early detection, and new bronchoscopic methods should eventually improve the ability to find very small tumors.

Fluorescent bronchoscopy is more sensitive than the traditional means of examination under white light for the detection of cancers. Kennedy and colleagues (2000) pointed out "the increased sensitivity [of fluorescent bronchoscopy] is associated with decreased specificity, resulting in many false positive biopsies" (p. 76S). A low specificity adds to the costs of using the fluorescent bronchoscope and increases the time of the procedure. Bias from overdiagnosis might also be introduced by the detection of very small cancers. Whether molecular or genetic markers in sputum, accompanied by bronchoscopic examination, can find curable lung cancers has yet to be shown.

FUTURE DIRECTIONS IN LUNG CANCER SCREENING

The promise of new technologies has led to the initiation of randomized controlled trials. Randomized studies of chest radiographs and spiral CT scanning for lung cancer screening are under way (Patz et al., 2000a). The Prostate, Lung, Colorectal, and Ovarian (PLCO) study has randomized 152,000 participants to receive screening chest radiographs or no screening (Simpson et al., 2000). The National Lung Screening Study, using a subset of the PLCO, will randomize 50,000 participants to chest radiographs or spiral CT screening. This NCI-sponsored trial is collaborating with the American College of Radiology Imaging Network (ACRIN) to enroll heavy smokers between the ages of 55 and 74. The trial will screen for 3 years with a 4-year follow-up, also collecting sputum samples in 10,000 participants. The trial will conclude data collection in 2009 (Sullivan, 2002).

How long before conclusive effectiveness data will be published? The NCI chest radiographic screening trials started in the early 1970s, and reports were published in the mid-1980s. Conclusive data for spiral CT may not be available for at least 5 to 10 years. Japan, in contrast to the United States, has already adopted spiral CT for lung cancer screening, despite a lack of evidence supporting its effectiveness. Ecological population data on the effect of widespread mass screening on lung cancer incidence and mortality rates could provide clues as to whether such screening is effective, although this type of data, due its limitations, usually does not provide sufficient evidence to recommend screening.

Already, techniques that are being used in practice are more advanced than those being considered in the most recent and ongoing studies. The initial spiral CT trials used single-detector CT technology, which is now outdated (National Cancer Institute and ACS, 2001). General Electric Medical Systems is selling multi-detector spiral CT scanners. Multi-detector scanners offer better resolution than prior machines and offer the option of magnifying parts of the lung without rescanning the participant. Within the next 5 to 10 years, even this technology will be updated (Fox, 2001). The NCI/ACRIN study, which is using multi-detector technology, is at risk of reporting data based on technology that will be considered obsolescent before the trial is completed.

These new scanners can detect 1- to 4-mm lesions called "ground glass opacities." These lesions are so small that they cannot be characterized as nodules. By improving the sensitivity of scanning, specificity is likely to decline so that false-positive results are likely to increase. The Mayo Clinic used multi-detector technology and found a higher rate of lung nodules than trials using single detector technology. Clinicians will face the challenge of distinguishing between false-positive and true-positive results in order to prevent unnecessary morbidity and mortality. On a short-term basis, antibiotic therapy can be administered followed by repeat scanning to see if the opacity was of an infectious etiology. Software that provides computer-aided diagnosis (CAD) can be used to enhance the accuracy of reading. Software algorithms can estimate the likelihood of a malignancy on the basis of certain characteristics of the lesion and the participant. CAD software can also double-check the readings of radiologists and pathologists. PAPNET, a CAD device for the reading of Pap smears, has been shown to reduce the number of smears with false-negative results (Halford et al., 1999). Similar software is being developed for mammograms and CT scans (National Cancer Institute and ACS, 2001).

CT imaging technology is also being used more widely. Virtual or three-dimensional means of bronchoscopy and colonoscopy imaging are being evaluated as noninvasive alternatives to conventional endoscopy (Black, 1999a). Spiral CT angiography evaluates arteriosclerosis without placing the individual at risk from the use of the contrast dye that is required by conventional angiography (Siegel and Evens, 1999). Spiral CT angiography has incidentally found lung cancers. Some radiology sites are offering screening by multiphasic imaging for cancer and arteriosclerosis (National Cancer Institute and ACS, 2001). If screening is not targeted, there is a high likelihood of finding many false-positive lesions.

Public and Policy Reactions to New Technologies

When the initial findings from the ELCAP study were reported in medical journals, major newspapers and weekly newsmagazines published articles about the findings. The articles mentioned that lung cancer death rates could be greatly reduced if smokers and former smokers were routinely given a CT test that can detect tumors when they are small enough to be cured (Brice, 2000). The public response to the news was dramatic. The voice mail systems at the hospital centers participating in the ELCAP study were overwhelmed, and at least 3,000 calls were placed to the Mayo Clinic by the next day. One ex-smoker whose husband died from lung cancer stated "I'm so grateful that the technology is present . . . lung cancer is just an awful, awful thing."

The public has long been worried about lung cancer. In an American Cancer Society survey that asked participants to "list the body sites susceptible to cancer that first come to mind," respondents most commonly mentioned the lung, breast, and skin (ACS, 1980b, p. 93). "About seven out of 10 smokers (71 percent) believe that if lung cancer is detected early, there is a good chance that it can be cured" (ACS, 1980b, p. 98). As lung cancer is a dreaded disease and screening is viewed as bringing hope for its detection and cure, it should come as no surprise that the ELCAP study results were enthusiastically received.

Some community physicians routinely perform screening chest radiographs, despite their lack of effectiveness as determined in clinical trials, and despite the lack of endorsement of their use by policy organizations (Black, 1999a). Adoption of CT technology by some providers is likely given their prior beliefs and practice patterns.

Radiology groups have adopted this technology and are advertising their use of the technology in local newspapers and on television and radio (Brice, 2000). One group in Skokie, Illinois,, found one cancer in 120 screening procedures. The average price per scan was $325, all of which was paid out of pocket by the screening participant. The premature promotion of spiral CT as a lung cancer screening tool raises many questions. Should spiral CT be promoted even though its effectiveness is not established? Does the public understand the consequences of having this screening test? How well informed is the public concerning the unwanted consequences of false-positive test results? What are the conflicts of interest when providers who could make financial gains by screening advertise on the promise of an unproven technology?

These reports suggest fast and too early adoption of this unproven technology. Cautions have been raised about spiral CT screening for lung cancer. Christine D. Berg of NCI's Division of Cancer Prevention and Suburban Cancer Hospital Center reported that "We had leeches in the 1800s, radium elixirs in the 1900s and radiation treatment for enlarged thyroids in the 1950s. A long list of medical fads have come and gone. Spiral CT has great promise. That's why it deserves further study" (Brice, 2000, p. 49). The Society of Thoracic Radiology, which included researchers of the Mayo trial and the ELCAP study, issued the following consensus statement: "It is the consensus of this committee that mass screening for lung cancer with CT is not currently advocated. Suitable subjects who wish to participate should be encouraged to do so in controlled trials, so that the value of CT screening can be ascertained as soon as possible" (Aberle et al., 2001, p. 65). The American College of Radiology has appointed a task force to evaluate spiral CT and withholds recommendation at the time of this writing (Zinninger MD, American College of Radiology, personal communication, 2001).

Although the initial results of evaluations of spiral CT scanning are encouraging, it is now known that radiographic detection of asymptomatic lung cancer provides no assurance that benefit in terms of the prevention of mortality from lung cancer will ensue. The same level of evidence that was available for chest X-ray and sputum cytology decades ago is now available for spiral CT, and any judgment on spiral CT as a screening modality should await the findings of trials and the availability of mortality rate data. Therefore, at this time, the evidence does not support a recommendation for either widespread screening or the screening of selective high-risk groups for lung cancer. This conclusion is based on the historical record and its lessons, the potential for harm from widespread screening, and the lack of proven effectiveness from current evidence on spiral CT.

Given that spiral CT is already in use, what specific policy recommendations can be implemented now? Public education, mutual decision-making, and a focus on primary prevention are needed to aid consumers, providers, researchers, payers, and policy makers.

Consumers

Smokers, current or former, are at far greater risk of lung cancer than those who have never smoked. However, the absolute risk of developing lung cancer among even the at-risk smoker groups is relatively low. SEER Program data show that the incidence rate of lung cancer among those age 65 and older is about 3 to 6 per 1,000 persons per year. Given the relatively low incidence rates, any decision to be screened for lung cancer by spiral CT should be made with full consideration of the rates of true-positive versus false-positive results and the attendant benefits and risks. Knowledgeable providers must adequately communicate these complexities so that patients can weigh the risks and benefits of screening. Educational materials that clearly explain risk can assist with informed decision-making.

Consumers who choose to undergo screening by spiral CT, despite the current lack of evidence, should be informed of the chance of finding true disease and the attendant risks of screening. Topics that should be covered include the costs of initial and follow-up tests, the potential physical harms from radiation and invasive secondary testing and surgery, and the potential psychological harms from misdiagnosis or mislabeling. An informed-consent form detailing these facts should be administered before the scan is performed. Consumers should be informed of the possibility that screening may result in their knowing of cancer early without lowering risk of death. In other words, they could be living longer with a diagnosis but not necessarily really living longer. Examples from past screening studies can be used to illustrate this point.

Providers

Current clinical practice guidelines advise against routine lung cancer screening. Neither chest radiographic nor spiral CT screening should be offered on a routine basis. Preferably, a primary care provider or specialty physician familiar with lung cancer screening and its likely limitations should appropriately counsel patients who desire testing. Consumers who lack primary care or who bypass their primary care provider and go directly to radiology groups should receive appropriate counseling before undergoing the procedure. Radiologists will need to arrange for appropriate follow-up care. If comorbid conditions such as heart disease or emphysema are present and could prevent eligibility for surgical resection, screening should be delayed until an appropriate evaluation is completed.

Radiology groups endorsing or advertising their use of spiral CT scanning should acknowledge its experimental nature and should clearly state the current lack of evidence. Follow-up mechanisms for individuals with indeterminate results should be established so that noncompliance is minimized. To ensure the highest standards of care, professional organizations and provider groups should develop guidelines on the management of pulmonary nodules.

Researchers

Since there is substantial uncertainty about spiral CT's effectiveness, resources should be made available for research. A randomized controlled trial will provide the clearest, most convincing evidence of possible effectiveness, and the level of evidence from trials with this design is considered the strongest for policy development. Others have called such trials unethical (Henschke and Yankelevitz, 2000), as this would be the case if spiral CT were clearly efficacious and such trials were simply testing a new or altered protocol. At present, however, randomized controlled trials of screening are ethically sound; the evidence about screening by spiral CT (or other modalities) has not yet been tipped to favor screening. Since observational studies are subject to selection bias and uncontrolled confounding, uncertainty often clouds observational evidence of effectiveness, leaving the question of whether the benefit was due to the intervention or to some unmeasured difference between groups. Observational studies are useful for evaluations of the natural history of disease, tumor doubling times, and biomarker analysis and should be done for these purposes. Neither study design—randomized or observational—would provide a result faster since mortality from the disease is the common and appropriate endpoint. While waiting for trial results, researchers could evaluate decision support models that simulate the natural history of disease and spiral CT. These models can identify important disease and test thresholds at which screening can be a viable option.

Additional research is needed to find high-risk participants most likely to benefit from lung cancer screening, find methods to improve compliance with cancer screening, risk stratify the numerous lung nodules that are found on screening, and prevent harms induced by screening.

Policy Makers and Payers

For coverage decisions, policy makers will want to know the cost-effectiveness of spiral CT. David Eddy (1981) estimated that primary prevention by smoking cessation is over 400 times more effective than screening by chest radiography. The direct costs to provide chest radiographic screening to 100,000 40-year-old smokers were estimated to be $500 million in 1980 dollars. Clearly, if resources are limited, primary prevention is more cost-effective. Given that the cost of spiral CT screening is higher than chest radiographs, the budgetary impact to implement systematic screening is likely to be much higher today.

During periods of uncertainty, policies should be implemented that educate consumers, providers, and policy makers of the risks of early adoption. Widespread mass screening for lung cancer has not been endorsed by professional organizations, given the history of past attempts and the difficulties with present attempts. Rapid dissemination of screening technology before establishment of its effectiveness and prior to establishment of quality control standards could result in more harm than benefits. Currently, for every three cancers detected by spiral CT screening, two false-positive participants will undergo invasive procedures and potential subsequent harm.

CONCLUSIONS

Lung cancer is a dreaded disease with a difficult and frequently fatal course. It is now the leading cause of cancer death in the United States. Smoking prevention and cessation can prevent most cases. Yet, one-quarter of adults in the United States are still regular smokers, and youths continue to experiment with tobacco and often become addicted. Although rates of smoking have declined, continuation of the current lung cancer epidemic can be anticipated for decades to come. In addition, lung cancer death rates will soon surge in the developing world (Hoel et al., 1992; Pandey et al., 1999; Parkin et al., 1999).

Logically, investigators have looked for approaches other than tobacco control to reduce the numbers of deaths from lung cancer. Screening was first attempted in the 1950s, soon after the scope of the lung cancer epidemic was recognized. The use of chest X-rays for screening appeared to be appropriate at the time and fit with the approach already in use for tuberculosis. Sputum cytology added another screening tool that also appeared promising, as the abnormalities in expectorated cells mirrored the abnormalities in the respiratory epithelium where they originated.

The first studies were observational rather than experimental in design. Although the randomized clinical trial is now the standard means for the assessment of screening tests, it had not yet been used for that purpose in the 1950s. The first studies of screening tests used a design equivalent to a demonstration project, inviting participants to have the screening test and then monitoring them over time. Viewed by today's standards, those studies had poor quality control measures, inaccurate standardization and poor means of interpretation of test results, and high rates of noncompliance with the screening regimen by participants. The designs of the studies were also flawed because they did not include randomization to a control group and one or more screening modalities; in fact, comparison or control groups were lacking in several of the studies.

In the 1970s four randomized controlled trials on lung cancer screening using chest radiography and sputum cytology were performed. Unfortunately, these randomized controlled trials of lung cancer screening showed no evidence of early detection of lung cancers by these tests (Fontana et al., 1991; Melamed et al., 1984; Tockman, 1986). The numbers of early-stage and late-stage cancers did not meaningfully differ between the study groups. Most disappointing was that on follow-up, the rates of mortality were the same among the screened and the unscreened participants.

An effective screening test for lung cancer has not yet been identified, therefore organizations that develop screening guidelines do not recommend screening for it (Aberle et al., 2001; Biesalski et al., 1998; Eddy, 1980a; Eddy, 1980b). Although the studies of screening to date have failed to show mortality reduction, the lessons learned from these trials can pave the way for future research with newer technologies such as spiral CT scans. The conceptual framework for cancer screening illustrates its complexity and provides criteria for the evaluation of new technologies such as spiral CT. Future studies need to account for biases when measuring survival data. These biases are lead-time bias, length bias, and overdiagnosis bias (described in Chapter 5). Future studies not only must show evidence that screening can detect smaller cancers but also must show evidence that screening can produce stage shifts, including both more early cancers and fewer late cancers, followed by lower lung cancer mortality rates (Patz et al., 2000a).

Potential concerns related to the psychological and physical harms from the finding of positive results and the management of patients with positive results need to be considered, as there is strong demand for screening by spiral CT and spiral CT has been adopted into practice, despite the uncertain and incomplete scientific evidence.

Clinicians and the public are eager to have new approaches to the prevention of lung cancer; consequently, any new tool for prevention is likely to be hailed and perhaps not receive a sufficiently critical evaluation. The lessons learned from past experience with lung cancer screening call for restraint in the use of spiral CT screening. Findings from uncontrolled trials conducted to date do not provide the level of evidence required to endorse systematic screening with spiral CT scans.

8

Professional Education and Training

Health care providers appear to be falling short of expectations that they counsel their patients regarding smoking, diet, and exercise and offer recommended screening tests to detect cancer early (see Chapters 4 and 6). According to recent studies, for example, less than half of adults who smoke cigarettes report that their physician inquired about smoking at their last visit, and among women eligible for breast cancer screening, roughly 20 to 30 percent report that they did not receive advice to have a mammogram. Improving professional education and training would seem an obvious remedy to this lack of counseling and screening advice, but evidence suggests that although improved education and training are necessary, these improvements by themselves are not sufficient to improve practice. Instead, education and training need to be coupled with other interventions so that practitioners are supported in their efforts with office systems that prompt them to adhere to guidelines, adequate reimbursement for behavioral interventions and screening services, and quality assurance systems that instill accountability. Enhancing professional education and training nevertheless remains one of the essential ingredients of a package of reforms needed to achieve national goals for cancer prevention and early detection set forth in *Healthy People 2010* (US DHHS and Office of Disease Prevention and Health Promotion, 2000). Providers have recognized their limitations in this area and generally express interest in furthering their training (Block et al., 2000; Costanza et al., 1993).

This chapter begins with a discussion of the challenges of providing professional education and training; assesses the status of education and training with a focus on physicians, nurses, and dentists; and concludes with a review of federal and private funding resources available to support education and training efforts.

CHALLENGES OF PROVIDING PROFESSIONAL EDUCATION AND TRAINING

Who Should Be Trained?

The education and training of health care providers occur on dual fronts, each of which has a unique set of challenges. First, those in training must be exposed to course work and clinical experience that reflect current evidence-based guidelines for cancer prevention and early detection interventions. Although updating of curricula would at first appear to be straightforward, such changes can be very difficult to make because of the competing demands among the various medical disciplines, each vying for the limited training time available. The second, and perhaps more daunting charge is providing continuing education to practitioners who are already trained but who have deficits in prevention education. As of 1997, most physicians (55 percent) had graduated from medical school before 1980 (American Medical Association, 1999), long before the publication of the U.S. Preventive Services Task Force's *Guide to Clinical Preventive Services* in 1989 and the availability of comprehensive smoking cessation guidelines.

In 1999 the United States had an estimated 9 million health care practitioners and health care technical and support staff (Bureau of Labor Statistics, http://stats.bls.gov), but this number does not capture fully those who may need to be trained in cancer prevention and early detection. Health plan managers not directly involved in hands-on care may need information on cancer screening guidelines to assess a proposed quality improvement program, and insurance company analysts may need up-to-date information on the costs and benefits of smoking cessation interventions to accurately price their package of benefits. Likewise, administrators who establish curriculum guidelines for public school systems and health educators who work in community-based social services settings may all require cancer-related education and training. Although this chapter recognizes the diversity of needs for education and training, the focus is on the education and training needs of direct providers of ambulatory health care services.

Among direct health care providers, answers to the questions of who should be trained and how they should be trained depend in part on who has regular contact with patients and the environment of contemporary practice. Where do individuals go for their routine or preventive care? In 1998, the vast majority of individuals relied on doctor's offices and health maintenance organizations (69.7 percent) and clinics or health centers (15.6 percent) for their care. Clearly, efforts to improve cancer prevention and early detection practices will have to focus on these ambulatory care settings.

Assessments of whom to train also require answers to questions about the number of providers who need to be trained and the appropriate roles for which physician and nonphysician providers of prevention services need to be prepared. The specter of a lack of provider capacity has arisen as the large baby boom cohort ages and falls into the age groups for whom regular screening is recommended. The need for qualified mammography providers, for example, will likely increase as the population ages and as more providers and women adopt screening recommendations. The number of women eligible for breast cancer screening is expected to increase by 46 percent from 2000 to 2020 (U.S. Census middle projections, www.census.gov/population/projections). The 2001 Institute of Medicine (IOM, 2001b) report *Mammography and Beyond* cites anecdotal reports that inadequate numbers of mammographers and mammography technologists are being trained to fill current and future needs, but it also notes that good data to support such claims are lacking. The IOM committee that prepared that report recommended that a study be conducted to assess provider supply.

Likewise, the demand for colorectal cancer screening could easily outpace the number of physicians trained to conduct the tests recommended in colorectal cancer screening guidelines (e.g., sigmoidoscopy and colonoscopy) if gains in the rate of acceptance of such screening tests are coupled with the aging of the baby boom cohort (Schoenfeld, 1999). Increased demand for tests could renew long-standing calls for greater involvement of nonphysician providers in screening programs. However, despite evidence suggesting that appropriately trained nurses can perform flexible sigmoidoscopy with the same degrees of accuracy and safety as physicians (Fletcher and Farraye, 1999; Maule, 1994; Schoenfeld, 1999; Schoenfeld et al., 1999), they have not uniformly been accepted as providers within health care systems (Floch, 1999). Nevertheless, several professional societies (e.g., the American Society for Gastrointestinal Endoscopy and the British Society of Gastroenterology) have endorsed the performance of flexible sigmoidoscopy by nurses, but 16 of 50 U.S. state boards of nursing expressly prohibit registered nurses from performing screening flexible sigmoidoscopy (Cash et al., 1999).[1] In 1996 the U.S. Preventive Services Task Force included a recommendation that flexible sigmoidoscopy be used to screen asymptomatic adults age 50 and older, and since 1998 Medicare has provided reimbursement for screening flexible sigmoidoscopy, but only physicians are

[1]Fifteen of 16 of these states allow nurse practitioners, but not registered nurses, to perform screening flexible sigmoidoscopy (Cash, 1999). Among U.S. institutions with gastroenterology fellowship programs, 15 percent (24 of 164 programs) were using paramedical personnel to perform flexible sigmoidoscopy (Cash, 1999).

reimbursed "to ensure that [the procedures] are performed as safely and accurately as possible" (Health Care Financing Administration, 1997).[2]

The demand for personnel to provide smoking cessation interventions should be very high given that an estimated one-quarter of the U.S. adult population smokes cigarettes. Physicians are important providers of smoking cessation interventions, but nonphysician personnel can be as effective as physicians as providers of interventions aimed at ending tobacco dependence and can do so at lower cost (US DHHS, 2000a). According to smoking cessation guidelines, multiple types of clinicians are effective and should be used. Well-established evidence-based guidelines are available for providers, but too few smokers are getting appropriate counseling and referrals to smoking cessation programs, according to assessments of provider practice (see Chapter 4). In general, less than half of smokers report on surveys that they received advice to quit smoking at their last physician visit (Doescher and Saver, 2000; Jaen et al., 1997). Smoking cessation guidelines include recommendations for the prescription of medications for certain individuals, but limitations on nonphysician practitioners' authority in this area could limit their role as primary providers of smoking cessation interventions. Most state practice laws limit prescriptive authority to physicians, dentists, and certain advanced practice providers such as nurse practitioners.[3]

One counseling strategy would be to have a medical clinician or a health care clinician deliver messages about health risks and benefits and deliver pharmacotherapy (e.g., bupropion or a nicotine patch) and to have nonmedical clinicians deliver additional psychosocial or behavioral interventions (US DHHS, 2000a). Some have advocated a stepped care approach for the treatment of nicotine dependence in which more intensive services are targeted to those with higher degrees of addiction or with comorbid conditions such as mental illness (Abrams, 1993). According to this model, a highly motivated smoker might require minimal assistance and be effectively treated with a brief intervention from a physician, nurse, or other health care provider within the course of a routine health care contact. A heavy smoker discouraged by a history of poor success with

[2]Although Health Care Financing Administration guidelines prohibit Medicare reimbursement of professional fees to nonphysicians for the performance of screening flexible sigmoidoscopy (and many national insurance agencies follow these guidelines), no policy prohibits the reimbursement of a facility fee when flexible sigmoidoscopy is performed by nonphysicians (when screening flexible sigmoidoscopy is performed in an outpatient setting, however, a facility fee is reimbursed only if a biopsy is performed) (Schoenfeld, 1999).

[3]All states provide some authority for nurse practitioners to prescribe noncontrolled substances such as those recommended in smoking cessation guidelines (e.g., certain nicotine replacement products or bupropion). In most states, prescriptive authority is granted only while the nurse practitioner is working in collaboration with a physician (National Conference of State Legislatures, American Nursing Association, www.ncsl.org/programs/health/Nurseaut.htm).

attempts at quitting might require referral to more intensive specialized treatment with follow-up. The tobacco user who is clinically depressed or who is also alcohol- or drug-dependent might best be served by a licensed mental health professional or an alcohol or drug addiction professional (Pbert et al., 2000). In terms of program intensity, evidence suggests that the counseling session length should be longer than 10 minutes, there should be four or more sessions, and the total contact time should be longer than 30 minutes (US DHHS, 2000a). Given evidence that current ambulatory care practices do not accommodate these recommendations very well (e.g., visits are short and contacts with nurses are limited), there appear to be opportunities to develop innovative models that integrate nonphysician providers and specialized referral services into office-based practices.

What Needs to Be Learned?

Perhaps the most important component of any education and training program is a clear statement of what is expected of the student following completion of the course of study. A set of expectations of health care providers regarding cancer prevention and early detection has been set forth in the objectives of *Healthy People 2010* (US DHHS and Office of Disease Prevention and Health Promotion, 2000) (Box 8.1). Having a clear set of objectives provides useful guidance to educators regarding the didactic materials that need be covered in the curriculum and the clinical experiences that are needed to ensure competency.

BOX 8.1 Selected *Healthy People 2010* Cancer Objectives

Behavioral Interventions

- Increase the proportion of physicians and dentists who counsel their at-risk patients about smoking and tobacco use cessation, physical activity, and cancer screening to at least 85 percent.

Cancer Screening

- Increase the proportion of women age 18 and older who received a Pap test within the preceding 3 years to 90 percent.
- Increase the proportion of adults age 50 and older who have received a fecal occult blood test within the preceding 2 years to 50 percent.
- Increase the proportion of adults age 50 and older who have ever received a sigmoidoscopy to 50 percent.
- Increase the proportion of women age 40 and older who have received a mammogram within the preceding 2 years to 70 percent.

SOURCE: US DHHS and Office of Disease Prevention and Health Promotion (2000).

This chapter focuses on the education and training needs of ambulatory care providers for whom knowledge in a variety of areas and a diverse set of skills must be acquired. The knowledge and skills needed for cancer prevention and early detection span population science (e.g., epidemiology and biostatistics), behavioral science (e.g., psychology and counseling), and basic science (e.g., pathology and molecular biology). The effective practice of cancer prevention and early detection can also depend on knowledge of and patient referral to community-based resources and support services. The disciplines of cancer prevention and early detection, like other areas of medicine, are subject to innovation, new technology, changing and conflicting guidelines, and controversy surrounding what constitutes best practice. Being able to provide good counsel to patients requires staying abreast of developments and knowing where to go for sources of credible information. Furthermore, education and training programs need to promote evidence-based practices and impart evaluative skills to students so that they can judge when to incorporate new interventions into their practices.

Although much of the counsel offered by providers of cancer prevention and early detection services can be prescriptive (e.g., advice to quit smoking), much of it cannot be because not enough is known about the benefits (and potential harms) of interventions. Men considering prostate-specific antigen testing to screen for prostate cancer, for example, should be informed of the relative benefits and harms related to screening and subsequent follow-up procedures and outcomes. Similarly, patient values and preferences should be considered along with information about the risk of cancer and the risk of testing to determine the most appropriate colorectal cancer screening method (Woolf, 2000a,b). Counseling patients about the relative risks and benefits of screening and eliciting information from patients regarding their concerns and values are time-consuming and require skill, however. Likewise, facilitation of a patient's behavioral change by a health care provider is a complex process and involves a cycle of assessment, assistance, reiteration, and continuing support. Professional education and training in the areas of cancer prevention and early detection would be incomplete if counseling skills and familiarity with the challenges (and rewards) of behavioral interventions were not core parts of the curriculum and clinical training experience (Ockene et al., 1990).

There are glaring disparities in the rates of cancer morbidity and mortality between socioeconomic groups, insured and uninsured individuals, and certain racial and ethnic groups (see Chapter 1). Lack of health insurance coverage is a key predictor of lower rates of use of cancer screening tests, but other sociocultural factors may also be at play. In a nation of increasing diversity, health care providers must be trained to accommodate language differences in their practices and must be aware of cultural values and beliefs that might need to be addressed during discussions of cancer prevention and early detection.

Education and training programs aimed at health care providers need to emphasize evidence that systemwide approaches are most effective in promoting disease prevention and health promotion and that providers are an integral part of that system. Providers can develop integrated approaches that use community-based resources to extend the impacts of their messages delivered in the health care context. For example, an extensive array of community-based smoking cessation programs (e.g., programs offered through the American Lung Association or the American Cancer Society) can supplement services provided in an office-based practice. Given the reality of time constraints in ambulatory care practice, referral to community-based specialists may be the most appropriate way to provide treatment services. Likewise, for patients who lack health insurance (or for patients who are underinsured), certain cancer screening services are available in community-based clinics at no cost or at a reduced fee (e.g., the Centers for Disease Control and Prevention's [CDC's] Breast and Cervical Cancer Early Detection Program).

Prevention services are most effectively integrated into ambulatory care when office systems are in place to remind providers of a patient's smoking status or eligibility for cancer screening. Furthermore, efforts to improve rates of adherence to evidence-based guidelines increasingly include quality improvement models that inform practitioners of their performance relative to those of their peers or accepted standards (see Chapter 9). Education and training programs should include didactic and clinical experiences that incorporate these systems of accountability.

In summary, professional education and training programs focused on cancer prevention and early detection can be offered to a range of providers in a variety of settings. Some programs may be housed within an individual medical or dental school, some may be organized regionally under the auspices of a state comprehensive cancer plan, whereas others may be sponsored nationally by representatives of professional societies or a particular federal program. Wherever they are offered and however they are organized, professional education and training programs ideally would include the following key components:

- a focus on established goals and objectives, such as those established as part of *Healthy People 2010* (US DHHS and Office of Disease Prevention and Health Promotion, 2000);
- an emphasis in the curriculum on evidence-based interventions and the interpretation of evidence in the context of population-based medicine;
- interdisciplinary didactic material and training experiences spanning the disciplines of the basic, population, and behavioral sciences;
- development of skills to integrate community-based resources into office practice;
- training and experience in providing services to special populations;

• continuing education to ensure maintenance of up-to-date knowledge and skills; and

• experience with systems approaches to promote quality care and accountability.

STATUS OF PROFESSIONAL EDUCATION AND TRAINING

The previous section of this chapter explored in some detail the National Cancer Policy Board's vision of who should be trained to provide cancer prevention and early detection services and what should be learned in education and training programs. This section examines how this ideal can be approached by reviewing the status of health promotion and disease prevention education and training in medical, nursing, and dental schools. Of note, at the time of this assessment there were few systematic reviews of curricula, texts and educational materials, training experiences, and continuing education opportunities related to cancer prevention and early detection.

Medical Schools

There is a general consensus that physicians are not adequately trained to deliver cancer prevention and control interventions (Brink et al., 1994; Costanza et al., 1993; Glanz et al., 1995; Kushner, 1995; Ockene, 1987; Ockene and Zapka, 1997, 2000; Ockene et al., 1996; Strecher et al., 1991). Practicing physicians themselves identify their lack of training and confidence as barriers to the delivery of cancer prevention and control interventions (Ashford et al., 2000; Becker and Janz, 1990; Berman et al., 1997; Brink et al., 1994; Costanza et al., 1993; Gilpin et al., 1993; Manley et al., 1992). This section of the report describes efforts to address shortcomings in both undergraduate and graduate medical school training and examines the availability of training opportunities in two areas, tobacco cessation and nutrition.

Undergraduate Medical Student Training

Attempts to improve the coverage of health promotion and disease prevention in the medical school curriculum have had a long history and have largely been led by professional organizations (Box 8.2).

As early as 1945, the American Association of Medical Colleges (AAMC) recommended that each medical school establish a department of preventive medicine (Association of American Medical Colleges, 1945). In a major report issued nearly 40 years later, an AAMC panel recommended that "the emphasis on preparing medical students to care for individuals

BOX 8.2 Professional Organizations with a Focus on Health Promotion and Disease Prevention

Association of American Medical Colleges

The **Association of American Medical Colleges** (AAMC) is a nonprofit association founded in 1876 to work for reform in medical education. AAMC represents the 125 accredited U.S. medical schools, 400 major teaching hospitals and health systems, 90 academic and professional societies representing nearly 100,000 faculty members, and the nation's medical students and residents. The AAMC works with its members to set a national agenda for medical education, biomedical research, and health care. AAMC assists its members by providing services at the national level, services that facilitate the accomplishment of their missions (www.aamc.org/about/start.htm).

Association of Teachers of Preventive Medicine

The **Association of Teachers of Preventive Medicine** (ATPM), a national professional association, is dedicated to advancing health promotion and disease prevention in the education of physicians and other health professionals. ATPM publishes curriculum guidelines (e.g., *Teaching Prevention Throughout the Curriculum: Multidisciplinary Perspectives on Enhancing Disease Prevention and Health Promotion in Undergraduate Medical Education* (Association of Teachers of Preventive Medicine, 2000), directories of programs in public health and preventive medicine, and the *American Journal of Preventive Medicine.* ATPM is developing, in partnership with the Centers for Medicare and Medicaid Services (formerly the Health Care Financing Administration) and the Centers for Disease Control and Prevention, a series of distance learning modules for health care providers called Improving Provider Education on Federal Health Programs. The educational program is aimed at health care providers and administrators, particularly those who serve minority populations, to inform them about the range of clinical and prevention services and administrative requirements for Medicaid and the State Children's Health Insurance Program.

American Association for Cancer Education

The **American Association for Cancer Education** (AACE), founded in 1947, provides a forum to address cancer education at the undergraduate, graduate, continuing professional, and paraprofessional levels. The association is involved in educational issues throughout the cancer continuum, from prevention, early detection, and treatment to rehabilitation. A group of AACE members participates in a cancer prevention education section. AACE's membership of approximately 400 includes the faculties of schools of medicine, dentistry, osteopathy, education, pharmacy, nursing, public health, and social work. AACE encourages projects for the training of paramedical personnel and educational programs for the general public, populations at risk, and patients with cancer. AACE publishes the *Journal of Cancer Education* and the *Cancer Education Newsletter.*

American Society of Preventive Oncology

The **American Society of Preventive Oncology** (ASPO), a 25-year-old professional organization with roughly 400 members, aims to promote the exchange and dissemination of information relating to cancer prevention and early detection; to identify

(continued on next page)

BOX 8.2 *(continued)*

and stimulate new research; and to support the implementation and evaluation of national, state, and local programs and policies (www.aspo.org, accessed December 13, 2000). Membership is largely from academic settings and is diverse, with representatives from anthropologists, communications specialists, biostatisticians, epidemiologists, medical oncologists, and psychologists. ASPO, in cooperation with the American Association for Cancer Research, publishes the journal *Cancer Epidemiology, Biomarkers and Prevention.*

SOURCES: http://rpci.med.buffalo.edu/aace/aacef1.html, accessed December 6, 2000; Judy Bowser, ASPO executive director, personal communication, December 13, 2000; www.atpm.org/education/IMPROVIN.htm, accessed January 3, 2001.

with acute illnesses . . . be balanced by an equivalent emphasis on promoting health and preventing disease" (Muller, 1984, p. 6).

A panel of the Association of Teachers of Preventive Medicine (ATPM) proposed in 1989 minimum requirements for curricular content related to health promotion and disease prevention, including recommendations for course timing, duration, and sequencing during medical school. In 1990, another expert ATPM panel recommended incorporation of the *Guide to Clinical Preventive Services* (U.S. Preventive Services Task Force, 1989) into both the undergraduate and postgraduate medical education (Altekruse et al., 1991; Collins et al., 1991).

An effort to improve medical schools' disease prevention and health promotion curricula and the ability to evaluate medical students' knowledge of disease prevention and health promotion principles and their application was launched in 1994. The effort was called the Prevention Curriculum Assistance Program (PCAP) and was funded by ATPM and the federal government's Health Resources and Services Administration (HRSA). Between 1997 and 1999 PCAP surveyed medical schools regarding their curricula and means of evaluation of students. A prevention self-assessment analysis inventory was created to allow comparison of existing curricula with recommended standards. The inventory covered four areas (Garr et al., 2000):

1. clinical prevention services,
2. quantitative methods,
3. community dimensions of medical practice, and
4. health services organization and delivery.

Virtually all (96 percent) of the responding programs expected medical students to be able to identify the age- and sex-specific recommendations for screening tests, prevention counseling, immunizations, and chemoprophylaxis. Less than one-third of the programs (31 percent) were satisfied with the quality of the evaluations they were using to assess students' abilities in clinical prevention services, and 41 percent of the programs expressed a desire to receive assistance with the design of their curricula or evaluation methods relating to clinical prevention services (Garr et al., 2000). With recognition that "evaluation drives learning," recommendations on how best to evaluate the competence of medical students in prevention have been outlined (Blue et al., 2000).

In another recent development, AAMC established the Medical School Objectives project to set forth program-level learning objectives that medical school deans and faculties could use as guides in reviewing and then improving their medical student education programs. Among the educational objectives recommended by the AAMC Population Health Perspective Panel is that medical students be able to "incorporate principles of disease prevention and behavioral change appropriate for specific populations of patients within a community" (Association of American Medical Colleges, 1999, p. 139). Suggestions designed to facilitate the development of a curriculum in population health, which would logically include the principles and practice of cancer prevention and early detection, included the following:

- Medical schools should develop an explicit list of mechanisms by which population health objectives are to be met.
- Teaching faculty should be identified.
- Liaisons should be formed with others who can help (e.g., the American Board of Preventive Medicine and Teachers of Preventive Medicine).
- The AAMC Liaison Committee on Medical Education should require that schools show evidence that they have developed objectives, designed and delivered a curriculum, and tested students for their competencies in population health.
- Competencies in population health should be tested in the examinations of the National Board of Medical Examiners.

The panel further suggested that AAMC take steps to facilitate and reinforce movement toward more effective teaching of population health by (Association of American Medical Colleges, 1999, p. 141):

- clearly articulating to the medical school leadership and constituency the priority of ensuring instruction in and supporting a population health curriculum;
- providing a clearinghouse of curricular materials and experts who can help schools develop their curricula and encouraging the development of an in-school infrastructure that links the functions of the schools of medicine

and public health, as well as those of the schools of nursing, pharmacy, and health services administration, in a way that creates interests and opportunities for teaching, research, and learning in population health;

• including specific curricular elements, objectives, processes, and outcomes for population health on the annual AAMC curriculum survey and listing the schools that have developed a population health curriculum in the AAMC curriculum directory;

• developing an explicit list of expectations of how teaching and learning at the undergraduate level should fit with postgraduate education programs; and

• encouraging public and private funding agencies to balance biomedical research funding with that provided for health services and public health research.

An *Inventory of Knowledge and Skills Relating to Disease Prevention and Health Promotion* has been developed jointly by the Bureau of Health Professions of the Health Resources and Services Administration, the Association of Teachers of Preventive Medicine, and the Medical School Objectives Project of the Association of American Medical Colleges. In 1998, these groups developed a set of core competencies in preventive medicine for undergraduate medical education (Pomrehn et al., 2000) so that students could:

• identify recommended clinical prevention services including screening tests (e.g., the Pap test and mammography) and prevention counseling (e.g., smoking cessation, dietary modification, and physical activity);

• demonstrate the skills necessary to perform screening tests and conduct preventive counseling; and

• understand the features of health systems (e.g., reminder systems for providers) that promote the integration of disease prevention interventions into clinical practices.

Emphasis was placed not only on teaching about prevention but also on providing opportunities to show students how to apply prevention interventions to patient care.

How do medical students view their training in disease prevention and health promotion? According to the Medical School Graduation Survey performed by AAMC, there has been a steady increase in the proportion of graduates reporting that an "adequate" amount of time in the curriculum is spent on health promotion and disease prevention, from 54 percent in 1993 to 76 percent in 1997 (Pomrehn et al., 2000).

There has also been a long history of critical evaluation of cancer education in medical school, although much of the focus has been on the curricula pertaining to cancer diagnosis and treatment rather than cancer prevention and early detection. In the late 1970s, the National Cancer Institute (NCI) funded what is known as the Cancer Education Survey I. This comprehensive assessment involved an educational resources questionnaire, a faculty and curriculum questionnaire, a student questionnaire, and site visits to 44 medical schools. Findings from this effort led to three recommendations (Bakemeier et al., 1992):

1. cancer education grant programs needed to be continued and expanded,
2. cancer education objectives should be defined, preferably on a nationwide basis, and
3. improved evaluation mechanisms should be developed and applied by all schools in a program of internal self-assessment of their cancer education programs.

After publication of the results of Cancer Education Survey I in 1981, the American Association for Cancer Education (AACE) in 1986 published *Cancer Education Objectives for Medical Schools* (Bakemeier and Edwards, 1986) and guidance on how to apply them (Bakemeier et al., 1992). A few years later, in 1989, AACE published nutrition cancer education objectives (Bakemeier et al., 1989). A follow-up survey, Cancer Education Survey II, was conducted in 1989–1990 and was funded by the American Cancer Society (Bakemeier et al., 1992; Gallagher et al., 1992; O'Donnell et al., 1992). Eight recommendations emanated from the second survey (Gallagher et al., 1992, pp. 97–101):

1. Cancer educators should receive training in the process of instructional planning.
2. The Cancer Education Objectives developed by AACE should be evaluated for currency and adaptability by a wide range of cancer teaching programs (very few faculty surveyed used the teaching objectives).
3. Formal studies are needed to clarify the conditions under which formal written cancer education objectives enhance the teaching and learning process.
4. Each institution should examine the appropriateness of the teaching method(s) being used to achieve each of its cancer education objectives.
5. High-quality, learning-validated, computer-assisted instruction programs that are useable in a wide range of institutions and settings should be developed.
6. Formal studies on how best to use computer-assisted instruction should be undertaken and reported in the cancer education literature.
7. Model demonstration teaching programs that exemplify effective cancer teaching practices in outpatient care settings should be designed and

formally studied. Successful programs should be described and disseminated in the cancer education literature.

8. Model demonstration teaching programs that exemplify effective cancer education instruction and that use cancer tumor registries should be designed and formally studied. Successful educational practices should be described and disseminated in the cancer education literature.

Recurring themes in evaluations of both health promotion and disease prevention curricula and cancer education curricula in medical schools are the need to identify educational objectives, the need to ensure resources and mechanisms to attain objectives, and the need to encourage change through dissemination activities (e.g., of best practices) and accountability.

It is difficult to judge the extent to which cancer prevention and early detection are addressed in medical schools without a careful review of detailed course outlines and clinical training opportunities. More cursory reviews of medical school curricula suggest that cancer prevention education is not prominently mentioned in the available descriptive materials. For example, in a recent assessment based on literature reviews, a survey of medical school websites, and contacts with listservs, only 15 medical schools had explicit cancer prevention offerings (Herl et al., 1999). Similarly, a review of the curricular content listed in the AAMC curriculum database, CURRMIT, revealed relatively few offerings (Johnson L, Association of American Medical Colleges, personal communication to M. Hewitt, 2001). Surveys of students enrolled in some medical schools indicate that cancer prevention is getting too little emphasis. In a recent assessment conducted at Boston University Medical School, for example, more than half of all the students surveyed indicated that cancer prevention was given too little emphasis in their curriculum (Geller et al., 1999). Some medical schools have integrated prevention-related counseling skills into their curricula. At the University of Massachusetts, for example, medical students are exposed to behavioral medicine and risk factor counseling skills at multiple points in the curriculum (Ockene et al., 1990). Although few comprehensive assessments of cancer prevention and early detection education and training in medical school are available, focused reviews of training in smoking cessation and nutrition have been conducted.

Training in Smoking Cessation in Undergraduate Medical Education

According to Cancer Education Survey II conducted in 1989–1990, only a third of medical schools taught smoking prevention and cessation methods in lectures, and less than a third of schools provided instruction on these topics by another mode (Chamberlain et al., 1992; Gallagher et al., 1992). An expert panel convened by NCI in 1992 recommended that by 1995 smoking cessation and prevention interventions be mandatory components of undergraduate medical education (Fiore et al., 1994). According to the NCI panel, curricula that teach smoking and tobacco use cessation interventions contain 12 essential elements. These are outlined in Box 8.3.

An assessment of the U.S. undergraduate medical school curricula in 1996–1997 revealed that 55 percent of medical schools had incorporated the six recommended basic science content areas into their basic science curricula but that only 4 percent of schools included the 6 recommended clinical science content areas into their clinical science curricula. Most medical schools (69 percent) did not require clinical training in smoking cessation techniques, but 23 percent offered additional experience as an elective course. Investigators recommended that a model core smoking and tobacco use cessation curriculum be developed and implemented in all U.S. medical schools (Ferry et al., 1999). The importance of this recommendation is further emphasized by the fact that some assessments suggest that medical students have positive attitudes toward health promotion (Bellas et al., 2000) and that when they are provided training they can achieve high levels of confidence in their ability to help patients quit smoking (Zapka et al., 2000a).

Educational interventions during formal medical training, in particular, opportunities for hands-on practice, improve trainees' ability to deliver smoking cessation interventions and in some cases increase smoking cessation rates, according to some evaluations of these interventions. Significant

BOX 8.3 Recommended Content Areas for a Smoking and Tobacco Use Cessation Intervention Curriculum

Basic Science

- Cancer risk from smoking and tobacco use
- Health effects (smoking- and tobacco-related diseases)
- Effects of passive smoking
- Cigarette smoke contents (nicotine, tar, carbon monoxide)
- Nicotine withdrawal symptoms
- High-risk groups with the most difficulty quitting (e.g., teens, pregnant women, and individuals with psychiatric disorders)

Clinical Science

- Clinical interventions (five A's: anticipate, ask, advise, assist, and arrange)
- Relapse prevention
- Pharmacological agents (nicotine replacement or antidepressant therapy)
- Smoking cessation techniques in artificial setting with no patients
- Smoking cessation techniques in clinical setting with patients
- Smoking cessation techniques in clinical setting with patients and evaluation of performance

SOURCE: Ferry et al. (1999).

improvements were found, for example, in family practice and internal medicine residents' knowledge of smoking risks, perception that they could affect patients' behavior, and counseling skills after a 3-hour training program that showed residents how to offer brief, patient-centered smoking cessation counseling (Ockene et al., 1988). After implementation of the program, patients' smoking cessation rates were shown to increase significantly. Allen and colleagues (1990) built on this work by testing a 2-hour workshop for second-year medical students. Trained students reported greater confidence in their ability to help patients stop smoking and performed better on an objective structured clinical examination than students in a control group. The investigators concluded that the use of specific instruction and opportunities for practice were important for students to successfully translate the smoking cessation skills knowledge into clinical practice (Allen et al., 1990; Ockene et al., 1988). The use of simulated patients has also been shown to improve the smoking cessation skills of medical students (Coultas et al., 1994). One randomized study of 261 internal medicine, family practice, and pediatric residents showed that educational interventions improved trainees' behavior but did not lead to subsequent changes in smoking behavior among patients seen by the trainees (Strecher et al., 1991).

Nutrition Education in Undergraduate Medical Education

The public sees physicians as the prime source of information on nutrition, so physicians have an obligation to be prepared to encourage healthy dietary practices and to refer patients to nutrition specialists when indicated (Levin, 1999). Dietary counseling in the context of primary care is needed not only to reduce the risk of cancer but also to counter the obesity epidemic in the United States and to reduce the risk of a number of chronic conditions associated with poor dietary practices, such as heart disease and diabetes. As with smoking cessation interventions, physicians can be effective agents of dietary change for patients when training in nutrition counseling is coupled with a supportive office environment (Ockene et al., 1996, 1999). Health care providers do not appear to be addressing dietary problems among the patients in their practices, however. In a 1996 survey, for example, less than half (42 percent) of obese individuals reported that their health care professional had advised them to lose weight during a visit for routine care made within the last year (Galuska et al., 1999).

A 1985 National Academy of Sciences survey of nutrition education in U.S. medical schools found that only 22 percent of medical schools had a clearly defined course in nutrition and 50 percent of the medical schools taught less than 20 hours of nutrition-related materials in their required curricula (National Research Council, 1985). One obstacle to nutrition literacy among physicians is the limited number of nutrition specialists on medical school faculties who can effectively advocate for change in medical school and residency curricula and who can serve as role models for the incorporation of nutrition counseling into patient care (Intersociety Professional Nutrition Education Consortium, 1998).

Considerable grant support to improve nutrition education in medical schools has led to some increased attention to nutrition in the medical school curriculum. In particular, NCI R25 training education grants have funded nutrition education development and innovations at selected medical schools since the late 1980s:

- The University of Nevada School of Medicine developed a required 20-hour freshman course, Medical Nutrition; elective courses in nutrition for juniors and seniors; and for seniors, an assignment in nutrition and cancer during a rural rotation with faculty preceptors. Funding also supported integration of nutrition education into the basic science courses, patient care courses, and specialty clerkships (Ashley et al., 2000).
- The University of North Carolina at Chapel Hill developed an interactive CD-ROM that teaches nutrition and nutritional biochemistry to medical students. By 1999 it had been distributed to all U.S. medical schools and was in use in 76 of them (Plaisted et al., 2000).
- The University of California, Los Angeles, School of Medicine developed a coordinated, vertically integrated, 2-year nutrition education curriculum to address identified proficiencies in nutrition education (Hodgson et al., 2000).
- The University of Arizona College of Medicine assessed its nutrition education curriculum, developed and evaluated specific course content, and moved toward comprehensive prevention-based nutrition education (Thomson et al., 2000).
- The University of Colorado Health Sciences Center developed a nutrition elective, Nutrition and Cancer, for students of the health professions and a section on nutrition was incorporated into the biochemistry course (Bakemeier, 2000).
- The University of Alabama at Birmingham supported predoctoral and postdoctoral trainees to address the shortage of health care professionals trained in the nutritional aspects of cancer prevention (Heimburger et al., 2000).
- The New York Academy of Medicine developed a minifellowship in clinical nutrition for primary care physicians to improve the availability of faculty to serve as role models and clinical preceptors for medical students (Deen et al., 2000).

Despite these and other investments, evidence suggests continued deficits in medical school nutrition education. For example, only 23 percent of medical school graduates surveyed by AAMC in 2000 reported that they had received adequate experience in clinical nutrition, but perceptions of training varied by clinical situation. Nearly half of the students surveyed (49 percent) believed that they were adequately trained to assess patients with type II diabetes nutritionally, and 58 percent believed that they were adequately trained to assess patients with coronary heart disease. On the other hand, only 26 percent felt comfortable assessing obesity or undernutrition, and only 23 percent believed that preceptors with whom they had worked during their clerkships served as appropriate role models in their provision of clinical nutrition services (Lockwood et al., 2000). Methods that can be used to improve training in nutrition in medical school have been suggested and include the following: curriculum analysis, the use of computer-aided instruction modules, Internet Websites, case-based tutorial discussions, physician nutrition specialists and dietitians, administratively separate nutrition units, and observed structured clinical examinations, and faculty development (Lo, 2000).

Graduate Medical Education

Preventive medicine specialists often teach cancer prevention and early detection courses within medical schools or provide the needed leadership in state health departments to oversee population-based prevention programs. By one estimate, there were roughly 6,000 certified specialists in preventive medicine in 2000 (Lane et al., 2000), but these represent less than 1 percent of the total number of physicians in the United States (American Medical Association, 1999). The total number of residents training in primary care has remained relatively constant in recent years, but concerns have been raised about the adequacy of the supply of preventive medicine specialists. Some attribute the declines in the number of trainees to diminishing support for residency training through the government's Title VII program (support provided by HRSA) (Lane et al., 2000). As of 1999, there were 88 certified programs in preventive medicine (an additional 6 internal medicine programs offered a subspecialty in preventive medicine) (http://www.ama-assn.org/cgi-bin/freida.cgi).

In some cases, special curricula have been developed to provide additional training in cancer prevention to residents in primary care programs. One such example is the Recommendations for Cancer Prevention program developed at the University of Texas M. D. Anderson Cancer Center. The curriculum consisted of a series of seven 1-hour presentations. A test of the curriculum among 21 primary care residents showed relatively poor knowledge about cancer prevention before the training program and modest gains in knowledge after the program (Chamberlain et al., 1995; Spitz et al., 1992).

According to one survey of primary care residents, 40 percent reported that the residency was preparing them to provide nutrition counseling and education services, 79 percent reported that the residency should be preparing them to provide nutrition counseling and education services, and 65 percent planned to offer nutrition counseling and education services. Even though the residents rated nutrition counseling as important, they had only fair confidence in their ability to conduct it (Orleans et al., 1985; Rosen et al., 1984; Walsh et al., 1999; Wells et al., 1986).

Educational interventions targeted to medical residents have increased confidence in the ability to provide counseling and have increased counseling activity according to the few assessments that have been published. Most studies on improvements in the nutrition knowledge and counseling skills of medical residents have focused on cardiovascular disease or general health promotion. One study, for example, assessed 130 internal medicine residents to determine if an educational and prompting intervention improved dietary counseling practices (Evans et al., 1996). Residents participated in two 1-hour sessions to improve their skills and confidence in dietary counseling. The education materials included a contract for the patient and physician, a dietary assessment tool with matching dietary advice, a wallet card for the patient, a recipe book, and pamphlets. At the 10-month follow-up, residents reported increased confidence in providing dietary counseling.

A significant increase in dietary counseling (12 to 94 percent) by residents as measured by chart audit was achieved after implementation of a practice-based teaching model aimed at improving compliance with U.S. Preventive Services Task Force guidelines (Geiger et al., 1993; U.S. Preventive Services Task Force, 1996). In contrast, no significant change in self-reports of counseling for nutrition and diet modification was observed after an educational intervention that involved making patient education booklets available and participation in several grand rounds (Madlon-Kay et al., 1994).

According to one assessment, physicians had received little to no training in physical activity counseling, and most did not believe that they had the knowledge or the skills needed to effectively counsel their patients about physical activity (Scott et al., 1992). One intervention to change residents' attitudes and behaviors about physical activity counseling led to improvements in physician confidence in physical activity counseling and self-reported counseling rates (over 3 months), but did not result in changes in physical activity levels among their patients with chronic diseases (Eckstrom et al., 1999). The residents were trained in two 2-hour workshops where they learned counseling skills specific to populations with chronic diseases, participated in a problem-solving session, and received educational handouts and information about community resources.

In another study, family practice residents randomly assigned to a group that was trained in approximately 15 minutes to give 2 to 3 minutes of exercise advice gave exercise advice to patients almost twice as often as those in the control groups, and the patients who received the advice significantly increased their exercise durations but not their exercise frequencies (Lewis and Lynch, 1993). In addition to the advice, the residents in the experimental group distributed an educational handout and advised the patient that a staff member would call in 1 month. An educational handout on the patient's chart prompted the physicians.

Schools of Nursing

Nursing represents the largest segment of the nation's health care workforce. In 2000, an estimated 2.2 million registered nurses were employed full- or part-time nationwide (Health Resources and Services Administration, 2001). In terms of level of training, most (57 percent) registered nurses have received less than a baccalaureate degree[4] as their highest nursing-related educational preparation, and 9 percent (196,300) have had formal preparation to practice in advanced nursing positions (e.g., nurse practitioner or nurse anesthetist) (Health Resources and Services Administration, 2001).

Despite their apparent potential role in cancer prevention and early detection, there is scant information about what role nurses are playing in this area. A 1992 comprehensive review of the literature on nurses' involvement in cancer prevention (with most of the papers in the literature published in the late 1980s) provides examples of nurse-led initiatives in patient and community education, prevention-related intervention, and research (Frank-Stromborg and Rohan, 1992). Other literature describes the roles of nurse practitioners in risk assessment, teaching, patient advocacy, and cancer screening programs aimed at early detection (Leslie, 1995). With few national surveys of nurses' practice activities, however, it is difficult to judge the level of nurses' involvement in cancer prevention. Some state assessments suggest that nurses rarely perform cancer prevention services. Nurses responding to a 1992 statewide survey in Florida, for example, reported performing screening examinations or counseling about lifestyle changes with less than 20 percent of their patients (Entrekin and McMillan, 1993).[5]

Current information on the settings in which nurses practice suggests that the role of nursing in primary care may be limited, insofar as relatively few nurses work in ambulatory and community-based settings, the places most associated with cancer prevention activities. In 2000, most

[4]Among the three primary types of education that allow a person to enter an entry-level position in nursing (diploma, associate degree, baccalaureate), the education required for a baccalaureate, with its broader, more scientific curriculum, provides a foundation from which a nurse may move into graduate education.

[5]Although an attempt was made to reach a representative sample of nurses in the state, the survey response rate was only 36 percent, limiting the ability to interpret the study's findings.

registered nurses (59 percent) worked in hospitals, an estimated 18 percent (402,900) worked in public or community health settings (e.g., state and local health departments and community health centers), and 9 percent (209,200) worked in ambulatory care settings. In these settings, evidence suggests that nurses do not routinely interact with patients—in 1998, an estimated 20 percent of ambulatory care visits involved a nurse (a registered nurse or an advanced practice nurse) or a physician's assistant spending time with patients. A study of African-American nurses conducted in 1990 suggested that nurses are performing cancer prevention activities on a voluntary basis rather than on the job (Olsen and Frank-Stromborg, 1994). The barriers to providing cancer prevention activities reported by nurses include time limitations and a lack of specialized knowledge (Genovese and Wholihan, 1995).

The National Council of State Boards of Nursing administers licensure examinations and periodically conducts a national practice analysis of newly licensed registered nurses to ensure a match between the contents of the licensure examinations and contemporary practices. The 1999 practice analysis found that the majority of newly licensed registered nurses were employed in hospitals (87 percent) and that less than 5 percent were employed in community-based settings. Results of the activity analysis suggest that in these settings newly licensed nurses are completing health risk assessments (83.0 percent), counseling clients regarding risk behaviors (77.9 percent), teaching clients about health risks and health promotion (73.0 percent), and performing age-specific screening examinations (41.7). They are less likely to be involved in community-based activities such as participating in health promotion programs (35.5 percent) or helping to determine health promotion needs (10.8 percent). An estimated 4 to 10 percent of the licensure examination is devoted to prevention and early detection of disease (section B4 of the examination) (http://www.ncsbn.org/files/diagnostic/pndefin.asp).

Nurses' level of interest in continuing education in cancer prevention, when it has been assessed, has not been high. According to an oncology education needs survey of 3,714 registered nurses in Texas, to which 378 nurses responded, training in prevention and screening was rated lowest in terms of priority relative to treatment-related topics (e.g., issues and trends in cancer care and investigational or new drug developments), even though perceived skill levels in prevention and screening were relatively low. This is likely explained by the fact that most of the nurses responding to the survey worked in hospital settings (Becker et al., 1995). Nursing workforce projections suggest that the hospital will remain the major employer of registered nurses but that in the future, because of a shift of care to outpatient settings and the aging of the population, nurses will need to focus on primary care and health promotion (http://bhpr.hrsa.gov/dn/bwrepex.htm).

Nurse Training

Approximately 95,000 nurses graduate each year from about 1,500 programs for registered nurses at schools of nursing, and approximately 3,500 nurse practitioners graduate annually from more than 150 certificate- or master's-level educational programs nationwide (National League for Nursing, 1997; Reed and Selleck, 1996). Master's degree programs in advanced practice oncology nursing are also available (Brown and Hinds, 1998), and as of 1997 the Oncology Nursing Society had certified an estimated 19,000 nurses as oncology nurses and 1,300 as advanced oncology nurses (J. Mills, ONS, personal communication, March 28, 2002). Although most oncology nurses work in clinical settings, some are involved in community-based education programs focused on prevention. The Oncology Nursing Society's Statement on the Scope and Standards of Oncology Nursing Practice (Oncology Nursing Society, 1996) and its Standards of Oncology Nursing Education (Oncology Nursing Society, 1995) include an emphasis on prevention, early detection, and health promotion.

At the time of writing of this chapter, there were no comprehensive reviews of nursing curricula, texts, or continuing educational opportunities in the area of cancer prevention and early detection. A few descriptions of attempts at integrating cancer prevention into nursing curricula (Mundt, 1996) and attempts to address the needs of certain groups of nurses are available. In recognition of the potential role of African-American nurses in promoting cancer prevention, for example, a cancer prevention and early detection program for nurses working with African Americans was developed. The curriculum includes learning objectives, detailed content outlines, lists of resources for professional and public education, and instruments for program evaluation (Underwood, 1999). One survey of African-American nurses who had enrolled in an NCI or Oncology Nursing Society workshop suggested that the majority of nurses were not participating in cancer prevention or screening activities before workshop participation (Olsen and Frank-Stromborg, 1994). In one assessment, nurse practitioners rated their clinical skills as excellent but rated their skills in patient education and counseling about cancer risk lower (Tessaro et al., 1996).

Training in Smoking Cessation in Nursing Education

Most oncology nurses who participated in a 1998 survey (38 percent response rate) could not recall whether they had received information about smoking or tobacco use prevention or cessation in their nursing curricula. Of those who did recall their student experience, most reported an absence of curricular content on prevention or the cessation of smoking or tobacco use. The majority of respondents said that they assessed and documented the smoking or tobacco use status of their patients and had assessed their patients' readiness to quit, but few went on to provide interventions. Common barriers reported by oncology nurses included a perceived lack of patient motivation and the nurse's lack of time and skills (Sarna et al., 2000). Most stated that they needed additional training. A survey of nursing programs in Minnesota indicated that cancer prevention and early detection components were addressed at various levels of depth (Post-White et al., 1993). A resource for nurses is a World Wide Web-based smoking and tobacco use cessation information program created by the American Nurses Foundation (http://www.con.ohio-state.edu/tobacco/).

Dental Schools

Dental providers are second only to physicians in having high rates of access to the population: in 1998, nearly two-thirds (63 percent) of adults reported that they had seen a dental provider in the previous year. Many oral conditions, including oral cancer and periodontitis, are attributed to smoking and tobacco use, and so the prevention of smoking and the use of smokeless tobacco, as well as the treatment of nicotine addiction, are major concerns in dental practice. Dental patients, perhaps more so than medical patients, represent a "captive audience" for which there are "teachable moments" (Jones, 2000). Regularly scheduled dental hygiene visits also provide oral health care professionals with a unique opportunity to reiterate smoking-related messages and provide support for patients attempting to quit (Severson et al., 1998).

Like physicians, dentists are not routinely advising their patients who smoke to quit (http://www.ada.org/public/media/newsrel/9905/nr-03.html; Chisick, 2000; Hastreiter et al., 1994; Martin et al., 1996; Tomar et al., 1996). According to a 1994 national survey of oral health care providers, for example, only one-third of dentists and one-quarter of dental hygienists said that they asked most or nearly all of their patients if they smoked. Among the dentists surveyed, 66 percent reported that they advised most or nearly all of their patients who reported smoking to stop. Only 20 percent of dentists surveyed believed that they were well prepared to assist patients in stopping smoking and tobacco use, and only 14 percent of dentists had completed formal training in the provision of tobacco use cessation services. The training experiences cited included continuing education courses, pharmaceutical company-sponsored educational programs, the dental school curriculum, and organized study clubs. Those who reported having had some training in smoking and tobacco use cessation were more likely to report providing services in their practices (Dolan et al., 1997).

In 1991 and 1992 the American Association of Dental Schools published curriculum guidelines recommending that dental and dental hygiene students be educated about the effects of tobacco on oral health and that students be able to conduct primary prevention counseling, assist with elimination of harmful habits, and assess compliance (Barker and Williams, 1999). More recently, a national strategic planning conference working group on professional education and practice recommended the development of health care curricula requiring competency in prevention, diagnosis, and multidisciplinary management of oral cancers, including the prevention and cessation of tobacco and alcohol use (CDC, 1998b). A 1998 review of the curricula in 47 of the nation's 52 dental schools revealed that only 33 percent of the schools taught smoking cessation as part of the curriculum. Continuing education in cancer for community dentists was provided by 60 percent of the schools. Lack of funding was cited by 57 percent of the schools as the primary reason why continuing education was not being offered. In 1998, very few (15 percent) dental schools reported that they had received financial support from NCI, representing a significant decline relative to that in 1981, when half (51 percent) of dental schools received such support (Rankin et al., 1999). Another survey assessed smoking and tobacco use cessation activities in U.S. dental and dental hygiene student clinics and found that 47 percent of dental schools incorporated clinical practices in smoking and tobacco use cessation in their student clinics (Barker and Williams, 1999). A study of fourth-year dental students at one school that did not have formal didactic or clinical programs specifically devoted to training in smoking and tobacco use cessation suggested that the lack of training lowers the rate of tobacco use counseling (Yip et al., 2000).

Training in Smoking and Tobacco Use Treatment Among Providers Outside of Medical, Nursing, and Dental Schools

Voluntary organizations have a long history of training volunteers (both health care professionals and laypeople) to provide smoking and tobacco use cessation education and counseling services, often in group settings. The American Lung Association (ALA) has, for example, offered its Freedom from Smoking Cessation Clinics for more than 20 years, and it has recently launched a new program targeted to teens (C. Pruitt, ALA, personal communication. February 22, 2001). The clinics are staffed by individuals who undergo a day-and-a-half educational program. Another, more advanced program is available to train trainers. ALA recently placed its cessation program online (www.lungusa.org).

A few states have organized training programs that certify smoking and tobacco use treatment providers (Box 8.4). Massachusetts has developed a rigorous program aimed at training providers skilled in treating more complex cases. Arizona provides certification at two levels: a basic skills course for those interested in providing brief interventions and a specialist course for those providing more intensive services. Mississippi is among the states

BOX 8.4 Examples of State Efforts to Train Smoking and Tobacco Use Treatment Providers

Massachusetts

Since 1993, the Massachusetts Tobacco Control Program (MTCP) has funded smoking and tobacco use treatment providers through the Massachusetts Department of Public Health to provide treatment services throughout the state. In 1997, MTCP contracted with the University of Massachusetts Medical School to develop a comprehensive statewide training and certification program for smoking and tobacco use cessation (Pbert et al., 2000) and a training program for tobacco treatment specialists was finalized in 1999. The training entails a basic 2-day training course, an intensive 6-day core certification training course, and a set of required continuing education courses after certification. To be eligible for certification, those completing the course work must document 2,000 hours of experience in smoking and tobacco use treatment; pass a written examination; and demonstrate integration of knowledge, skills, and experience by passing an oral defense of a case study presented to a review committee (Pbert et al., 2000; Ewy B., University of Massachusetts Medical School, personal communication, February 27, 2001).

Arizona

The Arizona Cessation Training and Evaluation Program offers two curriculum tracks (www.tepp.org/actev/training/right.html):

1. Smoking Use and Tobacco Cessation Skills Certification training is offered at three levels:
   - Basic skills—A 4-hour course open to anyone interested in helping individuals reduce tobacco dependency. Those certified in basic skills deliver brief interventions appropriate to a client's readiness to quit and give clients advice about the use of nicotine replacement and help them create a simple quit plan. Since April 1999, more than 800 individuals have been certified in basic skills.
   - Specialist—A 16-hour course offered to health care and human services professionals experienced in smoking and tobacco use cessation. Those certified as a Tobacco Cessation Specialist are able to offer intensive smoking and tobacco use cessation services within the structure of an existing program, as well as to act as a resource for other professionals. More than 100 persons are certified as Tobacco Cessation Specialists in Arizona.
   - Trainer—The trainer curriculum, which is under development, will train individuals to develop or manage smoking and tobacco cessation programs and act as leaders in their communities and organizations.
2. Systems training for individuals in health care, workplace, and school settings. The focus in this 16-hour course is on policy change, analysis of case studies, and review of best practice standards.

The Arizona Tobacco Education and Prevention Program posts tobacco cessation service providers' compliance with guidelines of the Agency for Healthcare Research and Quality on the World Wide Web.

Mississippi

Since 1998, Mississippi has used its tobacco settlement money to provide training to more than 1,000 physicians and allied health care providers throughout the state. Smoking cessation products have recently been approved for reimbursement under the Medicaid program, but reimbursement for Medicaid providers awaits implementation of a certification process for smoking cessation providers (T. Payne, University of Mississippi Medical Center, personal communication, February 21, 2001).

that are in the process of planning a certification for smoking and tobacco use treatment providers.

There have been calls for a nationwide certification program for smoking and tobacco use treatment specialists or at least a core curriculum that states could adapt for their needs. Concerns raised by requiring certification for smoking and tobacco use treatment providers include the cost of obtaining certification, the potential to exclude uncertified health care professionals from delivering basic smoking and tobacco use treatment, and integration of services in the health care delivery systems and the community (Pbert et al., 2000). Potential benefits of certification include quality assurance (e.g., providing services consistent with accepted guidelines), enhanced opportunities for reimbursement, and improved access to and recognition of smoking and tobacco use treatment.

Continuing Education

Health care providers who completed their training 10 or more years ago are unlikely to have been adequately trained in cancer prevention and early detection. In the early 1990s, for example, relatively few medical schools had any training in smoking cessation. Therefore, reaching providers after they have completed their training with continuing medical education (CME) programs is vital to improving the practice of cancer prevention and early detection.

Physicians seem to be interested in learning more about improving their office management of cancer prevention and screening activities. In a CME needs assessment survey conducted among primary care physicians in Massachusetts in 1990, this topic was the first preference of internists, family practitioners, and gynecologists. Almost all physicians (91 percent) indicated that they would find useful a comprehensive course on cancer prevention and early detection, with an emphasis on practical matters and with an opportunity to upgrade their clinical skills in physical examinations and counseling. Appealing to practitioners was a 1-day course that would lead to accreditation in screening and prevention and to reductions in malpractice premiums (Costanza et al., 1993).

A number of approaches have been used to provide continuing education to physicians, nurses, and dentists:

- Online continuing education. Web-based continuing medical education courses are convenient, relatively inexpensive, and can reach providers that may live far from medical schools or sites of traditional programs. Some evidence suggests that online CME is of interest to physicians (Richardson and Norris, 1997), but Internet use among physicians is not yet universal (Chin, 2001). There are examples of excellent free CME offerings in cancer prevention and early detection (e.g., An Evidence-Based Approach to Screening Breast, Prostate, & Colon Cancer [www.uwcme.org]), but they are difficult to locate, as there are few organized listings of online CME course offerings available to health care providers.

• Point-of-care education. Patient-specific cancer prevention reminders that physicians see immediately before or as they see their patients provide immediate guidance to physicians and, when coupled with educational interventions, have resulted in the increased use of some prevention services (McPhee et al., 1991).

• Academic detailing. Modeled after drug detailing developed by the pharmaceutical industry, academic detailing is an effort to provide continuing education in office practices. Such methods have been used to improve cancer prevention and early detection practices and have met with some success (Sheinfeld Gorin et al., 2000; Williams et al., 1994). In one example, educational visits to 221 inner-city physicians in Philadelphia led to substantial increases in cancer screening and prevention activities, as well as an increased confidence in counseling skills, as expressed by the physicians (Daly et al., 1993).

• Supervised skill training. Acquiring the necessary skills to incorporate unfamiliar or new technologies into practice usually requires some hands-on supervised experience as well as didactic education. As part of a community-based demonstration and education project, primary care physicians in one community were offered skills training in flexible sigmoidoscopy. Their patients were those age 50 and older who had never had a sigmoidoscopy and who responded to an invitation to have the procedure at a reduced fee (Renneker and Saner, 1995).

• Train the trainer. In 1989 NCI developed a 3-hour course for physicians and nurses and collaborated with organizations to reach providers in a train-the-trainer model of delivery (Manley et al., 1991). The goal of the program was to train 100,000 physicians.

• Multimethods. Multimethod CME approaches have been used to reach larger numbers of physicians through preferred (and perhaps different) learning styles. One such effort to improve compliance with mammography guidelines was based at a community hospital and was directed at physicians with hospital staff appointments engaged in fee-for-service office practice in the community. Educational interventions included formal CME conferences, a physician newsletter, breast examination skills training, a breast cancer CME monograph, primary care office visits, patient education materials, and a "question of the month" at hospital staff meetings. The package of interventions available to physicians increased referrals of asymptomatic women ages 50 to 75 (Lane et al., 1991).

• Development of educational materials. Put Prevention into Practice, a program sponsored by the Office of Disease Prevention and Health Promotion of the U.S. Public Health Service, was a multifaceted educational initiative consisting of a variety of printed materials made available in 1994 to providers, to patients, and in the office setting (Gemson et al., 1996). Consistent with other studies, the simple availability of a kit of materials is not sufficient to enhance the delivery of prevention services. Additional strategies for dissemination and implementation are needed, such as providing external consultation services to practices and adopting reminder systems (Goodson et al., 1999; Kikano et al., 1997; Medder et al., 1997; Weingarten, 1999).

A recent review of the effectiveness of approaches to CME suggests that interactive CME sessions that enhance participant activity and that provide the opportunity to practice skills can effect change in professional practice and, on occasion, health care outcomes (Davis et al., 1999). Performance-based learning, such as role playing and use of simulated or standardized patients, are especially effective in improving performance (Carney et al., 1995; Davis et al., 1999; Ockene and Zapka, 1997). Academic detailing, in which educators provide face-to-face education in an interactive manner within the practice setting, has been found to be effective (Daly et al., 1993; Davis et al., 1995a) and addresses the issue of limited provider time. Traditional continuing medical education strategies of lectures, grand rounds, or brief noon or morning reports can improve physicians' knowledge and awareness, but when used alone, they generally do not change a physician's clinical practice (Davis et al., 1999; Haynes et al., 1984; U.S. Preventive Services Task Force, 1996).

CME in cancer has been critiqued as being "off target" too often with too little emphasis on smoking cessation, for which there is ample evidence that providers are not trained. It has also been critiqued for not giving physicians opportunities to learn about office management or organizational interventions that could improve compliance with cancer prevention and early detection recommendations (Love, 1993). Some evidence suggests that provider training alone is not enough. Training of physicians in smoking cessation interventions appears to be most effective when it is paired with changes in the use of other systems, such as staff education and clinic reminder systems (US DHHS, 2000a). Several randomized clinical trials demonstrate, for example, the efficacy of physician training in combination with the implementation of office system innovations for smoking cessation (e.g., placement of stickers in the charts of smokers) (Cohen et al., 1987, 1989; Cummings et al., 1989a,b; Gilbert et al., 1992; Janz et al., 1987; Kottke et al., 1989; Lindsay et al., 1994; Ockene et al., 1991b; Manley et al., 1991; Wilson et al., 1988; Chang et al., 1995).

Similar findings have emerged from studies of educational interventions to improve physicians' provision of dietary counseling (Dietrich et al., 1992; Ockene et al., 1996; Tziraki et al., 2000) and physical activity counseling (Marcus et al., 1997; Pinto et al., 1998). Other research suggests that the development and implementation of office systems by themselves can substantially improve provision of cancer detection and early prevention services (Dietrich et al., 1992; McPhee et al., 1991). In fact, some have suggested that the major vehicle for improved clinical prevention services is the establishment of office systems that are conducive to meeting prevention needs during the course of normal patient care (Solberg et al., 1997a).

SUPPORT FOR PROFESSIONAL EDUCATION AND TRAINING

Public Programs

National Cancer Institute

A number of education and training opportunities are supported through NCI's Office of Centers, Training, and Resources. The Cancer Training Branch of this office plans, develops, administers, and evaluates the extramural, grant-supported research training and health professional education programs of NCI in the form of fellowships and institutional grants. Additional education and training opportunities at NCI exist through other programs such as the Cancer Centers Program and the Cancer Prevention Fellowship Program. Through the Office of Centers, Training, and Resources, NCI provided roughly $30 million in fiscal years 2000 and 2001 to support education and training in cancer prevention and early detection (Brian Kimes, director, Office of Centers, Training, and Resources, personal communication to Maria Hewitt, Institute of Medicine, November 14, 2001). Support is available both to training institutions and to individuals pursuing graduate and postgraduate training (Table 8.1).

The R25 grant has been used as a training instrument by NCI for years, but it has a varied history. NCI began awarding R25 grants to medical schools in 1948 on a noncompetitive basis to provide more education on cancer and to encourage faculty to pursue oncology. Between 1966 and 1983, medical schools competed for grants. In the 1980s, the R25 training grant program was cut because of NCI budget reductions, and an estimated one-third of medical schools lost funds. For some schools not able to find alternative funding sources, the number of cancer education faculty declined (Chamberlain et al., 1992). When support was assessed in 1989–1990 in Cancer Education Survey II, 66 of 125 medical schools had been the recipients of an NCI R25 training grant. NCI R25 training grant support was viewed as instrumental in maintaining key elements of the cancer education program, such as cancer education coordinators, cancer education committees, and student assistantships and fellowships (Chamberlain et al., 1992; Gallagher et al., 1992). In 1999, the NCI R25 grant was revamped as a training instrument with a new focus on preparing scientists who can work in multidisciplinary, team research settings. This newest version of the R25 grant is called the R25T grant and can support both

TABLE 8.1 National Cancer Institute Research Training and Career Development Opportunities for Prevention, Control, Behavioral, and Population Scientists

Program	Description	Support Level
Cancer Education and Career Development Program (R25T grants)	Institutional award for education and training predoctoral and postdoctoral candidates in multidisciplinary research settings	Up to 5 years of support, not to exceed $500,000 in direct costs per year (can exceed this level with special permission); grants are renewable
Cancer Prevention, Control, Behavioral and Population Sciences Career Development Award (K07 grant)	Institutional award for postdoctoral training	Annual salaries up to $75,000 plus fringe benefits and other costs up to $30,000; up to 5 years of support available; grants are not renewable
Transition Career Development Award (K22 grant)	Award to clinician-scientists or prevention control, behavioral, and population scientists to provide "protected time" to develop independent cancer research	Annual salaries up to $75,000 plus fringe benefits and other costs up to $50,000; up to 3 years of support available; grants are not renewable
Established Investigator Award in Cancer Prevention, Control, Behavioral, and Population Research (K05 grant)	Award to institutions for scientists with outstanding track records in research and who need protected time to devote to their research and to act as mentors for new investigators	Annual salaries up to 50 percent of the maximum allowable federal salary plus fringe benefits and other research costs up to $25,000; grants are renewable for one additional 5-year period
Cancer Education Grant Program (R25E grant)	Award to organizations for innovative education programs (e.g., academic short courses, national forums, and hands-on workshops)	Up to $300,000 in direct costs for any single year

SOURCE: http://cancertraining.nci.nih.gov/research/prevention/pr25t.html, accessed December 5, 2000.

predoctoral students and postdoctoral fellows for up to 5 years, with a cap of $500,000 in direct costs per year (http://cancertraining.nci.nih.gov/research/prevention/pr25t. html). The R25T grant is particularly adaptable to training cancer prevention and control and population scientists. One recent example of a program awarded an R25T grant is the Tobacco Research Training Program, in which individuals are trained in multidisciplinary research settings and have more than one mentor during the course of their training.

The other large organizational award that uses the R25 grant mechanism is the traditional Cancer Education Grant Program, which provides R25E grants at funding levels of up to $300,000 per year. The following are among the projects that have been funded through this mechanism (http://cancertraining.nci.nih.gov/cancerEd/cancered.html):

- a project that provides short introductory research opportunities for health professionals;
- a project that designs, implements, and evaluates new curricula of special significance to cancer (e.g., nutrition);
- a project that develops a curriculum for health care professionals in cancer pain management and palliative care;
- programs that offer outreach to the lay community; and
- workshops, national forums, short courses, and hands-on experiences (e.g., minority health initiatives, courses on state-of-the art basic research techniques).

One recent specific example of work funded by an NCI R25E grant is an effort to improve cancer prevention education across Texas. A consortium of eight Texas medical schools has charged 50 faculty "champions" with developing instructional resources, sharing their expertise, and leading the way in making changes to the curricula in their local institutions. Goals are to progress toward longitudinal integrated curricula, performance-based education, and competency-based testing (www.catchum.utmd.edu/catchum-goals.htm).

A number of other special programs at NCI provide support for individuals to pursue training in cancer prevention and early detection:

- The Cancer Prevention Fellowship Program provides multidisciplinary training in cancer prevention and early detection.
- The NCI Scholars Program provides for up to 4 years of research support in the laboratories or clinics of NCI for investigators who are ready to begin independent research careers.
- The Division of Cancer Epidemiology and Genetics offers fellowships and summer internships.

Centers for Disease Control and Prevention

CDC's federally mandated National Breast and Cervical Cancer Early Detection Program, in addition to providing screening services to women, supports public and professional education. Examples of state-initiated activities that are offered through this program include the following (CDC, 1998a):

- A self-study kit in Kentucky helps primary care physicians increase their use of and improve their practice of routine breast and cervical cancer screening. The program features a videotape that discusses communication strategies, physical examination recommendations and techniques, risk management, and office reminder systems. Physicians who complete the study are awarded incentives including a 5 percent malpractice insurance premium reduction (CDC, 2000c).

- A 3-day interactive course offered through the West Virginia Breast and Cervical Cancer Screening Program certifies public health nurses (primarily in county health departments and primary care centers) to perform breast self-examination education, clinical breast examinations, and pelvic examinations and Pap smears (S. Pickering, CDC, personal communication, March 20, 2001).
- The development and distribution of a video-based self-study packet, Follow-up of Abnormal CBE [clinical breast examination] and Mammographic Findings, designed by the CDC National Breast and Cervical Cancer Early Detection Program ensures that primary care providers are aware of current protocols and practice standards for the follow-up of abnormal clinical breast examination and mammographic findings. The packet includes a two-part video and self-study manual, and CME credits are offered through CDC (S. Pickering, senior program consultant, CDC, personal communication, March 20, 2001).
- A 2-hour satellite training conference for Alabama nurses and nurse practitioners provides training on follow-up of abnormal breast examinations. Continuing education credit is offered for this course (S. Pickering, CDC, personal communication, March 20, 2001).
- An educational outreach to mammography facility staff assists with compliance with the Mammography Quality Standards Act (Public Law 102-539) in rural North Carolina (Pisano et al., 1998a).
- Native Web was developed to enhance American Indian nurses' clinical breast examination skills.
- The Ohio Department of Health and the Ohio Breast & Cervical Cancer Project, in collaboration with the Medical College of Ohio, developed a CD-ROM, Cultural Competence in Breast Cancer Care, to enhance the capacity of primary health care providers (physicians and others) to effectively screen, evaluate, and manage breast cancer in culturally and ethnically diverse patient populations. The CD-ROM meets accreditation-contract and regulatory requirements for CME (S. Pickering, CDC, personal communication, March 20, 2001).

As part of an effort to generate a greater awareness among primary care providers of the importance of prevention and early detection of colorectal cancer, CDC staff have made available online a slide presentation, A Call to Action: Prevention and Early Detection of Colorectal Cancer (www.cdc.gov/

cancer/colorctl/calltoaction/index.htm). Speakers from CDC are available to deliver the training slides at national or regional professional conferences.

In fiscal year 2001 CDC funded two initiatives to provide education on prostate cancer screening for primary health care providers, including potential benefits and harms, fundamentals of effective patient counseling, and informed decision making (http://www.cdc.gov/od/pgo/funding/01094.htm).

Health Resources and Services Administration

HRSA is one of eight agencies of the U.S. Public Health Service. Its programs cover Community and Migrant Health Centers, national maternal and child health needs, placement of physicians in medically underserved areas through the National Health Service Corps, and community-based human immunodeficiency virus infection and AIDS services. Through its Bureau of Health Professions, HRSA attempts to promote and maintain the nation's supply of health professionals by supporting faculty to meet current health care challenges, designing new curricula, and providing student loans and scholarships to encourage lower-income, disadvantaged, and minority individuals to become health care professionals (Sampson, 1995). HRSA also funds primary care offices in each state health department and funds primary care associations to build statewide coalitions for primary care health delivery systems (Health Resources and Services Administration, 2000b).

As part of its charge, HRSA supports preventive medicine residency training. In 1998, HRSA provided $1.6 million to 11 schools to further advanced training (www.bhpr.hrsa.gov/dadphp/prevmed.htm). HRSA also supports public health traineeships to alleviate shortages of public health professionals in medically underserved areas or populations (www.bhpr.hrsa.gov/dadphp/phtrain.htm). In 1999, HRSA awarded 34 grants totaling $2.2 million to schools, and in 2000, HRSA awarded 33 noncompeting continuation grants totaling $1.8 million to schools. Innovations in curriculum in areas such as population health and providing primary care services to vulnerable, underserved populations will be supported by HRSA as part of a 5-year demonstration project, Undergraduate Medical Education for the 21st Century (www.aacom.org/UME/AboutUME).

HRSA oversees Area Health Education Centers (AHECs), which are programs housed within accredited schools of medicine and nursing that have the following objectives:

- to form linkages between health care delivery systems and educational resources in underserved communities;
- to create collaborative community-based education and training opportunities for health care professionals, students, and primary care resident physicians;

- to create systems for learning and networks for information dissemination;
- to support multidisciplinary and interdisciplinary training in response to community needs; and
- to provide technical assistance to educators and others.

In 2000, HRSA provided about $40 million to 39 AHECs and 40 AHEC programs (www.bhpr.hrsa.gov). Some examples of cancer prevention-related education and training offered through AHECs follow:

- A 2-day training session on cancer prevention and screening for nurses practicing in rural areas was designed in Colorado and delivered through AHECs. According to evaluation measures, it was successful in improving nurses' knowledge, attitudes, and skills (Howell et al., 1998).
- Continuing education on early detection of breast cancer was provided to 22 rural hospitals and clinics in Arkansas through interactive television linkages. The mammography seminar was attended by 136 mammographers, 40 clinics were provided breast examination training, and 40 nurse practitioners received training (CDC, 2000d).

HRSA also provides direct support for individual education and training:

- HRSA and the Centers for Medicare and Medicaid Services support a health policy fellowship program for preventive medicine physicians through a cooperative agreement with the Association of Teachers of Preventive Medicine (www.atpm.org/news/press4.htm).
- HRSA, in collaboration with CDC and the Association of State and Territorial Directors of Nursing, has developed a distance learning tool to teach core public health competencies. Called Waldtrek, the project has had three broadcasts and has enrolled an estimated 3,000 nurses (Carole Gassert, Division of Nursing, Bureau of Health Personnel, Health Resources and Services Administration personal communication to Maria Hewitt, January 2001). The broadcasts have covered principles of population health but nothing specifically related to cancer prevention.

HRSA's Cancer Action Plan has proposed means of improving cancer prevention and early detection services (Health Resources and Services Administration, 2000a). The initiatives include:

- the creation and dissemination of systematic training modules for primary care clinicians to increase their knowledge of cancer screening procedures (e.g., colonoscopy, colposcopy, endometrial biopsy, and fine-needle biopsy) and

• strengthening the cancer prevention, screening, and access-to-care content of Division of Nursing training grants to nurse practitioner and nurse midwifery training programs.

Agency for Healthcare Research and Quality

Although the training opportunities provided by the Agency for Healthcare Research and Quality (AHRQ) are not specific to cancer, AHRQ provides several training opportunities in health services research of potential interest to clinical and behavioral and social scientists (www.ahcpr.gov/fund/training/trainix.htm):

- Health Services Research Dissertation Awards (R03 grants)
- Independent Scientist Awards (K02 grants) (career development support for promising new investigators)
- Individual Postdoctoral Fellowship Awards (F32 grants)
- Institutional Training Awards (T32 grants) (National Research Service Award grants to institutions for predoctoral and postdoctoral training)
- Institutional Training Innovation Incentive Awards (R25 grants) (support for design and implementation of new models of health services research training)
- Kerr White Visiting Scholars Program (intramural opportunities for junior, mid-career-level, and senior researchers)
- Mentored Clinical Scientist Development Awards (K08 grants)
- Opportunities for Minority Students
- Predoctoral Fellowship Awards for Minority Students (F31 grants)
- Summer Intern Program.

AHRQ also supports health services research, including methods to improve physicians' preventive health practices.

Private Programs

American Cancer Society

The American Cancer Society (ACS) has spent an estimated $2 million to $3 million annually in recent years on training and career development in cancer prevention, representing roughly 20 percent of ACS's total spending for training and career development (Ginger Krawiec, ACS, personal communication to Maria Hewitt, Institute of Medicine, April 11, 2001). Opportunities for support available through ACS are described in Table 8.2.

Some ACS-funded programs have been described in the literature. With funding from an ACS professional education grant, for example, nurses at

TABLE 8.2 Training and Career Development Opportunities, American Cancer Society

Program	Description	Support Level
Postdoctoral fellowships	Awards to individuals for research training (basic, preclinical, clinical, psychosocial, behavioral, and epidemiological research)	One- to 3-year awards with stipends of up to $40,000 per year plus a $2,000 per year institutional allowance[a]
Clinical research training grants for junior faculty	Awards to individuals to conduct mentored clinical, epidemiological, psychosocial, behavioral, or health policy and outcomes research	Up to 3 years for up to $150,000 per year, including 25 percent indirect costs; renewable once for a 2-year period
Cancer control career development awards for primary care physicians	Awards to academic physicians pursuing a career in cancer control research, teaching, and practice	Three-year award for up to $60,000 per year
Physician training awards in preventive medicine	Awards to institutions to support physician training in accredited preventive medicine residency programs	Four-year awards in the total amount of $300,000 based on an average of $50,000 per year for resident training
Master's and post-master's training grants in clinical oncology social work	Awards to institutions (master's level) and individuals (postdoctoral level)	One- to 3-year awards with annual funding from $12,000 (master's) to $20,000 (doctorate)
Master's and doctoral degree scholarships in cancer nursing	Awards to individuals	Up to two year (master's) and four year (doctorate) awards with a stipend of $10,000 (master's) or $15,000 (doctorate) per year

[a]Top-ranked fellows receive 3-year fellowships with an award amount of $138,000.
SOURCE: wysiwyg: //40http://www2.cancer.org/research/index.cfm?sc=1, accessed December 5, 2000.

the Bronx Veterans Affairs Medical Center formed the VANAC (VA Nurses Against Cancer) team. After an intensive orientation, nurses participated in a wide range of educational activities, including patient education, staff seminars, and community presentations (Genovese and Wholihan, 1995). A hospitalwide Breast Health Awareness Team was organized as an offshoot of the VANAC team, and some funded activities were maintained after the cessation of grant support (e.g., school of nursing presentations were continued).

American Association of Health Plans

In 1997, the American Association of Health Plans (AAHP), the professional organization representing managed care plans, with support from the Robert Wood Johnson Foundation, CDC, and AHRQ, established the National Technical Assistance Office (NTAO) to help managed care organizations integrate smoking and tobacco use cessation activities into routine health care. NTAO's mission is to (www.aahp.org/atmc/ntaosum.htm):

- develop a comprehensive network of key contacts in health plans who are responsible for smoking cessation and health promotion;
- establish a clearinghouse of smoking and tobacco use prevention information gathered from academic and professional journals, conferences, newsletters, and white papers;
- provide technical assistance to health plans in developing smoking and tobacco use prevention and cessation programming, including the development and dissemination of a newsletter, a regularly updated annotated bibliography, an NTAO website, and phone and online consultations;
- conduct a benchmarking awards program highlighting exemplary initiatives by health plans in smoking and tobacco use prevention and cessation;
- distribute an annual survey to health plans to determine the current status of smoking and tobacco use cessation initiatives and to evaluate best practices; and
- promote best practices in smoking and tobacco use cessation and prevention through a series of training workshops, national and regional conferences, and a managed care smoking and tobacco use prevention and cessation tool kit.

According to a survey of health plans conducted in 2000, 24 percent had employed a full- or part-time staff person specifically for smoking and tobacco use control activities, and 22 percent were implementing provider training programs for smoking and tobacco use cessation counseling (Anne Cahill, program manager, Prevention Programs, AAHP, personal communication, March 6, 2001).

American Legacy Foundation

The American Legacy Foundation, set up to administer funds from the Tobacco Master Settlement Agreement, has included as part of its strategic plan increases in the number of health professional schools that include training and education in smoking and tobacco use cessation in their curricula (www.americanlegacy.org/overview/strategic.html).

SUMMARY AND CONCLUSIONS

Despite numerous calls to improve the education and training of health care professionals in health promotion and disease prevention, there is evidence of programmatic deficits in medical, dental, and nursing schools. A problem of greater magnitude is upgrading the knowledge and skills of practicing clinicians whose performance reflects their lack of training. The demand for behavioral and early detection services will increase as the population ages, placing new strains on ambulatory care providers. Some solutions follow:

- requirements that educational institutions meet established curriculum guidelines (e.g., the population health guidelines of AAMC),
- inclusion of cancer prevention and early detection questions on national board and licensure examinations,
- assurances that adequate continuing education opportunities are available through training institutions and professional organizations,
- applications of new learning technologies (e.g., distance learning and online CME),
- assessments of the adequacy of the future supply of providers, and
- research and demonstrations to test different delivery models to clarify who should be trained and how interventions can be best be delivered.

Although education alone is not sufficient to change the behaviors of providers, it remains an important factor in ensuring the delivery of evidence-based standard practices for cancer prevention and control. Many reciprocal factors can affect provider and patient behaviors at the health care plan and organizational levels. Structure and process characteristics, such as the availability of automated clinical reminder systems and quality improvement expectations, can enable and reinforce the practice of providing the needed prevention services. Required educational programs coupled with a system that identifies at-risk patients and that reminds the provider to intervene will produce increases in providers' rates of provision of counseling (Adams et al., 1998; Fiore et al., 1996, US DHHS, 2000a; Ockene et al., 1996).

9

Federal Programs That Support Cancer Prevention and Early Detection

Opportunities to promote cancer prevention and early detection span several sectors of society including health systems and providers, educational institutions, social services agencies, employer and labor organizations, and consumer groups. From a public policy perspective, actions to foster change can be taken by the federal government, states, and local entities (e.g., county and city governments and school boards). This chapter briefly describes the federal role in support of cancer-related prevention services in five important areas:

1. national objectives and guideline development,
2. information dissemination,
3. monitoring and surveillance,
4. facilitation of statewide program planning and evaluation, and
5. provision of and payment for services.

The federal government's role in education and training is described in Chapter 8, and its role in research is described in Chapter 10. Previous chapters highlight the significant roles of state and local entities (both public and private) in carrying out important functions to incorporate cancer prevention and early detection programs into community-based programs (Chapters 4 and 6).

NATIONAL OBJECTIVES AND GUIDELINE DEVELOPMENT

Explicit national health-related goals and objectives have been set as part of the *Healthy People 2010* initiative (U.S. DHHS, Office of Disease

Prevention and Health Promotion, 2000), and efforts are under way to chart the nation's progress toward those goals. Such objectives provide invaluable guidance to policy makers, and assessments of the achievement of these objectives often provide the impetus needed to stimulate systematic changes. Cancer-related objectives from *Healthy People 2010* are shown in Box 9.1.

Evidence-based guidelines for clinical and community practice also provide maps for action. The U.S. Preventive Services Task Force (USPSTF) periodically conducts rigorous assessments of the effectiveness of clinical

BOX 9.1 Cancer-Related *Healthy People 2010* Objectives

- Reduce the overall cancer death rate and death rates for lung cancer, breast cancer, cancer of the uterine cervix, colorectal cancer, oropharyngeal cancer, prostate cancer, and melanoma (Objectives 3-1 to 3-8).
- Increase the proportion of persons who use at least one of the following protective measures that may reduce the risk of skin cancer: avoid the sun between 10 a.m. and 4 p.m., wear sun-protective clothing when exposed to sunlight, use sunscreen with a sun-protective factor (SPF) of 15 or higher, avoid artificial sources of ultraviolet light (Objective 3-9).
- Increase the proportion of physicians and dentists who counsel their at-risk patients about tobacco use cessation, physical activity, and cancer screening (Objective 3-10).
- Increase the proportion of women who receive a Pap test (Objective 3-11).
- Increase the proportion of adults who receive a colorectal cancer screening examination (Objective 3-12).
- Increase the proportion of women aged 40 years and older who have received a mammogram within the preceding 2 years (Objective 3-13).
- Increase the number of states that have a statewide population-based registry that captures case information on at least 95 percent of the estimated number of reportable cancers (Objective 3-14).
- Increase the proportion of cancer survivors who are living 5 years or longer after diagnosis (Objective 3-15).
- Increase the proportion of local health departments that have established culturally appropriate and linguistically competent community health promotion and disease prevention programs (Objective 7-11)
- Increase the proportion of adults who are at a healthy weight (Objective 19-1).
- Reduce the proportion of adults who are obese (Objective 19-2).
- Increase the proportion of oral and pharyngeal cancers detected at the earliest stage (Objective 21-6).
- Increase the proportion of adults who, in the past 12 months, report having had an examination to detect oral and pharyngeal cancers (Objective 21-7).
- Reduce the proportion of adults who engage in no leisure-time physical activity (Objective 22-1).

SOURCE: US DHHS and Office of Disease Prevention and Health Promotion, 2000 (www.health.gov/healthypeople).

prevention services, and the U.S. Task Force on Community Preventive Services is assessing the effectiveness of interventions aimed at communities. USPSTF is an ad hoc independent panel of private-sector experts in primary care and prevention convened by the U.S. Public Health Service's Agency for Healthcare Research and Quality (AHRQ). USPSTF evaluates scientific evidence of the effectiveness of clinical prevention services (e.g., screening tests, counseling, immunization, and chemoprophylaxis) and produces age- and risk factor-specific recommendations for the services that should be included in a periodic health examination. USPSTF is supported by outside experts, two Evidence-Based Practice Centers (groups that systematically synthesize available literature), and liaisons from the major primary care societies and from U.S. Public Health Service agencies. Currently, the third USPSTF, convened in 1998, is issuing recommendations updating its *1996 Guide to Clinical Preventive Services* (www.ahrq.gov/clinic/cps3dix.htm).

The 15-member independent, nonfederal Task Force on Community Preventive Services first met in 1996 and issued a number of reports, among them *Recommendations Regarding Interventions to Reduce Tobacco Use and Exposure to Environmental Tobacco Smoke* (Task Force on Community Preventive Services, 2001).

Other agencies within the federal government such as the Centers for Disease Control and Prevention (CDC) and AHRQ have been at the forefront in identifying effective prevention intervention strategies. CDC, for example, has issued three guidelines aimed at improving the health of school-age children: (1) CDC's *Guidelines for School Health Programs: Promoting Lifelong Healthy Eating* (www.cdc.gov/nccdphp/dash/nutguide.htm), (2) *Guidelines for School and Community Programs to Promote Lifelong Physical Activity Among Young People* (CDC, 1997a), and (3) *Guidelines for School and Community Health Programs Preventing Tobacco Use and Addiction* (www.cdc.gov/nccdphp/dash/ptuaaag.htm). In 2000 AHRQ helped issue an update of its 1996 smoking cessation guideline that provides exhaustive information on best practices for clinicians (http://www.surgeongeneral.gov/tobacco/systems.htm). Another activity that has provided guidance regarding certain cancer prevention interventions is the National Cancer Institute's (NCI's) Consensus Development Conference process. Here, expert panels convene for a few days to review a synthesis of the literature and produce a consensus statement. In the area of cancer prevention and early detection, recent statements are available for breast cancer screening for women ages 40 to 49 (1997),[1] cervical cancer (1996), and ovarian cancer screening, treatment, and follow-up (1994) (http://odp.od.nih.gov/consensus/cons/cancer.htm).

[1]The controversy surrounding this statement is described in Chapter 4.

The federal government also plays an active role in guideline dissemination. The AHRQ Put Prevention into Practice (PPIP) initiative is designed to help implement the recommendations of USPSTF by supplying health care providers with easy-to-use materials to prompt adherence to the guidelines (http://www.ahrq.gov/clinic/ppipix.htm). Roughly 20 percent of the services considered by USPSTF and PPIP relate to cancer detection or prevention.

Another federally sponsored guideline dissemination activity is CONQUEST (Computerized Needs-Oriented Quality Measurement Evaluation System), which consists of a database of performance measures (conditions, diseases, and procedures), measure sets (measures with a common purpose and developer), and conditions (with detailed epidemiological information). CONQUEST includes measures related to the management of several cancers (i.e., colorectal, lung, prostate, and breast cancer), the use of screening tests (i.e., mammography and Pap smear), and cigarette use (www.ahrq.gov/qual/conquest.htm).

INFORMATION DISSEMINATION

NCI is at the center of federal efforts to disseminate cancer-specific information to individuals and health care providers. By telephone, individuals can receive up-to-date cancer information in English or Spanish through the Cancer Information Service (1-800-4-CANCER). Over 390,000 calls are received each year, with 79 percent from cancer patients and their families and the balance from the general public and health care professionals (http://cis.nci.nih.gov/about/underserved.html, accessed January 30, 2002). Through the World Wide Web (www.nci.nih.gov/cancerinfo/index.html), individuals can get information about the basics of cancer; treatment options; clinical trials; genetics, causes, risk factors, and prevention; screening; and information about support and other resources. Information about cancer trials and how to access them is available through a dedicated clinical trial website (http://cancertrials.nci.nih.gov).

In an effort to learn more about the public's access to and use of cancer-related health information, the NCI is conducting a national survey, the Health Information National Trends Survey. Other research-oriented activities that are a part of NCI's cancer communications initiative are described in Chapter 10.

PDQ (Physician Data Query) is NCI's comprehensive cancer database originally designed for use by physicians. The database contains peer-reviewed summaries on cancer treatment, screening, prevention, genetics, and supportive care. These summaries are updated monthly by specialized editorial boards. There are two versions of the screening and detection summaries. One is for health professionals and contains current data, by cancer site, on screening interventions, levels of evidence for statements regarding screening, and the significance and evidence of benefit for the statements. Another version is available for patients and is written in non-technical language (http://cancernet.nci.nih.gov/pdqfull.html). Provider- and consumer-oriented prevention summaries are also available. In addition to these summaries, PDQ includes an online registry of approximately 1,800 open and 10,300 closed clinical trials from around the world. An additional resource is directories of health professionals and organizations involved in cancer care, and professionals who provide genetics services (e.g., cancer risk assessment, genetic counseling, genetic susceptibility testing).

The Centers for Disease Control and Prevention also supports information dissemination, often targeted to states and localities. Tobacco Information and Prevention Source (TIPS) is a Web portal that provides an array of tobacco control information and links to resources (http://www.cdc.gov/tobacco/issue.htm). The site provides access to guides to tobacco cessation; educational materials for parents, educators, professional and youth leaders; state information, such as best practices; and information of interest to children and young adults (sports initiatives, celebrities against smoking). Also online at CDC's site is information about obesity and overweight, including guidelines and recommended strategies to prevent chronic diseases and obesity, and programs to support state health departments and their partners (www.cdc.gov/nccdphp/dnpa/obesity/index.htm). In October 2000, CDC's Division of Nutrition and Physical Activity initiated a program to support state health departments and their partners in developing and implementing targeted nutrition and physical activity interventions in an effort to prevent chronic diseases, especially obesity. Twelve states funded in FY 2000 and 2001 were encouraged to use a social marketing approach in designing their population-based strategies, particularly policy-level and environmental interventions. Information about cancer screening is also available at CDC's website, including a series of "At-a-Glance" publications focusing on the importance of early detection (www.cdc.gov/health/cancer.htm).

The Office of the Surgeon General has issued a series of reports regarding the health consequences of tobacco (Box 9.2).

MONITORING AND SURVEILLANCE

Several federally supported surveys and administrative record systems provide the data needed to assess progress toward reaching the nation's cancer prevention and early detection goals (Box 9.3).

The National Health Interview Survey (NHIS) is the principal source of information on the health of the civilian noninstitutionalized population of the United States (http://www.cdc.gov/nchs/about/major/nhis/hisdesc.htm) and provides national estimates of a number of cancer-related health behaviors including tobacco use and use of cancer screening tests. The NCI supports periodic supplements to the NHIS on cancer control (most re-

BOX 9.2 Surgeon General's Reports on Tobacco Control

Date	Topic
1964	Reducing the Health Consequences of Smoking
1981	The Health Consequences of Smoking: The Changing Cigarette
1982	The Health Consequences of Smoking: Cancer
1986	The Health Consequences of Involuntary Smoking
1988	The Health Consequences of Smoking: Nicotine Addiction
1989	Reducing the Health Consequences of Smoking
1990	The Health Benefits of Smoking Cessation
1994	Preventing Tobacco Use Among Young People
1998	Tobacco Use Among U.S. Racial/Ethnic Minority Groups
2000	Reducing Tobacco Use
2001	Women and Smoking

cently, in 2000) to assess knowledge, attitudes, and practices concerning cancer-related health behaviors and cancer screening (Stacey Vandor, Planning Officer, NCI, personal communication to Maria Hewitt, February 11, 2002). The NHIS involves personal interviews in homes to gather information on household members. The NCI also supports a smoking supplement to the Current Population Survey (CPS), a household survey of 60,000 households conducted by the Bureau of Census for the Bureau of Labor Statistics. The CPS provides data on the U.S. labor force and employment statistics (http://www.bls.gov/cps/cps_over.htm#overview).

State-based estimates of preventive health behaviors, knowledge, and attitudes are available through CDC's Behavioral Risk Factor Surveillance

BOX 9.3 Selected Examples of Cancer Prevention and Early Detection Surveillance Tools

Sponsor	Surveillance Tool
Centers for Disease Control and Prevention	• National Health Interview Survey (national estimates) • Behavioral Risk Factor Surveillance System (state-based estimates) • Youth Risk Behavior Surveillance System • National Ambulatory Medical Care Surveys (provider practices) • National Health and Nutrition Examination Survey (clinical measures and assessments)
Centers for Medicare and Medicaid Services	• Medicare Beneficiary Survey • Claims analyses (estimates of use of services)
U.S. Department of Veterans Affairs	• Veterans surveys • Medical records and administrative records

System. This telephone survey is conducted by states among adults age 18 and older. States generally use a core survey instrument and may add additional items to meet local informational needs.

A number of data systems provide information on important subpopulations. Estimates of rates of tobacco use and levels of access to cigarettes among youth, for example, are available through CDC's Youth Risk Behavior Surveillance System (CDC, Division of Adolescent and School Health, http://www.cdc.gov/nccdphp/dash/yrbs/), and estimates of cancer screening practices among Medicare beneficiaries are available through the Medicare Beneficiary Survey.

National surveys of ambulatory care practices help gauge the extent to which physicians are delivering preventive health services such as counseling on diet, nutrition, and exercise. Two surveys sponsored by CDC, the National Ambulatory Medical Care Survey and the National Hospital Ambulatory Medical Care Survey, collect data from a representative sample of physicians' offices and hospital outpatient departments and provide national estimates of the number of ambulatory care visits, reasons for visits (e.g., diagnoses associated with visits and use of selected preventive health interventions), and actions taken during visits (e.g., counseling, ordering of tests, prescriptions for medication).

The National Health and Nutrition Examination Survey, sponsored by CDC, collects information about the health and diet of people in the United States. NHANES is unique in that it combines a home interview with health tests that are done in a mobile examination center (www.cdc.gov/nchs/nhanes.htm). Results of the survey have been used to monitor trends in overweight and obesity (see Chapter 3, figure 3.1).

Some data systems are unique to a system of care. The U.S. Department of Veterans Affairs (VA), for example, uses both survey data and formal audits of medical records to assess progress in cancer prevention and early detection (see Tables 9.3 and 9.4).

FACILITATING STATEWIDE PROGRAM PLANNING AND EVALUATION

National organizations may set guidelines and policy for cancer prevention and control, but implementation of public health measures to reduce the burden of cancer largely falls to state and local health departments, along with their partners, which include consumer and advocacy organizations, universities, and area health care providers. Wide state-level variations in the prevalence of cancer-related risk factors are alarming but provide opportunities to target interventions and achieve gains in health (Box 9.4).

CDC would like to build the capacities of states—and, in turn, their local partners—to both develop and implement comprehensive cancer control plans. As part of CDC's National Comprehensive Cancer Control

BOX 9.4 State-Level Variations in Cancer Risk Factors

Tobacco smoking. The rates of smoking among adults in the 10 states with the lowest smoking rates and the 10 states with the highest smoking rates were 19 and 28 percent, respectively, in 1999. Closing this gap, alone, could reduce lung cancer rates by a third in the 10 states with the highest smoking rates.

Breast cancer screening. The rate of adherence to current recommendations for screening mammography by women age 50 and older was 84 percent in the 10 states with the highest screening rates in 1999, but the rate was only 70 percent in the 10 states with the lowest rates. Closing this gap could reduce breast cancer mortality rates by 5 percent in the 10 states with the lowest rates.

Colorectal cancer screening. The gap between the 10 states with the highest colorectal cancer screening rates and the 10 states with the lowest screening rates is wide (39 versus 30 percent), but much more important is the observation that screening rates are low in all states. Screening for colorectal cancer has a very high potential for saving lives, as it has proven effectiveness, yet it is being applied to only a small proportion of the population.

SOURCE: Byers, University of Colorado School of Medicine, unpublished analyses of data from CDC's Behavioral Risk Factor Surveillance System.

Program, such plans have been defined as those with an integrated and coordinated approach to reducing the incidence and the rates of morbidity and mortality from cancer through prevention, early detection, treatment, rehabilitation, and palliation (CDC, 2001a; www.cdc.gov/cancer/ncccp/index.htm).

CDC has identified a useful framework for the establishment of a state cancer control program and has provided various models for comprehensive planning and evaluation. Essential elements of a comprehensive plan include (Abed et al., 2000a,b) the following:

- strategies and mechanisms for developing and maintaining partnerships,
- assessments and surveillance,
- infrastructure development,
- public education,
- professional education,
- policy and legislative activities, and
- evaluation and monitoring.

Phases of implementation of a comprehensive state plan include setting optimal objectives that are data-driven, determining optimal strategies that are science-driven, establishing feasible priorities given the capacity, and implementing effective strategies that are assessed by evaluations of outcomes (Abed et al., 2000b).

Many states have in place some of the essential elements of a comprehensive program. Nearly half of the states, for example, have cancer registries that achieve the standards of completeness, timeliness, and coverage to provide accurate cancer incidence data for planning and evaluation. State data on the prevalence of cancer-related risk factors such as smoking are available through the Behavioral Risk Factor Surveillance System (CDC, Division of Adult and Community Health, http://www.cdc.gov/nccdphp/brfss/) and the Youth Risk Behavior Surveillance System (CDC, Division of Adolescent and School Health, 1999, http://www.cdc.gov/nccdphp/dash/yrbs/index.htm). In the area of early detection, all states have in place CDC-funded breast and cervical cancer screening programs targeted to low-income and underserved women (CDC, The National Breast and Cervical Cancer Early Detection Program, http://www.cdc.gov/cancer/nbccedp/about.htm).

NCI has also promoted the development of state cancer control capacity through its Surveillance, Epidemiology, and End Results Program and through special grants (see the discussion of research initiatives in Chapter 10).

According to a recent CDC assessment, however, only 13 states have comprehensive state plans that are being implemented (or that are ready to be implemented), 14 states and the District of Columbia are creating a new plan (or are updating an old plan), and 23 states have no plan or one that is outdated (Figure 9.1).

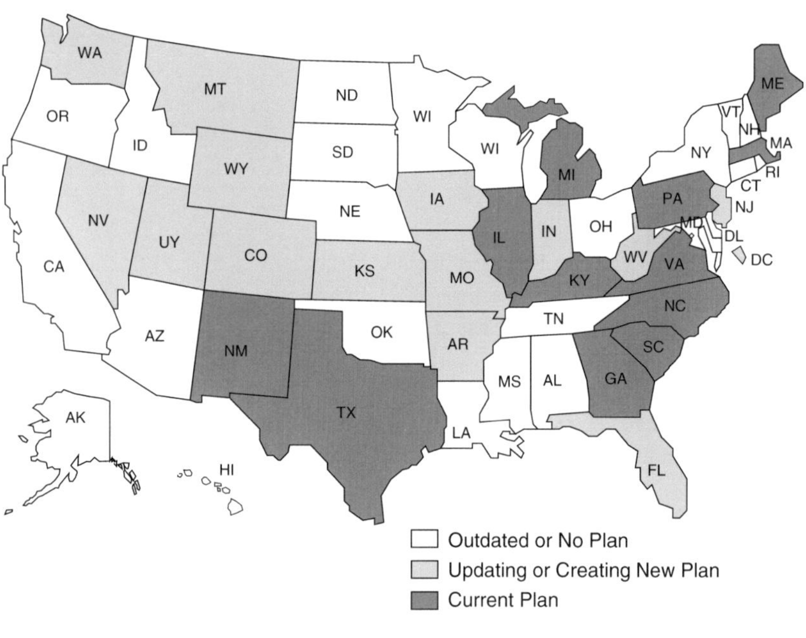

FIGURE 9.1 Comprehensive cancer control plans, 2001.

Although considerable variations in state capacities have been observed and certain barriers to implementation have been identified, it is unclear what levels and types of investments are needed to build state and local capacities and how these needs may vary across the nation. CDC's Division of Cancer Prevention and Control spends an estimated \$250 million on cancer control and prevention annually, but much of the money is categorically targeted to specific activities (e.g., cancer registries), populations, or cancer sites (see Chapter 10). Since 1998, 19 states and 1 tribal organization have received grant support totalling approximately \$37 million from CDC to develop and implement a comprehensive cancer control (CCC) plan. In addition, states and tribal organizations have been provided technical assistance regarding CCC plans with \$1 million from the CDC (Leslie Given, Division of Cancer Prevention and Control, CDC, personal communication to Maria Hewitt, IOM, September 9, 2002). The CDC-funded states are developing programs that are varied, depending on the needs and organizational preferences of each state. The key to each program is, however, the same: fostering collaborative efforts among many sectors within the states to increase individual and organizational awareness of the state's cancer burden and achieve objectives that will lead to future reductions in that burden (Byers, University of Colorado School of Medicine, unpublished). Resources appear to be inadequate to meet the need for CCC plan development and implementation. In 2002, for example, CDC had resources to support only half of the requests for assistance from states, territories, and Indian tribes in response to its National Cancer Prevention and Control Program Announcement (Leslie Given, Division of Cancer Prevention and Control, CDC, personal communication to Maria Hewitt, IOM, August 26, 2002). The CDC estimates that \$30 million per year would be needed before states would have plans developed and implementation in progress by 2005 (Leslie Given, Division of Cancer Prevention and Control, CDC, personal communication to Maria Hewitt, IOM, August 26, 2002).

CDC also provides guidance to states regarding comprehensive approaches to risk reduction. The CDC's Office on Smoking and Health, for example has described essential elements of a comprehensive tobacco control program (CDC, 1999d). The extent to which states have such comprehensive programs is discussed in Chapter 11. Guidelines for comprehensive state programs to promote healthy eating and physical activity are forthcoming.

The National Governors Association has launched a website, State Best Practices in Cancer Prevention and Control, to help states communicate their successes and learn from the experience of other states (National Governors Association, http://www.nga.org/center/divisions/1,1188,C_ISSUE_BRIEF^D_1913,00.html). The website also provides basic cancer statistics by state, and summaries of relevant state legislation.

PROVIDING AND PAYING FOR SERVICES

This section reviews the role of the following selected federal programs in the provision of (or reimbursement for) prevention services:

Direct Providers of Services

- Health Resources and Services Administration programs (Community and Migrant Health Centers)
- Veterans Health Administration
- Indian Health Service
- Centers for Disease Control and Prevention (National Breast and Cervical Cancer Early Detection Program)
- Office of Family Planning, US DHHS

Indirect Providers of Services (Payers)

- Centers for Medicare and Medicaid Services (formerly the Health Care Financing Administration)
- Medicaid
- Office of Management and Budget (which oversees federal employee health benefits)

Direct Providers of Services

Health Resources and Services Administration

Sometimes called the "access" agency, the Health Resources and Services Administration (HRSA) oversees a number of direct service and training programs that provide primary care and other services to vulnerable and underserved populations. HRSA's Bureau of Primary Health Care (BPHC) programs serve more than 12 million people in roughly 4,000 primary care sites including Community and Migrant Health Centers, Black Lung Clinics, and clinics along the United States-Mexico border. BPHC programs further bolster the public health infrastructure through training and educational programs, placement of clinicians in areas with shortages of health care professionals, and support of primary care offices in state health departments and independent primary care associations that attempt to build statewide coalitions for primary care health delivery systems. In 1999, BPHC launched the "100% Access and 0 Health Disparities Campaign" to support community leaders in setting and achieving access and disparity goals (Health Resources and Services Administration, 2000a).

Community and Migrant Health Centers HRSA's largest direct service program is the Community Health Center (CHC) and Migrant Health Center (MHC) Program. In 1998 the program had approximately 700 health centers with nearly 3,000 clinics providing services to more than 9 million people (Health Resources and Services Administration, 2001; www. hrsa.gov). Most clients of such centers are uninsured or are insured by Medicaid. In 1998, HRSA-funded health centers served approximately 9 percent of Medicaid beneficiaries, 8 percent of uninsured Americans, and 20 to 25 percent of the poor and near-poor uninsured Americans (Health Resources and Services Administration, 2001; Institute of Medicine, 2000d). The majority of BPHC health center patients are from racial or ethnic minority groups (Health Resources and Services Administration, 2001). Health centers must meet certain criteria to be designated federally qualified health centers (FQHCs); for example, they must provide culturally competent, comprehensive primary care services to all age groups, offer services on a sliding scale based on income, and provide services regardless of ability to pay. HRSA's fiscal year 2001 appropriation for the CHC program is $1.169 billion, and that for the MHC program, $98.9 million.

Rates of Pap smears, screening mammography, and clinical breast examinations among women served in CHCs exceeded those identified as *Healthy People 2000* goals when they were examined in 1995 (Regan et al., 1999). Efforts are under way to complete a Health Center Primary Care Effectiveness Review to support continuous quality improvement of health center programs funded by the Bureau of Primary Health Care (www.hrsa.gov). Among the measures included in the review are the availability of written protocols for cancer screening, whether screening intervals are defined, use of patient tracking and recall systems, follow-up for abnormal screening tests, and evidence in medical records of adherence to protocols.

A number of research and demonstration projects have been conducted within CHCs to improve cancer screening (Hedegaard et al., 1996; Kohatsu et al., 1994; Lacey et al, 1993; Lipkus et al., 1996; Paskett et al., 1998; Polednak and Flannery, 1994; Rimer et al., 1996a; Valdini and Cargill, 1997; Yarnall et al., 1998; Zapka et al., 1993) or promote smoking cessation (Lipkus et al., 1999; Tessaro et al., 1997; Yarnall et al., 1998; Zapka et al., 2000b).

BPHC has requested $19.3 million to support several new initiatives to improve its cancer prevention programs (Health Resources and Services Administration, 2000a):

- launch culturally appropriate prevention campaigns in collaboration with CDC;
- hire full-time community outreach workers at selected health centers to distribute educational materials in homes, churches, and other community settings;
- develop training modules on cancer screening and diagnostic procedures for primary care clinicians;

- establish linkages between primary care sites and cancer treatment facilities to facilitate referral;
- identify models of success and replicate the models across BPHC programs;
- fund full-time clinical coordinators in each of the 50 state primary care associations to track primary cancer care performance, exchange information about successful initiatives among member sites, establish and expand linkages between primary care sites and tertiary cancer care centers, support cancer educational initiatives, and coordinate with CDC state cancer coordinators;
- develop and implement the Cancer Health Disparities Collaborative for BPHC-supported health centers in conjunction with the Institute for Health Care Improvement to address screening, diagnosis, and referral for treatment and follow-up care; and
- study factors that affect health care access and outcomes among vulnerable populations with breast cancer.

Veterans Health Administration

The Veterans Health Administration (VHA) is one of the nation's largest integrated health care systems, with 173 medical centers, 771 ambulatory care and community-based clinics, 134 nursing homes, 42 domiciliaries, and 206 counseling centers and other facilities (www.va.gov). These facilities are organized regionally into 22 Veterans Integrated Service Networks (VISN). Each year, VHA, with a budget of more than $20 billion, serves approximately 3.6 million veterans, an estimated 15 percent of the total veteran population (www.va.gov/vetdata). Only about 12 percent of those treated at VA facilities are treated for a service-connected disability. The majority are poor and without other sources of health care (Institute of Medicine, 2000d). Each year, an estimated 50,000 new cases of cancer are diagnosed and 170,000 cancer patients are cared for within the VHA system (www.va.gov/cancer). A national cancer strategy articulated in 1997 addresses the need for high-quality cancer prevention, detection, and treatment services (Box 9.5)

Health promotion and disease prevention practices within VHA are guided by formal recommendations established by the VHA National Center for Health Promotion and Disease Prevention (Veterans Health Administration, 1999). Recommendations regarding counseling for cancer-related behavioral risk factors and cancer screening are summarized in Tables 9.1 and 9.2.

VHA has in place a management system for the implementation of prevention services. Each facility has a designated preventive medicine program coordinator, a health education coordinator, and a smoking cessation coordinator. VHA-wide efforts are facilitated by an individual who provides

Box 9.5 VHA National Cancer Strategy Policy Objectives

1. Ensure that the quality of VHA cancer care will meet or exceed accepted national standards of practices
2. Improve cancer patients' access to care
3. Provide appropriate cancer management expertise to each patient as promptly as possible
4. Provide for the continual monitoring and improvement of the outcomes of therapy
5. Provide clinically useful prevention, screening, and early detection services
6. Improve the quality of life of cancer patients
7. Provide compassionate and humane care that clearly demonstrates respect for the patients' dignity
8. Ensure that the care provided derives from shared decision making between the patient and treatment personnel

SOURCE: U.S. Department of Veterans Affairs VHA Directive 97-050 (www.va.gov/cancer).

TABLE 9.1 VHA Cancer-Related Behavioral Risk Factor Counseling Recommendations

Service	Target Condition	Recommendation
Tobacco use screening and counseling	Cancer and pulmonary and cardiovascular diseases	All veterans should be screened annually for tobacco use, and counseling should be offered to those who use tobacco.
Problem drinking and alcohol moderation counseling	Problem alcohol drinking	Veterans should be asked each year to describe their use of alcohol. The use of a standardized screening questionnaire is recommended. High risk patients (those who consume three or more drinks daily) should receive alcohol counseling.
Weight control and nutrition screening and counseling	Cardiovascular disease, hypertension, hyperlipidemia, obesity, osteoporosis, and neural tube defects	All veterans should receive height and weight measurements every 2 years. All veterans should have access to counseling to limit dietary intake of fat and cholesterol, maintain caloric balance, and emphasize the consumption of foods containing fiber. Female veterans should be advised to consume adequate amounts of calcium. Female veterans younger than age 50 years should be advised to take daily multi-vitamins containing folic acid.
Physical activity screening and counseling	Cardiovascular disease, hypertension, obesity, and diabetes mellitus	All veterans should be encouraged annually to engage in a program of physical activity tailored to their health status and personal lifestyles. All veterans should have access to counseling regarding optimizing their level of physical activity.

SOURCE: Veterans Health Administration (1999).

TABLE 9.2 VHA Cancer Screening Recommendations

Cancer Site	Target Group	Recommendation
Cervical	Female veterans age 65 and under	Pap smear testing is recommended every 3 years until age 65 for all women who are or who have been sexually active.
Breast	All female veterans	All female veterans age 50 to 69 years should receive a mammogram every 1 to 2 years unless it is medically not indicated. Female veterans age 40 to 49 years should be counseled regarding the risks and benefits of screening, and those desiring mammography will receive that service.
Colon-Rectum	All veterans age 50 and older	All persons aged 50 years and older should receive an annual fecal occult blood test or should undergo a sigmoidoscopy every 5 years.
Prostate	All male veterans age 50 and older	All male veterans aged 50 years and older should receive annual counseling regarding potential benefits and hazards of prostate-specific antigen testing.

SOURCE: Veterans Health Administration (1999).

field liaison activities, for example, conducting regularly scheduled telephone conference calls with facility and VISN representatives. These contacts, in addition to active e-mail communications, provide opportunities to disseminate information on VHA polices and new research findings and to hear from providers about service-related issues, needs, and barriers. Special-interest groups interested in prevention topics such as nutrition and obesity have been established, and the members of those groups communicate via e-mail. Smoking cessation coordinators also have a group whose members communicate via e-mail.

Many VHA facilities have an electronic medical record system with the capability to provide reminders to clinicians regarding prevention services. Adherence to recommendations is monitored through ongoing independent chart reviews of each facility and periodic surveys of the health of veterans who use VA services. Independent chart audits provide objective evidence of the provision of service but do not detect the prevention services that a veteran may have received outside the VA system (e.g., tobacco counseling from a community-based program). The veterans health survey can capture such out-of-system uses of prevention services and may identify services that were provided within the VA system but not recorded in the chart. A comparison of some results regarding cancer-related prevention services from the 1999 chart audit and the veterans health survey shows somewhat higher rates of adherence to recommendations from the chart review than from the veterans health survey (Tables 9.3 and 9.4). Some of the discrepancy might be due to a failure of patients to recall events that occurred during a health care visit, for example, remembering that a physician asked about alcohol use. The chart audit was for care provided in 1999, whereas the survey reported on care that may have been provided in the prior year.

TABLE 9.3 Preventive Health Practices, Veterans Health Survey, 1997–1999

Preventive Practice and Group	Goals for Year 2000[a]	VHA Rate (percent)[b] 1997	1998	1999
Tobacco use counseling				
• Men who are current tobacco users	15	30	30	27
• Women who are current tobacco users	15	27	27	25
• Men tobacco users offered counseling	75	73	79	79
• Women tobacco users offered counseling	75	78	82	84
Problem drinking and alcohol moderation counseling				
• Men asked about/screened for problem drinking and alcohol use this year	75	29	39	38
• Women asked about/screened for problem drinking and alcohol use this year	75	21	29	30
Weight control and nutrition counseling				
• Men receiving nutrition counseling this year	75	49	50	50
• Women receiving nutrition counseling this year	75	45	47	48
Physical activity counseling				
• Men receiving activity counseling this year	50	57	60	61
• Women receiving activity counseling this year	50	55	58	59
Cervical cancer detection				
• Women under age 65 with Pap test in past 3 years	85	89	89	87
Breast cancer detection				
• Women ages 50 to 69 receiving a mammogram in the past 2 years	60	85	87	86
Colorectal cancer detection[c]				
• Women over age 50 receiving a fecal occult blood test this year	50	33	56	61
• Men over age 50 receiving a fecal occult blood test this year	50	29	51	55

[a]*Healthy People 2000* goals as stated in VHA Handbook 1101.8.
[b]Weighted as appropriate; 95 percent confidence interval for VHA is less than ±1 percent. Sample size for 1997 = 44,304; sample size for 1998 = 42,625; sample size for 1999 = 45,037.
[c]The figures for 1997 measure fecal occult blood test in the last year; the figures for 1998 and 1999 also include sigmoidoscopy within the last 5 years.
SOURCE: VHA National Center for Health Promotion and Disease Prevention Veterans Health Survey, 1997–1999, June 4, 2001.

TABLE 9.4 Preventive Health Practices, Results of Chart Audit, External Peer Review Program, 1999

Preventive Service	VHA Rate (percent)
Tobacco use screening	95
Smoking counseling	
One or more times per year	93
Three times per year	49
Alcohol use screening	69
Cancer screening	
Screening for colorectal cancer	74
Mammography	91
Cervical cancer	94
Prostate cancer	66

SOURCE: VHA, 1999 Network Performance Report; Ron Sorrell, administrative officer, National Center for Health Promotion, personal communication, June 4, 2001.

Top-performing programs for prevention services, identified through the chart audit program and veterans health survey, were contacted in 1999 to identify best practices to be shared across the program. Acceptance from clinical staff, the involvement of primary care staff in program planning, and the active involvement of nursing staff as part of multidisciplinary teams were among the elements believed to contribute to program success (Burdick, 1999).

As part of a special initiative in 1997, a directive called for all VHA facilities to implement a strategic plan based on the Agency for Health Care Policy and Research smoking cessation recommendations. According to a 1997 assessment of smoking cessation activities within the 147 VA medical centers that provide primary care services, virtually all facilities offered access to smoking cessation programs (145 of 147 medical centers) and had tobacco user identification systems in place (143 of 147). Among the centers with access to treatment programs, the treatments offered to smokers included brief encouragement during routine office visits (129 of 145 medical centers), intensive tobacco use cessation program (129 of 145 medical centers), and brief tobacco use cessation skills education program (80 of 145 medical centers) (Burdick, 1998). This systemwide review of capacity identified some deficits and has led to program development and improvement (Burdick, M, VA National Center for Health Promotion and Disease Prevention, personal communication, May 31, 2001). Although virtually all medical centers have a smoking cessation program, their contents vary widely, and some recommended services are not available (Oliver Par, VHA, personal communication, May 31, 2001). Nicotine inhalers, for example, although recognized as effective interventions for smoking cessation, are not listed on the national VA formulary and so are not routinely available throughout the VA system. Under development in collaboration with the U.S. Department of Defense is a smoking cessation "tool kit" which will demonstrate models of excellence in two areas: smoking cessation provided in the context of primary care and specialized intensive services (Burdick, personal communication, May 31, 2001). The program will be disseminated through a satellite conference. As part of the program, an actual tool kit for providers will be made widely available and will include aids to counseling, for example, pocket cards to assist in referrals and playing cards for patients that include smoking informational messages (Oliver Par, VHA, personal communication, May 31, 2001).

Indian Health Service

The Indian Health Service (IHS), an agency within the US DHHS, is responsible for providing health services to American Indians and Alaska Natives. With $2.6 billion in federal appropriations in 2001, IHS serves individuals who are members of any of the 556 federally recognized tribes located in 35 states. The majority (55 percent) of American Indians and Alaska Natives eligible for IHS services rely on IHS as their sole provider of health care.

Care is provided by nearly 15,000 IHS employees in 49 hospitals, 221 health centers; and more than 300 clinics, health stations, and residential treatment centers. In locations where IHS does not have its own facilities or is not equipped to provide a needed service, IHS contracts with local hospitals, state and local health agencies, tribal health institutions, and individual health care providers. Since 1968, IHS has trained American Indian and Alaska Native community health representatives. More than 1,400 community health representatives are employed and supervised by their tribes and communities to provide early intervention and case finding and, in some cases, direct primary care and follow-up services. In addition to direct health services, IHS provides environmental health and engineering services (e.g., occupational health and safety services and pollution control services), and school-based programs (e.g., health education).

IHS serves 1.5 million individuals who reside on or near reservations and 330,000 individuals living in urban areas. Estimates are that 60 percent of the 2.5 million American Indians and Alaska Natives identified in the 1990 census are both eligible for services from IHS by virtue of their tribal affiliation and reside in or proximate to an IHS service area. Most American Indians live in urban areas, and there are concerns that the cancer needs of urban American Indians are not being met (Burhansstipanov, 2000; Michalek et al., 1996).

American Indians and Alaska Natives have historically had very low rates of cancer, in part because of competing causes of death (e.g., infectious diseases like tuberculosis) but, possibly, also because of their diets, physical activity patterns, and limited tobacco use. There is evidence, however, that the cancer incidence rates of American Indians and Alaska Natives are underestimated because of misclassification of American Indian or Alaska Native status on case reports to cancer registries (Partin et al., 1999; Sugarman et al., 1996).

American Indians have the poorest rate of survival from cancer of any racial or ethnic group, but it is unclear what is responsible for the disparity. In one case-control study, survival differences between Montana American Indians and non-American Indians could not be explained by differences in the cancer stage at diagnosis or the type of treatment received (Dennis, 2000). In another study, poorer survival among American Indians than among whites in western Washington State could not be explained by age, differences in stage at diagnosis, lack of cancer treatment, or residence in nonurban counties (Sugarman et al., 1994).

Although many American Indian cultures traditionally use tobacco ceremonially, habitual smoking is a relatively recent development, and its practice is reflected in rising lung cancer rates among American Indians. Smoking rates among Indian people nationwide are now about twice as high as those among the general population (www.ihs.gov).

Rates of use of screening tests among American Indian and Alaska Native women tend to be low. Mammography within the past 2 years was reported by 65 percent of American Indian and Alaska Native women age 50 and older during the period from 1992 to 1997 in the Behavioral Risk Factor Surveillance System (Coughlin et al., 1999). Studies of the rate of screening mammography use among selected groups of American Indian women—Navajo Indian women (Strauss et al., 1997); Sioux Indian women (Mahmoodian, 1997); American Indian women in Albuquerque, New Mexico (Gilliland et al., 2000); American Indian women in Phoenix, Arizona (Risendal et al., 1999b); and American Indian and Alaska Native women with diabetes (Giroux et al., 2000)—indicated that it is well below the recommended levels. One study suggested that lay health advisers, "Native Sisters," are effective in motivating American Indian women to have mammograms (Burhansstipanov, 2000).

Cervical cancer rates among American Indian and Alaska Native women are higher than the rates among the U.S. general population. Rates of use of Pap tests among American Indian and Alaska Native women from 1992 to 1997 were relatively high: 83 percent according to the Behavioral Risk Factor Surveillance System (Coughlin et al., 1999). However, among women screened for cervical cancer as part of the National Breast and Cervical Cancer Early Detection Program from 1991 to 1998, American Indian or Alaska Native women were more likely than others to report never having had a prior Pap test and to have had the highest proportion of abnormal Pap tests among those screened for the first time as part of the program (Benar et al., 2001). Limited access to health care, lower than recommended levels of provider referrals, and a lack of knowledge about Pap smears were identified as barriers to Pap smear use among American Indian women residing in Phoenix, Arizona (Risendal et al., 1999a,b).

Very high rates of alcohol-related disease and injury, diabetes, and mental health conditions among American Indians and Alaska Natives may diminish the emphasis placed on cancer control among programs administered by tribal health directors (Michalek et al., 1996).

Centers for Disease Control and Prevention

Since 1991 CDC has administered the National Breast and Cervical Cancer Early Detection Program (NBCCEDP) to provide screening services to medically underserved women, including older women, women with low incomes, and women of racial and ethnic minority groups. The program has provided more than 2.7 million screening examinations and diagnosed more than 8,600 breast cancers, more than 39,400 precancerous cervical lesions, and more than 660 cervical cancers (CDC, The National Breast and Cervical Cancer Early Detection Program, http://www.cdc.gov/cancer/nbccedp/about.htm).

The program operates in all 50 states, the District of Columbia, 6 U.S. territories, and as part of 12 American Indian and Alaska Native organizations. Fiscal year 2001 appropriations of $174 million enabled CDC to increase its education and outreach programs for women and health care providers, improve quality assurance measures for screening, and improve access to screening and follow-up services (CDC, The National Breast and Cervical Cancer Early Detection Program, http://www.cdc.gov/cancer/nbccedp/about.htm). The program covers postscreening diagnostic services, such as surgical consultation and biopsy, but does not cover treatment. As of July 2002, 43 states had expanded their Medicaid benefits after enactment of the Breast and Cervical Cancer Prevention and Treatment Act of 2000 (PL 106-354; http://www.cdc.gov/cancer/nbccedp/law106-354.htm# actions), a law that gives states the option to provide medical assistance through Medicaid to eligible women who are screened for and found to have breast or cervical cancer (including precancerous conditions) through NBCCEDP.

Estimates are that only 15 percent of women eligible for services receive care through NBCCEDP. Although NBCCEDP operates in all states, coverage within a state may be far from complete. In Louisiana, for example, three of nine regions in the state lack NBCCEDP screening services because of difficulties in recruiting providers in regions outside of major metropolitan areas. Plans are to close this gap by contracting with community primary care centers in underserved areas (Lynn Buggage, Women's Preventive Health Program, New Orleans, LA, personal communication, to Vivien Chen, Louisiana State University Medical Center, August 21, 2001). The Institute of Medicine Committee on the Early Detection of Breast Cancer recommended in its report, *Mammography and Beyond*, that the program be expanded to reach at least 70 percent of the program's target population (Institute of Medicine, 2001b).

Office of Family Planning, U.S. Department of Health and Human Services

The National Family Planning Program was created in 1970 as Title X of the Public Health Service Act (PL 910572). Grants made under Title X provide funding for comprehensive family planning and preventive reproductive health services (www.os.dhhs.gov/opa/titlex/ofp.html). The Office of Family Planning had appropriations of $238.9 million in fiscal year 2000 and supports services offered through a network of 4,600 clinics nationwide. Grantees include states, family planning councils, Planned Parenthood affiliates, and other public and private entities that provide family planning services. In 1994 an estimated 4.2 million family planning clients were served by clinics administered by Title X-supported agencies (www.agi-usa.org/pubs/ib16.html). In addition to contraceptive services, Title X clinics provide basic reproductive health care such as screening for breast and cervical cancer; screening for sexually transmitted diseases including human immunodeficiency virus infection; and general health education, counseling, and referrals. Services are provided on a sliding scale based on income, with persons whose incomes are at or below the federal poverty level receiving services at no cost. An estimated 97 percent of the population served by Title X clinics are female, 85 percent are from low-income households, and 60 percent are younger than age 25. Family planning clinics are often an entry point into the health care system for young adults and for low-income persons.

Title X clinics are very important sources of Pap testing for women of reproductive age who are uninsured or covered by Medicaid. According to the 1995 National Survey of Family Growth, Pap tests were obtained in the past year by 61.9 percent of women of reproductive age (ages 15 to 44). Women who were uninsured or who had Medicaid coverage were significantly less likely than privately insured women to have been tested at private doctors' offices or health maintenance organizations (HMOs) and were significantly more likely to have been tested at Title X and other clinics (Table 9.5).[2]

Indirect Service Providers

Centers for Medicare and Medicaid Services

Programs administered by the Centers for Medicare and Medicaid Services (CMS; formerly the Health Care Financing Administration [HCFA])

[2]The name of the clinic or health care provider reported by respondents was used by survey sponsors to identify clinics as Title X sites.

TABLE 9.5 Percentage (95% confidence interval) of Reproductive-Age Women Reporting Pap Testing in the Past Year, by Location of Test and Health Insurance Coverage, National Survey of Family Growth, 1995

		Health Insurance Coverage		
Test or Test Site	All Women	Some Private	Medicaid	None
Pap test	61.9 (60.7–63.1)	64.6 (63.2–66.0)	61.1 (58.2–64.1)	46.6 (43.3–49.8)
Testing site	100.0	100.0	100.0	100.0
Private doctor's office/HMO	78.9 (77.5–80.3)	86.2 (84.7–87.7)	47.6 (44.0–51.3)	57.0 (52.6–61.4)
Clinic, Title X	8.0 (7.1–8.9)	4.7 (4.0–5.4)	22.5 (19.2–25.1)	17.8 (14.4–21.3)
Clinic, other	10.2 (8.9–11.5)	6.9 (6.8–7.0)	25.1 (21.8–28.3)	19.5 (15.8–23.2)
Hospital, school, other	2.8 (2.4–3.3)	2.2 (1.8–2.7)	4.8 (3.3–6.2)	5.7 (3.7–7.6)

NOTE: The numbers in the columns may not total 100 percent because of rounding. Sample size = 10,847.
SOURCE: National Cancer Policy Board staff analyses, National Survey of Family Growth, Cycle V 1995, CD-ROM, Series 23(3), issued November 1997, SETS Version 1.22a, National Center for Health Statistics, CDC, DHHS.

include Medicare, Medicaid, the State Children's Health Insurance Program, and the End-Stage Renal Disease Program. This section focuses on prevention services provided as part of Medicare and Medicaid.

Medicare Medicare enrollment in 2001 was estimated to be 40.3 million individuals, most (86 percent) of whom are age 65 and older. Most Medicare beneficiaries (94 percent) have both hospital insurance and supplemental insurance coverage and report relatively high levels of access to routine care. Having had a routine checkup in the past year, for example, was reported by from 74 to 92 percent of Medicare beneficiaries, according to surveys conducted in all 50 states and the District of Columbia (Health Care Financing Administration, 2000a). Most Medicare beneficiaries obtain care in the traditional fee-for-service system. As of 1999 only 18 percent of Medicare beneficiaries were enrolled in managed care plans. Total outlays for Medicare benefit payments were $210.1 billion in 1998, representing an estimated 13 percent of the total federal budget (Health Care Financing Administration, 2000b).

CMS has several mechanisms in place to ensure the quality of care for the beneficiaries it serves. In 1992, CMS initiated the Health Care Quality Improvement Program to address shortcomings in the health care received by its beneficiaries. Although the quality improvement program was initially focused on acute myocardial infarction, CMS has expanded its quality improvement efforts to include five other clinical priority areas (breast cancer, diabetes, heart failure, pneumonia, and stroke) and reductions in disparities in health care (www.cms.hhs.gov/qio/1a1.asp). Much of CMS's quality improvement work is carried out by its national network of 53 Quality Improvement Organizations (formerly called peer review organizations or PROs) (http://www.cms.hhs.gov/qio/default.asp). A number of national performance goals, including increased rates of receipt of a screening mammography, have been set to hold CMS accountable for improvements in care pursuant to the Government Performance and Results Act of 1993 (PL 103-62). Medicare managed care organizations are required to adopt the quality, access, and utilization performance measures of the National Committee for Quality Assurance's Health Plan Employer Data and Information Set (http://www.ncqa.org/Programs/HEDIS/), and CMS is in the process of developing performance measures in its fee-for-service program that serves the majority of beneficiaries. Preliminary results of research in this area suggest that measures of screening for breast cancer by mammography could be applied at the national, small geographic, and large group practice levels (www.hcfa.gov/quality/docs/ffs2-es.htm). The Balanced Budget Act of 1997 (PL 105-33) required CMS to provide comparable information regarding performance in both fee-for-service and managed care settings.

Medicare Screening Benefits Until recently, preventive services were explicitly excluded from Medicare coverage. As it was originally conceived, the Medicare program was to limit its coverage to hospital, physician, and certain other services that are "reasonable and necessary for the diagnosis or treatment of illness or injury or to improve the functioning of a malformed body member" (section 1862 of the Social Security Act). Since the program's inception in 1965, the U.S. Congress has expanded coverage to screening for breast, cervical, colorectal, and prostate cancer (Table 9.6). The coverage is not entirely consistent with recommendations of the U.S. Department of Health and Human Service's USPSTF. For example, prostate cancer screening by digital rectal examinations or by detection of tumor markers in serum (e.g., prostate-specific antigen) is a Medicare benefit, but screening is not recommended by USPSTF (U.S. Preventive Services Task Force, 1996).

Some of the out-of-pocket costs associated with cancer screening are defrayed by some sort of supplemental coverage through the Medicaid program, private insurance, or an employer-sponsored benefit program. Medicare beneficiaries who receive their care through managed care plans may obtain additional benefits that include prevention services (Centers for Medicare and Medicaid Services, 2002). Estimates of mammography use among female Medicare beneficiaries are shown in Table 9.7

The Mammography Campaign was launched by CMS in 1995 to improve female beneficiaries' knowledge of breast cancer screening and awareness of Medicare's annual screening mammography benefit (before 1998, the benefit covered mammography every 2 years). Educational materials for distribution to beneficiaries have been developed in partnership with NCI's Office of Communications. Both beneficiaries and providers have been targeted for outreach by CMS's peer review organizations.

The overall rate of use of colorectal cancer screening and diagnostic services among Medicare beneficiaries is generally low, even though more than 70 percent of new cases of colorectal cancer occur among those age 65 and older (Ries et al., 2000b). The rate of use has not changed significantly since 1995, despite the issuance of a clinical practice guideline in 1997 and the expanded Medicare benefit that became effective in 1998. In 1999, only 14.1 percent of beneficiaries age 50 and older used one or more of the covered services for screening or diagnosis of colorectal cancer. The overall rate of use in 1999 was roughly equivalent to the rate in 1995, when 13.6 percent of beneficiaries used any of these services (U.S. General Accounting Office, 2000). In 1999, the rates of use of colorectal cancer screening tests among beneficiaries age 50 and older were 9.1 percent for the fecal occult blood test, 1.9 percent for sigmoidoscopy, 1.9 percent for flexible sigmoidoscopy, and 3.8 percent for colonoscopy. These low levels of screening occur even though nearly all older Americans report having a regular source of health care and a large majority report receiving routine checkups. In

TABLE 9.6 Coverage for Cancer Screening Tests Under Original Medicare Plan, Centers for Medicare and Medicaid Services

				Extent of Coverage	
Cancer	Test	Individuals Covered	Test Frequency	Coinsurance (percent)	Deductible[a]
Breast	Mammogram[b]	Women age 40 and older	Annual	20	None
		Women ages 35 to 39	One-time baseline exam	20	None
	Clinical breast exam	All women	Every 2 years	20	None
Cervical	Pap test	All women	Every 2 years, annual for high-risk women	None for lab, 20 for collection	None
	Pelvic exam	All women	Every 2 years, annual for high-risk women	20	None
Prostate	Digital rectal exam	Men age 50 and older	Annual	20	Yes
	Prostate-specific antigen (PSA)	Men age 50 and older	Annual	None	None
Colorectal	Colonoscopy	Individuals age 50 and older; at high risk, no minimum age	Every 10 years, but not within 4 years of a screening flexible sigmoidoscopy. Every 2 years for high-risk individuals	20[c]	Yes
	Fecal occult blood test	Individuals age 50 and older	Annual	None	None
	Flexible sigmoidoscopy	Individuals age 50 and older	Every 4 years	20[c]	Yes
	Barium enema	Alternative to sigmoidoscopy or colonoscopy		20	Yes

[a]The Part B deductible is $100 per year.
[b]Medicare also covers new digital technologies for mammogram screening.
[c]Beneficiary pays 25% of the Medicare-approved amount if sigmoidoscopy or colonoscopy is performed in an ambulatory surgical center or hospital outpatient department.
SOURCE: Centers for Medicare and Medicaid Services (2002).

TABLE 9.7 Mammography Use Within Past 2 Years

	Survey-Based Estimates 1997 (Women Age 65 and Older) % (95% confidence interval)	Claims-Based Estimate 1997–1999 (Women Ages 52 to 69) %
Rate in median state	70	56
Rate range	57–83	47–66
Alabama	76 (70–81)	55
Alaska	72 (57–87)	52
Arizona	76 (69–83)	57
Arkansas	57 (51–64)	50
California	78 (74–83)	54
Colorado	72 (65–79)	55
Connecticut	75 (69–81)	60
Delaware	74 (69–80)	59
District of Columbia	82 (75–89)	52
Florida	80 (76–83)	62
Georgia	72 (65–79)	52
Hawaii	79 (73–85)	52
Idaho	63 (58–67)	53
Illinois	67 (61–73)	54
Indiana	58 (51–65)	54
Iowa	61 (57–66)	60
Kansas	68 (62–74)	58
Kentucky	66 (62–70)	53
Louisiana	70 (63–78)	50
Maine	76 (70–83)	66
Maryland	76 (70–81)	58
Massachusetts	75 (68–82)	63
Michigan	77 (72–82)	64
Minnesota	68 (64–72)	61
Mississippi	62 (56–69)	47
Missouri	68 (61–74)	54
Montana	71 (65–77)	59
Nebraska	60 (55–66)	56
Nevada	64 (50–77)	50
New Hampshire	75 (67–82)	63
New Jersey	69 (63–75)	50
New Mexico	67 (60–74)	51
New York	75 (70–80)	56
North Carolina	72 (67–76)	57
North Dakota	71 (65–77)	64
Ohio	69 (64–75)	56
Oklahoma	59 (52–65)	49
Oregon	77 (73–82)	59
Pennsylvania	70 (65–75)	56
Rhode Island	83 (78–88)	58
South Carolina	76 (71–81)	55
South Dakota	70 (64–75)	57
Tennessee	69 (64–74)	53
Texas	65 (58–72)	51

TABLE 9.7 (continued)

	Survey-Based Estimates 1997 (Women Age 65 and Older) % (95% confidence interval)	Claims-Based Estimate 1997–1999 (Women Ages 52 to 69) %
Utah	70 (63–77)	55
Vermont	70 (65–76)	63
Virginia	68 (62–75)	55
Washington	69 (64–74)	59
West Virginia	66 (61–71)	55
Wisconsin	69 (63–75)	60
Wyoming	70 (64–76)	55

SOURCES: Jencks et al. (2000) and Health Care Financing Administration, state-specific estimates (2000a).

general, higher rates of colorectal screening test use were seen among women than among men, higher rates were seen among whites than among members of racial or ethnic minority groups, and higher rates were seen among beneficiaries ages 70 to 79 than among younger and older beneficiaries (Table 9.8).

Uncertainty remains regarding the benefits of screening for breast cancer at older ages. Resolving these uncertainties is of paramount importance to the Medicare program because nearly half (47 percent) of beneficiaries are age 75 and older.

Smoking Cessation Benefits Within the Medicare Program The rate of current smoking among Medicare beneficiaries age 65 and older varies markedly by state, with the range being from 3.7 percent in Utah to 20.6 in Nevada. Estimates of the share of smokers who have attempted to quit smoking range from 16.7 percent in Arizona to 59.3 percent in Alabama (Health Care Financing Administration, 2000a). According to one estimate, a person who smokes more than 20 cigarettes a day and who quits at age 65 can expect to increase his or her life expectancy by 2 to 3 years (Sachs, 1986). Even though evidence supports the health and quality-of-life benefits of smoking cessation at older ages, Medicare does not provide coverage for smoking cessation programs or products. As part of CMS's Healthy Aging Initiative, a literature review of the evidence of the effectiveness of interventions to promote smoking cessation in the Medicare population has been completed (DHHS, HCFA, undated). In addition, a demonstration program testing the effects of various benefit enhancements on smoking cessation is in progress. The three benefit options being compared with usual care (smoking cessation information) in the seven-state Medicare Stop Smoking Program are (www.hcfa.gov/healthyaging/1b.htm):

TABLE 9.8 Medicare Beneficiaries' Rates of Use (Percent) of Tests for Colorectal Cancer Screening and Diagnostic Services, 1995–1999[a]

Characteristic	1995	1996	1997	1998	1999
Total	13.6	13.2	12.6	13.1	14.1
Sex					
Male	12.8	12.4	11.9	12.1	13.2
Female	14.2	13.8	13.2	13.8	14.8
Race or ethnicity					
White	14.2	13.8	13.3	13.9	14.9
Black	9.0	8.9	8.5	8.4	9.1
Asian	11.8	11.2	8.9	11.2	12.6
Hispanic	8.0	8.2	5.9	7.7	8.1
Other and unknown	10.5	10.5	11.9	9.0	10.6
Age					
Younger than 65	4.6	4.6	4.5	4.5	4.9
65–69	15.0	14.6	13.7	14.7	15.6
70–74	16.6	16.2	15.6	16.3	17.6
75–79	16.8	16.4	15.7	16.4	17.9
80–84	15.2	14.8	14.4	14.8	15.9
85 and older	10.9	10.5	10.3	10.0	11.0

[a]Rates represent the percentage of Medicare beneficiaries who had a fecal occult blood test, flexible sigmoidoscopy, colonoscopy, or barium enema for screening, diagnostic, and, in the case of colonoscopy, treatment purposes. Rates are based on analyses of Medicare claims.
SOURCE: McMullan M, HCFA Center for Beneficiary Services, Testimony before the Special Committee on Aging, U.S. Senate (March 6, 2000).

1. reimbursement for provider counseling only,
2. reimbursement for provider counseling and Food and Drug Administration-approved prescription or nicotine replacement pharmacotherapy, and
3. a telephone counseling quit line and reimbursement for nicotine replacement therapy.

The program commenced in the summer of 2001 and is expected to be completed in 2003.

Medicaid Medicaid is a joint federal and state program that provides essential medical and medically related services to the nation's most vulnerable populations (HCFA, 2000d). Three types of health protection are available through Medicaid:

1. health insurance for low-income families with children and people with disabilities;
2. long-term care for older Americans and individuals with disabilities; and

3. supplemental coverage for low-income Medicare beneficiaries for services not covered by Medicare and Medicare premiums, deductibles, and cost sharing.[3]

Each state establishes its own eligibility standards, benefits package, payment rates, and program administration under broad federal guidelines. Many variations exist among state Medicaid programs regarding not only which services are covered but also the amount, duration, and scope of services. Each state Medicaid program must cover "mandatory services" identified by statute and have the discretion to cover additional "optional services." Early and Periodic Screening, Diagnosis, and Treatment services are mandatory for individuals under age 21, whereas screening and prevention services are optional for older enrollees (Health Care Financing Administration, 2000d).

The population enrolled in the Medicaid program is dynamic, with individuals entering and leaving the program at fairly high rates, but at any point in time an estimated 12 percent of the U.S. population is enrolled, with most of these individuals consisting of low-income women and children. In 1998, Medicaid enrollment was 41.4 million, with children under age 21 making up 54 percent of Medicaid enrollment (HCFA, 2000d). In 1998 it was estimated that one in five U.S. children was served by the Medicaid program.[4] Total outlays for Medicaid medical assistance payments were $96.4 billion in 1998.

Throughout the 1990s states significantly expanded the enrollments in Medicaid managed care programs.[5] By 1998, more than half (54 percent) of the Medicaid population was enrolled in some type of managed care plan. Medicaid managed care penetration varies greatly by state: 2 states (Alaska, Wyoming) have no beneficiaries enrolled in managed care plans, whereas 12 states (Arizona, Colorado, Delaware, Georgia, Hawaii, Iowa, Montana, New Mexico, Oregon, Tennessee, Utah, and Washington) have more than 75 percent of their beneficiaries enrolled in such plans. As of 1998, 35 states and the District of Columbia operated Freedom of Choice

---

[3]In 1998 about 6 million persons were enrolled in both Medicare and Medicaid.

[4]In 1997, the U.S. Congress created the State Children's Health Insurance Program (SCHIP) to address the growing number of uninsured children. By 1999 nearly 2 million children were enrolled in one of the 53 SCHIP plans (3 plans were not yet in operation). Most states use a Medicaid expansion as part of the SCHIP plans, either solely or in combination with a separate program.

[5]Medicaid managed care contractors include comprehensive health maintenance organization (HMO) plans, Medicaid-only HMO plans, prepaid health plans (i.e., an entity that provides a noncomprehensive set of services on either a capitated risk basis or a nonrisk basis or an entity that provides comprehensive services on a nonrisk basis), and primary care case management plans (i.e., a program in which the state contracts directly with primary care providers who agree to be responsible for the provision or coordination of medical services to Medicaid beneficiaries under their care).

waivers [84 Section 1915(b)] to mandatorily enroll beneficiaries in managed care programs, provide additional services via the savings produced from managed care, or create a "carve-out" system for the delivery of specialty care (e.g., behavioral health).[6]

Smoking rates tend to be higher among the Medicaid population, and 5 million or more adult smokers were estimated to be covered by the program in 1999 (Schauffler et al., 2001a). Only half of the states, however, cover even one smoking cessation treatment for their Medicaid recipients, according to a review of Medicaid coverage for treatments for tobacco dependence in 1998 (Schauffler et al., 2001a). State Medicaid programs were most likely to cover pharmacotherapy for tobacco dependence, including bupropion, the nicotine patch, nicotine gum, and a nicotine nasal spray (Table 9.9). Six states (Delaware, Maine, Maryland, Minnesota, New Mexico, and Oregon) offered comprehensive Medicaid benefits for the treatment of tobacco dependence (all forms of nicotine replacement therapy, bupropion, and both group and individual counseling). Even in states whose Medicaid programs did provide coverage for treatments for tobacco dependence, the programs made little effort to inform smokers of the availability of these benefits or how to access and use them. Only four state Medicaid programs (those in Arizona, Maine, Rhode Island, and Wyoming) reported offering any special programs designed to assist women who are pregnant or breast-feeding to quit smoking, despite the strong evidence that the cessation of smoking during pregnancy reduces the incidence of low birth weight.

Cancer screening rates among Medicaid beneficiaries appear to be similar to those among privately insured individuals, according to recent studies (Potosky et al., 1998; Hewitt et al., 2002).

Office of Management and Budget

In 1997, a presidential executive order established smoke-free environments for the more than 1.8 million civilian federal employees and members of the public visiting or using federal facilities. In 2001, federal departments and agencies were directed to establish a policy that provides up to 4 hours of excused absence each year, without a loss of pay or a charge to leave, for participation in preventive health screenings. Agencies were also directed to develop or expand programs offered at the worksite to help employees understand their risks for disease, obtain preventive health services, and make healthy lifestyle choices. The Office of Personnel Management has issued guidance for a model smoking cessation program and is

---

[6]In addition, 17 states operated statewide comprehensive research and demonstration projects to test substantially new ideas with potential policy merit.

TABLE 9.9 Medicaid Program Coverage of Pharmacotherapy and Counseling—United States,[a] 2000

State	Any treatment	Over-the-counter medication		Prescription Medication		
		Gum	Patch	Any	Spray	Inhaler
Arizona	•[b]	•	•			
Arkansas	•			•		
California[c]	•	•	•	•	•	•
Colorado[c]	•	•	•	•	•	•
Delaware[c]	•	•	•	•	•	•
District of Columbia	•			•	•	
Florida	•	•	•	•		
Hawaii	•			•	•	•
Illinois[c]	•	•	•	•	•	•
Indiana[c]	•	•	•	•	•	•
Kansas	•		•	•		
Louisiana	•			•	•	•
Maine[c]	•	•	•	•	•	•
Maryland	•			•	•	•
Massachusetts	•					
Michigan	•	•	•	•		
Minnesota[c]	•	•	•	•	•	•
Montana	•	•	•	•		
Nevada[c]	•	•	•	•	•	•
New Hampshire[c]	•	•	•	•	•	•
New Jersey[c]	•	•	•	•	•	•
New Mexico[c]	•	•	•	•	•	•
New York[c]	•	•	•	•	•	•
North Carolina	•			•	•	•
North Dakota	•	•	•	•		
Ohio	•	•	•	•		•
Oklahoma	•			•		
Oregon[d]	•	•	•	•	•	•
Rhode Island	•					
Texas[c]	•	•	•	•	•	•
Vermont	•	•	•	•	•	•
Virginia	•			•	•	•
West Virginia[c]	•	•	•	•	•	•
Wisconsin	•			•	•	•
No. states in 2000	34	22	23	31	23	23
% states in 2000	67	43	45	61	45	45

[a]Covered treatment.
[b]States offering no coverage were Alabama, Alaska, Connecticut, Georgia, Idaho, Iowa, Kentucky, Mississippi, Missouri, Nebraska, Pennsylvania, South Carolina, South Dakota, Tennessee, Utah, Washington, and Wyoming.
[c]Offered all pharmacotherapy recommended in *Public Health Service Clinical Practice Guideline for Treating Tobacco Use and Dependence.*
[d]Offered all treatments.
[e]Covers pregnant women only.
SOURCE: Adapted from CDC, 2001e.

Prescription Medication			Counseling			
Zyban	Wellbutrin	Bupropion	Any	Group	Individual	Telephone
			•	•	•	
•	•					
•	•	•				
•	•	•				
•	•	•				
•	•	•				
•						
•	•	•				
•	•	•				
•	•	•	•		•	
•	•	•	•	•	•	
•	•	•				
•	•	•	•	•	•	
•	•	•	•[e]	•[e]	•[e]	
			•	•	•	
•	•					
•	•	•	•	•	•	
•						
•	•	•				
•	•	•	•	•	•	
•	•	•				
•	•	•	•[e]	•[e]	•[e]	•[e]
•	•	•				
•	•	•				
•	•	•				
•	•	•				
•	•	•				
•	•	•	•	•	•	•
			•	•	•	
•	•	•				
•	•	•				
•	•	•				
•	•	•	•		•	•
•	•	•	•		•	
31	29	27	13	10	13	3
61	57	53	26	20	26	6

compiling a list of best practices to be shared with agencies. Agencies can pay the costs incurred by employees participating in agency-authorized smoking cessation programs, including payment for nicotine replacement therapy when it is purchased as part of an agency's smoking cessation program (www.opm.gov/ehs).

SUMMARY AND CONCLUSIONS

The federal government provides many opportunities to further cancer prevention and early detection by promulgating national goals and objectives, issuing clinical guidelines, disseminating information, carrying out monitoring and surveillance activities, facilitating statewide program planning and evaluation, and providing or paying for services.

Explicit national cancer-related goals and objectives have been set as part of the *Healthy People 2010* initiative (US DHHS and Office of Disease Prevention and Health Promotion, 2000), and efforts are under way to chart the nation's progress toward those goals. Federally sponsored evidence-based guidelines for clinical and community practice provide clinicians and public health providers with the information they need to achieve these goals. NCI is the lead federal agency in the dissemination of cancer-related information to clinicians, consumers, and the public health community through a number of channels including its telephone Cancer Information Service, its websites, and PDQ, a comprehensive cancer information database. Tracking the successes of these and other efforts in reaching cancer prevention and early detection goals often relies on federally sponsored surveys and surveillance systems that assess the prevalence of risk behaviors, levels of access to services, and health behaviors among the general and selected members of the U.S. population. Federal safety net providers including Community and Migrant Health Centers and Title X family planning clinics are key to closing the gap in service use and, ultimately, in reducing the unequal burden of cancer observed among poor and disadvantaged populations.

Although some federal programs are at the forefront of promoting effective cancer prevention and early detection interventions, there appears to be much room for improvement. In particular, policies are needed to improve coverage of evidence-based smoking cessation interventions within the Medicare and Medicaid programs. Such policies could greatly reduce the burden of cancer. In addition, the significant variations in the rates of use of screening services among beneficiaries served by the Medicare and VHA programs suggest that interventions are needed to improve rates of adherence to evidence-based guidelines.

10

Research Trends and Opportunities

The United States is at a crossroads in cancer prevention research. Basic science and epidemiology are advancing knowledge in a number of areas, from the relationship between cancer and modifiable behavioral risk factors all the way down to the molecular pathways that mediate the actions of those risk factors. At the same time applied research is illustrating how the already vast amount of available evidence can be better used to more rapidly reduce cancer rates. To effectively reduce the cancer burden in the United States, however, there needs to be greater emphasis on action-oriented research (Colditz, 1997, 2001; Wegman, 1992). Knowledge about health problems and their causes does not automatically guarantee that appropriate actions are taken. Only when etiological knowledge is linked to evidence on the effectiveness of behavioral change strategies, and, in turn, to public awareness and policy support can the potential to reduce the burden of cancer be realized.

In this chapter the National Cancer Policy Board describes the range of research activities in the field of cancer prevention and early detection, with a focus on translational research—the research needed to move the fruits of research into provider and community practice. The chapter also presents estimates of the level of cancer prevention and early detection research through an analysis of publication trends in cancer prevention and control and a description of the current research portfolios of selected federal and private research sponsors.

DEFINING TRANSLATIONAL RESEARCH IN CANCER PREVENTION AND EARLY DETECTION

Research on ways to promote the widespread adoption of evidence-based prevention and early detection interventions generally falls under the rubric of cancer control research, health services research, or, more specifically, applied or translational research. The definition of cancer control research has evolved over time but generally involves behavioral, social, and population sciences and spans the continuum of interventions aimed at cancer, from dietary recommendations for the prevention of cancer to the use of palliative care services to alleviate suffering at the end of life (Box 10.1).

Health services research is a multidisciplinary field of inquiry, both basic and applied, that examines the use, costs, quality, accessibility, delivery, organization, financing, and outcomes of health care services to increase knowledge and understand the structure, processes, and effects of health services for individuals and populations (Institute of Medicine, 1995a). Both cancer control and health services research can be defined broadly to include behavioral and psychological research, evaluations of programs that may fall outside the purview of the traditional health care systems (e.g., school-based health programs), and randomized controlled clinical trials (e.g., studies of the effectiveness of health care technologies in situations representative of community practice).

Other disciplines and research frameworks such as those from sociology, anthropology, economics, and political science are also relevant to cancer prevention and early detection. A hallmark of such research is its

BOX 10.1 Evolving Definition of Cancer Control Research

- Cancer research seeks to find the means for combating cancer, whereas cancer control is concerned with identifying, community testing, evaluating, and promoting the application of cancer control means that are found (1975).
- Cancer control research is the reduction of cancer incidence, morbidity, and mortality through an orderly sequence from research on interventions and their impacts in defined populations to the broad, systematic application of the research results (1985).
- Cancer control encompasses a full spectrum of research in the behavioral, social, epidemiological, and population sciences aimed at creating or enhancing interventions that, by themselves or in combination with biomedical approaches, reduce cancer risk, incidence, morbidity, and mortality, and improve quality of life (2000).

SOURCE: Hiatt and Rimer (1999) and National Cancer Institute (2000b).

TABLE 10.1 Types of Research Necessary to Improve the Application of Evidence-Based Cancer Prevention and Early Detection Interventions

Question	Example	Examples of Types of Research Needed
1. What do we know?	• Smoking causes cancer	• Basic biomedical research • Epidemiological research
2. What works?	• Behavioral counseling, pharmacological interventions, and policies to increase the price of cigarettes to reduce smoking	• Intervention research (e.g., clinical trials) • Surveillance research • Program evaluation • Health services research • Meta-analyses
3. Where are we?	• Certain populations are at high risk for cancer (e.g., 35 percent of adolescents smoke) • Effective interventions are not being applied (e.g., half of primary care providers are not asking smokers about their habit)	• Surveillance systems (e.g., national behavioral risk surveys) • Health services research (e.g., patterns of care studies)
4. How can we do better?	• Physicians provided with continuing education and office reminder systems improve their smoking-related practices • States with multilevel programs have observed increased rates of smoking cessation among certain populations • Improved access to insurance increases access to smoking cessation services	• Intervention research • Community trials • Program evaluation • Policy research • Epidemiology • Meta-analyses
5. What is the impact?	• Significant declines in smoking-related diseases have occurred following the passage of laws to raise the price of cigarettes	• Health services research • Surveillance research • Policy research

SOURCE: Adapted from Hiatt and Rimer (1999) and the Advisory Committee on Cancer Control, National Cancer Institute of Canada (1994).

interdisciplinary nature. For the purposes of this report, the Board chose to focus on research that improves understanding of how to implement and disseminate interventions known to be effective. Such applied or translational research builds on epidemiological research, surveillance research, and the conduct of community trials and program evaluations. Such research focuses on questions posed in steps three and four of the stages of inquiry described in Table 10.1.

STATUS OF TRANSLATIONAL RESEARCH IN CANCER PREVENTION AND EARLY DETECTION

This section first describes publication trends in cancer prevention and early detection and then summarizes the support for such research provided by the following organizations:

Federally Sponsored Research

- U.S. Department of Health and Human Services
- National Institutes of Health (National Cancer Institute, National Institute on Aging)
- Centers for Disease Control and Prevention
- Agency for Healthcare Research and Quality
- Centers for Medicare and Medicaid Services (formerly the Health Care Financing Administration)
- U.S. Department of Defense
- U.S. Department of Veterans Affairs

Privately Sponsored Research

- American Cancer Society
- Foundations (e.g., Robert Wood Johnson Foundation and the Legacy Foundation)

Although these organizations are not the only sponsors of research on cancer prevention and early detection, they represent the major funding sources for such research. Excluded from this review are health services research supported by health plans, insurers, pharmaceutical companies, and other private organizations. Much of the research done in those settings is proprietary.

Publication Trends

The evaluation of trends in research publications is one way to assess the level of activity within a discipline. A resource that can be used to track such studies is the National Library of Medicine's PubMed database, which stores information about individual citations including index terms used to characterize each article (articles are indexed according to a dictionary of medical subject headings called MESH terms). The PubMed database includes citations from MedLine, HealthStar, and other bibliographical databases.

The volume of articles on cancer prevention and control appears to have increased markedly from 1985 to 2000, from 548 to 2,193 (Figure 10.1). Although the number of research citations on cancer prevention and control increased during this period, by 2000 they represented less than 5 percent of all cancer-related citations indexed in the medical literature (Figure 10.2). These trends reflect articles written in the English language, but not necessarily by U.S. investigators. Figures 10.1 and 10.2 therefore reflect trends in the general medical literature, not necessarily trends in the United States. These trends must be interpreted with caution because they may

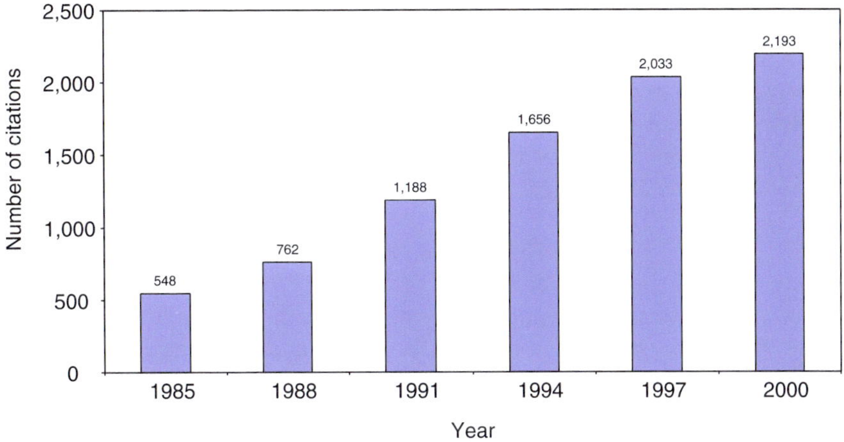

FIGURE 10.1 PubMed citations for cancer-related prevention and control research, 1985–2000.

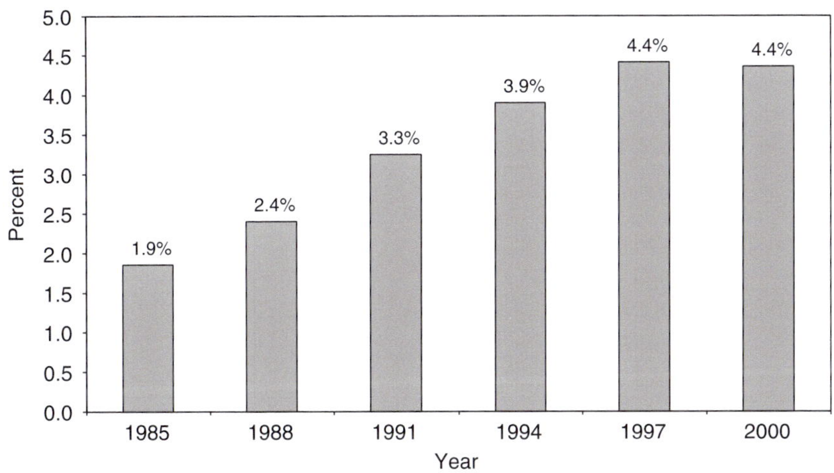

FIGURE 10.2 PubMed citations for cancer-related prevention and control research as a percentage of all cancer-related citations, 1985–2000.

reflect changes in the ways in which MESH headings were applied to index the literature rather than real increases in cancer-related research. The term "prevention and control," the MESH subheading used to identify citations, refers to prevention and control of environmental hazards and social factors that lead to disease and preventive measures taken by individuals (National Library of Medicine, 2001).

Research Support

A more direct way to assess the status of U.S.-based prevention and early detection research is to describe current topics of investigation and levels of research spending. No one comprehensive source of information on cancer prevention and early detection exists. As part of its review, the National Cancer Policy Board relied on the following sources:

- review of agency websites (e.g., those of the National Cancer Institute [NCI] and the U.S. Department of Defense);
- reviews of annual reports of the research arms of certain agencies (e.g., those of the U.S. Department of Veterans Affairs and the Health Care Financing Administration, now the Centers for Medicare and Medicaid [CMS]);
- informal contacts with agency representatives known to be involved in related research (e.g., those from CMS and U.S. Department of Veterans Affairs Centers of Excellence);
- meetings with senior agency representatives (e.g., those from NCI);
- information catalogued in the Health Services Research Project database, which is maintained by the National Library of Medicine and which includes brief descriptions of ongoing extramural research sponsored by federal and state agencies, foundations, and other organizations;
- the Research and Development in the United States (RADIUS) database maintained by the RAND Corporation; this database includes information on the research and development activities of the U.S. government, including activities indexed in the Computer Retrieval of Information on Scientific Projects database maintained by the National Institutes of Health (NIH; http://radius.rand.org).
- the Foundation Center's online directory (www.fconline.fdncenter. org);
- publications of Grantmakers in Health (e.g., Prevention Strategies for All Ages: Findings from the Grantmakers in Health Resource Center) (Grantmakers in Health, 2000); and
- announcements of research support in prevention-related newsletters and listservs (e.g., Health Behavior Information Transfer and the Susan G. Komen Breast Cancer Foundation's Newsletter).

Despite the best efforts of the Board, the description of selected agencies' research portfolios that follows may under- or overestimate the actual level of research. Organizations varied in how they defined cancer prevention and early detection, and consequently, there is likely some inconsistency in what was included (or excluded) as a relevant research activity. An attempt was made to limit the search to applied or translational research, but it was not always possible to distinguish projects that fit this description. Furthermore, some research activities may have been missed because of limitations of research tracking systems. This review is limited to sources of research support that are national in scope; however, the Board recognizes that there are many significant sources of support for cancer prevention-related research at the state and regional levels (e.g., the California Department of Health Services, the California HealthCare Foundation, the Colorado Trust, the Kansas Health Foundation, and the Paso del Norte Health Foundation). The review was conducted in 2001 and is limited, for most organizations, to research projects active at that time.

Federally Sponsored Research

U.S. Department of Health and Human Services

National Institutes of Health, National Cancer Institute NCI spent 12 percent of its fiscal year (FY) 2001 operating budget on cancer control ($459.5 million of $3.7 billion) (Stacey Vandor, Planning Officer, Office of the Director, Division of Cancer Control and Population Sciences, National Cancer Institute, personal communication to Maria Hewitt, Institute of Medicine, February 11, 2002). The U.S. Congress directed NCI to appropriate 10 percent of its budget to its Cancer Prevention and Control Program in the Revitalization Act of 1993 (National Institutes of Health, 1998). NCI supports a large portfolio of basic and applied research. In FY 2001, for example, NCI let 510 grants and contracts for basic and applied research related to tobacco totaling $128 million. Behavioral research grants and contracts on obesity and physical activity totaled over $25 million and there were 37 grants totaling $15 million in the Behavioral Research Applied Cancer Screening grants portfolio. Listed below are selected NCI-supported grants that represent applied or translational research active in 1999 according to the RADIUS database.[1]

Tobacco

- Enhanced self-help interventions for smoking cessation
- Individualized relapse prevention among female smokers
- Accelerating progress of smoking cessation during pregnancy
- A new channel for smoking cessation: visiting nurses
- Nicotine patch and self-help treatment for those who use smokeless tobacco
- Interventions targeting tobacco use

[1]This list of NCI-supported research is meant to provide examples of grant support to illustrate the breadth and scope of applied research. The list may not be complete because of limitations to the search of the RADIUS database for relevant research. Keywords used in the search included "human," "cancer," "smoking" or "tobacco," "diet" or "nutrition," "physical activity," "obesity," "screening," and "prevention and control."

- Smoking cessation among childhood cancer survivors
- Spousal influence on tobacco use after cancer diagnosis
- Smoking cessation outcomes in individuals on methadone maintenance
- Tobacco use prevention multimedia system for children (application of CD-ROM and World Wide Web lessons and activities on tobacco use prevention)
- Tobacco advocacy at the state level (case studies of activities of the tobacco industry and tobacco control advocates).

Diet and Nutrition

- Five-a-Day Power Plus Program (assessment of a school cafeteria-focused intervention for promoting increased consumption of vegetables and fruit among elementary school children to reduce the risk of cancer)
- Five-a-Day achievement badge for urban Boy Scouts (intervention to increase fruit and vegetable consumption among youth)
- Five-a-Day WIC promotion program (intervention to improve consumption of fruits and vegetables among participants of the Special Supplemental Nutrition Program for Women, Infants, and Children [WIC] in Maryland)
- Goal setting for health-related behavioral changes among children (intervention to improve consumption of fruits and vegetables)
- Reducing cancer-related dietary risk behaviors in adolescents (school-based program targeting multiethnic students from families of lower socioeconomic status, their families, and their school environment to increase student consumption of fruits and vegetables and to reduce their intake of total calories from fat)
- Reaching rural residents with nutrition strategies.

Obesity, Physical Activity

- Cancer risk factor prevention for high-risk youth (focus on diet, physical activity, and obesity among Hispanic Americans)
- Fitness as a means of fighting cancer among African-American women
- Weight control to prevent cancer in African-American women.

Screening

- Increasing use of mammography among older, minority, and rural women
- Increasing use of screening mammography through urban churches
- Breast cancer screening in a triracial rural population
- Reducing barriers to the use of breast cancer screening
- Screening of older minority women

- Population-based approach to increased mammography use
- Interactive multimedia to promote breast cancer screening
- Multimedia breast cancer education kiosks for Latinos
- Breast cancer risk and symptom care in African-American women ages 40 to 49
- Breast and cervical cancer screening among Filipino women
- Promotion of breast cancer screening among indigent women
- Cancer screening of low-income and minority women
- Increasing adherence to follow-up of breast abnormalities
- Single-visit cervical cancer prevention program
- Intergroup cancer prevention research units: screening of first-degree relatives for colorectal cancer
- Informed decision making in prostate cancer screening (test methods of unbiased patient education).

Community-Based Interventions

- Accelerating the process of change for cancer prevention (evaluation of multiple intervention channels to enhance cancer prevention and control)
- Northern Appalachian Leadership Initiative on Cancer (development of community-based coalitions to develop, implement, maintain, and evaluate long-range, comprehensive, multidisciplinary, and community-wide projects in West Virginia, Pennsylvania, New York, Ohio, Maryland, and Virginia)
- Tristate Appalachian Leadership Initiative on Cancer (consortium of cooperative extension services, universities, and a hospital system in North Carolina, South Carolina, and Georgia to create a network of community cancer control coalitions, mobilize community lay and professional leaders, develop and disseminate cancer control interventions, and evaluate the effectiveness of the initiative)
- County-based cancer control in northern Appalachia (consortium development in Pennsylvania, Maryland, and New York)
- Central highlands Appalachian Leadership Initiative on Cancer (consortium development in Kentucky, Tennessee, and Virginia)
- Capacity building for public education (effort to transfer cancer education and prevention information and educational skills from health professionals to community-based lay health promoters and successor groups)
- Community outreach model for cancer control (community analysis and implementation of an educational program by a comprehensive cancer center)
- Worksite-based cancer prevention (Wellworks-2)
- Worksite-based smokeless tobacco-related behaviors.

Provider Practices

- Female physicians health study—cancer prevention (examines whether physicians' personal health practices help predict their counseling behaviors)
- Cancer prevention in primary care—patient activation (randomized, controlled trial to test the efficacies of two computer-tailored, stage-based interventions to address multiple cancer risk behaviors and screening use)
- Cancer prevention in primary care—practice activation (quasi-experimental study of 68 primary care practices in two cities in North Carolina to evaluate an office system for cancer prevention)
- New health assessment methods for cancer prevention (assessment of a dissemination model termed "physician-directed, customized delivery")
- Breast cancer education in north Manhattan (focus on physicians through "academic detailing" and patients through office-based health educators)
- Direct observation of primary care-cancer prevention trial (focus on increasing rates of adherence to prevention guidelines)
- Patient-focused cancer control in a health maintenance organization (HMO) population
- Promoting cancer prevention and control with message framing (evaluation of methods to convey health information in terms of individual gains and losses).

Special Populations

- Colorectal disease prevention in multiethnic populations
- Cancer prevention for the underserved (training home attendant as a community educator)
- Economically disadvantaged youth and cancer prevention
- Cancer prevention in rural youth—teaching health goals
- Preventing cancer in Hispanic communities (5-year program to establish and maintain the National Hispanic Leadership Initiative on Cancer).
- Reducing cancer risk in migrant Hispanic adolescents
- Community-based randomized trial of cancer prevention in the Hispanic population
- Community-based outreach for high-risk Mexican-American women (focus on cervical cancer screening, safe sex practices, and smoking)
- *Por la Vida* intervention model in cancer education (focus on community-based health promotion among Hispanics)
- National African-American Leadership Initiative on Cancer (development and support of community coalitions in the African-American community)

- Improving cancer risk communication (focus on risk perception and interventions to improve decision making among African Americans and women in their 50s and 60s regarding smoking and mammography use)
- Cultural methods to decrease cancer fatalism among African-American elders
- Network radio health care program for African Americans (development of a talk show to deliver cancer prevention and control information and offer opportunities to call in with questions).
- Cancer control in North American Chinese women (focus on cervical cancer screening and dietary behavior)
- Cervical cancer control in a Cambodian population (focus on cervical cancer screening)
- Cancer control needs among Native American Samoans
- Health promotion for women at risk for breast cancer.

NCI's Division of Cancer Control and Population Sciences (DCCPS) is the main locus for NCI-sponsored applied cancer prevention and early detection research. The five major research areas overseen by DCCPS include epidemiology and genetics research, behavioral research, applied research, cancer surveillance research, and survivorship research (Figure 10.3) (http://cancercontrol.cancer.gov). Through its research activities, the DCCPS aims to understand the causes and distribution of cancer in populations, support the development and implementation of effective interventions, and monitor and explain cancer trends in all segments of the population. Cancer control research is also supported through other areas of NCI including the Division of Cancer Prevention and the Center to Reduce Cancer Health Disparities. In addition, the Cancer Information Service, an important dissemination arm, is housed within the Office of Communications (see Chapter 9).

In FY 2001, DCCPS funded 733 research grants totaling $332.7 million. The areas receiving the most support were epidemiology and genetics (54 percent, or $180.3 million) and behavioral research (34 percent, or $113.5 million) (Table 10.2).

Within the behavioral research portfolio, tobacco control research received 47 percent of the total amount of funding devoted to research ($52.9 million of $113.5 million) (Figure 10.4).

NCI supports several priority areas of prevention and early detection research including tobacco, cancer communications, health disparities, quality of care, and dissemination and diffusion.

Tobacco-Related Research. In its plan and budget proposal for 2003, research on tobacco use and tobacco-related cancers and cancer communication were identified as "extraordinary opportunities for investment"

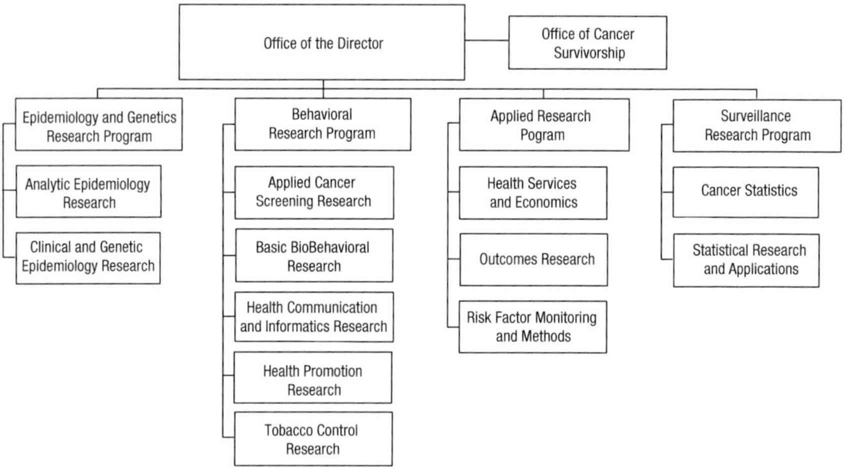

FIGURE 10.3 Organizational chart for NCI's DCCPS.

(http://plan.cancer.gov).[2] In the area of control of tobacco use, a budget increase of $67 million was requested for 2003, with $24 million to be used to develop, test, and disseminate more effective interventions to prevent and treat tobacco use and tobacco-related cancers. Collaborative and interdisciplinary research in this area is being fostered by the Transdisciplinary Tobacco Use Research Centers, launched in 1999 under the joint sponsorship of NCI, the National Institute on Drug Abuse, and the Robert Wood Johnson Foundation (http://www.partnerstturc.com).

A variety of cross-cutting applied research activities are being sponsored through NCI (http://tobaccocontrol.cancer.gov):

- youth prevention and cessation research;
- studies on tobacco use and addiction among women; and
- state and community research and evaluation (http://dccps.nci.nih.gov/TCRB/scrfa.html).

Cancer-Related Communications. NCI has identified cancer-related communications as an "extraordinary opportunity" for investment and has outlined an extensive research agenda to take advantage of the remarkable advances in communication technology and opportunities to improve the

[2] In 1996, NCI began to systematically identify areas in which focused efforts and increased resources could help reduce the burden of cancer. "Extraordinary opportunities" are large-scale, multicomponent initiatives that reflect NCI's highest priorities (Behavioral Research Program, National Cancer Institute, undated).

TABLE 10.2 Distribution of Cancer Control and Population Sciences Grants Funded in FY 2001, by Program

Program	No. of Grants	Funding Amount (dollars)	Percentage of Total DCCPS Grants	Percentage of Total DCCPS Funding
Epidemiology and genetics	378	$180,315,942	52	54
Behavioral research	246	113,466,498	34	34
Applied research	46	24,631,812	6	7
Survivorship research	48	11,478,279	7	3
Surveillance research[a]	15	2,777,382	2	1
Total	733	332,669,913	100	100

[a]DCCPS has a sizable research contracts portfolio that includes the Surveillance, Epidemiology, and End Results Program and rapid response surveillance studies.

public's understanding of cancer-related issues. Among the activities in progress are the following:

- the nationally representative Health Information National Trends Survey to assess the public's access to and use of cancer-related health information;
- research projects to test strategies to increase access to and use of online and other interactive cancer communications by underserved populations;

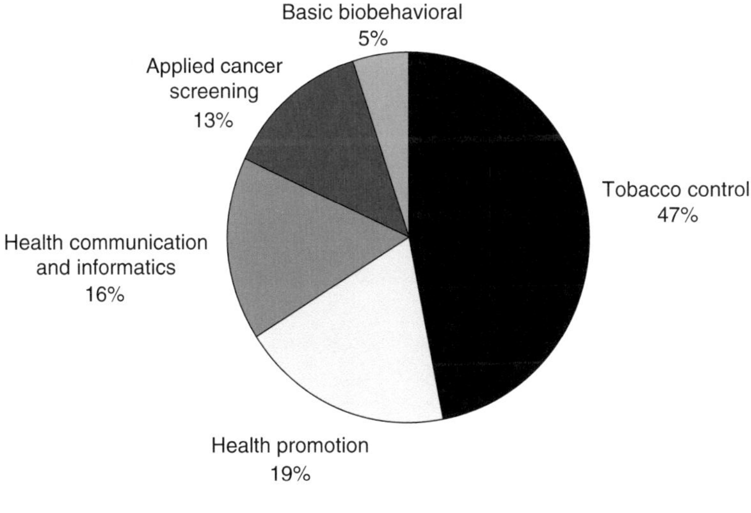

FIGURE 10.4 Distribution of research dollars (not the number of grants) spent in DCCPS behavioral research portfolio, FY 2001 (total amount, $113.5 million).

• studies of innovative strategies for communicating cancer information to diverse populations (e.g., message tailoring);

• creation of Centers of Excellence in Cancer Communications Research (http://cancercontrol.cancer.gov/communicationcenters);

• research on applications of multimedia technology such as smoking and tobacco use cessation interventions, decision-making programs, information products for professionals, innovative alternative teaching methods, and educational and training tools (supported with Small Business Innovation Research and Small Business Technology Transfer grants) (http://cancercontrol.cancer.gov/hcirb/sbir/); and

• a review in collaboration with the Agency for Healthcare Research and Quality (AHRQ) of the research evidence on cancer-related "decision aids," interventions designed to help people make specific and deliberate choices by providing information on options and outcomes specific to a person's health status.

A budget increase of $19.1 million for 2003 was requested to support cancer-related communications.

Reducing Health Disparities. NCI established the Center to Reduce Cancer Health Disparities in December 2000 to direct the implementation of NCI's Strategic Plan to Reduce Health Disparities (Box 10.2) (http://www.cancer.gov/announcements/healthdisp.html). A budget increase of $52.7 million for FY 2003 was requested to support this activity.

NCI has set aside $30 million in a 5-year effort to establish Special Populations Networks for Cancer Awareness, Research, and Training (SPNs).

BOX 10.2 Objectives of NCI Strategic Plan to Reduce Health Disparities

Objective I: Expand the capacity to conduct fundamental cancer control and population research to elucidate the determinants of cancer-related health disparities.

Objective II: Expand the ability to define and monitor cancer-related health disparities.

Objective III: Support intervention research in prevention, early detection, treatment, and communications that may reduce cancer-related health disparities.

Objective IV: Expand the channels for research dissemination and diffusion and foster collaborations with allied agencies and organizations to facilitate the translation of evidence into practice.

Objective V: Strengthen training and education in health disparities research and increase the number of minority scientists working in cancer control science.

SOURCE: The NCI Strategic Plan to Reduce Health Disparities (http://www.cancer.gov/announcements/healthdisp.html).

It is anticipated that SPNs will help create a sustainable infrastructure to promote cancer awareness and the conduct of research and cancer control activities within minority and underserved communities (http://ospr.nci.nih.gov/networks.html). Centers for Population Health and Health Disparities are planned to conduct interdisciplinary research to identify the causes of health disparities and to develop effective interventions to reduce them (http://plan.cancer.gov/). Opportunities for minorities in cancer research are promoted through NCI's Comprehensive Minority Biomedical Branch (http://minorityopportunities.nci.nih.com).

Quality of Care. In 1999, NCI began a 4-year, $16 million project, the Cancer Research Network, to study ways to increase effective cancer prevention and control efforts among enrollees in HMOs. Ten HMOs that are members of the HMO Research Network participate in the project.[3] These HMOs have large integrated health care systems that facilitate research. Projects under way include analyses of the effectiveness of system-wide smoking cessation policies and services, analyses of barriers to cancer screening, and studies of the efficacy of preventive strategies such as mammography and prophylactic mastectomy (http://healthservices.cancer.gov/hmo.html).

NCI is engaged in a number of collaborative research efforts related to quality of care with other federal agencies including the Department of Veterans Affairs, Centers for Medicare and Medicaid Services, and Health Resources and Services Administration.

Dissemination and Diffusion. NCI provides financial support for grant supplements to fund the dissemination of promising intervention programs and products (http://grants1.nih.gov/grants/guide/notice-files/not-ca-02-007.html). Descriptions of NCI's information dissemination activities are provided in Chapter 9 (e.g., the Cancer Information Service).

Cancer Intervention and Surveillance Modeling Network. Another important initiative within NCI is the development of a network of investigators who apply statistical modeling techniques to assess the effects of interventions such as primary prevention, screening, and treatment on population-based cancer trends (http://srab.cancer.gov/cisnet.html). Investigators have evaluated the impacts of population changes in smoking, diet, physical activity, weight status, and use of screening tests on cancer incidence and mortality rates (Eric

---

[3]The HMO Research Network was established in 1996 to create opportunities for researchers to collaborate on multisite projects; to respond to the national imperative to develop more efficient, effective, and high-quality health care delivery systems; and to provide a forum for HMO researchers to discuss methodology and disseminate research findings (www.hmoresearchnetwork.org/about.htm).

Feuer, NCI, Division of Cancer Control and Population Sciences, personal communication to Maria Hewitt, Institute of Medicine, May 18, 2001).

Other Institutes of NIH Other institutes of NIH support some research related to cancer prevention and early detection. Selected projects identified in the RADIUS database are listed below, by institute.

National Institute on Aging

- Cancer prevention videos in a community setting: family and the health of elderly African-American individuals (a pilot project to assess the value of a video intervention on breast cancer knowledge, attitudes, self-concept, and screening behavior)
- Cancer screening guideline adherence for underserved elders (study of barriers to regular ongoing participation in screening mammography and tests of nurse-based community outreach).

National Institute of Nursing Research

- Perceived risk of inherited susceptibility to cancer
- Factors associated with colorectal cancer screening (examination of the relationship of selected predisposing, reinforcing, and enabling factors on stages of adoption of screening)
- Wellness Circles—An American Indian Approach (randomized trial of a "Wellness Talking Circle" intervention among clinics for American Indians in rural California).

National Institute on Drug Abuse

- Cancer risk and preventive health for marijuana users
- Dietary interventions in African-American and Hispanic women
- Prevention of cigarette smoking in youth with attention deficit and hyperactivity disorder.

National Human Genome Research Institute

- Counseling strategies for women at risk of breast cancer (evaluation of different strategies for counseling female relatives of women with breast cancer)
- Psychosocial aspects of genetic testing for hereditary nonpolyposis colon cancer
- Beliefs and attitudes toward hereditary prostate cancer
- Psychosocial risks of gene tests for colon cancer
- History of breast cancer risk, 1900 to present

• Outcomes of education and counseling for testing for mutations in *BRCA1* and *BRCA2* genes.

Centers for Disease Control and Prevention

Much of the cancer-related prevention research supported by the Centers for Disease Control and Prevention (CDC) is funded through the National Center for Chronic Disease Prevention and Health, Division of Cancer Prevention and Control. The division plans and conducts epidemiological studies and evaluations to identify the feasibility and effectiveness of cancer prevention and control strategies. Other activities include the provision of technical assistance to states, local public health agencies, and other health care provider organizations. Research activities can be difficult to distinguish from programmatic activities because research and evaluation are often integrated into educational and service-related activities.

In 2001, chronic disease prevention and health promotion activities (administrative, programmatic, and research activities) received 17.8 percent of CDC's total appropriation ($749.8 million of $4,202.2 million). Cancer prevention and control activities made up the largest single unit within the chronic disease prevention and health promotion area, receiving one-third of total CDC support for chronic disease prevention and health promotion ($245.3 million of $749.8 million). The National Breast and Cervical Cancer Early Detection Program is administered within the chronic disease prevention and health promotion budget. Activities related to cancer (e.g., tobacco use, nutrition, physical activity and obesity, health promotion, youth media campaign, and prevention centers) made up a large share of the chronic disease prevention and health promotion budget (Table 10.3).

Several cooperative agreements are being supported to address the focus area of cancer described in *Healthy People 2010* (US DHHS and Office of Disease Prevention and Health Promotion, 2000):

• *Physical activity.* As part of its National Youth Media Campaign, CDC provided approximately $625,000 in FY 2001 to national health, education, and social services organizations to promote healthy physical activity among youth ages 9 to 13, their parents and other primary caregivers, and others who can influence preteens (e.g., teachers and coaches). Each funded organization is obliged to evaluate its own program. Another effort to promote physical activity is the cooperative agreement program, Redesigning Cities and Suburbs for Public Health. One award of approximately $100,000 was granted in FY 2001 to plan and evaluate projects that attempt to create healthier communities through better design and use of buildings and the natural environment or through policies and practices related to physical activity (e.g., urbanization, transportation, business location, employment, education, and recreation) (www. cdc.gov/od/pgo/funding/01121.htm).

TABLE 10.3 Centers for Disease Control and Prevention FY 2001 Appropriation

Budget Activity	Funding Amount (in thousands of dollars)	Percentage of Total
Total	$4,202,180	100.0
Chronic disease prevention and health promotion	749,773	17.8
Preventive health and health services block grant	135,030	3.2
Chronic disease prevention and health promotion	749,773	100.0
Cancer prevention and control	245,340	32.7
Youth media campaign	125,000	16.7
Tobacco	101,971	13.6
School health	58,467	7.8
Diabetes	57,715	7.7
Safe motherhood and infant health	51,000	6.8
Heart disease and stroke	34,702	4.6
Prevention centers	23,132	3.1
Arthritis and other chronic diseases	17,188	2.3
Nutrition, physical activity, and obesity	15,997	2.1
Health promotion	10,083	1.3
Oral health	9,178	1.2

SOURCE: www.cdc.gov/fmo/fmogybudget.htm, accessed July 2, 2001.

- *Cancer screening.* Approximately $2.9 million was made available in FY 2001 to support research on interventions to improve rates of screening for breast and cervical cancer, colorectal cancer, and prostate cancer. Interventions targeted for research included those applied in communities or health care systems (e.g., through the media, individual and small group education, incentives, reminders, laws, screening in nonclinical settings, and reimbursement policies) and those aimed at health care providers (e.g., incentives, reminders, checklists, and assessment and feedback). Researchers are encouraged to assess the effects of multicomponent interventions (www.cdc.gov/of/pgo/funding/01099.htm).
- *Racial and ethnic health disparities.* CDC awarded $9.4 million to 32 community coalitions in 18 states to help address racial and ethnic disparities in health. The demonstration projects, called Racial and Ethnic Approaches to Community Health (REACH 2010), target six health priority areas including cancer (www.raceandhealth.hhs.gov/sidebars/sbwhats1.htm). Targeted populations include African Americans, American Indians, Alaska Natives, Hispanic Americans, Asian Americans, and Pacific Islanders. Five of the 32 REACH 2010 projects funded will focus on breast and cervical cancer (www.raceandhealth.hhs.gov).
- *Comprehensive cancer control plans and their implementation.* Since 1994, CDC has encouraged the development of comprehensive state plans

and their implementation as an approach to address the lack of coordination and collaboration across cancer control programs (see Chapter 9). CDC defines comprehensive cancer control as an integrated and coordinated approach to reduce the rates of cancer incidence, morbidity, and mortality through prevention, early detection, treatment, rehabilitation, and palliation. The six building blocks for comprehensive control planning identified by CDC include (1) assessing and addressing the cancer burden, (2) using data and research, (3) mobilizing support, (4) building partnerships, (5) enhancing the infrastructure, and (6) conducting evaluation. As of 2001, 13 states re-ported having a current comprehensive cancer control plan, 14 states were creating their first plan or were updating an old plan, and 23 states had no plan or had an outdated plan with no plans to revise it.

• *Community health programs.* A $4.4 million grant program administered in FY 2001 supports seven community-based health programs, for example, the Center for Chronic Disease in the Baltimore City Health Department (www.cdc.gov/od/pgo/funding/01052.hrm).

Educational and community-based programs are also supported through CDC's Health Promotion and Disease Prevention Research Centers. These programs focus on the major causes of death and disability, including cancer, and attempt to improve public health practice within communities and promote more effective state and local public health programs (http://www.cdc.gov/od/pgo/funding/01101.htm, accessed May 22, 2001).

Partnering with Employers for Prevention General Motors (GM) has formed a partnership with CDC to increase the use of priority clinical prevention services among employees, improve overall health status, increase worker productivity, and ultimately, decrease health care costs. GM is the largest private provider of health insurance in the United States, with 1.25 million enrollees. GM contracts with more than 120 HMOs, 80 fee-for-service (FFS) carriers, and with an equal number of preferred provider organizations. As part of the Partnering with Employers for Prevention initiative, health claims have been linked to personnel data to identify potential barriers to cancer screening tests. Initial findings showed that hourly employees in FFS plans were underutilizing screening services, probably because they did not have office visits as a covered benefit (Friedman, C, Sixth Annual HMO Research Network Conference, 2000).

The U.S. Department of Health and Human Services (DHHS) recently announced "microgrants" to community organizations for activities that support the goals of *Healthy People 2010* (US DHHS and Office of Disease Prevention and Health Promotion, 2000). The grants aim to foster effective prevention efforts at the community level. The 2-year pilot program will commit a total of between $500,000 and $700,000 in funding, and each grant will be worth up to $2,010. If the pilot phase is successful, the plans will be expanded nationally (www.hhs.gov/news/press/2001pres/20010716.html).

Agency for Healthcare Research and Quality

AHRQ is the lead agency within DHHS charged with supporting research on health care quality, outcomes, cost, utilization, and access. The agency supports intramural research as well as an extramural grants program with a budget of $269.9 million (FY 2001 appropriation) (www.ahrq.gov). Nearly 80 percent of AHRQ's budget is awarded as grants and contracts to researchers at universities and other research institutions. Support for intramural and extramural cancer-related health services research grants active since FY 1999 totals $5.2 million, roughly $1.7 million per year. An additional $650,000 was awarded to support the update of the smoking cessation guideline (FYs 1998 to 2001), nearly $1 million in contracts was awarded to support evidence-based practice reports (FYs 1999 to 2001), and $1 million in contracts was awarded in support of the U.S. Preventive Services Task Force (FYs 1999 to 2001) (Wendy Perry, Agency for Health Care Policy and Research [AHCPR], personal communication to Maria Hewitt, Institute of Medicine, August 7, 2001).

Ongoing extramural research grants supported by AHCPR active since FY 1999 are listed in Table 10.4.

Evidence-Based Practice Centers AHRQ's 13 Evidence-Based Practice Centers conduct systematic, comprehensive analyses and syntheses of the scientific literature to develop evidence-based reports and technology assessments on clinical topics that are common and expensive and that present challenges to decision makers (www.ahcpr.gov/clinic/epc11.htm). Since December 1998, more than 30 evidence-based reports have been released. Cancer-related topics have included modification of dietary behavior related to cancer risk, cervical cytology, advanced prostate cancer, and management of pain associated with cancer (www.ahrq.gov/about/ahrqfact.htm). Forthcoming analyses will include assessments of the impact of cancer-related decision aids and the diffusion and dissemination of evidence-based cancer-related information, both of which will be funded by NCI (W. Perry, personal communication to Maria Hewitt, August 3, 2001).

National Guideline Clearinghouse AHRQ no longer develops treatment guidelines, but in 2000 it served as part of a consortium of seven federal government and nonprofit organizations that issued guidelines published by the U.S. Public Health Service, *Treating Tobacco Use and Dependence,* an update of a 1996 Agency for Health Care Policy and Research clinical practice guideline on smoking cessation (US DHHS, 2000a). AHRQ

TABLE 10.4 AHRQ-Supported Research Grants, FYs 1999 to 2001

Grant	Description	Level of Support (dollars)
Racial and ethnic variations in medical interactions	Assessment of contribution of doctor-patient communication to variations in the use of medical services including breast cancer screening	62,826
Cancer—reaching medically underserved populations	Support of conference and information dissemination on literacy and cultural barriers that affect cancer prevention and treatment in minority and medically underserved populations	31,000
Understanding and reducing native elder health disparities	Interventions to improve participation in clinical prevention services, including cancer detection and smoking cessation	171,956
Health disparities in minority adult Americans	Interventions to improve use of prevention services including a study of patient provider communication regarding cancer screening	149,614
University of California at Los Angeles/Charles R. Drew University of Medicine and Science/RAND program to address disparities in health	Assessments of barriers to effective care including missed opportunities for colon cancer detection among African Americans	52,362
Promoting effective communication and decision making in diverse populations	Development of decision-making tools, including those for cancer screening, taking into account perception of risk and using different ways to convey risk and benefit	252,145
Dissemination of a quit smoking program	Assessment of program adoption including staff perceptions, organizational support, coverage, and factors associated with success	84,526
Rural emergency department as access point for teen smoking intervention	Randomized controlled trial of an intervention to help a low-income teen population quit smoking	340,069
Smoking control in maternal and child health clinics: dissemination strategies	Randomized study to test effectiveness of a centralized counseling service and academic detailing	637,805
Practice profiling to increase rates of tobacco use cessation	Randomized controlled trial of effectiveness of personalized data feedback on physician performance	351,932
A trial of two decision aids for colon cancer screening	Randomized controlled trial pilot study to compare decision-making aids on the process and outcome of decision making	52,409

TABLE 10.4 continued

Grant	Description	Level of Support (dollars)
A two-stage model for colorectal cancer screening	Study of physician recommendations and communication, patient barriers, and patient decision making	70,245
Understanding variability in community mammography	Assessment of factors associated with variability in radiologists' interpretations of mammograms	768,484
Mammography and detection, controlled estimation	Analysis of underlying causes of false-positive and false-negative mammograms	66,537
The efficacy of colposcopy by telemedicine	Intervention to improve follow-up of minority rural women with abnormal Pap test results	560,676
Shared decision making, prostate cancer screening by couples	Randomized controlled trial of a computerized, interactive decision-making tool tailored for high-risk individuals (African-American men)	462,452
Prostate cancer detection, treatment, and outcomes in two Surveillance, Epidemiology, and End Results Program areas: A natural experiment	Assessment of effect of prostate-specific antigen screening and treatment among Medicare beneficiaries in two geographic areas with different practice patterns	357,619
Translating prevention research into practice	Randomized trial comparing a nursing intervention with physician reminders to improve prevention services (including cancer screening) in a low-income population	643,021
Cancer patients' attitudes toward cancer trials	Assessment of positive and negative attitudes toward cancer trials with a focus on prevention trials	32,296
Health communication over the Internet	Development of an electronic Web-based intervention to improve informed decision making for colorectal cancer screening	100,858

SOURCE: Wendy Perry, AHCPR, personal communication to Maria Hewitt, Institute of Medicine, August 3, 2001.

issued a technical review of colorectal cancer screening in 1998 (www.ahrq.gov). In addition, AHRQ, in collaboration with the American Medical Association and the American Association of Health Plans, has developed a National Guideline Clearinghouse accessible on the Internet (www.guideline.gov). The Website contains information on available guidelines, permits comparisons of the recommendations found in various guidelines, and facilitates communication among those involved in guideline development and dissemination. As of mid-2001, 289 guidelines were related to cancer, and 179 of those were accessed by use of "cancer and prevention" (www.guideline.gov).

CONQUEST CONQUEST (Computerized Needs-Oriented Quality Measurement Evaluation System) is a database of performance measures (conditions, diseases, and procedures), measure sets (measures with a common purpose and developer), and conditions (with detailed epidemiological information). CONQUEST includes measures related to the management of several cancers (i.e., colorectal, lung, prostate, and breast cancer), the use of screening tests (i.e., mammography and Pap smear), and cigarette use.

U.S. Preventive Services Task Force and Put Prevention into Practice Since the 1980s, the U.S. Preventive Services Task Force (USPSTF) has evaluated scientific evidence for the effectiveness of clinical prevention services (e.g., screening tests, counseling, immunization, and chemoprophylaxis) and produced age- and risk factor-specific recommendations for the services that should be included in a periodic health examination. The USPSTF *Guide to Clinical Preventive Services* (2nd edition) was published in 1996 (U.S. Preventive Services Task Force, 1996). The work of USPSTF is supported by the AHRQ Evidence-Based Practice Centers. An evidence-based review on screening for skin cancer was published in 2001 (U.S. Preventive Services Task Force, 2001b). Put Prevention into Practice is designed to help implement the recommendations of USPSTF. Roughly 20 percent of the services considered by USPSTF and Put Prevention into Practice relate to cancer detection or prevention.

Translating Research into Practice AHRQ funds translational research and demonstrations through Translating Research into Practice (TRIP). The first round (TRIP-I) supported 14 studies that addressed a variety of health care problems, primarily through randomized controlled trials. Two TRIP-I projects were related to cancer prevention and early detection: (1) practice profiling to increase rates of tobacco cessation and (2) dissemination strategies for smoking control programs in maternal and child health clinics. Building on earlier initiatives, TRIP-II is aimed at applying and assessing strategies and methods that were developed in idealized practice settings or that are in current use but that have not been previously or rigorously evaluated. TRIP-II focuses on implementation techniques and factors—such as organizational and clinical characteristics—associated with the successful translation of research findings into diverse applied settings. Two TRIP-II projects are related to cancer prevention and early detection: (1) implementation of adolescent preventive guidelines and (2) translation of prevention research into practice (www.ahrq.gov/research/trip2fac.htm).

Office of Priority Populations AHRQ established the Office of Priority Populations to ensure that the needs of special populations are addressed throughout AHRQ's intramural and extramural research portfolio. Beginning in FY 2003, AHRQ will release an annual report on prevailing disparities in health care delivery as it relates to selected priority populations (e.g., low-income groups, minorities, women, children, elderly individuals, and individuals with special heath care needs) (www.ahrq/about/profile.htm).

Quality Interagency Coordination Task Force The Quality Interagency Coordination (QuIC) Task Force was established in response to the final report of the President's Advisory Commission on Consumer Protection and Quality in the Health Care Industry (1998). QuIC's goal is to ensure that all federal agencies involved in purchasing, providing, researching, or regulating health care services are working in a coordinated way toward the common goal of improving quality of care. AHRQ coordinates QuIC activities for the 12 federal agencies that comprise this task force (www.ahrq.gov).

Intramural Research Projects Some of the research conducted by AHRQ staff concerns cancer-related prevention services (e.g., variations in preventive service use among insured and uninsured individuals).

Centers for Medicare and Medicaid Services (formerly the Health Care Financing Administration)

The Office of Strategic Planning of the Centers for Medicare and Medicaid Services (CMS) oversees a research and demonstration program that supports projects to develop, test, and implement new health care financing and payment policies and to evaluate the impacts of CMS's programs on its beneficiaries, providers, states, and other customers and partners (www.hcfa.gov/research). Many of CMS's extramural research and demonstration activities are funded through contracts, but CMS does award grants and cooperative agreements under several focused grants programs.

The following are some active CMS-supported research and demonstration projects related to cancer prevention and early detection (Health Care Financing Administration, 2001):

- Study on expansion or modification of preventive benefits provided to Medicare beneficiaries (included skin cancer screening) ($1,333,656, September 1998–February 2000)
- Researching and identifying the most effective provider education efforts for encouraging the use of Medicare prevention services ($325,812, September 1999–September 2000)

- Survey of colorectal cancer screening practices in health care organizations ($816,642, September 1998–July 2001)
- Medicare quality monitoring system (measuring the effectiveness of peer review organizations' Health Care Quality Improvement Project that includes activities focused on breast cancer) ($1,173,065, September 2000–January 2001)
- Provision of early and periodic screening, diagnosis, and treatment services in state Medicaid plans and Medicaid managed care contracts ($49,241, August 1999–January 2001)
- Utilization of health care services related to cancer prevention for women in the Medicaid program ($233,440, September 2000–September 2001)
- Mauli Ola (Spirit of Life) Project, an outreach and preventive health demonstration project targeted to native Hawaiians ($704,055, September 2000–September 2005)
- Community health advocate program, which uses lay health workers to reach vulnerable populations (general focus, not specific to cancer) ($500,000, August 2000–July 2002)
- Health Promotion in the African-American Community, a computer-based nutrition program ($120,754, September 2000–September 2001)
- Increasing breast cancer screening in African-American women, a community pilot project ($124,990, September 2000–September 2001)
- Cervical and breast cancer screening for post-reproductive-age Hispanic women residing near the U.S.-Mexico border ($263,281, September 2000–September 2001)
- A systematic approach to improving Pap smear screening rates among Hispanic and Latino women in managed Medicaid systems ($124,450, September 2000–September 2001)

As part of CMS's Healthy Aging Initiative, a literature review has been completed of the evidence of the effectiveness of prevention services (e.g., screening and smoking cessation programs) in the Medicare population. In addition, a demonstration program is in progress to test the effects of various benefit enhancements on smoking cessation. The three benefit options being compared with usual care (smoking cessation information) in the seven-state Medicare Stop Smoking Program are (www.hcfa.gov/healthyaging/1b.htm):

1. reimbursement for provider counseling only,
2. reimbursement for provider counseling and Food and Drug Administration-approved prescription or nicotine replacement pharmacotherapy, and
3. a telephone counseling quit line and reimbursement for nicotine replacement therapy.

The program began in 2001 and is expected to be completed in 2003.

Much of CMS's quality improvement work is carried out by its national network of 53 Quality Improvement Organizations (see Chapter 9 for a description of efforts to improve the use of mammography screening).

U.S. Department of Defense

The U.S. Department of Defense (DoD) administers extramural grant programs for research related to cancer of the breast, prostate, and ovary through the U.S. Army Medical Research and Materiel Command office of the Congressionally Directed Medical Research Programs (CDMRP) (Table 10.5). CDMRP strives to identify gaps in funding and provide award opportunities that will enhance program research objectives without duplicating existing funding opportunities. Funding is available for research, infrastructure, and training. A Special Populations Program was established in FY 1998 to help boost the participation of minority scientists and to support research on health disparities within the other programs of CDMRP.

Very few awards available through CDMRP support prevention-related translational research. In FYs 1999 and 2000, 5 of 584 research awards were for breast cancer-related health services research (http://cdmrp.army.mil):

1. factors affecting African-American women's participation in screening,
2. remote patient management for screening mammography in underserved areas,
3. screening of older, disadvantaged women,
4. mammography follow-up of women ages 40 to 49, and
5. exercise and breast cancer prevention.

TABLE 10.5 Congressionally Directed Medical Research Programs of the U.S. Department of Defense

	Appropriations (in millions of dollars)[a]		Number of Awards	
Research Area	Pre-FY 2000[b]	FY 2001	Pre-FY 2000[b]	FY 2000
Breast cancer	$1,043	$174	2,290	553
Prostate cancer	$210	$100	297	140
Issues pertinent to military forces	$44.5	$50.0	16	14

[a]Additional funds ($3.1 million as of FY 2001) are available for breast cancer research through the sales of the breast cancer postage stamp.

[b]Funding for prostate cancer research began in 1997. Funding for the Peer-Reviewed Medical Research Program to promote research on issues pertinent to the military forces began in 1999.

SOURCE: http://cdmrp.army.mil.

In FYs 1999 and 2000, 6 of 185 research awards were for prostate cancer-related health services research (http://cdmrp.army.mil):

1. screening among African-American men,
2. informed consent for prostate-specific antigen testing,
3. utility assessment for prostate cancer screening among African-American men,
4. tracking system to improve screening and follow-up,
5. changing attitudes and behaviors of African-American men for screening for prostate cancer, and
6. pharmacists as health educators and risk communicators in the prevention of prostate cancer.

Smoking cessation is 1 of 18 prioritized areas of the DoD Peer-Reviewed Medical Research Program, but only one award for smoking cessation research has been made since the program's inception in 1999. The funded program aimed to develop a model DoD smoking cessation program.

U.S. Department of Veterans Affairs

The U.S. Department of Veterans Affairs (VA) Office of Research and Development had a FY 2001 budget of $351 million and supports intramural biomedical, rehabilitation, and health services research (Veterans Administration, Office of Research and Development, 2000). Health services research focuses on conditions that are common among veterans, including cancer (especially prostate and lung cancer). Much of the VA's health services research is carried out in its 12 Centers of Excellence. Each center was contacted regarding its cancer prevention and early detection research. Table 10.6 describes the VA-funded prevention research carried out at some of these centers.

In 1998, the VA launched its Quality Enhancement Research Initiative (QUERI) to provide a systematic approach to quality improvement. Eight clinical areas were initially targeted that were of particular significance to veterans (i.e., chronic heart failure, diabetes, human immunodeficiency virus infection and AIDS, ischemic heart disease, mental health, spinal cord injury, stroke, and substance abuse), and subsequently, health services research was funded in these areas (Veterans Administration Office of Research and Development, Health Services Research and Development Service, 2000). In 2001, a Cancer QUERI Center was established with support from NCI (Veterans Administration Office of Research and Development, Health Services Research and Development Service, 2001).

The VA's Cooperative Studies Program (CSP) is a large multicenter clinical trial program that determines the effectiveness of interventions. A

TABLE 10.6 VA-Supported Cancer Prevention and Early Detection Research at VA Centers of Excellence

VA Center of Excellence	Research Activity in Prevention and Early Detection
1. Center for Health Services Research in Primary Care	• Cost utility analysis of alternative strategies for screening for colorectal cancer • Identification of factors prognostic of late-stage disease, particularly those that are modifiable
2. Center for the Study of Health Disparities	• Barriers and facilitators for colorectal cancer screening in VA and non-VA settings
3. Center for the Study of Health Care Provider Behavior	• Smoking cessation, prevention in the elderly, exercise
4. Houston Center for Quality of Care and Utilization Studies	• Barriers to colorectal screening • Hepatitis C screening and surveillance patterns

recent CSP trial demonstrated that colonoscopy may be the best method of screening for colon cancer for asymptomatic individuals.

Privately Sponsored Research

American Cancer Society

The American Cancer Society (ACS) is the largest private, not-for-profit source of funds for cancer research in the United States ($97.3 million in FY 1999–2000) (www2.cancer.org). ACS focuses its research spending on beginning investigators and a program of targeted research, and in recent years it has enhanced its commitment to psychosocial and behavioral, health services, health policy, epidemiological, clinical, and cancer control research. In response to identified needs in clinical oncology, ACS also sponsors grants in support of training for health care professionals seeking to develop their clinical expertise or their ability to conduct independent research. (Training and educational support are described in Chapter 8.) ACS prioritizes investigator-initiated proposals and funds proposals by a peer-review process.

In FYs 1999 to 2000, relatively little ACS research funding was devoted to prevention (14 percent) and detection (15 percent) relative to that devoted to the causes or etiology of cancer (70 percent) or cancer treatment (33 percent) (Table 10.7).

TABLE 10.7 ACS Research Funding (Intramural and Extramural), FYs 1999 to 2000

Area of Research	Amount Awarded (dollars)	Percentage of Total[a]
Total	$97,299,000	100
Prevention	13,675,000	14
Detection	14,272,000	15
Treatment	31,784,000	33
Causes and etiology	68,411,000	70
Psychosocial and behavioral	11,473,000	12
Poor and underserved populations	7,711,000	8

[a]Categories are not mutually exclusive (e.g., a grant that is related to both prevention and detection is counted twice). Dollar amounts are rounded off to the nearest $1,000.
SOURCE: www2.cancer.org.

Robert Wood Johnson Foundation

As part of its philanthropic activities the Robert Wood Johnson Foundation (RWJF) has prioritized reducing the harm caused by substance abuse including tobacco, alcohol, and illicit drugs. In 2000, RWJF provided $83.4 million in support for initiatives related to that priority, with roughly $33 million in support provided for smoking and tobacco use cessation-related research (Julie Painter, proposal management associate, RWJF, personal communication to Maria Hewitt, Institute of Medicine, July 7, 2001). The following were among the projects related to smoking and tobacco use control funded by RWJF(www.rwjf.org):

- Addressing Tobacco in Managed Care is a program that promotes the integration of effective smoking cessation interventions into the basic health care provided by managed care organizations. RWJF makes available grants for studies that evaluate the effectiveness of replicable organizational strategies that lead health care providers, practices, and plans to adopt and adhere to the recommendations of the AHCPR Smoking Cessation Clinical Practice Guideline. Projects funded under this initiative examine the impacts of organizational strategies (including clinical, financial, and administrative practices) on such outcomes as smoker identification, tobacco use reduction among patients, rates of clinician intervention, and costs of intervention efforts.
- National Center for Tobacco-Free Kids is a program that supports a national campaign to reduce youth tobacco use through the establishment of a center that develops a national strategy, serves as a media center, provides technical assistance, and broadens organizational support to reduce youth tobacco use.

• Partners with Tobacco Use Research Centers, Advancing Transdisciplinary Science and Policy Studies, provides support for an NCI-National Institute on Drug Abuse program to apply and integrate advances in molecular biology, neuroscience, genetics, and behavioral science to the challenge of tobacco use control. RWJF funds dissemination and policy research and analysis efforts and supports efforts to communicate scientific breakthroughs in language that policy makers, the public, and the media can understand.

• Research Network on the Etiology of Tobacco Dependence is a program that brings together leading researchers from a variety of perspectives and disciplines to work collaboratively in the study of the etiology of tobacco dependence.

• Smoke-Free Families: Innovations to Stop Smoking During and Beyond Pregnancy uses a multicomponent strategy to improve current clinical practice and advance the smoking and tobacco use cessation field into the next generation of smoking cessation techniques for childbearing women.

• Smokeless States: National Tobacco Policy Initiative is a program that supports the development and implementation of comprehensive statewide strategies to reduce tobacco use through education, treatment, and policy initiatives.

The American Legacy Foundation

The American Legacy Foundation is a national, independent, public health foundation established to reduce tobacco use in the United States (www.americanlegacy.org). The Foundation is supported with funds from tobacco manufacturers as dictated by the 1998 Tobacco Master Settlement Agreement. Through this agreement, a coalition of 46 state attorneys general successfully reached agreement with tobacco companies, which will pay $206 billion over 25 years. As outlined in the 1998 Tobacco Master Settlement Agreement, the Foundation supports educational programs and research to (1) reduce tobacco product use by youth and (2) prevent diseases associated with the use of tobacco products.

In early December 2001, Legacy launched its "Great Start" educational, counseling and marketing campaign to help pregnant women quit smoking. The foundation has budgeted $7.5 million to run and promote this initiative. American Legacy Foundation funds a national grants program with an annual budget of approximately $30 million which provides support for state and local tobacco use prevention, education, and cessation programs and provides small grants to fund innovative approaches and programs to reduce or eliminate tobacco use. Legacy is addressing disparities in access to tobacco cessation and prevention service among various ethnic and cultural groups through its Priority Populations Initiative. This program is providing $21 million over three years to support capacity-building grants, innovative projects, and applied research grants. Legacy has also provided over $200 million over the last two years to support a major tobacco use prevention and education advertising campaign targeted at young people, called truth[sm] (Christine Fritz, Accounting Manager, American Legacy Foundation, personal communication to Maria Hewitt, Institute of Medicine, February 11, 2002).

Several other selected large foundations support cancer prevention and early detection research and dissemination activities (Table 10.8).

The Cochrane Collaboration

The Cochrane Collaboration is an international nonprofit organization that "aims to help people make informed decisions about health care, by reviewing and promoting the best available evidence on the effects of interventions and treatments" (www.cochraneconsumer.com). Review groups, organized by area of health care (e.g., breast cancer and tobacco addiction), conduct systematic reviews of evidence, emphasizing results from published

TABLE 10.8 Other Selected Foundations Supporting Cancer Prevention and Early Detection Research

Foundation[a]	Total Amount Given (dollars)	Priority Area(s)	Type of Support
American Institute for Cancer Research	$4,924,212	Diet, nutrition, and cancer	Collaborative research grants, investigator-initiated grants, matching grants, postdoctoral grant awards
Federated Department Stores Foundation	11,513,341	Breast cancer	Local agency support to develop projects that affect their communities
General Mills Foundation	15,009,937	Health and nutrition	Promotion of healthy lifestyles in underserved communities
Susan G. Komen Breast Cancer Foundation	23,497,426	Breast cancer	Basic, clinical, and translational research; fellowships; professorships
Metropolitan Life Foundation	13,186,931	Health education	National programs aimed at youth
Robertson Foundation	5,410,959	Cancer	Organizational unrestricted support

[a]The foundations listed are those included in the Foundation Center database that (1) gave total amounts in excess of $4 million in the most recent year for which data were available, (2) listed a focus on cancer prevention or a cancer-related risk factor (e.g., diet, nutrition, or smoking), and (3) did not restrict their support to one or a few local areas or states.

SOURCE: Foundation Center, www.fconline.fdncenter.org, accessed May 2001.

and unpublished randomized clinical trials. Available evidence is reviewed systematically (www.canet.org/rationale.htm) by:

- using an explicit, detailed search strategy to find as many reports of relevant trials as possible;
- carrying out the review according to a written protocol;
- using explicit prespecified inclusion and exclusion criteria;
- using standard methods to assess trial quality;
- employing two people to independently extract the data;
- analyzing by synthesis of the actual numerical results, where possible (a technique known as meta-analysis); and
- presenting the review in a detailed, clear, and transparent fashion so that readers can see how conclusions were reached.

Since 1996, the Cochrane Cancer Network (www.canet.org) has coordinated the work of cancer site-specific groups. Systematic reviews included in the Cochrane Library and relevant to cancer prevention and early detection are listed in Box 10.3.

The Cochrane Cancer Network is developing a specialized database for cancer, the Cancer Library, which will serve as a comprehensive source of information about cancer for consumer groups and other members of the cancer community (www.update-software.com/cancer/about-cancer.html).

Translational Research Models

A hallmark of translational cancer prevention and control research is its interdisciplinary nature and potential for broad application to the practices of individuals, clinicians, educators, social service providers, and community-based programs. An ideal research program would therefore reflect this wide scope and crosscutting nature of the practice of cancer prevention and early detection.

Collaborative and interdisciplinary research are supported by several mechanisms. Transdisciplinary Tobacco Use Research Centers (TTURCs), for example, jointly sponsored by NCI and the National Institute on Drug Abuse, involve researchers with a wide range of perspectives to aid further understanding of tobacco use and nicotine addiction. These novel centers are designed to bridge disciplinary barriers, establish new conceptual frameworks and methods to understand and treat tobacco use, speed the transfer of innovative approaches to communities nationwide, and create a core of new tobacco control researchers (http://www.partnerstturc.com). The affiliated Partners program is funded by the Robert Wood Johnson Foundation to support tobacco-related policy research and communications activities at the funded TTURCs (http://www.partnerstturc.com/overview/index.htm).

BOX 10.3 Cochrane Reviews Related to Cancer Prevention and Early Detection

Breast cancer
- Strategies for increasing participation of women in community breast cancer screening
- Screening for breast cancer with mammography

Colorectal cancer
- Screening for colorectal cancer by the fecal occult blood test (Hemoccult)

Gynecological cancer
- Interventions for encouraging sexual lifestyles and behaviors intended to prevent cervical cancer

Tobacco addiction
- Acupuncture for smoking cessation
- Antidepressants for smoking cessation
- Anxiolytics for smoking cessation
- Aversive smoking therapy for smoking cessation
- Clonidine for smoking cessation
- Community interventions for prevention of smoking in young people
- Exercise interventions for smoking cessation
- Group behavior therapy programs for smoking cessation
- Hypnotherapy for smoking cessation
- Individual behavioral counseling for smoking cessation
- Interventions for prevention of smoking in public places
- Interventions for prevention of tobacco sales to minors
- Interventions for smoking cessation in hospitalized patients
- Lobeline for smoking cessation
- Mass media interventions for prevention of smoking in young people
- Mecamylamine (a nicotine antagonist) for smoking cessation
- Nicotine replacement therapy for smoking cessation
- Nursing interventions for smoking cessation
- Physician advice for smoking cessation
- Self-help interventions for smoking cessation
- Silver acetate for smoking cessation
- Telephone counseling for smoking cessation
- Training health professionals in smoking cessation

SOURCE: www.update-software.com, accessed June 28, 2001.

Other interesting models for the conduct of translational research can be found in the areas of diabetes and mental health. Translational research for the prevention and control of diabetes is being supported through a public-private collaboration of the National Institute of Diabetes and Digestive and Kidney Diseases, the National Eye Institute, the National Institute of Nursing Research, and the American Diabetes Association (http://grants.nih.gov/grants/guide/pa-files/PA-01-069.htm). The purpose of the program is to learn more about how to translate recent advances in the prevention and treatment of diabetes into clinical practice for individuals and communities at risk. Targets for funding are studies that will develop and test improved methods of delivery of health care to patients with or at risk of diabetes as well as cost-effective community-based strategies to promote healthy lifestyles that will reduce the risk of diabetes and obesity. The program is based on the principle that strategies are needed to achieve objectives that have already been proved to be beneficial or to enhance behaviors that are expected to improve health outcomes. Of particular interest also are interventions that focus on the translation of new advances into practice for underserved and minority populations. Research is supported through the NIH research demonstration and dissemination project award mechanism (R18 grants). This mechanism is designed to support the testing and evaluation of interventions and activities that lead to the application of existing knowledge to disease control and prevention. Awards are made for up to 5 years.

Translational Research Centers in Behavioral Science (TRCBSs) are being supported by the National Institute of Mental Health to "transcend the barriers of disciplines, research settings, and institutions in order to harness the full range of modern behavioral science to the service of the nation's critical mental health needs" (http://grants.nih.gov/grants/guide/pa_files/PAR-01-027.html). A TRCBS is funded through the NIH Center Grant mechanism (P50 grants), which provides support for multidisciplinary and multi-investigator approaches to the investigation of specific and complex research problems requiring the application of diverse expertise and methodologies. Support is available for periods of up to 5 years, followed by a competitive renewal application for a second 5-year period. TRCBSs are expected to be organized around a specific and focused set of hypotheses, in which one or more areas of basic behavioral science are applied to clinical issues in mental disorders or mental health services delivery.

SUMMARY

The major government sponsors of cancer prevention and early detection translational research are the National Cancer Institute, the Agency for Healthcare Research and Quality, and the Centers for Disease Control and Prevention. Private sponsors making significant contributions to research include the ACS and, for smoking-related research, the Robert Wood Johnson Foundation and the American Legacy Foundation.

When it could be ascertained, the share of total research spending devoted to cancer prevention and early detection is relatively low: 12 percent at the National Cancer Institute (this estimate includes the entire spectrum of cancer prevention and control), roughly 12 percent at the Centers for Disease Control and Prevention ($500 million of $4,202 million),[4] and 14 percent at the ACS. A very limited cancer prevention research portfolio exists within the U.S. Department of Defense's Congressionally Directed Medical Research Programs.

The spectrum of cancer prevention and research activity appears to be wide, but notably absent was much applied cancer-related research related to obesity and physical activity. More research in this area is needed in light of the emergence of an epidemic of obesity in the United States. Specific recommendations for research are outlined in Chapter 11.

[4]This estimate includes the following chronic disease prevention and health promotion areas: cancer prevention and control; tobacco; nutrition, physical activity, and obesity; health promotion; and the youth media Campaign (see Table 10.3).

11

Findings, Policy Implications, and Recommendations

The nation needs new strategies to prevent cancer and, when cancer occurs, to catch it at its earliest stages. The failure to implement proven methods of cancer prevention and early detection results in more than 60,000 premature deaths each year. Behavioral interventions and cancer screening work; but they have not been fully adopted by individuals, physicians, health care systems, and society at large.

Much of the recent decline in U.S. cancer death rates is a result of cancer prevention and early detection, but more progress is possible by simply implementing known interventions. A 19 percent decline in the rate at which new cancer cases occur and a 29 percent decline in the rate of cancer deaths could potentially be achieved by 2015 if efforts to help people change their behaviors that put them at risk were stepped up and if behavioral change were sustained. Smoking, obesity, sedentary lifestyles, alcohol use, and failure to get screened for cancer all contribute to the excess burden of cancer. The possible reductions in cancer incidence are particularly striking for certain cancers: accelerated changes in risk behavior of a magnitude that is feasible by the application of current knowledge could reduce the number of colorectal cancer cases by up to 33 percent and halve the number of smoking-related cancer cases such as lung cancer. The health benefits of such behavioral change extend well beyond cancer, however. Significant reductions in the rates of cardiovascular disease and diabetes would also occur with the adoption of healthier lifestyles.

To save the most lives from cancer, health care providers, health plans, insurers, employers, policy makers, and researchers should be concentrating their resources on helping people to stop smoking, maintain a healthy weight and diet, exercise regularly, keep alcohol consumption at low to moderate levels, and get screening tests for cancer that have proven effectiveness. Doing so could shift the balance away from the current devotion of attention and resources to the treatment of advanced disease to more effective prevention (Woolf, 1999).

In this chapter, the National Cancer Policy Board summarizes the evidence presented in the report to address four questions:

1. What lifestyle and health care behaviors contribute to the burden of cancer?
2. What share of new cases of cancer and cancer deaths could be prevented with changes in lifestyle and health care behavior?
3. What interventions work to bring about health-enhancing behavioral change?
4. What steps can be taken to overcome barriers to using effective interventions and to improve what we know about cancer prevention and early detection?

WHAT LIFESTYLE AND HEALTH CARE BEHAVIORS CONTRIBUTE TO THE BURDEN OF CANCER?

The Board recognized that a number of personal and health care behaviors are known to contribute to the burden of cancer but limited its review to tobacco use, obesity, physical activity, diet, alcohol use, and the use of screening tests. Examples of behaviors known to contribute to cancer risk but not considered in this report, include exposure to sun and exposure to cancer-causing viruses through sexual activity (e.g., human papillomavirus) and blood contact such as through intravenous drug use (e.g., hepatitis B virus).

Tobacco Use

Tobacco is responsible for approximately 30 percent of cancer deaths in the United States, an estimated 170,000 deaths in 2002 (ACS, 2002a). A causal link between smoking and lung and laryngeal cancer was first made public in the 1964 Surgeon General's report, *Smoking and Health* (U.S. Department of Health Education and Welfare, 1964). Since then convincing evidence has accumulated to support smoking as a cause of several cancers including cancers of the oral cavity, esophagus, bladder, kidney, pancreas, cervix, colon, and stomach, and leukemia.

Smoking increases the risk of lung cancer 10- to 20-fold and the risk of other cancers up to 5-fold, depending on an individual's smoking habits and history. Although the lung cancer risk in former smokers never quite returns to that for individuals who have never smoked, it is drastically reduced. There are substantial health benefits for smokers who quit. A person who quits smoking before age 50, for example, has, on average, half the mortality risk of dying in the next 15 years compared with the risk for those who continue to smoke.

Obesity

Overweight, as indicated by a body mass index (BMI; weight [in kilograms] divided by height [in meters] squared) of 25.0 to 29.9, and obesity, as indicated by a BMI of ≥30.0, contribute an estimated 10 percent to the cancer mortality rate among men and 15 to 20 percent to the cancer mortality rate among women. There is convincing evidence that obesity contributes to a higher incidence of esophageal, breast, endometrial, colon, and kidney cancer. The high risk of esophageal cancer associated with obesity is likely due to its relationship with gastroesophageal reflux, a risk factor for esophageal adenocarcinomas. Obesity—or more precisely, excess body fat (adiposity)—affects levels of female hormones, which are known to affect the risk for breast and uterine cancers. Obesity may also modify insulin pathways, which, in turn, may affect colon cancer. The degree to which obesity elevates risk varies by cancer site. The elevation in risk is very large (a fivefold increase in risk) in the case of esophageal cancer, large (a two- to fourfold increase in risk) for cancers of the breast and uterus, and moderate (a 35 percent to twofold increase in risk) for colon cancer.

Physical Activity

Physical activity is associated with a 10 to 25 percent reduction in the risk for breast cancer and a potential 25 to 50 percent reduction in the risk for colon cancer. Although an association between cancer and physical activity is established, the mechanisms whereby physical activity reduce risk of cancer are not fully known.

Diet

There is clear and convincing evidence that a diet rich in plant foods and moderate in animal products lowers the risk of cardiovascular disease, diabetes, and other important outcomes, but evidence linking specific aspects of the diet to cancer risk is inconsistent. Recent evidence from large prospective studies, for example, has not consistently shown a reduced risk of cancer for those who consume large amounts of fruits and vegetables or small amounts of red meat, although a large number of case-control studies have shown those relationships. There is a growing body of evidence that certain nutritional components of foods affect cancer risk (e.g., calcium or folate and colorectal cancer), but further research is needed to confirm these specific associations.

Alcohol

A downward shift in the population distribution of alcohol intake could lead to decreases in the incidence of cancer and injuries, but it could also lead to higher rates of cardiovascular disease because consumption of moderate amounts of alcohol confers some protection against cardiovascular disease. Public education campaigns must focus on reductions in hazardous drinking and encouraging those who choose to drink to do so moderately.

Use of Cancer Screening

A core consensus has emerged about the appropriateness of some methods of cancer screening. There is essentially universal agreement across organizations that all adults age 50 and older should be screened for colorectal cancer, that all women should receive mammograms every 1 to 2 years beginning at least by age 50, and that cervical cancer screening should occur regularly in all sexually active women with a cervix. Appropriate use of screening could reduce the rate of mortality from colorectal cancer by 30 to 80 percent (among adults age 50 and older), reduce the rate of mortality from breast cancer by 25 to 30 percent (among women age 50 and older), and reduce the rate of mortality from cervical cancer by 20 to 60 percent (among women age 18 and older).

WHAT SHARE OF NEW CASES OF CANCER AND CANCER DEATHS COULD BE PREVENTED WITH CHANGES IN LIFESTYLE AND HEALTH CARE BEHAVIORS?

Projections of the precise number of cancer cases and cancer deaths that could be averted with changes in individuals' health behaviors are difficult to make, but recent estimates suggest that if current trends toward a decline in the prevalence of cancer risk factors continue over the next decade, by the year 2015 one could expect a 13 percent decline in cancer incidence rates and a 21 percent decline in cancer mortality rates below those in 1990. With redoubled efforts to reduce the prevalence of known cancer risk factors further, by the year 2015, cancer incidence rates could be reduced by 19 percent and cancer mortality rates could be reduced by 29 percent. Such redoubled efforts would equate to the prevention of approximately 100,000 cancer cases and 60,000 cancer deaths each year by the year 2015 (Byers et al., 1999).

More than half of the estimated future gains are attributable to projected reductions in tobacco use. Although it is difficult to predict the future success of public health measures to reduce tobacco use, much progress has already been made. The rate of smoking among adult males has been nearly halved, to 26 percent in 1998 from 51 percent in 1965. Among adult females during this period, the prevalence of smoking has dropped to 22 percent in 1998 from 34 percent in 1965 (National Center for Health Statistics, 2000). It is these trends that are largely responsible for the recent declines in the numbers of deaths from all cancers—the first such decline ever recorded. Following years of steady decline, rates of smoking among adults appear to have leveled off in the 1990s, however.

Smoking cessation has major and immediate health benefits for men and women of all ages and for those who smoke at all levels. There is alarming evidence, however, that the rate of smoking is increasing among adolescents, giving rise to a new generation of adults whose health will be at risk. In 1999, as many as 35 percent of adolescents in grades 9 to 12 smoked (US DHHS and Office of Disease Prevention and Health Promotion, 2000) (Figure 11.1). Almost half of adolescents who continue smoking regularly will eventually die from a smoking-related illness.

As America becomes increasingly diverse, lifestyle trends within some subpopulations are troubling. After years of declining rates of smoking

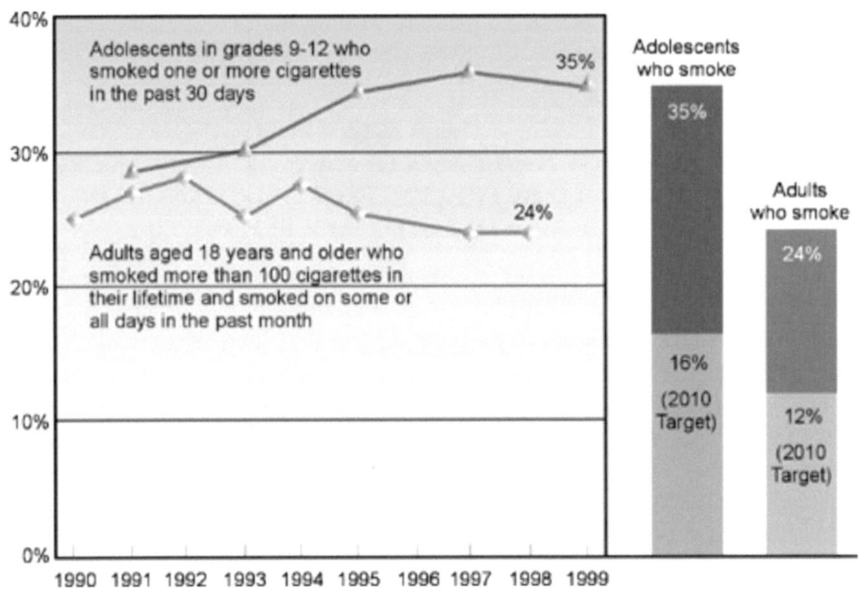

FIGURE 11.1 Cigarette smoking, United States, 1990–1999.
SOURCE: US DHHS and Office of Disease Prevention and Health Promotion, 2000.

among adolescents during the 1970s and 1980s, rates of cigarette smoking among white, African-American, and Hispanic high school students increased in the 1990s (US DHHS and Office of Disease Prevention and Health Promotion, 2000). In 1999, 39 percent of white high school students smoked cigarettes, whereas the rates were 33 percent for Hispanics and 20 percent for African Americans.

Among adults, American Indians and Alaska Natives, blue-collar workers, and military personnel have the highest rates of smoking (US DHHS and Office of Disease Prevention and Health Promotion, 2000). Lower incomes and lower levels of educational attainment are also linked to higher smoking rates among adults. Hispanic adults have relatively low rates of smoking, but analyses of smoking patterns by immigration status suggest that rates of smoking will likely increase among Hispanics because, over time, migrants tend to adopt the poorer health habits of the U.S. general population.

The levels of physical inactivity among Americans also pose a great threat to health. More than 60 percent of American adults are not regularly physically active (28 percent are not active at all), and physical activity levels continue to decline dramatically even in adolescents (US DHHS, 1996; CDC, 2001b). Groups with relatively low rates of physical activity include women, individuals with lower incomes and less education, African Americans, Hispanics, and elderly people. The major barriers that most people face when trying to increase physical activity are lack of time, lack of access to convenient facilities, and lack of safe environments in which to be active (US DHHS and Office of Disease Prevention and Health Promotion, 2000).

More than 1 in 10 children and more than half of adults in the United States are overweight or obese, representing sharp increases in rates of obesity over the last three decades (US DHHS and Office of Disease Prevention and Health Promotion, 2000). Trends are particularly alarming for children and adolescents (Figure 11.2).

Obesity is a result of a complex array of social, behavioral, cultural, environmental, physiological, and genetic factors and is especially prevalent among those with lower incomes. The prevalence of obesity is very high among African-American and Mexican-American women. The proportion of adolescents from poor households who are overweight or obese is twice that of adolescents from middle- and high-income households.

Many aspects of U.S. culture and society over the past few decades have discouraged youth physical activity, including the following (CDC, Division of Adolescent and School Health, 2000):

- Community designs centered around the automobile have discouraged walking and bicycling and have made it more difficult for children to get together to play.

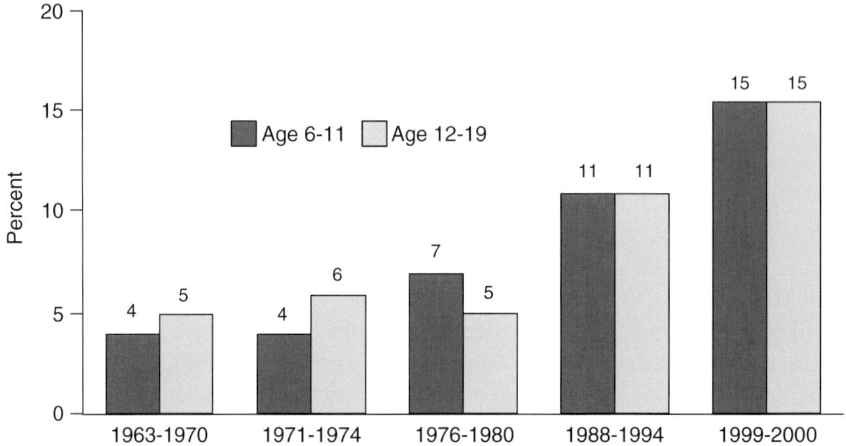

FIGURE 11.2 Prevalence of overweight among children and adolescents: United States, 1963–1970 to 1999–2000.
NOTE: Excludes pregnant women starting with 1971-1974. Pregnancy status not available for 1963-1965 and 1966-1970. Data for 1963-1965 are for children 6-11 years of age; data for 1966-1970 are for adolescents 12-17 years of age, not 12-19 years.
SOURCE: http://www.cdc.gov/nchs/products/pubs/pubd/hestats/overwght99.htm.

- Increased concerns about safety have limited the times and places available to children to play outside.
- New technology has conditioned young people to be less active, whereas new electronic media (e.g., video and computer games and cable and satellite television) have made sedentary activities more appealing.
- States and school districts have reduced the amounts of time that students are required to spend in physical education classes.
- Communities have failed to invest adequately in physical activity facilities (e.g., parks and recreation centers) close to places where children live.

The potential benefits of cancer screening in the United States fall far short of being achieved, costing health and lives. The lost opportunities take several forms: a substantial proportion of eligible people are never screened or are screened too infrequently to achieve early detection, those who are screened are not screened well, and the follow-up steps for abnormal results are often inadequate. Inadequate screening occurs more commonly among certain segments of the population. Insurance status, age, socioeconomic status, race, ethnicity, and education account for marked disparities in the access of Americans to cancer screening tests. Rates of screening of women for breast and cervical cancer are relatively high. Recent estimates are that more than 60 percent of women age 50 and older have had a mammogram in the past year and that more than 80 percent of women age 18 and older have had a Pap test in the past 3 years. In contrast, only 40 percent of adults ages 50 and older report ever having had a screening test for colorectal cancer.

WHAT INTERVENTIONS WORK TO BRING ABOUT HEALTH-ENHANCING BEHAVIORAL CHANGE?

In its review of the literature on the effectiveness of interventions to change health behaviors, the Board encountered a recurring theme: programs are most successful if they intervene at multiple levels. To effectively make populationwide improvements in the major behavioral risk factors, changes must occur on many different social levels, and the policy recommendations in this report reflect this fact. They aim to create a prevention-oriented environment that makes risk reduction behaviors easier for individuals to choose. It is not enough, however, to assume that individuals who are educated about their cancer risk will modify their behavior to lower their risk (US DHHS, 1994).

Barriers to behavioral change exist not only at the individual level but also at the community level and within the broader social milieu. Broad social movements are needed if health behavioral changes are to be stimulated and sustained at the population level. Because U.S. society is heterogeneous, composed of persons of different racial, ethnic, and socioeconomic backgrounds, these social movements will of necessity be heterogeneous as well. It is only through such large-scale movements that barriers to healthy behavior (including economic, social, political, cultural, and psychological barriers) can be eliminated at the population level.

A comprehensive program to change a population's cancer risk profile should engage individuals, health care providers, organizations, and whole communities. This finding reiterates a conclusion reached by the Institute of Medicine's Committee on Capitalizing on Social Science and Behavioral Research to Improve the Public's Health. In its 2000 report, *Promoting Health: Intervention Strategies from Social and Behavioral Research* (Institute of Medicine, 2000b), the committee concluded that "interventions on social and behavioral risk factors should link multiple levels of influence, individual, interpersonal, institutional, community, and policy levels" (Institute of Medicine, 2000b, p. 7).

Tobacco Use

Certain states such as California and Massachusetts have implemented comprehensive tobacco control programs and have achieved some important milestones: sharp reductions in smoking and declines in rates of chronic illnesses associated with smoking such as cardiovascular disease and, more recently, lung cancer. Further reductions in the cancer burden are expected as the programs are in place for longer periods. The Board concluded in its 2000 report, *State Programs Can Reduce Tobacco Use*, that such programs are successful and should serve as models for other states (Institute of Medicine, 2000e).

A general consensus on what works in tobacco control has been reached by several organizations charged with reviewing the evidence of program effectiveness (e.g., the Task Force on Community Preventive Services, the Office of the Surgeon General, the U.S. Preventive Services Task Force, the Agency for Healthcare Research and Quality) (Hopkins et al., 2001a; Wasserman, 2001) (Box 11.1).

BOX 11.1 Interventions Recognized as Effective Against Smoking and Promoted by National Organizations

To reduce youth initiation of smoking:
- Increase the unit price for tobacco products, particularly through increases in state and federal excise taxes.
- Develop extensive and extended mass media campaigns, particularly when they are the centerpiece along with other strategies.

To decrease the effects of environmental tobacco smoke:
- Develop laws and regulations to restrict or ban tobacco consumption in workplaces and general areas used by the public.

To assist with smoking cessation from a population orientation:
- Use broadcast and print media to encourage people to quit along with other strategies.
- Increase the unit price of tobacco products.
- Use provider education and have providers implement self-reminder systems to ensure that this issue is raised during the clinical examination.
- Provide telephone counseling and support services along with treatments offered by other strategies.
- Reduce patient out-of-pocket costs for effective cessation treatments.

To assist with smoking cessation from a clinical perspective:
- Screen patients for tobacco use.
- Deliver brief advice or more intense or frequent counseling to quit.
- Use pharmacological treatments (nicotine replacement therapy or bupropion as first-line therapies).

SOURCE: Wasserman (2001) and Hopkins et al. (2001a,b).

Physical Activity and Healthy Weight and Diet

Relative to tobacco use, less is known about what interventions work to maintain a healthy diet, increase levels of activity, and reduce obesity, and there is less experience with such interventions. Efforts to maintain a healthy weight should start early in childhood and continue throughout adulthood, as this is likely to be more successful than efforts to lose substantial amounts of weight and maintain weight loss once obesity is established. It is also recognized that a healthy diet and regular physical activity are both important for the maintenance of a healthy weight. Over time, even a small decrease in the numbers of calories consumed and a small increase in physical activity can help prevent weight gain or facilitate weight loss.

It is recommended that obese individuals who are trying to lose substantial amounts of weight seek the guidance of a health care provider (US DHHS and Office of Disease Prevention and Health Promotion, 2000). Worksite fitness programs have resulted in increased levels of physical activity among employees, and it is recognized that environmental policies related to zoning, land use, safety, and transportation greatly affect opportunities for exercise. Among youth, school policies regarding physical education requirements and the availability of after-school recreational programs and facilities affect rates of participation in exercise before and after school.

It is clear that efforts targeted only to individuals cannot be fully effective to prevent or manage obesity or increase physical activity. Governments, the food industry, international agencies, the media, communities, and individuals all need to work together to modify the environment so that it is less conducive to weight gain and more supportive of physical activity (World Health Organization, 1998).

Cancer Screening

To enhance the use of screening, multilevel approaches are also recommended. Optimizing the delivery of effective cancer screening services and reducing inappropriate testing lie in changing the behaviors of

- systems of care, to make cancer screening services available to eligible populations;
- health care providers, to perform cancer screening as recommended, on time, and with skill when they encounter patients eligible for screening; and
- individuals, to obtain recommended screening tests and pursue follow-up.

The elimination of financial and access barriers to screening improves screening rates. These barriers can be reduced, for example, through health insurance coverage, reduced cost sharing, and the availability of free screening at public clinics. In addition, certain organizational innovations are tied to improved screening performance, such as the implementation of systems to prompt providers to recommend screening, facilitate referrals, and remind patients and providers of the need for rescreening. Other opportunities to improve screening rates, particularly among underserved populations, include outreach and education, case management, and facilitation of referrals.

WHAT STEPS CAN BE TAKEN TO OVERCOME BARRIERS TO USING EFFECTIVE INTERVENTIONS AND TO IMPROVE WHAT WE KNOW ABOUT CANCER PREVENTION AND EARLY DETECTION?

The Board recommends that the following steps be taken to increase the rate of adoption, the reach, and the impacts of evidence-based cancer prevention and early detection interventions.

Recommendation 1: The U.S. Congress and state legislatures should enact and provide funding for enforcement of laws to substantially reduce and ultimately eliminate the adverse public health consequences of tobacco use and exposure.

Tobacco is the greatest contributor to deaths from cancer, and reduction in tobacco use offers the greatest opportunity to reduce the incidence, morbidity, and mortality of cancer. Specific actions that would be effective include the following:

- Taxation is the single most effective method of reducing the demand for tobacco (IOM 2000a). States should set sufficiently high levels of excise taxation on tobacco products to discourage tobacco use, but levels should not be so high that they encourage significant tax avoidance activities.
- States should allocate sufficient funds from the Tobacco Master Settlement Agreement[1] and tobacco excise taxes to support comprehensive, state-based tobacco control efforts consistent with guidelines of the Centers for Disease Control and Prevention (CDC).

The CDC's Office on Smoking and Health has identified nine essential

[1]The Master Settlement Agreement signed in 1998 transferred $246 billion from tobacco firms to states over 25 years.

elements of a state-level comprehensive tobacco control program (CDC, 1999d):

1. community programs to reduce tobacco use,
2. chronic disease programs to reduce the burden of tobacco-related diseases,
3. school programs,
4. enforcement,
5. statewide programs,
6. countermarketing,
7. cessation programs,
8. surveillance and evaluation, and
9. administration and management.

The estimated annual costs of implementing such a comprehensive program range from $7 to $20 per capita in smaller states (those with populations of less than 3 million), $6 to $12 per capita in medium-sized states (those with populations of 3 million to 7 million), and $5 to $16 per capita in larger states (those with populations of more than 7 million). California and Massachusetts, two states with large-scale and sustained tobacco control programs, fund the program using excise tax revenues and Tobacco Master Settlement Agreement funds. Only eight states (Arizona, Hawaii, Maine, Maryland, Massachusetts, Minnesota, Mississippi, and Ohio) meet these CDC guidelines on recommended levels of support for tobacco control (CDC, 1999d, 2002a). Recent estimates are that only 5 percent of the tobacco settlement monies have been invested in prevention (National Conference of State Legislatures, 2001).

Not all states are contributing money to tobacco control. In at least five states (Connecticut, North Carolina, North Dakota, Pennsylvania, and Tennessee) and the District of Columbia, federal and private funds are the only funds being invested in tobacco control. In at least 20 states, funding from the federal government and the private sector makes up 50 percent or more of the funds being invested. For the country as a whole, the combined resources available in fiscal year 2001 to fund tobacco use prevention and control programs in states total almost $1 billion, but this amount is less than one-sixth of the $8.2 billion that the tobacco industry spent annually in 1999 on promoting and advertising its products (National Conference of State Legislatures, 2001; CDC, 2002b).

Tobacco products cannot by law be sold to those under age 18, but local governments charged with imposing the law generally do not have adequate resources for monitoring and enforcement activities. (www.samhsa.gov/programs/content/brief2001/01csapsynar.htm).

- States should improve compliance with the provisions of the 1992

Synar amendment, which requires that states have sales-to-minor rates of no greater than 20 percent in order to receive federal Substance Abuse Prevention and Treatment Block Grant awards. By 2000, only 25 states had achieved this level of compliance.

- States should impose tobacco-licensing requirements for merchants selling tobacco products, as recommended in the 2000 report of the Surgeon General (U.S. Department of Health and Human Services and Office of Disease Prevention and Health Promotion, 2000). The threat of revocation of the license as a consequence of selling tobacco products to minors could provide a strong incentive for merchants to comply with existing laws. Further, requiring that merchants pay for a license to sell tobacco could provide needed funds for monitoring and enforcement.
- Internet sales of tobacco products are not covered by the Synar amendment, which leaves a significant opening for minors to have access to tobacco. More than 90 websites sell cigarettes in the United States, and the number is expected to grow. Furthermore, tobacco products sold over the Internet are often not subject to state sales taxes, making them much less expensive than their counterparts sold in retail stores. Congress should therefore act to prohibit the promotion, sale, and distribution of tobacco products over the Internet to individuals under the age of 18.
- Regulations at the state level vary greatly across the country. Until the passage of federal legislation, state and local legislatures should increase their regulatory efforts related to environmental tobacco smoke by establishing smoke-free indoor workplaces, public buildings, and restaurants. Eight states still have no restrictions on state government worksites, and 30 states have no restrictions on smoking in nongovernmental workplaces. For local jurisdictions, clean air legislation may be difficult to enact because of state preemption rules that make it unlawful for local governments to enact clean air restrictions that are more stringent than those imposed at the state level. If a state has no restrictions on worksite smoking, for example, it may be impossible for a local community to ban smoking in restaurants or other workplaces. Preemption laws need to be overturned to give local governments the right to protect their communities.
- Further restrictions are needed to reduce tobacco promotion and advertising, which compromises youth tobacco prevention efforts. Restrictions now in place include a mix of voluntary agreements, restrictions resulting from settlements of law suits, and prohibitions defined by state or local ordinances, but some efforts have been hampered by protection of commercial speech (Bayer et al., 2002; Morrison, 2002). The Board urges renewed national consideration of how to address these issues.

The Board's proposed recommendations are consistent with meeting the tobacco-related objectives outlined in *Healthy People 2010* (US DHHS and Office of Disease Prevention and Health Promotion, 2000) (Box 11.2).

BOX 11.2 Summary of Objectives to Reduce Illness, Disability, and Death Related to Tobacco Use and Exposure to Secondhand Smoke Outlined in *Healthy People 2010*

Objective Number	Objective Short Title
Tobacco Use in Population Groups	
27-1	Reduce the rate of tobacco use by adults
27-2	Reduce the rate of tobacco use by adolescents
27-3	Reduce the rate of initiation of tobacco use among children and adolescents (developmental)
27-4	Increase the average age of first use of tobacco products by adolescents and young adults
Cessation and Treatment	
27-5	Increase smoking cessation attempts by adult smokers
27-6	Increase rates of smoking cessation during pregnancy
27-7	Increase smoking cessation attempts by adolescents
27-8	Increase insurance coverage for evidence-based treatment for nicotine dependency
Exposure to Secondhand Smoke	
27-9	Reduce the proportion of children who are regularly exposed to tobacco smoke at home
27-10	Reduce the proportion of nonsmokers exposed to environmental tobacco smoke
27-11	Increase the area of smoke-free and tobacco-free environments in schools, including all school facilities, property, vehicles, and school events
27-12	Increase the proportion of worksites with formal smoking policies that prohibit smoking or limit it to separately ventilated areas
27-13	Establish laws on smoke-free indoor air that prohibit smoking or limit it to separately ventilated areas in public places and worksites
Social and Environmental Changes	
27-14	Reduce the rate of illegal sales of tobacco products to minors through enforcement of laws prohibiting the sale of tobacco products to minors
27-15	Increase the number of states, including the District of Columbia, that suspend or revoke state retail licenses for violations of laws prohibiting the sale of tobacco to minors
27-16	Eliminate tobacco advertising and promotions that influence adolescents and young adults (developmental)
27-17	Increase the level of adolescent disapproval of smoking
27-18	Increase the number of tribes, territories, and states, including the District of Columbia, with comprehensive, evidence-based tobacco control programs
27-19	Eliminate laws that preempt stronger tobacco control laws
27-20	Reduce the toxicity of tobacco products by establishing a regulatory structure to monitor toxicity (developmental)
27-21	Increase the average federal and state taxes on tobacco products

SOURCE: US DHHS and Office of Disease Prevention and Health Promotion (2000).

Recommendation 2: A national strategy should be developed and coordinated by the U.S. Department of Health and Human Services to address the epidemic of obesity, unhealthy diet, and physical inactivity in America, which are all significant risk factors for cancer and other diseases. Effective interventions need to be identified and broadly applied to reduce cancer risk among the general population and among populations at higher risk.

Dietary interventions to prevent cancer have, to date, focused primarily on particular components such as the consumption of fruits and vegetables, fiber, and fats. Obesity and physical inactivity have recently joined unhealthy diet as leading risk factors for cancer. Interventions aimed at maintaining a healthy weight and diet and increasing levels of physical activity can reduce the burden of cancer and other chronic illnesses such as cardiovascular disease and diabetes.

A comprehensive set of recommendations, the Recommendations for Public Health Action on Weight Control and Physical Activity to Promote Cancer Prevention, has been proposed by the International Agency for Research on Cancer (IARC), an agency within the World Health Organization (2002) (Box 11.3). The National Cancer Policy Board endorses these recommendations for action.

BOX 11.3 Recommendations for Public Health Action on Weight Control and Physical Activity to Promote Cancer Prevention, IARC, WHO

Governmental and Nongovernmental Organizations

1. Public education should provide timely and accurate information on the epidemic of obesity and inactivity and on ways this can be addressed.
2. Governments at local and national levels should ensure that schoolchildren at all stages have proper access at school to healthy meals and to recreation and sports facilities.
3. Governments at local and national levels, as well as nongovernmental organizations, should provide adequate funding for effective physical education programs in schools.
4. Communities and buildings should be designed to encourage use of stairs and walking. A proportion of transportation budgets should be allocated for development of bicycle and pedestrian facilities, notably in urban areas.
5. In developing countries there are dietary traditions, behavioral patterns, and infrastructures that potentially could aid weight gain prevention programs. Efforts should be made to prevent the loss of cultural traditions that promote healthy diets and physical activity.

(continued on next page)

BOX 11.3 continued

Worksites and Schools

1. Employers should encourage physical activity and weight control by all employees. Methods can include provisions for exercise areas at work; showers; and financial incentives to walk, bicycle, or use public transportation rather than cars.
2. School curricula include adequate teaching of food, nutrition, and health and on the importance of active living.
3. Schools should include 1 hour of physical education on most days.

Health Professionals and Educators

1. Health professionals should counsel individuals about a healthy range of body weights. For persons currently within the healthy range, it is recommended that weight gain during adult life not exceed 5 kilograms (11 pounds).
2. Medical schools and other health science professional programs should make the study of food, nutrition, and physical activity and their relation to health and disease an integral part of the training of health care professionals.
3. Physicians and health care providers should counsel their patients on the need for an active lifestyle for the prevention of cancer and other noncommunicable diseases.
4. Health care providers and educators should set a personal example by engaging in regular physical activity and controlling their weight to the best of their ability.
5. Health care providers and teachers should take an active role in their communities to support regular physical activity and weight control.
6. Maternal and child health programs can provide a suitable context for promoting awareness of the need for physical activity and preventing weight gain, particularly in developing countries.

Families and Individuals

1. Prevention of overweight and obesity should begin early in life. It should be based on the development of lifelong healthy eating and physical activity patterns. However, it is never too late to benefit from starting to be more active.
2. Individuals should be encouraged to maintain physical activity to promote energy balance and weight control. The primary goal should be to perform continuous physical activity on most days of the week. A total of 1 hour of moderate-intensity activity such as walking may be needed each day to maintain a healthy body weight, particularly for people with sedentary occupations. More vigorous activity, such as fast walking, several times a week may give some additional benefits regarding cancer prevention. Therefore, planned vigorous activities such as sports should be undertaken according to individual interests and capabilities.
3. Individuals should, where possible, give priority to the more active alternatives in their daily lives.
4. Parents and individuals should limit the purchase and availability at home of high-energy foods and beverages with low nutritional value, such as soda beverages and baked snacks, and instead should provide healthy foods, in particular, an abundant supply of fruits and vegetables and whole-grain products.

Of special concern are the nation's youth. Many children and adolescents are not engaged in recommended levels of physical activity and are increasingly overweight or obese. These trends, in addition to the prevalence of smoking among adolescents, threaten the recent gains made in reducing cancer deaths. Comprehensive school physical education and health programs have the potential to help students establish lifelong, healthy physical activity and eating patterns, thereby avoiding overweight and obesity.

The Board endorses the following 10 strategies designed to promote lifelong participation in enjoyable and safe physical activity and sports identified in *Promoting Better Health for Young People Through Physical Activity and Sports, A Report to the President from the Secretary of Health and Human Services and the Secretary of Education* (CDC, Division of Adolescent and School Health, 2000):

1. Include education for parents and guardians as part of youth physical activity promotion initiatives.
2. Help all children, from prekindergarten through grade 12, receive quality, daily physical education. Help all schools have certified physical education specialists; appropriate class sizes; and the facilities, equipment, and supplies needed to deliver quality, daily physical education.
3. Publicize and disseminate tools to help schools improve their physical education and other physical activity programs.
4. Enable state education and health departments to work together to help schools implement quality, daily physical education and other physical activity programs:
    - with a full-time state coordinator for school physical activity programs,
    - as part of a coordinated school health program, and
    - with support from relevant governmental and nongovernmental organizations.
5. Enable more after-school care programs to provide regular opportunities for active, physical play.
6. Help provide access to community sports and recreation programs for all young people.
7. Enable youth sports and recreation programs to provide coaches and recreation program staff with the training they need to offer developmentally appropriate, safe, and enjoyable physical activity experiences for young people.
8. Enable communities to develop and promote the use of safe, well-maintained, and close-to-home sidewalks, crosswalks, bicycle paths, trails, parks, and recreation facilities and community designs that feature mixed-use development and a connected grid of streets.

9. Implement an ongoing media campaign to promote physical education as an important component of a quality education and long-term health.

10. Monitor youth physical activity, physical fitness, and school and community physical activity programs in the nation and each state.

Most states do not adhere to these recommendations. As of 2001, for example, although 48 states had mandates for physical education, only Illinois required daily physical education for all students in kindergarten through grade 12 (Alabama required daily physical education for all students in kindergarten through grade 8). In states with mandatory physical education, many elementary and middle school students are spending relatively little time in physical education classes, and most high school students take physical education for only 1 of their 4 years (http://www.aahperd.org/naspe/pdf_files/shape_nation.pdf, assessed July 24, 2002).

Establishing healthy eating habits at a young age is critical because changing poor eating patterns in adulthood is difficult. Schools can help young people improve their eating habits by implementing effective policies and educational programs. CDC has issued guidelines for school health programs to promote lifelong healthy eating, including four attributes of effective school-based nutrition education programs (http://www.cdc.gov/nccdphp/dash/nutguide.htm):

1. help young people learn skills (not just facts);
2. give students repeated chances to practice healthy eating;
3. make nutrition education activities fun; and
4. involve teachers, administrators, families, community leaders, and students in delivering strong, consistent messages about healthy eating as part of a coordinated school health program.

The CDC guidelines provide schools with strategies to improve nutrition education programs through policies, curriculum, instruction, program coordination, staff training, family and community involvement, and program evaluation.

The 2001 Surgeon General's Call to Action to Prevent and Decrease Overweight and Obesity proposed a framework, CARE: Communication, Action, Research, and Evaluation to address the problem (US DHHS, 2001b). Recognizing the need for interventions at multiple levels, the Surgeon General's report outlines needed action within five settings: families and communities, schools, health care, media and communications, and worksites.

Recommendation 3: The U.S. Congress should provide sufficient appropriations to the Centers for Disease Control and Prevention to support innovative public and private partnerships to develop, implement, and evaluate comprehensive community-based programs in cancer prevention and early detection. Every state should have and implement a comprehensive cancer control plan.

No coordinated infrastructure involving public and private efforts to launch multilevel interventions known to be effective in bringing about behavioral change exists at the federal or state levels. CDC is the federal link to the nation's public health infrastructure, principally through state and local health departments. It is most often at these levels that multilevel cancer prevention and early detection interventions are carried out. The network that makes up the public health infrastructure is vast and includes 59 state and territorial health departments, more than 3,000 county and city health departments, more than 3,000 local boards of health, tribal health departments, and other federal and private organizations. This network generally engages the support of partners including consumer and advocacy organizations, universities, and area health care providers. This network of systems and organizations is essential to the public health mission of health promotion and disease prevention, but it is fragile, under stress, and underfunded (Box 11.4) (Institute of Medicine, 2003).

CDC's Center for Chronic Disease Prevention and Health Promotion is an important locus for activity to improve the nation's and individual states' capacities to provide comprehensive cancer control services. CDC's Office of Smoking and Health, for example, provides technical assistance to states and monitors progress in reaching tobacco-related goals outlined in *Healthy People 2010* (US DHHS and Office of Disease Prevention and Health Promotion, 2000). Other programs at CDC address other risk factors, for example, the Division of Nutrition and Physical Activity promotes healthy diet, weight control, and physical activity, and the Division of Cancer Prevention and Control oversees the National Breast and Cervical Cancer Early Detection Program that operates in all states to provide screening and follow-up services to underserved women.

CDC also supports states in the development and implementation of comprehensive cancer control plans. State efforts in cancer prevention and early detection are in many cases piecemeal and are organized around categorically funded programs. CDC needs to build the capacities of states—and in turn, their local partners—to both develop and implement comprehensive cancer control plans. As part of CDC's National Comprehensive Cancer Control Program, cancer control plans have been defined as those with an integrated and coordinated approach to reduce the rates of incidence, morbidity, and mortality of cancer through prevention, early detec-

BOX 11.4 Public Health's Mission and Services

Public Health Mission

- Prevent epidemics and the spread of disease
- Protect against environmental hazards
- Prevent injuries
- Promote and encourage healthy behaviors
- Respond to disasters and assist communities in recovery
- Ensure the quality and accessibility of health services

Essential Public Health Services

- Monitor health status to identify and solve community health problems
- Diagnose and investigate health problems and health hazards in the community
- Inform, educate, and empower people about health issues
- Mobilize community partnerships and action to solve health problems
- Develop policies and plans that support individual and community health efforts
- Enforce laws and regulations that protect health and ensure safety
- Link people to needed personal health services and ensure the provision of health care when otherwise unavailable
- Ensure a competent workforce (public health and personal care)
- Evaluate effectiveness, accessibility, and quality of personal and population-based health services
- Research new insights and innovative solutions to health problems

SOURCE: Public Health Functions Steering Committee, Public Health in America, July 1995 (www.health.gov/phfunctions/public.htm assessed July 24, 2002).

tion, treatment, rehabilitation, and palliation (CDC, 2001a; www.cdc.gov/cancer/ncccp/index.htm) (see Chapter 9).

Roughly half of the states (27 states) report having a comprehensive cancer control plan, but the plans are in various stages of implementation. CDC is supporting states in developing and implementing such plans, but the available support has been modest (less than $37 million since 1998) (see Chapter 9). The CDC estimates that $30 million per year would be needed before states would have plans developed and implementation in progress by 2005 (Leslie Given, Division of Cancer Prevention and Control, CDC, personal communication to Maria Hewitt, IOM, September 9, 2002).

Many states have in place some of the essential elements of a comprehensive program. Approximately half of them, for example, have cancer registries that achieve the standards of completeness, timeliness, and coverage to provide accurate cancer incidence data for planning and evaluation. All states monitor the prevalence of cancer-related risk factors such as smoking, and all states have in place CDC-funded breast and cervical cancer screening programs targeted to low-income and underserved women.

State and local health departments can play important roles in instituting and coordinating comprehensive cancer prevention programs. Health departments can, for example:

- monitor and publicize state trends in cancer and cancer-related behaviors;
- support media campaigns to promote healthy behaviors;
- target interventions to low income and racial/ethnic groups at high risk for cancer, e.g., by providing breast, cervical, and colorectal cancer screening services to medically uninsured and medically underserved populations;
- develop and distribute best-practice guidelines to major employer human resources departments to encourage smoking cessation programs, wellness programs, on-site healthy eating and exercise facilities, flexible time for employees to allow alternative means of commuting (e.g., by bicycle or foot), and use of preventive health services (e.g., screening and smoking cessation programs);
- collaborate with school systems to develop cancer prevention-related educational curricula and programs;
- collaborate with public and private organizations to provide incentives for physical activity, healthy eating, and participation in weight loss programs (e.g., reduced fees for fitness clubs, on-site weight control groups, employer nonautomotive commuting programs);
- track state use of funds available through the 1998 Transportation Equity Act for the 21st Century (Public Law 105-178), which provides federal funds to construct sidewalks and bicycle trails and to integrate mass transit, roads, and pedestrian and bicycle facilities into a comprehensive transportation plan;
- support free and reduced-fee health clinics organized through local health departments and other community-based programs; and
- evaluate the effectiveness of services and programs.

Despite the evidence of success of tobacco control efforts, the effort to support comprehensive plans to further a wide range of cancer prevention activities remains a promising but untested approach. Rigorous assessments of this approach, with an eye to defining essential components, innovative delivery systems, and model programs, need to be integrated into the plans themselves. Key to success is also the incorporation at the outset of broad community input into the plans, especially from important constituencies such as minority groups, elderly people, parents, and the advocacy community. Successful implementation of plans will depend on collaborative public-private partnerships because in many areas, state and local health departments lack the infrastructure needed to fully carry out a comprehensive plan. With these components in place, the Board recommends further support to allow states to develop and implement comprehensive state plans.

The National Dialogue on Cancer (NDC), an initiative spearheaded by the American Cancer Society, has since 1999 provided a forum for leaders in both the public and private sectors to foster and support efforts to overcome cancer. In the area of prevention and early detection, NDC has convened an issue team to address primary cancer prevention and a team to formulate a strategy for ensuring the development and implementation of cancer prevention and early detection plans in every state (www.ndoc.org). NDC has recently recommended that all states have a comprehensive plan in place by 2003 and that implementation of the plan be in progress by 2005.

Recommendation 4: Public and private insurers and providers should consider evidence-based cancer prevention and early detection services to be essential benefits and should provide coverage for them. These services at a minimum should include interventions recommended in the 2000 U.S. Public Health Service's clinical practice guideline on treating tobacco use and dependence, screening for breast cancer among women age 50 and older, screening for cervical cancer among all sexually active women with an intact cervix, and screening for colorectal cancer among adults age 50 and older.

Public and private health insurers and providers who want to improve the health of their beneficiaries should include in their benefit packages coverage for evidence-based interventions for cancer prevention and early detection. Nicotine replacement therapy, treatment with certain antidepressants (i.e., Bupropion SR), and counseling, for example, are effective in helping individuals quit smoking. Very few insurers or health maintenance organizations cover the cost of pharmaceutical treatment for smoking cessation and health education and preventive counseling are usually not defined benefits. In one innovative program funded by the Robert Wood Johnson Foundation, health plans are collaborating to examine ways to provide coverage for smoking cessation services.

States have mandated coverage for some cancer prevention and early detection interventions. As of 1998, for example, 43 states and the District of Columbia mandated coverage of cancer screening tests. Such mandates, however, do not always apply broadly to all insured individuals. Employers that are self-insured, for example, are usually exempt from such mandates (Rathore et al., 2000).

For insurers that offer coverage for preventive services, the reduction or elimination of cost sharing (e.g., coinsurance and copayments) can address a financial deterrent to seeking services and can improve the rate of service use (Solanki et al., 1999, 2000). The specifics of an insurer's coverage policy may be dictated broadly by the insurer or plan, or they may be negotiated with employers or other group purchasers. In the latter case, employer benefits managers informed of the effectiveness of cancer prevention services might be motivated to obtain more comprehensive coverage for their employees.

Just as preventive services of proven effectiveness should be covered under insurance plans, services for which evidence of benefit is lacking should be excluded from coverage. Population-based or routine screening of smokers for lung cancer using spiral or helical computed tomography (CT) scans, for example, does not yet meet standards of evidence to support their coverage under health insurance plans. Evidence was not sufficient to include a recommendation regarding mandated reimbursement for interventions to increase physical activity, improve diet, and reduce obesity as a general cancer prevention strategy, though optional offerings by insurers should be encouraged.

There are many opportunities for employers, business coalitions, and other large purchasers of health insurance to exert influence to encourage the use of cancer prevention and early detection services. Employers can provide coverage for preventive services as part of their insurance benefit packages, give discounts to employees who choose plans with more extensive prevention services, and can create financial incentives for health plans to meet performance goals. The Pacific Business Group on Health (PBGH), for example, is a nonprofit coalition of 45 large health care purchasers in California and Arizona representing 3 million insured individuals who account for $3 billion in annual health care expenditures (www.pbgh.org). PBGH also oversees a small business purchasing group that includes more than 9,500 small businesses. PBGH collects and analyzes health plan and provider performance data to produce report cards for consumers, promotes shared treatment decision making between providers and consumers, and promotes value-based buying decisions among its purchasers (Castles et al., 1999; Schauffler and Rodriguez, 1996; President's Advisory Commission, 1998; www.pbgh.org).

Working with health plans in California, an agreement was reached to follow a uniform set of minimum preventive care guidelines based on the US Preventive Services Task Force recommendations (Partnership for Prevention, 1997). In 2000, PBGH approved new benefits for treatment to aid smoking cessation, including behavioral interventions and over-the-counter pharmacotherapy (Harris et al., 2001). PBGH was the first purchasing coalition to impose a condition on contracting plans whereby it would withhold 2 percent of the premium until the plans achieved specific goals for improving customer satisfaction and quality of care, including adherence to cancer screening guidelines. The Alliance, a health insurance purchasing cooperative in Denver, Colorado, subsequently adopted a similar approach (Darby, 1998). General Motors, the nation's largest private employer, has recently collaborated with CDC to examine barriers to the use of prevention services and to devise strategies to improve the rate of use of such services by its employees. Partnership for Prevention, a national nonprofit organization, provides guides for employers and health plans regarding highest value preventive health services (http://www.prevent.org/publications.htm).

Actions taken on behalf of federal employees in some areas of cancer control provide models that private-sector employers can emulate. In 1997, an executive order established smoke-free environments for the more than 1.8 million civilian federal employees and members of the public visiting or using federal facilities. In 2001, federal departments and agencies were directed to establish a policy that provides up to 4 hours of excused absence each year, without a loss of pay or a charge to leave, for participation in preventive health screenings. Agencies were also directed to develop or expand programs offered at the worksite to help employees understand their risks for disease, obtain preventive health services, and make healthy lifestyle choices. The Office of Personnel Management has issued guidance for a model smoking cessation program and is compiling a list of best practices to be shared with agencies. Agencies can pay the costs incurred by employees participating in agency-authorized smoking cessation programs, including payment for nicotine replacement therapy when purchased as part of an agency's smoking cessation program (www.opm.gov/ehs).

Other opportunities to encourage prevention include employer-sponsored wellness and physical fitness programs, either through on-site facilities or through discounts to local gymnasiums or fitness programs. Relatively few employers offer such benefits, and employees with the least access to them are blue-collar or service workers and those working for small firms.

Recommendation 5: The U.S. Congress should increase support for programs that provide primary care to uninsured and low-income people (e.g., Community and Migrant Health Centers and family planning programs of Title X of the Public Health Service Act). These programs increase the use of cancer prevention and early detection services among medically underserved populations.

A pervasive problem in the United States is poor access to health care because of a lack of health insurance. Persons with health insurance are more likely to have a primary care provider and to have received appropriate preventive care such as recent cancer screening tests. Adults with health insurance are twice as likely as adults without health insurance to receive a routine checkup. In 2001, an estimated 15 percent of the U.S. population (41.2 million individuals) was uninsured during the entire year (U.S. Census

Bureau, 2002). Many others are underinsured, with poor coverage for interventions that have been proven to be effective, such as smoking cessation counseling and products. In fact, smokers are more likely than nonsmokers to be uninsured, making them less able to gain access to effective programs.

Individuals who are uninsured (or underinsured) rely on a patchwork of public and private programs for primary care (IOM, 2000d). Community and Migrant Health Centers and Title X family planning clinics are vital sources of primary health care and are important providers of cancer prevention and early detection services (see Chapter 9). Full support for these programs enhances the nation's health care safety net and at the same time extends the availability of cancer prevention and early detection services to vulnerable populations. Even with increased program support, however, many people would likely remain underserved, given the fragmented and limited nature of the nation's health care safety net (Norton and Lipson, 1998).

Recommendation 6: Support for the Centers for Disease Control and Prevention's National Breast and Cervical Cancer Early Detection Program should be increased so that the program can reach all uninsured women using innovative delivery strategies. Support is also needed for a similar program at the CDC to provide screening for colorectal cancer for uninsured and low-income men and women.

Underfunding of CDC's National Breast and Cervical Cancer Early Detection Program (NBCCEDP) contributes to lost opportunities for prevention. This program provides screening services to uninsured and underinsured women, but the program reaches only 15 percent of eligible women because of limited financial support. This is especially unfortunate insofar as racial, ethnic, and socioeconomic disparities in cancer mortality can often be traced to poor use of screening services. Racial and ethnic disparities in cancer incidence could in fact widen if this gap in access to effective prevention services is not addressed. Despite its lack of coverage because of limited funding, NBCCEDP has succeeded in improving screening rates among medically underserved populations.

Because screening for colorectal cancer is also a proven strategy for reducing cancer mortality in people over 50 years of age, a similar program is needed to provide colorectal cancer screening to people who are uninsured and underinsured. The majority of individuals eligible for colorectal screening have not been screened, and screening rates are particularly low among minority and low-income populations.

Recommendation 7: The U.S. Department of Health and Human Services

should complete a comprehensive review to assess whether evidence-based prevention services are being offered and successfully delivered in federal health programs.

The federal government administers or funds Medicare; Medicaid; the Health Resources and Services Administration's Community and Migrant Health Centers; Title X family planning clinics; the U.S. Department of Agriculture's programs such as the Special Supplemental Nutrition Program for Women, Infants, and Children; the Indian Health Service; U.S. Department of Defense health programs; and Federal Employees Health Benefits Program. These programs do not always reflect best practices in cancer prevention and early detection.

The Medicare program, for example, does not cover any costs for smoking cessation treatment, and two-thirds of state Medicaid programs cover such treatments (Schauffler et al., 2001a). The lack of coverage for effective prevention services in public programs introduces a significant barrier to those most burdened by cancer: the uninsured population and members of racial and ethnic minority groups who often depend on federal programs for care. The availability of evidence-based prevention services should be ensured in these and other public programs. The Centers for Medicare and Medicaid Services (CMS, formerly the Health Care Financing Administration) is examining how a smoking cessation benefit might best be structured through a demonstration program.

Evidence-based prevention services should be available in these and other public programs. Therefore, a comprehensive review of the benefits being offered and the effectiveness of delivery systems is needed to identify opportunities to improve access to cancer prevention and early detection services in federal programs.

Recommendation 8: Programs are needed for health care providers to improve their education and training, monitor their adherence to evidence-based guidelines, and enhance their practice environments to support their provision of cancer prevention and early detection services.

Primary care providers in health care settings are effective agents of behavioral change. When counseled about smoking in clinical settings, 5 to 10 percent of individuals are able to quit. Evidence suggests, however, that physicians and other practitioners are not providing effective clinical interventions such as counseling and screening tests as often as would be beneficial. Fewer than half of adults who smoke cigarettes, for example, report that at their last visit the physician inquired whether they smoked.

Shortcomings in providers' delivery of clinical preventive services can, in part, be traced to a lack of education and training. There is evidence of programmatic deficits in medical, dental, and nursing schools, despite numerous calls to improve the education and training of health care professionals in health promotion and disease prevention. A problem of greater magnitude is upgrading the knowledge and skills of practicing clinicians whose performance reflects their lack of training. Health care providers who completed their training 10 or more years ago are unlikely to have been trained in cancer prevention and control. In the early 1990s, for example, relatively few medical schools offered any training in smoking cessation. Ensuring the inclusion of comprehensive prevention curricula in health professional schools is necessary, but the larger task is reaching providers who have completed their training. Continuing medical education programs can be made more accessible by applying new learning technologies (e.g., distance learning and online continuing medical education). Innovative alternative teaching methods are among the interventions being targeted as part of translational research in multimedia technology funded by the National Cancer Institute (2000a).

To address the deficits observed in medical schools, the Association of American Medical Colleges (AAMC) has developed population health guidelines to help ensure that medical students are able to "incorporate principles of disease prevention and behavioral change appropriate for specific populations of patients within a community" (Association of American Medical Colleges, 1999, p. 139). The AAMC Population Health Perspective Panel recommended that medical schools develop an action plan, identify teaching faculty, form liaisons with groups that can help (e.g., Teachers of Preventive Medicine), and show evidence of success. The panel also recommended that population health competencies be tested in the examinations of the National Board of Medical Examiners. Similar actions could be taken by dental, nursing, and other health professional schools to improve their inclusion of course work in cancer prevention and early detection in their curricula.

The Board recommends the following strategies for improving education and training:

- Professional education and training programs should adequately cover cancer prevention and early detection in their curricula.
- Training institutions and professional organizations should provide continuing education in cancer prevention and early detection. Continuing medical education programs can be made more accessible by applying new learning technologies (e.g., distance learning and online continuing medical education).
- Professional organizations representing primary care providers should promote their members' adherence to evidence-based cancer prevention and early detection guidelines.

Systems of care encounter a variety of infrastructure and operational barriers in the delivery of prevention services. The systems that health care providers need depend on supportive management structures; efficient patient-flow procedures; and information systems that support reminder systems, documentation of services, timely follow-up and referrals, and coordinated communication with providers and institutions across the community. Evidence consistently shows that such support systems improve physician and patient compliance with recommended preventive practices.

- Health systems should support the infrastructure needed to identify patients in need of intervention (e.g., smokers or those who are due for screening), remind providers to intervene, and track progress toward clinical goals.

Efforts to improve the quality of health care delivery have increasingly relied on monitoring the performance of health care providers and systems of care. Clinicians want to provide good care and need to know the effects of their actions and be in a position to respond to incentives (Center for the Advancement of Health, 2001). There are many opportunities to monitor performance and assist providers in improving their practices:

- CMS could examine provider performance regarding adherence to recommended cancer prevention and early detection recommendations. CMS has specified in the most recent scope of work for peer review organizations that the quality of breast cancer services is a priority area. Assessments of provider adherence to mammography guidelines could be undertaken.
- State health departments could use data from cancer registries to examine regions and population subgroups characterized by high rates of late-stage diagnoses of breast, cervical, and colorectal cancer, for which screening programs are available, to identify where to target outreach efforts.
- The National Committee for Quality Assurance could expand efforts to monitor preventive practices of managed care plans through its Health Plan Employer Data and Information Set system.
- Employers and other group benefit managers could define performance targets for health education and preventive counseling to hold health plans accountable for the provision of these services (Schauffler et al., 1999; Schauffler et al. 1996).
- The Joint Commission on the Accreditation of Healthcare Organizations could evaluate the availability of services to promote risk behavior change as part of its accreditation process.

Quality assurance systems must not only track the appropriate provision of services, but they must also assess the quality of the services provided. Clinicians, for example, need to collect samples properly, laboratories must adhere to standards in processing specimens and interpreting results, and rigorous follow-up must be carried out for patients with positive screening test results. Adherence to quality standards maximizes the benefits of prevention services.

The aging of the nation's population will sharply increase the demand for certain cancer prevention services such as screening. There may be an inadequate supply of personnel to meet these demands. There are uncertainties, for example, about the supply of gastroenterologists to perform colonoscopy for colorectal cancer screening programs and the adequacy of the numbers of mammography personnel (Institute of Medicine, 2001c). If such shortages are anticipated, policies to address them will need to be identified.

• The Health Resources and Services Administration should assess the adequacy of the future supply of providers of cancer prevention and early detection services.

Models of successful delivery of services are as essential as an adequate supply of trained providers. There is convincing evidence that nonphysician providers are just as effective as physician providers in delivering certain smoking cessation and screening services, but research is needed on how to integrate provision of prevention services by such providers into routine primary care.

• The Agency for Healthcare Research and Quality and other research sponsors should support demonstration programs to evaluate innovative models of prevention service delivery.

Recommendation 9: The U.S. Congress should provide sufficient support to the U.S. Department of Health and Human Services for the U.S. Preventive Services Task Force and the U.S. Task Force on Community Preventive Services to conduct timely assessments of the benefits, harms, and costs associated with screening tests and other preventive interventions. Summaries of recommendations should be made widely available to the public, health care providers, and state and local public health officials and policy makers.

Evidence-based guidelines for clinical and community practice provide maps for action. Rigorous assessments of the effectiveness of clinical prevention services are conducted periodically by the U.S. Preventive Services Task Force,[2] and the effectiveness of interventions aimed at communities

[2]The U.S. Preventive Services Task Force (USPSTF) is an independent panel of private-sector experts in primary care and prevention convened by the U.S. Public Health Service's Agency for Healthcare Research and Quality. USPSTF is supported by outside experts, two Evidence-Based Practice Centers (groups that systematically synthesize available literature), and liaisons from the major primary care societies and from U.S. Public Health Service agen-

are being assessed by the U.S. Task Force on Community Preventive Services.[3] These task forces are overseen by the Agency for Healthcare Research and Quality and CDC, respectively, federal agencies that have been at the forefront in identifying effective prevention intervention strategies. Widely accepted public health goals and objectives have been established through the *Healthy People 2010* initiative (US DHHS and Office of Disease Prevention and Health Promotion, 2000), and efforts are under way to chart the nation's progress toward those goals (see Chapter 9, Box 9.1).

Although there is a general consensus among public health scientists regarding interventions that work, many areas of controversy remain and evidence is inconsistently applied across federal, state, and private programs. There are examples of screening and other prevention interventions that were quickly adopted before adequate research had been completed to fully understand their potential benefits and harms. Screening for prostate cancer by prostate-specific antigen testing, for example, for which there is comparatively little evidence of effectiveness, is more commonly used than colorectal cancer screening, for which there is strong evidence of effectiveness. More recently, low-dose computed tomography scanning has been promoted as a screening test for lung cancer among high-risk individuals, with the scientific community divided on the merits of its effectiveness. The history of the rapid dissemination into practice of X-ray screening for lung cancer in the 1960s and 1970s and its later withdrawal after evidence from clinical trials showed that it did not reduce the rate of mortality from lung cancer provides a cautionary precedent for the use of computed tomography scanning as a routine screening test for lung cancer. It will be years before the results of clinical trials are available to answer questions about the test's effectiveness. Until definitive evidence is available to resolve the controversies, clear information should be available to the public on the potential benefits, harms, and costs of new technologies so that consumers and health care providers can make informed judgments.

The U.S. Preventive Services Task Force has provided comprehensive assessments of clinical prevention services, but the task force has, until recently, been convened only periodically. In 2001 it published selected updates of recommendations made in 1996 (U.S. Preventive Services Task Force 2001a,b, 2002). Assessments of prevention services are needed on a

---

cies. Currently, the third USPSTF, convened in 1998, is issuing recommendations updated from its 1996 *Guide to Clinical Preventive Services* (U.S. Preventive Services Task Force, 1996) (www.ahcpr.gov/clinic/uspstfaab.htm).

[3]The 15-member independent, nonfederal U.S. Task Force on Community Preventive Services first met in 1996 and has issued reports on improving vaccination coverage, reducing exposure to environmental tobacco smoke, and increasing physical activity (www.thecommunityguide.org).

continual basis to ensure that public health recommendations are current and incorporate the latest scientific evidence. The task force's main responsibility is making clinical recommendations, but its role should be expanded to also recommend priority areas for research on clinical preventive services.

The U.S. Community Services Task Force is relatively new and has the responsibility to identify interventions that work for communities. As state efforts to implement comprehensive cancer control plans gain momentum, guidance on the effectiveness of public health interventions will be critically needed.

The Board recommends that support for both task forces be sufficient for systematic syntheses and meta-analyses of data from the literature and to keep abreast of developments in both clinical and community disease prevention and health promotion. Greater investments in dissemination activities are also needed to reach health providers and the general public, both about areas of consensus among public health scientists regarding interventions that work, and about the areas of controversy that remain. Some evidence suggests that health care providers and the public are not very familiar with the recommendations of the U.S. Preventive Services Task Force. Likewise, individuals who make insurance coverage decisions for employers are unfamiliar with these recommendations (Partnership for Prevention, 1997).

A promising complementary development aimed at improving dissemination of evidence-based cancer control interventions has been initiated at the National Cancer Institute (NCI), Closing the Discovery to Delivery Gap: Translating Research into Improved Outcomes (TRIO). The effort aims to (National Cancer Institute, 2001):

- model and monitor the impacts of diffusion and dissemination efforts on the health promotion and cancer control objectives of *Healthy People 2010* (US DHHS and Office of Disease Prevention and Health Promotion, 2000);
- collaboratively promote adoption of evidence-based cancer control interventions by local, state, and national service organizations; and
- focus on eliminating cancer-related health disparities among medically underserved populations with cancer.

Recommendation 10: Public and private organizations (e.g., the National Cancer Institute, the American Cancer Society) should take steps to improve the public's understanding of cancer prevention and early detection with a focus on promoting healthy lifestyles and informed decision making about health behaviors and cancer screening.

Raising public awareness of the benefits of cancer prevention and early detection is central to reducing the cancer burden. Despite the public's keen interest in the potential hazards and benefits of various lifestyle factors, several barriers to effective communication exist. The first is the difficulty of dealing with media coverage that is often contradictory and based on questionable research. In some cases the results of a single study or preliminary laboratory findings are well publicized and their implications are overstated in the press. In other cases, lifestyle recommendations based on years of descriptive epidemiology are countered by new evidence from more robust studies, for example, clinical trials. The recommendation to consume fiber to prevent cancer, for example, was grounded in good evidence from descriptive population studies (e.g., studies of the health of migrants), but the recommendation was undermined by new scientific findings from clinical trials that showed that no clear benefit was associated with fiber consumption. The public is generally not equipped to interpret the seemingly conflicting advice, and confusion, skepticism, and cynicism may result.

The public's thirst for quick medical "miracles" and simple impatience also pose significant barriers to progress in cancer prevention and early detection. It can take many years to reap the benefits of behavioral change like smoking cessation and the rewards of many other interventions can take time to be realized. Significant reductions in breast cancer mortality rates as a result of screening programs have only recently been observed in the general population. The fascination of the American public with advanced technology and "getting tested," the commercial and marketing interests in servicing this demand, and the sense of urgency to take action in combating cancer set the stage for the premature adoption of interventions that are potentially ineffective or harmful. That screening can be harmful is itself an unfamiliar concept to the general public and many health care professionals. Cultivating a deeper awareness of the health risks of screening might promote more responsible choices about screening at both the individual and the population levels and undo the popular misconception that the only arguments against screening are economic (Woolf, 2001).

Increasingly, cancer screening guidelines incorporate the tenets of informed decision making. Rather than issuing prescriptive recommendations regarding prostate-specific antigen testing, for example, most organizations are suggesting that individuals discuss the relative benefits and harms of screening, weigh these factors according to their individual values and preferences, and decide whether or not to proceed with screening. Although this shared decision-making approach tends to be embraced by the well-educated health consumer, little is known regarding its acceptance among the general public and how best to incorporate it into the delivery of preventive services.

Improved understanding of cancer prevention by the general public is also critical to support for research in this area. Although the public is generally supportive of clinical medical innovations, it has less of an appreciation of the potential of public health interventions. Clinical interventions play an essential role in prevention, but public health programs can more effectively reach a broader audience and bring about shifts in behavior within a population. There is generally a failure to appreciate the significance of the levels of change achieved with current interventions. A program that helps 10 to 15 percent of individuals stop smoking has tremendous rewards in terms of reductions in morbidity and mortality rates. Likewise, support for cancer prevention may lag behind that for other interventions because many people do not acknowledge the difficulty of initiating behavioral change and the need for supportive systems to help individuals maintain healthy behavioral change.

Recognizing that society is in the midst of a communications revolution, NCI (2001) has found that an extraordinary opportunity to invest in communications about cancer exists at present. Effective communication can move people to engage in behaviors that will improve their health, can give people the information that they need to make informed cancer-related decisions, and may empower people by raising their awareness of health problems and recommended actions. The goals of the NCI initiative are to

- accelerate reductions in the U.S. cancer burden through the use of communications about cancer;
- integrate communications about cancer into the cancer care continuum so that it is an accepted and practiced component of quality care; and
- increase the demand for, access to, and use of communications about cancer by diverse populations including the public, high-risk persons, underserved and disabled populations, children, patients, survivors, and health care professionals.

Among the activities to be sponsored as part of this initiative are national surveys to assess public perceptions; monitoring of emerging information needs; creation of cancer-related communications centers of excellence; development of tool kits for the public, patients, underserved populations, advocacy groups, and others; and training of health communications scientists, researchers, and practitioners (National Cancer Institute, 2001).

The lessons learned from the research supported by this initiative will inform the educational programs of both public and private organizations. Knowledge of how to frame educational messages that will lead to both increased knowledge and health-promoting behaviors could, for example, be applied by the American Cancer Society in its community-based programs and by CMS in its beneficiary education campaigns.

Recommendation 11: Public and private initiatives to reduce disparities in the cancer burden (e.g., initiatives of the National Cancer Institute and the American Cancer Society) should be supported.

There are glaring disparities in rates of morbidity and mortality from cancer between socioeconomic groups, insured and uninsured populations, and certain racial and ethnic groups (IOM, 1999b). The differences among these various groups present both a challenge in terms of understanding the reasons and an opportunity in terms of reducing the burden of cancer (US DHHS and Office of Disease Prevention and Health Promotion, 2000). Lack of health insurance coverage is a key predictor of lower rates of use of cancer screening tests. Other psychological and sociocultural factors may also be at play. Personal barriers can include cultural differences, language barriers, not knowing what to do or when to seek care, or concerns about confidentiality or discrimination (US DHHS and Office of Disease Prevention and Health Promotion, 2000). In a nation of increasing diversity, interventions to improve cancer prevention and early detection must accommodate different languages, cultural values, and beliefs.

The elimination of racial and ethnic disparities in health is an overarching goal of *Healthy People 2010* (US DHHS and Office of Disease Prevention and Health Promotion, 2000), and an ongoing initiative involving agencies of the U.S. Department of Health and Human Services is in place. Cancer screening and management is one of six focus areas of the initiative (http://raceandhealth.hhs.gov/sidebars/sbinitOver.htm). The National Institutes of Health (NIH) has drafted a trans-NIH, 5-year Strategic Research Plan to Reduce and Ultimately Eliminate Health Disparities (www.nih.gov/about/hd/strategicplan.pdf), and in December 2000 NCI established the Center to Reduce Cancer Health Disparities (http://crchd.nci.nih.gov) to implement the NCI Strategic Plan to Reduce Health Disparities. Through this initiative, NCI aims to understand the causes of health disparities as they relate to cancer and develop effective interventions to eliminate these disparities. Specific initiatives and an action plan have been developed for each of the five objectives outlined in the strategic plan (http://www.cancer. gov/announcements/healthdisp.html):

1. expand the capacity to conduct fundamental cancer control and population research to elucidate the determinants of cancer-related health disparities;
2. expand the ability to define and monitor cancer-related health disparities;
3. support intervention research in prevention, early detection, treatment, and communications that may reduce cancer-related health disparities;
4. expand the channels for research dissemination and diffusion and

foster collaborations with allied agencies and organizations to facilitate the translation of evidence into practice; and

5. strengthen training and education in health disparities research and increase the number of minority scientists working in cancer control science.

The Board fully supports this NCI initiative and encourages NCI to collaborate with other private and public efforts to achieve success. Also needed are effective methods to evaluate and track the success of this and other initiatives.

Recommendation 12: Public and private sponsors of research including the National Institutes of Health, the Agency for Healthcare Research and Quality, the Centers for Medicare and Medicaid Services, the Centers for Disease Control and Prevention, the U.S. Department of Defense, and the American Cancer Society should expand their support of applied behavioral research and how best to disseminate evidence-based prevention interventions. Effective strategies are especially needed to encourage healthy behaviors among children and their families, medically underserved populations, and the public at large through multicomponent interventions.

The United States is at a crossroads in cancer prevention research. Basic science and epidemiology are advancing knowledge in a variety of areas, from the relationship between cancer and modifiable behavioral risk factors all the way down to the molecular pathways that mediate the actions of those risk factors. At the same time applied research is illustrating how the already vast amount of available evidence can be better used to more rapidly reduce cancer rates. To effectively reduce the cancer burden in the United States, however, there needs to be greater emphasis on action-oriented research (Colditz, 1997, 2001; Wegman, 1992). Knowledge about health problems and their causes does not automatically guarantee that appropriate actions are taken. Only when etiological knowledge is linked to evidence on the effectiveness of behavioral change strategies, and in turn to public awareness and policy support can the potential to reduce the burden of cancer be realized.

IDENTIFYING RESEARCH PRIORITIES

The Board has prioritized research to encourage healthy behaviors among children and their families, underserved populations, and the public at large through multicomponent interventions. In its review of the evidence regarding the effectiveness of cancer prevention and early detection, the Board identified specific research priorities in the major areas covered in this report: tobacco use, physical activity, obesity and diet-nutrition, and cancer screening. The research priorities in each of these areas are described in the following sections.

Tobacco Use

- Evaluate tobacco control programs, especially those that attempt to promote change through multiple channels including schools, community-based organizations, and the media. States need to know what works when allocating limited resources.
- Assess the Tobacco Master Settlement Agreement, in particular, industry adherence to its provisions and the success of these provisions in reducing youth smoking rates.
- Evaluate the effectiveness of channels for the delivery of smoking cessation services (e.g., workplaces, the Internet, families, health care providers, and peers) and other approaches to smoking cessation (e.g., restrictive smoking policies in schools and workplaces).
- Identify effective cessation strategies for youth and young adults. Although many programs are designed to prevent smoking in adolescents and young adults, few evidence-based programs are aimed at smoking cessation in this age group. Research is needed to identify effective strategies for smoking cessation in young people.
- Identify factors that increase demand for smoking cessation services. Researchers need to identify barriers to participation, factors that foster participation, and factors that promote sustained program participation.
- Identify factors related to disparities in tobacco use and success in quitting by gender, race-ethnicity, occupation, educational level, and socioeconomic status. Understanding the social contextual factors such as social support, social networks, social norms, cultural beliefs, language, and psychological stressors could further understanding of how underserved groups can be helped to quit smoking.
- Identify ways to help low-income smokers quit smoking. Applied research is needed into ways to make pharmacotherapy (e.g., nicotine replacement therapy) available and affordable for low-income groups.

Physical Activity

- Identify strategies to build community support for environmental changes to promote activity. The Centers for Disease Control and Prevention has established a blueprint for promoting physical activity in communities, but support for the implementation of the recommendations presented in that blueprint has not been forthcoming. Research is needed to identify strategies that promote physical activity at the local level and that are tailored to the needs of individual communities.

- Identify the optimal approaches to comprehensive health education programs for children and young adults to promote lifelong activity. Research is needed that provides a better understanding of the tracking of activity into the early adult years, the types of programs that foster lifelong activity, and the components of programs that foster adequate levels of physical activity to maintain a healthy weight through the adult years.
- Identify strategies to make the work environment and social environments conducive to increased activity.
- Identify how best to implement counseling for physical activity and weight management into routine, ongoing medical care.

Obesity and Diet-Nutrition

- Translate the health benefits of weight maintenance through the adult years into health messages that motivate population-based strategies for the maintenance of healthy weight.
- Identify strategies that can be used to reinforce behavioral changes that will promote and sustain a healthy weight.
- Conduct long-term clinical intervention studies to alter behavioral patterns that may influence weight gain.
- Identify the underlying causes of racial-ethnic and socioeconomic differences in obesity, and evaluate methods that deliver effective interventions to reduce disparities.
- Conduct community-based intervention studies involving public and private partners (e.g., employers, food and fitness industry) to prevent weight gain and promote healthy diet and physical activity.

Cancer Screening

- Develop useful methods for implementing shared decision making as applied to cancer screening. Given the growing number of cancer screening tests for which shared decision making is recommended, there is a growing need to answer questions surrounding the appropriateness, feasibility, and proper methods of this form of counseling.
- Identify the underlying causes of racial-ethnic and socioeconomic disparities in the use of screening tests, and evaluate methods for the delivery of screening tests to reduce such disparities.
- Encourage research to ensure that screening is performed well—with proper timing, technique, follow-up, and repeat screening—and that all eligible persons are screened.
- Examine opportunities to increase rates of access to cancer screening in non-clinical venues such as worksites.
- Evaluate the success of state and local health departments in using state and local estimates of screening use to target areas (and providers)

for improvement. Likewise, for Medicare beneficiaries, evaluate the success of peer review organizations in targeting areas (and providers) for improvement.

- Clarify the effectiveness of screening tests relative to the effectiveness of primary prevention and other clinical or public health interventions in lowering rates of morbidity and mortality. The findings from such research can guide decisions about resource allocation.

The Board aims, with this summary of research priorities, to motivate research sponsors to invest in research that will lead to the identification of interventions that work and dissemination strategies that effect behavioral changes in the population. Essential too are investments in basic research in both cancer biology and behavioral health that can lead to the development of improved methods for cancer prevention and control (IOM, 2001a). The Board concurs with IOM's Committee on Health and Behavior: Research, Practice and Policy when they concluded in their report, *Health and Behavior: The Interplay of Biological, Behavioral, and Societal Influences,* that "Most studies, though demonstrating the ability to alter behavior, either do not test, or when tested do not demonstrate, sustained behavior change. These factors present major challenges for the research and application of behavioral interventions and point to the need for long-term studies" (IOM, 2001a, page 334).

References

Abed J, Reilley B, Butler MO, Kean T, Wong F, Hohman K. 2000a. Comprehensive cancer control initiative of the Centers for Disease Control and Prevention: an example of participatory innovation diffusion. *J Public Health Manag Pract* 6(2):79–92.

Abed J, Reilley B, Butler MO, Kean T, Wong F, Hohman K. 2000b. Developing a framework for comprehensive cancer prevention and control in the United States: an initiative of the Centers for Disease Control and Prevention. *J Public Health Manag Pract* 6(2):67–78.

Aberle DR, Gamsu G, Henschke CI, Naidich DP, Swensen SJ. 2001. A consensus statement of the Society of Thoracic Radiology: screening for lung cancer with helical computed tomography. *J Thorac Imaging* 16(1):65–8.

Abrams DB. 1993. Treatment issues: towards a stepped-care model. *Tobacco Control* 2 (Suppl): S17–S29.

Abrams DB, Follick MJ. 1983. Behavioral weight-loss intervention at the worksite: feasibility and maintenance. *J Consult Clin Psychol* 51(2):226–33.

Abrams DB, Emmons KM, Linnan LA. 1995. Health behavior and health education: the past, present, and future. Glanz K, Lewis FM, Rimer BK, eds. *Health Behavior and Health Education: Theory, Research, and Practice*. San Francisco: Jossey-Bass. Pp. 453–478.

Adams A, Ockene JK, Wheller EV, Hurley TG. 1998. Alcohol counseling: physicians will do it. *J Gen Intern Med* 13(10):692–8.

Adolfsson J. 1993. Deferred treatment of low grade stage T3 prostate cancer without distant metastases. *J Urol* 149(2):326–9.

Adolfsson J, Steineck G, Whitmore WF Jr. 1993. Recent results of management of palpable clinically localized prostate cancer. *Cancer* 72(2):310–22.

Adolfsson J, Ronstrom L, Lowhagen T, Carstensen J, Hedlund PO. 1994. Deferred treatment of clinically localized low grade prostate cancer: the experience from a prospective series at the Karolinska Hospital. *J Urol* 152(5 Pt 2):1757–60.

Adolfsson J, Steineck G, Hedlund PO. 1999. Deferred treatment of locally advanced non-metastatic prostate cancer: a long-term followup. *J Urol* 161(2):505–8.

Advisory Committee on Cancer Control, National Cancer Institute of Canada. 1994. Bridging research to action: a framework and decision-making process for cancer control. *Can Med Assoc J* 151(8):1141–46.

Advisory Committee to the Surgeon General. 1986. *The Health Consequences of Using Smokeless Tobacco: a Report of the Advisory Committee to the Surgeon General.* Bethesda, MD: U.S. Public Health Service, U.S. Department of Health and Human Services.

Agency for Health Care Policy and Research. 1999. *Evaluation of Cervical Cytology*. AHCPR Pubication No. 99-E010. Rockville, MD: Agency for Health Care Policy and Research.

Agency for Health Care Policy and Research. 1996. *Smoking Cessation: Clinical Practice Guideline, No. 18*. AHCPR Pubication No. 96-0692. Rockville, MD: Agency for Health Care Policy and Research.

Agency for Healthcare Research and Quality. 2001a. *Evidence Report on the Efficacy of Interventions to Modify Dietary Behavior Related to Cancer Risk: Final Evidence Report*. Rockville, MD: Agency for Healthcare Research and Quality.

Agency for Health Care Research and Quality. 2001b. *Access and Experiences Regarding Medical Care, Fall 2000*. MEPS Statistical Brief #2. Rockville, MD: Agency for Health Care Research and Quality.

Agurs-Collins TD, Kumanyika SK, Ten Have TR, Adams-Campbell LL. 1997. A randomized controlled trial of weight reduction and exercise for diabetes management in older African-American subjects. *Diabetes Care* 20(10):1503–11.

Ahlquist DA, Skoletsky JE, Boynton KA, Harrington JJ, Mahoney DW, Pierceall WE, Thibodeau SN, Shuber AP. 2000. Colorectal cancer screening by detection of altered human DNA in stool: feasibility of a multitarget assay panel. *Gastroenterology* 119(5):1219–27.

Ahluwalia JS, Gibson CA, Kenney RE, Wallace DD, Resnicow K. 1999. Smoking status as a vital sign. *J Gen Intern Med* 14(7):402–8.

Albanes D, Blair A, Taylor PR. 1989. Physical activity and risk of cancer in the NHANES I population. *Am J Public Health* 79(6):744–50.

Alberts DS, Martinez ME, Roe DJ, Guillen-Rodriguez JM, Marshall JR, van Leeuwen JB, Reid ME, Ritenbaugh C, Vargas PA, Bhattacharyya AB, Earnest DL, Sampliner RE. 2000. Lack of effect of a high-fiber cereal supplement on the recurrence of colorectal adenomas. Phoenix Colon Cancer Prevention Physicians' Network. *N Engl J Med* 342(16):1156–62.

Albertsen P. 2000. When is a death from prostate cancer not a death from prostate cancer? *J Natl Cancer Inst* 92(8):590–1.

Albertsen PC, Fryback DG, Storer BE, Kolon TF, Fine J. 1995. Long-term survival among men with conservatively treated localized prostate cancer. *JAMA* 274(8):626–31.

Albertsen PC, Hanley JA, Gleason DF, Barry MJ. 1998. Competing risk analysis of men aged 55 to 74 years at diagnosis managed conservatively for clinically localized prostate cancer. *JAMA* 280(11):975–80.

Alexander FE, Anderson TJ, Brown HK, Forrest AP, Hepburn W, Kirkpatrick AE, Muir BB, Prescott RJ, Smith A. 1999. 14 years of follow-up from the Edinburgh randomised trial of breast-cancer screening. *Lancet* 353(9168):1903–8.

Allen SS, Bland CJ, Dawson SJ. 1990. A mini-workshop to train medical students to use a patient-centered approach to smoking cessation. *Am J Prev Med* 6(1):28–33.

Alpha-Tocopherol Beta Carotene Cancer Prevention Study Group. 1994. The effect of vitamin E and beta carotene on the incidence of lung cancer and other cancers in male smokers. *N Engl J Med* 330(15):1029–35.

Altekruse J, Goldenberg K, Rabin DL, Riegelman RK, Wiese WH. 1991. Implementing the Association of Teachers of Preventive Medicine's recommendations into the undergraduate medical school curriculum. *Acad Med* 66(6):312–6.

Altman DG, Wheelis AY, McFarlane M, Lee H, Fortmann SP. 1999. The relationship between tobacco access and use among adolescents: a four community study. *Soc Sci Med* 48(6):759–75.

American Academy of Family Physicians. 1998. Periodic health examination, Appendix F. In *AAFP Reference Manual 1997–1998*. Kansas City, MO: American Academy of Family Physicians.

American Academy of Family Physicians. 2000. AAFP summary of policy recommendations for periodic health examination. In *AAFP Reference Manual 1999–2000, Clinical Policies*. Kansas City, MO: American Academy of Family Physicians.

ACS (American Cancer Society). 1980a. *Guidelines for the Cancer-Related Checkup: Recommendation and Rationale*, p. 30. Atlanta: American Cancer Society.

ACS. 1980b. Public attitudes toward cancer and cancer tests. *CA Cancer J Clin* 30(2):92–8.

ACS. 1996. Guidelines on diet, nutrition, and cancer prevention: reducing the risk of cancer with healthy food choices and physical activity. The American Cancer Society 1996 Advisory Committee on Diet, Nutrition, and Cancer Prevention. *CA Cancer J Clin* 46(6):325–41.

ACS. 2001. *Cancer Prevention Studies*. [Online]. Available at: http://www.cancer.org/eprise/main/docroot/RES/RES_6?sitearea=RES&level=1 (accessed May, 2001).

ACS. 2002a. *Cancer Facts and Figures 2002*. Atlanta: American Cancer Society.

ACS. 2002b. *Cancer Prevention and Early Detection Facts and Figures 2002*. Atlanta: American Cancer Society.

American College of Obstetricians and Gynecologists. 2000. *ACOG Periodic Assessment Charts*, updated December 2000. Washington, DC: American College of Obstetricians and Gynecologists.

American College of Physicians. 1997. Screening for prostate cancer. *Ann Intern Med* 126(6): 480–4.

American College of Radiology. 1991. Resolution No. 36. Reston, VA: American College of Radiology.

American College of Radiology. 2000. *ACR Standards for the Performance of Screening Mammography*. Approved January 1, 2000. Reston, VA: American College of Radiology.

American Geriatrics Society Clinical Practice Committee. 2000. Breast cancer screening in older women. *J Am Geriatr Soc* 48(7):842–4.

American Medical Association. Pasko T, Seidman B. 1999. *Physician Characteristics and Distribution in the U.S.* Chicago: American Medical Association, Department of Survey and Planning, Division of Survey and Data Resources.

American Society of Clinical Oncology. 1996. Statement of the American Society of Clinical Oncology: genetic testing for cancer susceptibility, Adopted on February 20, 1996. *J Clin Oncol* 14(5):1730–40.

American Urological Association. 1992. Early detection of prostate cancer and use of transrectal ultrasound. In *American Urological Association 1992 Policy Statement Book*. Baltimore: American Urological Association.

American Urological Association. 2000. Prostate-specific antigen (PSA) best practice policy. *Oncology (Huntington)* 14(2):267–72, 277–8, 280.

Anda RF, Remington PL, Sienko DG, Davis RM. 1987. Are physicians advising smokers to quit? The patient's perspective. *JAMA* 257(14):1916–9.

Andersen MR, Yasui Y, Meischke H, Kuniyuki A, Etzioni R, Urban N. 2000. The effectiveness of mammography promotion by volunteers in rural communities. *Am J Prev Med* 18(3):199–207.

Andersen RE, Franckowiak SC, Snyder J, Bartlett SJ, Fontaine KR. 1998. Can inexpensive signs encourage the use of stairs? Results from a community intervention. *Ann Intern Med* 129(5):363–9.

Andersen RE, Wadden TA, Bartlett SJ, Zemel B, Verde TJ, Franckowiak SC. 1999. Effects of lifestyle activity vs structured aerobic exercise in obese women: a randomized trial. *JAMA* 281(4):335–40.

Anderson HA, Hanrahan LP, Schirmer J, Higgins D, Sarow P. 1991. Mesothelioma among employees with likely contact with in-place asbestos-containing building materials. *Ann NY Acad Sci* 643:550–72.

Anderson J, Dusenbury L. 1999. Worksite cholesterol and nutrition: an intervention project in Colorado. *AAOHN J* 47(3):99–106.

Anderson K, Potter JD, et al. 1996. Pancreatic cancer. In Schottenfeld D, Fraumeni JF. *Cancer Epidemiology and Prevention.* New York: Oxford University Press. Pp. xxi, 1521.

Anderson ML, Pasha TM, Leighton JA. 2000. Endoscopic perforation of the colon: lessons from a 10-year study. *Am J Gastroenterol* 95(12):3418–22.

Anderson P. 1995. Alcohol and risk of physical harm. In Holder H, Edwards G (eds.). *Alcohol: Evidence and Issues.* Oxford, United Kingdom: Oxford University Press. Pp. 82–113.

Anderson RN. 2001. Deaths: leading causes for 1999. *Natl Vital Stat Rep* 49(11):1–87.

Andersson I, Janzon L. 1997. Reduced breast cancer mortality in women under age 50: updated results from the Malmo Mammographic Screening Program. *J Natl Cancer Inst Monogr* (22):63–7.

Andersson SO, Wolk A, Bergstrom R, Adami HO, Engholm G, Englund A, Nyren O. 1997. Body size and prostate cancer: a 20-year follow-up study among 135,006 Swedish construction workers. *J Natl Cancer Inst* 89(5):385–9.

Andreasson S, Allebeck P, Romelsjo A. 1988. Alcohol and mortality among young men: longitudinal study of Swedish conscripts. *Br Med J (Clin Res Ed)* 296(6628):1021–5.

Andriole GL, Catalona WJ. 1993. Using PSA to screen for prostate cancer. The Washington University experience. *Urol Clin N Am* 20(4):647–51.

Andriole GL, Smith DS, Rao G, Goodnough L, Catalona WJ. 1994. Early complications of contemporary anatomical radical retropubic prostatectomy. *J Urol* 152(5 Pt 2):1858–60.

Anglian Breast Cancer Study Group. 2000. Prevalence and penetrance of BRCA1 and BRCA2 mutations in a population-based series of breast cancer cases. *Br J Cancer* 83(10):1301–8.

Anonymous. 1980. The Cardiff cervical cytology study. Enumeration and definition of population and initial acceptance rates. *J Epidemiol Community Health* 34(1):9–13.

Anonymous. 1986. Screening (lung cancer). *Chest* 89(4 Suppl):324S–6S.

Anonymous. 1990. 1989 survey of physicians' attitudes and practices in early cancer detection. *CA Cancer J Clin* 40(2):77–101.

Anonymous. 1995a. Community Intervention Trial for Smoking Cessation (COMMIT). I. Cohort results from a four-year community intervention. *Am J Public Health* 85(2):183–92.

Anonymous. 1995b. Community intervention trial for smoking cessation (COMMIT). II. Changes in adult cigarette smoking prevalence. *Am J Public Health* 85(2):193–200.

Anonymous. 2000. Dieting and the development of eating disorders in overweight and obese adults. *Arch Intern Med* 160(17):2581–9.

Ansari MZ, Costello AJ, Jolley DJ, Ackland MJ, Carson N, McDonald IG. 1998. Adverse events after prostatectomy in Victorian public hospitals. *Aust NZ J Surg* 68(12):830–6.

Apfelbaum M, Vague P, Ziegler O, Hanotin C, Thomas F, Leutenegger E. 1999. Long-term maintenance of weight loss after a very-low-calorie diet: a randomized blinded trial of the efficacy and tolerability of sibutramine. *Am J Med* 106(2):179–84.

Ashford A, Gemson D, Sheinfeld Gorin SN, Bloch S, Lantigua R, Ahsan H, Neugut AI. 2000. Cancer screening and prevention practices of inner-city physicians. *Am J Prev Med* 19(1):59–62.

Ashley JM, St Jeor ST, Veach TL, Mackintosh FR, Anderson JL, Perumean-Chaney SE, Krenkel JA, Scott BJ. 2000. Nutrition and cancer education: ten years of progress. *J Cancer Educ* 15(3):123–6.

Association of American Medical Colleges. 1945. Final Report of the Committee on the Teaching of Preventive Medicine and Public Health. *J Assoc Am Med Col* 20:152.

Association of American Medical Colleges. 1999. Contemporary issues in medicine—medical informatics and population health: report II of the Medical School Objectives Project. Acad Med 74(2):130–41.

Association of Teachers of Preventive Medicine. 2000. Teaching prevention throughout the curriculum: multidisciplinary perspectives on enhancing disease prevention and health promotion in undergraduate medical education. *Acad Med* 75(7): supplement.

Astrup A, Grunwald GK, Melanson EL, Saris WH, Hill JO. 2000. The role of low-fat diets in body weight control: a meta-analysis of ad libitum dietary intervention studies. *Int J Obes Relat Metab Disord* 24(12):1545–52.

Atkin WS, Morson BC, Cuzick J. 1992. Long-term risk of colorectal cancer after excision of rectosigmoid adenomas. *N Engl J Med* 326(10):658–62.

Atkin WS, Hart A, Edwards R, McIntyre P, Aubrey R, Wardle J, Sutton S, Cuzick J, Northover JM. 1998. Uptake, yield of neoplasia, and adverse effects of flexible sigmoidoscopy screening. *Gut* 42(4):560–5.

Aubin M, Godin G, Vezina I, Maziade J, Desharnais R. 1998. Hypercholesterolemia screening. Does knowledge of blood cholesterol level affect dietary fat intake? *Cancer Family Physician* 44:1289–97.

Auerbach O. 1969. Cancerous and precancerous lung changes: a slide review. *CA Cancer J Clin* 19(3):138–45.

Aus G. 1994. Prostate cancer. Mortality and morbidity after non-curative treatment with aspects on diagnosis and treatment. *Scand J Urol Nephrol Suppl* 167:1–41.

Aus G, Hermansson, CG, Hugosson J, Pedersen KV. 1993. Transrectal ultrasound examination of the prostate: complications and acceptance by patients. *Br J Urol* 71(4):457–9.

Auslander W, Haire-Joshu D, Williams JH, Houston C, Krebill H. 2000. The short-term impact of a health promotion program for African-American women. *Res Social Work Pract* 10:56–77.

Austin JH, Romney BM, Goldsmith LS. 1992. Missed bronchogenic carcinoma: radiographic findings in 27 patients with a potentially resectable lesion evident in retrospect. *Radiology* 182(1):115–22.

Austin OJ, Valente S, Hasse LA, Kues JR. 1997. Determinants of prostate-specific antigen test use in prostate cancer screening by primary care physicians. *Arch Fam Med* 6(5):453–8.

Australian Health Technology Advisory Committee. 1996. *Prostate Cancer Screening*. Canberra, Australia: Australian Health Technology Advisory Committee.

Baer DM, Wolf MM, Risley TR. 1968. Some current dimensions of applied behavior analysis. *J Appl Behav Anal* 1:91–7.

Bagshaw MA, Cox RS, Hancock SL. 1994. Control of prostate cancer with radiotherapy: long-term results. *J Urol* 152(5 Pt 2):1781–5.

Bailar JC III, MacMahon B. 1997. Randomization in the Canadian National Breast Screening Study: a review for evidence of subversion. *Can Med Assoc J* 156(2):193–9.

Bailey EJ, Erwin DO, Belin P. 2000. Using cultural beliefs and patterns to improve mammography utilization among African-American women: the Witness Project. *J Natl Med Assoc* 92(3):136–42.

Baillie AJ, Mattick RP, Hall W, Webster P. 1994. Meta-analytic review of the efficacy of smoking cessation interventions. *Drug Alcohol Rev* 13:157–70.

Bakemeier RF. 2000. Nutrition and cancer education at the University of Colorado Health Sciences Center. *J Cancer Educ* 15(3):148–50.

Bakemeier RF, Edwards MH. 1986. The American Association for Cancer Education: cancer education objectives for medical schools. *J Cancer Educ* 1:109–36.

Bakemeier RF, Anderson JJ, Brooks CM, Cairoli VJ, Chamberlain RM, Gallagher RE, Lopez A, Prout MN, Schapira DV, Shils ME. 1989. Nutrition and cancer education objectives of the American Association for Cancer Education. *J Cancer Educ* 4(4):241–53.

Bakemeier RF, Kupchella CE, Chamberlain RM, Gallagher RE, O'Donnell JF, Parker JA, Hill GJ, Brooks CM. 1992. Survey design and observations relating to cancer education funding. Cancer Education Survey II: cancer education in United States medical schools (conducted by The American Association for Cancer Education with the support of the American Cancer Society). *J Cancer Educ* 7(2):85–93.

Bandera EV, Freudenheim JL, Marshall JR, Zielezny M, Priore RL, Brasure J, Baptiste M, Graham S. 1997. Diet and alcohol consumption and lung cancer risk in the New York State Cohort (United States). *Cancer Causes Control* 8(6):828–40.

Bandura A. 1989. Human agency in social cognitive theory. *Am Psychol* 44(9):1175–84.

Bang KM, Kim JH. 2001. Prevalence of cigarette smoking by occupation and industry in the United States. *Am J Ind Med* 40(3):233–9.

Baranowski T, Henske J, Simons-Morton B, Palmer J, et al. 1990a. Dietary change for cardiovascular disease prevention among Black-American families. *Health Educ Res* 5(4): 433–53.

Baranowski T, Simons-Morton B, Hooks P, Henske J, Tiernan K, Dunn JK, Burkhalter H, Harper J, Palmer J. 1990b. A center-based program for exercise change among black-American families. *Health Educ Q* 17(2):179–96.

Baranowski T, Cullen KW, Baranowski J. 1999. Psychosocial correlates of dietary intake: advancing dietary intervention. *Annu Rev Nutr* 19:17–40.

Baranowski T, Davis M, Resnicow K, Baranowski J, Doyle C, Lin LS, Smith M, Wang DT. 2000. Gimme 5 fruit, juice, and vegetables for fun and health: outcome evaluation. *Health Educ Behav* 27(1):96–111.

Barker GJ, Williams KB. 1999. Tobacco use cessation activities in U.S. dental and dental hygiene student clinics. *J Dent Educ* 63(11):828–33.

Barry MJ. 1999. Involving patients in medical decisions: how can physicians do better? *JAMA* 282(24):2356–7.

Barry MJ, Roberts RG, Oesterling JE. 1996. Differences in how primary care physicians and urologists approach early detection of prostate cancer. *Journal of General Internal Medicine* 11(Suppl):62.

Barton MB, Harris R, Fletcher SW. 1999. Does this patient have breast cancer? The screening clinical breast examination: should it be done? How? *JAMA* 282(13):1270–80.

Bartsch G, Horninger W, Klocker H, Reissigl A, Oberaigner W, Schonitzer D, Severi G, Robertson C, Boyle P. 2001. Prostate cancer mortality after introduction of prostate-specific antigen mass screening in the Federal State of Tyrol, Austria. *Urology* 58(3): 417–24.

Battista RN, Mickalide AD. 1990. *Integration of Preventive Services into Primary Care: A Conceptual Framework for Implementation*. New York: Springer-Verlag.

Batty D, Thune I. 2000. Does physical activity prevent cancer? Evidence suggests protection against colon cancer and probably breast cancer. *BMJ* 321(7274):1424–5.

Bauer RL, Heller RF, Challah S. 1985. United Kingdom Heart Disease Prevention Project: 12-year follow-up of risk factors. *Am J Epidemiol* 121(4):563–9.

Bauman KE, Foshee VA, Ennett ST, Pemberton M, Hicks KA, King TS, Koch GG. 2001. The influence of a family program on adolescent tobacco and alcohol use. *Am J Public Health* 91(4):604–10.

Baumrind D. 1991. The influence of parenting style on adolescent competence and substance use. *J Early Adolesc* 11:59–95.

Baxter AP, Milner PC, Hawkins S, Leaf M, Simpson C, Wilson KV, Owen T, Higginbottom G, Nicholl J, Cooper N. 1997. The impact of heart health promotion on coronary heart disease lifestyle risk factors in schoolchildren: lessons learnt from a community-based project. *Public Health* 111(4):231–7.

Bayer R, Gostin LO, Javitt GH, Brandt A. 2002. Tobacco advertising in the United States: a proposal for a constitutionally acceptable form of regulation. *JAMA* 287(22):2990–5.

Bazinet M, Meshref AW, Trudel C, Aronson S, Peloquin F, Nachabe M, Begin LR, Elhilali MM. 1994. Prospective evaluation of prostate-specific antigen density and systematic biopsies for early detection of prostatic carcinoma. *Urology* 43(1):44–51.

Bechtel JJ, Petty TL, Saccomanno G. 2000. Five year survival and later outcome of patients with X-ray occult lung cancer detected by sputum cytology. *Lung Cancer* 30(1):1–7.

Beck JR, Kattan MW, Miles BJ. 1994. A critique of the decision analysis for clinically localized prostate cancer. *J Urol* 152(5 Pt 2):1894–9.

Becker HA, Chesley DA, Miller I. 1995. Oncology education needs survey of registered nurses in Texas. *J Cancer Educ* 10(1):41–7.

Becker MH, Janz NK. 1990. Practicing health promotion: the doctor's dilemma. *Ann Intern Med* 113(6):419–22.

Becona E, Vazquez FL. 2001. Effectiveness of personalized written feedback through a mail intervention for smoking cessation: a randomized-controlled trial in Spanish smokers. *J Consult Clin Psychol* 69:33–40.

Bedenne L, Faivre J, Boutron MC, Piard F, Cauvin JM, Hillon P. 1992. Adenoma-carcinoma sequence or "de novo" carcinogenesis? A study of adenomatous remnants in a population-based series of large bowel cancers. *Cancer* 69(4):883–8.

Beeker C, Kraft JM, Southwell BG, Jorgensen CM. 2000. Colorectal cancer screening in older men and women: qualitative research findings and implications for intervention. *J Community Health* 25(3):263–78.

Beemsterboer PM, Warmerdam PG, Boer R, de Koning HJ. 1998. Radiation risk of mammography related to benefit in screening programmes: a favourable balance? *J Med Screen* 5(2):81–7.

Begley S. 1997. The mammogram war. *Newsweek* 129(8):54–8.

Bell RA, Spangler JG, Quandt SA. 2000. Smokeless tobacco use among adults in the Southeast. *South Med J* 93(5):456–62.

Bellas PA, Asch SM, Wilkes M. 2000. What students bring to medical school: attitudes toward health promotion and prevention. *Am J Prev Med* 18(3):242–8.

Benar VB, Lee NC, Piper M, Richardson L. 2001. Race-specific results of Papanicolaou testing and the rate of cervical neoplasia in the National Breast and Cervical Cancer Early Detection Program, 1991–1998 (United States). *Cancer Causes Control* 12(1):61–8.

Benoit RM, Naslund MJ. 1997. The economics of prostate cancer screening. *Oncology (Huntington)* 11(10):1533–43.

Benson MC, Whang IS, Pantuck A, Ring K, Kaplan SA, Olsson CA, Cooner WH. 1992. Prostate specific antigen density: a means of distinguishing benign prostatic hypertrophy and prostate cancer. *J Urol* 147(3 Pt 2):815–6.

Beresford SA, Curry SJ, Kristal AR, Lazovich D, Feng Z, Wagner EH. 1997. A dietary intervention in primary care practice: the Eating Patterns Study. *Am J Public Health* 87(4):610–6.

Beresford SA, Thompson B, Feng Z, Christianson A, McLerran D, Patrick DL. 2001. Seattle 5 a Day worksite program to increase fruit and vegetable consumption. Prev Med 32(3):230–8.

Berkman LF, Kawachi I. 2000. *Social Epidemiology*. Oxford, United Kingdom: Oxford University Press.

Berlin NI, Buncher CR, Fontana RS, Frost JK, Melamed MR. 1984. The National Cancer Institute Cooperative Early Lung Cancer Detection Program. Results of the initial screen (prevalence). Early lung cancer detection: introduction. *Am Rev Respir Dis* 130(4):545–9.

Berman BA, Yancey AK, Bastani R, Grosser SC, Staveren A, Williams RA, Lee D. 1997. African-American physicians and smoking cessation counseling. *J Natl Med Assoc* 89(8): 534–42.

Bernstein J, Mutschler P, Bernstein E. 2000. Keeping mammography referral appointments: motivation, health beliefs, and access barriers experienced by older minority women. *J Midwifery Women's Health* 45(4):308–13.

Bernstein L, Henderson BE, Hanisch R, Sullivan-Halley J, Ross RK. 1994. Physical exercise and reduced risk of breast cancer in young women. *J Natl Cancer Inst* 86(18):1403–8.

Bero LA, Grilli R, Grimshaw JM, Harvey E, Oxman AD, Thomson MA. 1998. Closing the gap between research and practice: an overview of systematic reviews of interventions to promote the implementation of research findings. The Cochrane Effective Practice and Organization of Care Review Group. *BMJ* 317(7156):465–8.

Berry DA. 1998. Benefits and risks of screening mammography for women in their forties: a statistical appraisal. *J Natl Cancer Inst* 90(19):1431–9.

Berry DP, Clarke P, Hardcastle JD, Vellacott KD. 1997. Randomized trial of the addition of flexible sigmoidoscopy to faecal occult blood testing for colorectal neoplasia population screening. *Br J Surg* 84(9):1274–6.

Biener L, Harris JE, Hamilton W. 2000. Impact of the Massachusetts tobacco control programme: population based trend analysis. *BMJ* 321(7257):351–4.

Biesalski HK, de Mesquita BB, Chesson A, Chytil F, Grimble R, Hermus RJ, Kohrle J, Lotan R, Norpoth K, Pastorino U, Thurnham D. 1998. European Consensus Statement on Lung Cancer: risk factors and prevention. Lung Cancer Panel. *CA Cancer J Clin* 48(3): 167–76.

Biglan A, Duncan TE, Ary DV, Smolkowski K. 1995. Peer and parental influences on adolescent tobacco use. *J Behav Med* 18(4):315–30.

Biglan A, Ary DV, Smolkowski K, Duncan T, Black C. 2000. A randomised controlled trial of a community intervention to prevent adolescent tobacco use. *Tob Control* 9(1):24–32.

Bini EJ, Rajapaksa RC, Weinshel EH. 1999. The findings and impact of nonrehydrated guaiac examination of the rectum (FINGER) study: a comparison of 2 methods of screening for colorectal cancer in asymptomatic average-risk patients. *Arch Intern Med* 159(17):2022–6.

Bjurstam N, Bjorneld L, Duffy SW, Smith TC, Cahlin E, Erikson O, Lingaas H, Mattsson J, Persson S, Rudenstam CM, Sawe-Soderberg J. 1997. The Gothenburg Breast Cancer Screening Trial: preliminary results on breast cancer mortality for women aged 39–49. *J Natl Cancer Inst Monogr* (22):53–5.

Black W. 1999a. Lung Cancer. In Kramer BS, Prorok PC, Gohagan J. (eds.) *Cancer Screening: Theory and Practice*, Vol. 13. New York: Marcel Dekker, Inc.

Black WC. 1999b. Should this patient be screened for cancer? *Eff Clin Pract* 2(2):86–95.

Black WC. 2000. Overdiagnosis: an underrecognized cause of confusion and harm in cancer screening. *J Natl Cancer Inst* 92(16):1280–2.

Blackman DK, Bennett EM, Miller DS. 1999. Trends in self-reported use of mammograms (1989–1997) and Papanicolaou tests (1991–1997). Behavioral Risk Factor Surveillance System. *Morbid Mortal Wkly Rep CDC Surveill Summ* 48(6):1–22.

Blamey A, Mutrie N, Aitchison T. 1995. Health promotion by encouraged use of stairs. *BMJ* 311(7000):289–90.

Block DE, Hutton KH, Johnson KM. 2000. Differences in tobacco assessment and intervention practices: a regional snapshot. *Prev Med* 30(4):282–7.

Blot WJ, McLaughlin JK, Winn DM, Austin DF, Greenberg RS, Preston-Martin S, Bernstein L, Schoenberg JB, Stemhagen A, Fraumeni JF Jr. 1988. Smoking and drinking in relation to oral and pharyngeal cancer. *Cancer Res* 48(11):3282–7.

Blue AV, Barnette JJ, Ferguson KJ, Garr DR. 2000. Evaluation methods for prevention education. *Acad Med* 75(7 Suppl):S28–34.

Bobo JK, Lee NC, Thames SF. 2000. Findings from 752,081 clinical breast examinations reported to a national screening program from 1995 through 1998. *J Natl Cancer Inst* 92(12):971–6.

Boccignone G, Chianese A, Picariello A. 2000. Computer aided detection of microcalcifications in digital mammograms. *Comput Biol Med* 30(5):267–86.

Bocking A, Biesterfeld S, Chatelain R, Gien-Gerlach G, Esser E. 1992. Diagnosis of bronchial carcinoma on sections of paraffin-embedded sputum. Sensitivity and specificity of an alternative to routine cytology. *Acta Cytol* 36(1):37–47.

Bodiya A, Vorias D, Dickson HA. 1999. Does telephone contact with a physician's office staff improve mammogram screening rates? *Fam Med* 31(5):324–6.

Boer R, de Koning HJ, van der Maas PJ. 1999. A longer breast carcinoma screening interval for women age older than 65 years? *Cancer* 86(8):1506–10.

Boffetta P, Pershagen G, Jockel KH, Forastiere F, Gaborieau V, Heinrich J, Jahn I, Kreuzer M, Merletti F, Nyberg F, Rosch F, Simonato L. 1999. Cigar and pipe smoking and lung cancer risk: a multicenter study from Europe. *J Natl Cancer Inst* 91(8):697–701.

Bogardus ST Jr, Holmboe E, Jekel JF. 1999. Perils, pitfalls, and possibilities in talking about medical risk. *JAMA* 281(11):1037–41.

Borre M, Nerstrom B, Overgaard J. 1997. The natural history of prostate carcinoma based on a Danish population treated with no intent to cure. *Cancer* 80(5):917–28.

Bosch FX, Munoz N, de Sanjose S, Izarzugaza I, Gili M, Viladiu P, Tormo MJ, Moreo P, Ascunce N, Gonzalez LC, et al. 1992. Risk factors for cervical cancer in Colombia and Spain. *Int J Cancer* 52(5):750–8.

Botterweck AA, van den Brandt PA, Goldbohm RA. 1998. A prospective cohort study on vegetable and fruit consumption and stomach cancer risk in The Netherlands. *Am J Epidemiol* 148(9):842–53.

Botvin GJ, Griffin KW, Diaz T, Miller N, Ifill-Williams M. 1999. Smoking initiation and escalation in early adolescent girls: one-year follow-up of a school-based prevention intervention for minority youth. *J Am Med Women's Assoc* 54(3):139–43, 152.

Bouchard C, Tremblay A, Nadeau A, Dussault J, Despres JP, Theriault G, Lupien PJ, Serresse O, Boulay MR, Fournier G. 1990. Long-term exercise training with constant energy intake. 1. Effect on body composition and selected metabolic variables. *Int J Obes* 14(1):57–73.

Bowen D, Hickman KM, Powers D. 1997. Importance of psychological variables in understanding risk perceptions and breast cancer screening of African American women. *Women's Health* 3(3–4):227–42.

Boyd NF. 1997. The review of randomization in the Canadian National Breast Screening Study. Is the debate over? *Can Med Assoc J* 156(2):207–9.

Boyd NF, Martin LJ, Beaton M, Cousins M, Kriukov V. 1996. Long-term effects of participation in a randomized trial of a low-fat, high-carbohydrate diet. *Cancer Epidemiol Biomarkers Prev* 5(3):217–22.

Braddock CH III, Edwards KA, Hasenberg NM, Laidley TL, Levinson W. 1999. Informed decision making in outpatient practice: time to get back to basics. *JAMA* 282(24):2313–20.

Brasso K, Friis S, Juel K, Jorgensen T, Iversen P. 1999. Mortality of patients with clinically localized prostate cancer treated with observation for 10 years or longer: a population based registry study. *J Urol* 161(2):524–8.

Breen N, Wagener DK, Brown ML, Davis WW, Ballard-Barbash R. 2001. Progress in cancer screening over a decade: results of cancer screening from the 1987, 1992, and 1998 National Health Interview Surveys. *J Natl Cancer Inst* 93(22):1704–13.

Brennan P, Bogillot O, Cordier S, Greiser E, Schill W, Vineis P, Lopez-Abente G, Tzonou A, Chang-Claude J, Bolm-Audorff U, Jockel KH, Donato F, Serra C, Wahrendorf J, Hours M, T'Mannetje A, Kogevinas M, Boffetta P. 2000. Cigarette smoking and bladder cancer in men: a pooled analysis of 11 case-control studies. *Int J Cancer* 86(2):289–94.

Breslow L. 1999. From disease prevention to health promotion. *JAMA* 281(11):1030–3.

Breslow L, Fielding J, Herrman AA, Wilbur CS. 1990. Worksite health promotion: its evolution and the Johnson & Johnson experience. *Prev Med* 19(1):13–21.

Breslow RA, Graubard BI, Sinha R, Subar AF. 2000. Diet and lung cancer mortality: a 1987 National Health Interview Survey cohort study. *Cancer Causes Control* 11(5): 419–31.

Brett GZ. 1969. Earlier diagnosis and survival in lung cancer. *Br Med J* 4(678):260–2.

Bretton PR. 1994. Prostate-specific antigen and digital rectal examination in screening for prostate cancer: a community-based study. *South Med J* 87(7):720–3.

Brice J. 2000. Low-dose CT. The promise and the paradox of lung cancer screening. *Diagn Imaging (San Francisco)* 22(5):44–53.

Brink SG, Gottlieb NH, McLeroy KR, Wisotzky M, Burdine JN. 1994. A community view of smoking cessation counseling in the practices of physicians and dentists. *Public Health Rep* 109(1):135–42.

Brookoff D, O'Brien KK, Cook CS, Thompson TD, Williams C. 1997. Characteristics of participants in domestic violence. Assessment at the scene of domestic assault. *JAMA* 277(17):1369–73.

Brown AD, Garber AM. 1999. Cost-effectiveness of 3 methods to enhance the sensitivity of Papanicolaou testing. *JAMA* 281(4):347–53.

Brown DW, French MT, Schweitzer ME, McGeary KA, McCoy CB, Ullmann SG. 1999. Economic evaluation of breast cancer screening: a review. *Cancer Pract* 7(1):28–33.

Brown J, Buckley D, Coulthard A, Dixon AK, Dixon JM, Easton DF, Eeles RA, Evans DG, Gilbert FG, Graves M, Hayes C, Jenkins JP, Jones AP, Keevil SF, Leach MO, Liney GP, Moss SM, Padhani AR, Parker GJ, Pointon LJ, Ponder BA, Redpath TW, Sloane JP, Turnbull LW, Walker LG, Warren RM. 2000. Magnetic resonance imaging screening in women at genetic risk of breast cancer: imaging and analysis protocol for the UK multicentre study. UK MRI Breast Screening Study Advisory Group. *Magn Reson Imaging* 18(7):765–76.

Brown JK, Hinds P. 1998. Assessing master's programs in advanced practice oncology nursing. *Oncol Nurs Forum* 25(8):1433–4.

Brown LM, Swanson CA, Gridley G, Swanson GM, Schoenberg JB, Greenberg RS, Silverman DT, Pottern LM, Hayes RB, Schwartz AG, et al. 1995. Adenocarcinoma of the esophagus: role of obesity and diet. *J Natl Cancer Inst* 87(2):104–9.

Brownell KD. 1991. *The LEARN Program for Weight Control.* Dallas: American Health Publishing Company.

Brownell K, Wadden T. 1986. Behavior therapy for obesity: modern approaches and better results. In Brownell KB, Foreyt JP (eds.). *Handbook of Eating Disorders: Physiology, Psychology, and Treatment of Obesity, Anorexia and Bulimia.* New York: Basic Books. Pp. 180–98.

Brownell KD, Stunkard AJ, Albaum JM. 1980. Evaluation and modification of exercise patterns in the natural environment. *Am J Psychiatry* 137(12):1540–5.

Brownell KD, Kelman JH, Stunkard AJ. 1983. Treatment of obese children with and without their mothers: changes in weight and blood pressure. *Pediatrics* 71(4):515–23.

Brownell KD, Cohen RY, Stunkard AJ, Felix MR, Cooley NB. 1984. Weight loss competitions at the work site: impact on weight, morale and cost-effectiveness. *Am J Public Health* 74(11):1283–5.

Brownson RC, Baker EA, Housemann RA, Brennan LK, Bacak SJ. 2001. Environmental and policy determinants of physical activity in the United States. *Am J Public Health* 91(12): 1995–2003.

Brownson RC, Novotny TE, Perry MC. 1993. Cigarette smoking and adult leukemia. A meta-analysis. *Arch Intern Med* 153(4):469–75.

Brug J, Steenhuis I, van Assema P, de Vries H. 1996. The impact of a computer-tailored nutrition intervention. *Prev Med* 25(3):236–42.

Brug J, Glanz K, Van Assema P, Kok G, van Breukelen GJ. 1998. The impact of computer-tailored feedback and iterative feedback on fat, fruit, and vegetable intake. *Health Educ Behav* 25(4):517–31.

Brug J, Steenhuis I, van Assema P, Glanz K, De Vries H. 1999. Computer-tailored nutrition education: differences between two interventions. *Health Educ Res* 14(2):249–56.

Bucher HC, Guyatt GH, Cook DJ, Holbrook A, McAlister FA. 1999. Users' guides to the medical literature. XIX. Applying clinical trial results. A. How to use an article measuring the effect of an intervention on surrogate end points. Evidence-Based Medicine Working Group. *JAMA* 282(8):771–8.

Budenholzer B. 1998. Benefits of screening for colorectal cancer. *Am Fam Physician* 57(5): 947–8, 950.

Buehler SK, Parsons WL. 1997. Effectiveness of a call/recall system in improving compliance with cervical cancer screening: a randomized controlled trial. *Can Med Assoc J* 157(5):521–6.

Buller DB, Morrill C, Taren D, Aickin M, Sennott-Miller L, Buller MK, Larkey L, Alatorre C, Wentzel TM. 1999. Randomized trial testing the effect of peer education at increasing fruit and vegetable intake. *J Natl Cancer Inst* 91(17):1491–500.

Burack RC, Gimotty PA. 1997. Promoting screening mammography in inner-city settings. The sustained effectiveness of computerized reminders in a randomized controlled trial. *Med Care* 35(9):921–31.

Burack RC, Gimotty PA, George J, Simon MS, Dews P, Moncrease A. 1996. The effect of patient and physician reminders on use of screening mammography in a health maintenance organization. Results of a randomized controlled trial. *Cancer* 78(8):1708–21.

Burack RC, Gimotty PA, George J, McBride S, Moncrease A, Simon MS, Dews P, Coombs J. 1998. How reminders given to patients and physicians affected Pap smear use in a health maintenance organization: results of a randomized controlled trial. *Cancer* 82(12):2391–400.

Burack RC, George J, Gurney JG. 2000a. Mammography use among women as a function of age and patient involvement in decision-making. *J Am Geriatr Soc* 48(7):817–21.

Burack RC, Simon MS, Stano M, George J, Coombs J. 2000b. Follow-up among women with an abnormal mammogram in an HMO: is it complete, timely, and efficient? *Am J Manag Care* 6(10):1102–13.

Burdick MB. 1998. AHCPR Smoking Cessation Practices in the VA. *Veterans Health System Journal* Jul/Aug:83–84.

Burdick MB. 1999. Solutions: success stories in prevention. *Veterans Health System Journal* (Sept).

Burhansstipanov L. 2000. Urban native American health issues. *Cancer* 88(5 Suppl):1207–13.

Burhansstipanov L, Dignan MB, Wound DB, Tenney M, Vigil G. 2000. Native American recruitment into breast cancer screening: the NAWWA project. *J Cancer Educ* 15(1):28–32.

Burhenne LJ, Burhenne HJ. 1993. The Canadian National Breast Screening Study: a Canadian critique. *Am J Roentgenol* 161(4):761–3.

Burke W, Beeker C, Kraft JM, Pinsky L. 2000. Engaging women's interest in colorectal cancer screening: a public health strategy. *J Women's Health Gend Based Med* 9(4):363–71.

Burns KJ, Camaione DN, Chatterton CT. 2000. Prescription of physical activity by adult nurse practitioners: a national survey. *Nurs Outlook* 48(1):28–33.

Byers TE, Mouchawar J, Marks J, Cady B, Lins N, Swanson GM, Bal DG, Eyre H. 1999. The American Cancer Society challenge goals. How far can cancer rates decline in the U.S. by the year 2015? *Cancer* 86(4):715–27.

Byers T, Nestle M, McTiernan A, Doyle C, Currie-Williams A, Gansler T, Thun M. 2002. American Cancer Society guidelines on nutrition and physical activity for cancer prevention: Reducing the risk of cancer with healthy food choices and physical activity. *CA Cancer J Clin* 52(2):92–119.

Calfas KJ, Long BJ, Sallis JF, Wooten WJ, Pratt M, Patrick K. 1996. A controlled trial of physician counseling to promote the adoption of physical activity. *Prev Med* 25(3):225–33.

Calle EE, Miracle-McMahill HL, Moss RE, Heath CW Jr. 1994. Personal contact from friends to increase mammography usage. *Am J Prev Med* 10(6):361–6.

Cameron R, Brown KS, Best JA, Pelkman CL, Madill CL, Manske SR, Payne ME. 1999. Effectiveness of a social influences smoking prevention program as a function of provider type, training method, and school risk. *Am J Public Health* 89(12):1827–31.

Cameron R, Best JA, Brown KS. 2001. Re: Hutchinson Smoking Prevention Project: long-term randomized trial in school-based tobacco use prevention—results on smoking. *J Natl Cancer Inst* 93(16):1267–8.

Campbell MK, Demark-Wahnefried W, Symons M, Kalsbeek WD, Dodds J, Cowan A, Jackson B, Motsinger B, Hoben K, Lashley J, Demissie S, McClelland JW. 1999a. Fruit and vegetable consumption and prevention of cancer: the Black Churches United for Better Health project. *Am J Public Health* 89(9):1390–6.

Campbell MK, Honess-Morreale L, Farrell D, Carbone E, Brasure M. 1999b. A tailored multimedia nutrition education pilot program for low-income women receiving food assistance. *Health Educ Res* 14(2):257–67.

Canadian Task Force on the Periodic Health Examination. 1994. *The Canadian Guide to Clinical Preventive Health Care*. Ottawa, Ontario, Canada: Canada Communication Group.

Cantor SB, Spann SJ, Volk RJ, Cardenas MP, Warren MM. 1995. Prostate cancer screening: a decision analysis. *J Fam Pract* 41(1):33–41.

Caplan LS, Coughlin SS. 1998. Worksite breast cancer screening programs: a review. *AAOHN J* 46(9):443–51.

Caraballo RS, Giovino GA, Pechacek TF, Mowery PD, Richter PA, Strauss WJ, Sharp DJ, Eriksen MP, Pirkle JL, Maurer KR. 1998. Racial and ethnic differences in serum cotinine levels of cigarette smokers: Third National Health and Nutrition Examination Survey, 1988–1991. JAMA 280(2):135–9.

Cardinal BJ, Sachs ML. 1996. Effects of mail-mediated, stage-matched exercise behavior change strategies on female adults' leisure-time exercise behavior. *J Sports Med Phys Fitness* 36(2):100–7.

Carleton RA, Lasater TM, Assaf AR, Feldman HA, McKinlay S. 1995. The Pawtucket Heart Health Program: community changes in cardiovascular risk factors and projected disease risk. *Am J Public Health* 85(6):777–85.

Carney PA, Dietrich AJ, Freeman DH, Mott LA. 1995. A standardized-patient assessment of a continuing medical education program to improve physicians' cancer-control clinical skills. *Acad Med* 70(1):52–8.

Carney PA, Goodrich ME, O'Mahony DM, Tosteson AN, Eliassen MS, Poplack SP, Birnbaum S, Harwood BG, Burgess KA, Berube BT, Wells WS, Ball JP, Stevens MM. 2000. Mammography in New Hampshire: characteristics of the women and the exams they receive. *J Community Health* 25(3):183–98.

Carter HB, Pearson JD, Metter EJ, Brant LJ, Chan DW, Andres R, Fozard JL, Walsh PC. 1992. Longitudinal evaluation of prostate-specific antigen levels in men with and without prostate disease. *JAMA* 267(16):2215–20.

Carter HB, Epstein JI, Chan DW, Fozard JL, Pearson JD. 1997. Recommended prostate-specific antigen testing intervals for the detection of curable prostate cancer. *JAMA* 277(18):1456–60.

Carvalhal GF, Smith DS, Mager DE, Ramos C, Catalona WJ. 1999a. Digital rectal examination for detecting prostate cancer at prostate specific antigen levels of 4 ng/ml or less. *J Urol* 161(3):835–9.

Carvalhal GF, Smith DS, Ramos C, Krygiel J, Mager DE, Yan Y, Catalona WJ. 1999b. Correlates of dissatisfaction with treatment in patients with prostate cancer diagnosed through screening. *J Urol* 162(1):113–8.

Cash BD, Schoenfeld PS, Ransohoff DF. 1999. Licensure, use, and training of paramedical personnel to perform screening flexible sigmoidoscopy. *Gastrointest Endosc* 49(2): 163–9.

Castles A, Adams EK, Melvin CL, Kelsch C, Boulton ML. 1999. Effects of smoking during pregnancy. Five meta-analyses. *American Journal of Preventive Medicine* 16(3):208–15.

Catalona WJ. 1994. Conservative management of prostate cancer. *N Engl J Med* 330(25): 1830–1.

Catalona WJ, Avioli LV. 1987. Diagnosis, staging, and surgical treatment of prostatic carcinoma. *Arch Intern Med* 147(2):361–3.

Catalona WJ, Smith DS. 1998. Cancer recurrence and survival rates after anatomic radical retropubic prostatectomy for prostate cancer: intermediate-term results. *J Urol* 160(6 Pt 2):2428–34.

Catalona WJ, Smith DS, Ratliff TL, Dodds KM, Coplen DE, Yuan JJ, Petros JA, Andriole GL. 1991. Measurement of prostate-specific antigen in serum as a screening test for prostate cancer. *N Engl J Med* 324(17):1156–61.

Catalona WJ, Smith DS, Ratliff TL, Basler JW. 1993. Detection of organ-confined prostate cancer is increased through prostate-specific antigen-based screening. *JAMA* 270(8):948–54.

Catalona WJ, Richie JP, Ahmann FR, Hudson MA, Scardino PT, Flanigan RC, deKernion JB, Ratliff TL, Kavoussi LR, Dalkin BL, et al. 1994. Comparison of digital rectal examination and serum prostate-specific antigen in the early detection of prostate cancer: results of a multicenter clinical trial of 6,630 men. *J Urol* 151(5):1283–90.

Catalona WJ, Partin AW, Slawin KM, Brawer MK, Flanigan RC, Patel A, Richie JP, deKernion JB, Walsh PC, Scardino PT, Lange PH, Subong EN, Parson RE, Gasior GH, Loveland KG, Southwick PC. 1998. Use of the percentage of free prostate-specific antigen to enhance differentiation of prostate cancer from benign prostatic disease: a prospective multicenter clinical trial. *JAMA* 279(19):1542–7.

Catalona WJ, Carvalhal GF, Mager DE, Smith DS. 1999a. Potency, continence and complication rates in 1,870 consecutive radical retropubic prostatectomies. *J Urol* 162(2):433–8.

Catalona WJ, Partin AW, Finlay JA, Chan DW, Rittenhouse HG, Wolfert RL, Woodrum DL. 1999b. Use of percentage of free prostate-specific antigen to identify men at high risk of prostate cancer when PSA levels are 2.51 to 4 ng/mL and digital rectal examination is not suspicious for prostate cancer: an alternative model. *Urology* 54(2):220–4.

Catalona WJ, Southwick PC, Slawin KM, Partin AW, Brawer MK, Flanigan RC, Patel A, Richie JP, Walsh PC, Scardino PT, Lange PH, Gasior GH, Loveland KG, Bray KR. 2000. Comparison of percent free PSA, PSA density, and age-specific PSA cutoffs for prostate cancer detection and staging. *Urology* 56(2):255–60.

Cates C, Senn S. 2000. Screening mammography re-evaluated. *Lancet* 355(9205):750.

CDC (Centers for Disease Control and Prevention). 1993. Physician and other health-care professional counseling of smokers to quit—United States, 1991. *Morb Mortal Wkly Rep* 42(44):854–7.

CDC. 1995. Update: alcohol-related traffic crashes and fatalities among youth and young adults—United States, 1982–1994. *Morb Mortal Wkly Rep* 44(47):869–74.

CDC. 1996. Cigarette smoking before and after an excise tax increase and an antismoking campaign—Massachusetts, 1990–1996. *Morb Mortal Wkly Rep* 45(44):966–70.

CDC. 1997a. Guidelines for school and community programs to promote lifelong physical activity among young people. *Morb Mortal Wkly Rep Recomm Rep* 46(RR-6):1–36.

CDC. 1997b. Cancer screening offered by work sites—United States, 1992 and 1995. *MMWR* 46:421–24.

CDC. 1998a. Strategies for providing follow-up and treatment services in the National Breast and Cervical Cancer Early Detection Program—United States, 1997. *Morb Mortal Wkly Rep* 47(11):215–8.

CDC. 1998b. Preventing and Controlling Oral and Pharyngeal Cancer—Recommendations from a National Strategic Planning Conference. *Morb Mort Wkly Rep* 47(RR-14).

CDC. 1999a. Decline in cigarette consumption following implementation of a comprehensive tobacco prevention and education program—Oregon, 1996–1998. *Morb Mortal Wkly Rep* 48(7):140–3.

CDC. 1999b. Tobacco use—United States, 1900–1999. *Morb Mortal Wkly Rep* 48(43):986–93.

CDC. Janes GR, Blackman DK, Bolen JC, Kamimoto LA, Rhodes L, Caplan LS, Nadel MR, Tomar SL, Lando JF, Greby SM, Singleton JA, Strikas RA, Wooten KG. 1999c. Surveillance for use of preventive health-care services by older adults, 1995–1997. *Morb Mortal Wkly Rep CDC Surveill Summ* 48(8):51–88.

CDC. 1999d. *Best Practices for Comprehensive Tobacco Control Programs—August 1999.* Atlanta GA: U.S. Department of Health and Human Services, Centers for Disease Control and Prevention, National Center for Chronic Disease Prevention and Health Promotion, Office on Smoking and Health.

CDC. Bolen JC, Rhodes L, Powell-Griner EE, Bland SD, Holtzman D. 2000a. State-specific prevalence of selected health behaviors, by race and ethnicity—Behavioral Risk Factor Surveillance System, 1997. *Morb Mortal Wkly Rep CDC Surveill Summ* 49(2):1–60.

CDC. 2000b. Screening with the prostate-specific antigen test—Texas, 1997. *Morb Mortal Wkly Rep* 49:818–20

CDC. 2000c. *State and Federal Laws Relating to Cervical Cancer: Legislative Summary, January 1977 to May 2000.* Atlanta: U.S. Department of Health and Human Services, Centers for Disease Control and Prevention, Division of Cancer Prevention and Control.

CDC. 2000d. *CDP File.* Cancer Prevention and Control Database. Available on CD-ROM. Atlanta, GA: National Center for Chronic Disease Prevention and Health Promotion, Centers for Disease Control and Prevention.

CDC. 2001a. National Comprehensive Cancer Control Program. Atlanta: Centers for Disease Control and Prevention.

CDC. 2001b. Physical activity trends—United States, 1990–1998. *Morb Mortal Wkly Rep* 50(9):166–9.

CDC. 2001c. Trends in screening for colorectal cancer—United States, 1997 and 1999. *Morb Mortal Wkly Rep* 50(9):162–6.

CDC. 2001d. Increasing physical activity. A report on recommendations of the Task Force on Community Preventive Services. *MMWR Recomm Rep* 50(RR-18):1–14.

CDC. 2001e. State medicaid coverage for tobacco-dependence treatments—United States, 1998 and 2000. *Morb Mortal Wkly Rep* 50(44):979–82.

CDC. 2002a. *Tobacco Control State Highlights 2002: Impact and Opportunity.* Atlanta: Centers for Disease Control and Prevention, National Center for Chronic Disease Prevention and Health Promotion.

CDC. 2002b. Point-of-purchase tobacco environments and variation by store type—United States, 1999. *Morb Mortal Wkly Rep* 51(9):184–7.

CDC, Behavioral Risk Factor Surveillance System. 2000. *Surveillance Summary Report, 2000.* Atlanta: Centers for Disease Control and Prevention, National Center for Chronic Disease Prevention and Health Promotion.

CDC, Division of Adolescent and School Health. 1999. *Youth Risk Behavior Surveillance System.* [Online]. Available at: http://www.cdc.gov/nccdphp/dash/yrbs.

CDC, Division of Adolescent and School Health. 2000. *Promoting Better Health for Young People Through Physical Activity and Sports.* A Report to the President. Atlanta: Centers for Disease Control and Prevention, National Center for Chronic Disease Prevention and Health Promotion.

CDC, Division of Adult and Community Health. 1999. *Behavioral Risk Factor Surveillance System Online Prevalence Data, 1995–1999.* [Online]. Available at: http://www2.cdc.gov/nccdphp/brfss.

CDC, The National Breast and Cervical Cancer Early Detection Program. About the Program. May 2, 2001. [Online]. Available at: http://www.cdc.gov/cancer/nbccedp/about.htm (accessed June 11, 2001).

Center for the Advancement of Health. 2001. *Integration of Health Behavior Counseling in Routine Medical Care.* Washington, DC: Center for the Advancement of Health.

Centers for Medicare and Medicaid Services. 2002. *Medicare and You 2002.* Washington, DC: U.S. Department of Health and Human Services.

Chamberlain RM, Bakemeier RF, Gallagher RE, Kupchella CE, O'Donnell JF, Parker JA, Hill GJ, Brooks CM. 1992. Cancer prevention education in United States medical schools. Cancer Education Survey II: cancer education in United States medical schools. *J Cancer Educ* 7(2):105–14.

Chamberlain RM, Smith DW, Zhang JJ, Sider JG, Philips BU, Spitz MR. 1995. Improving residents' knowledge of cancer prevention: are physicians prepared for prevention? *J Cancer Educ* 10(1):9–13.

Chan JM, Rimm EB, Colditz GA, Stampfer MJ, Willett WC. 1994. Obesity, fat distribution, and weight gain as risk factors for clinical diabetes in men. *Diabetes Care* 17(9):961–9.

Chan JM, Giovannucci E, Andersson SO, Yuen J, Adami HO, Wolk A. 1998. Dairy products, calcium, phosphorous, vitamin D, and risk of prostate cancer (Sweden). *Cancer Causes Control* 9(6):559–66.

Chang HC, Zimmerman LH, Beck JM. 1995. Impact of chart reminders on smoking cessation practices of pulmonary physicians. *Am J Respir Crit Care Med* 152(3):984–7.

Chao A, Thun MJ, Jacobs EJ, Henley SJ, Rodriguez C, Calle EE. 2000. Cigarette smoking and colorectal cancer mortality in the Cancer Prevention Study II. *J Natl Cancer Inst* 92(23):1888–96.

Chapman S, Borland R, Scollo M, Brownson RC, Dominello A, Woodward S. 1999. The impact of smoke-free workplaces on declining cigarette consumption in Australia and the United States. *Am J Public Health* 89(7):1018–23.

Chassin L, Presson CC, Rose JS, Sherman SJ. 1996. The natural history of cigarette smoking from adolescence to adulthood: demographic predictors of continuity and change. *Health Psychol* 15(6):478–84.

Chen AH, Sallis JF, Castro CM, Lee RE, Hickmann SA, William C, Martin JE. 1998. A home-based behavioral intervention to promote walking in sedentary ethnic minority women: project WALK. *Women's Health* 4(1):19–39.

Chen HH, Tabar L, Fagerberg G, Duffy SW. 1995. Effect of breast cancer screening after age 65. *J Med Screen* 2(1):10–4.

Chin T. 2001, February 12. Doctors go online, but mostly from home not the office. *American Medical News*. Technology.

Chisick MC. 2000. Do military dentists advise tobacco users to quit? The patient's perspective. *Public Health* 114(2):129–32.

Chiu BC, Cerhan JR, Folsom AR, Sellers TA, Kushi LH, Wallace RB, Zheng W, Potter JD. 1996. Diet and risk of non-Hodgkin lymphoma in older women. *JAMA* 275(17):1315–21.

Chlebowski RT, Sayre J, Frank-Stromborg M, Lillington LB. 1992. Current attitudes and practice of American Society of Clinical Oncology-member clinical oncologists regarding cancer prevention and control. *J Clin Oncol* 10(1):164–8.

Chodak GW. 1998. Comparing treatments for localized prostate cancer—persisting uncertainty. *JAMA* 280(11):1008–10.

Chodak GW, Thisted RA, Gerber GS, Johansson JE, Adolfsson J, Jones GW, Chisholm GD, Moskovitz B, Livne PM, Warner J. 1994. Results of conservative management of clinically localized prostate cancer. *N Engl J Med* 330(4):242–8.

Choiniere R, Lafontaine P, Edwards AC. 2000. Distribution of cardiovascular disease risk factors by socioeconomic status among Canadian adults. *Can Med Assoc J* 162(9 Suppl): S13–24.

Chow WH, Blot WJ, Vaughan TL, Risch HA, Gammon MD, Stanford JL, Dubrow R, Schoenberg JB, Mayne ST, Farrow DC, Ahsan H, West AB, Rotterdam H, Niwa S, Fraumeni JF Jr. 1998. Body mass index and risk of adenocarcinomas of the esophagus and gastric cardia. *J Natl Cancer Inst* 90(2):150–5.

Christiansen CL, Wang F, Barton MB, Kreuter W, Elmore JG, Gelfand AE, Fletcher SW. 2000. Predicting the cumulative risk of false-positive mammograms. *J Natl Cancer Inst* 92(20):1657–66.

Chyou PH, Nomura AM, Hankin JH, Stemmermann GN. 1990. A case-cohort study of diet and stomach cancer. *Cancer Res* 50(23):7501–4.

Circling the Mammography Wagons (editorial). 2002, February 6. *The New York Times*. p. A20.

Clark LC. 1985. The epidemiology of selenium and cancer. *Fed Proc* 44(9):2584–9.

Clark LC, Combs GF Jr, Turnbull BW, Slate EH, Chalker DK, Chow J, Davis LS, Glover RA, Graham GF, Gross EG, Krongrad A, Lesher JL Jr, Park HK, Sanders BB Jr, Smith CL, Taylor JR. 1996. Effects of selenium supplementation for cancer prevention in patients with carcinoma of the skin. A randomized controlled trial. Nutritional Prevention of Cancer Study Group. *JAMA* 276(24):1957–63.

Clarke VA, Lovegrove H, Williams A, Machperson M. 2000. Unrealistic optimism and the Health Belief Model. *J Behav Med* 23(4):367–76.

Clemow L, Costanza ME, Haddad WP, Luckmann R, White MJ, Klaus D, Stoddard AM. 2000. Underutilizers of mammography screening today: characteristics of women planning, undecided about, and not planning a mammogram. *Ann Behav Med* 22(1):80–8.

Coates RJ, Bowen DJ, Kristal AR, Feng Z, Oberman A, Hall WD, George V, Lewis CE, Kestin M, Davis M, Evans M, Grizzle JE, Clifford CK. 1999. The Women's Health Trial Feasibility Study in Minority Populations: changes in dietary intakes. *Am J Epidemiol* 149(12):1104–12.

Cockburn J, Pit S, Redman S. 1999. Perceptions of screening mammography among women aged 40–49. *Aust NZ J Public Health* 23(3):318–21.

Coffield AB, Maciosek MV, McGinnis JM, Harris JR, Caldwell MB, Teutsch SM, Atkins D, Richland JH, Haddix A. 2001. Priorities among recommended clinical preventive services. *Am J Prev Med* 21(1):1–9.

Cohen MM, Kaufert PA, MacWilliam L, Tate RB. 1996. Using an alternative data source to examine randomization in the Canadian National Breast Screening Study. *J Clin Epidemiol* 49(9):1039–44.

Cohen SJ, Christen AG, Katz BP, Drook CA, Davis BJ, Smith DM, Stookey GK. 1987. Counseling medical and dental patients about cigarette smoking: the impact of nicotine gum and chart reminders. *Am J Public Health* 77(3):313–6.

Cohen SJ, Stookey GK, Katz BP, Drook CA, Smith DM. 1989. Encouraging primary care physicians to help smokers quit. A randomized, controlled trial. *Ann Intern Med* 110(8): 648–52.

Colditz GA. 1995. The nurses' health study: a cohort of US women followed since 1976. *J Am Med Womens Assoc* 50(2):40–4.

Colditz GA. 1997. Epidemiology—future directions. *Int J Epidemiol* 26(4):693–7.

Colditz GA. 2001. Cancer culture: epidemics, human behavior, and the dubious search for new risk factors. *Am J Public Health* 91(3):357–9.

Colditz GA, Frazier AL. 1995. Models of breast cancer show that risk is set by events of early life: prevention efforts must shift focus. *Cancer Epidemiol Biomarkers Prev* 4(5):567–71.

Colditz GA, Gortmaker SL. 1995. Cancer prevention strategies for the future: risk identification and preventive intervention. *Milbank Q* 73(4):621–51.

Colditz GA, Willett WC, Rotnitzky A, Manson JE. 1995. Weight gain as a risk factor for clinical diabetes mellitus in women. *Ann Intern Med* 122(7):481–6.

Colditz GA, DeJong D, et al. 1996. Harvard Report on Cancer Prevention. Volume 1: Causes of human cancer. *Cancer Causes Control* 7 Suppl 1:S3–59.

Colditz GA, Cannuscio CC, Frazier AL. 1997. Physical activity and reduced risk of colon cancer: implications for prevention. *Cancer Causes Control* 8(4):649–67.

Coley CM, Barry MJ, Fleming C, Fahs MC, Mulley AG. 1997. Early detection of prostate cancer. Part II. Estimating the risks, benefits, and costs. American College of Physicians. *Ann Intern Med* 126(6):468–79.

Collins TR, Goldenberg K, Ring A, Nelson K, Konen J. 1991. The Association of Teachers of Preventive Medicine's recommendations for postgraduate education in prevention. *Acad Med* 66(6):317–20.

Compas BE, Haaga DA, Keefe FJ, Leitenberg H, Williams DA. 1998. Sampling of empirically supported psychological treatments from health psychology: smoking, chronic pain, cancer, and bulimia nervosa. *J Consult Clin Psychol* 66(1):89–112.

Cooner WH, Mosley BR, Rutherford CL Jr, Beard JH, Pond HS, Terry WJ, Igel TC, Kidd DD. 1990. Prostate cancer detection in a clinical urological practice by ultrasonography, digital rectal examination and prostate specific antigen. *J Urol* 143(6):1146–52.

Cooper GS, Fortinsky RH, Hapke R, Landefeld CS. 1998. Factors associated with the use of flexible sigmoidoscopy as a screening test for the detection of colorectal carcinoma by primary care physicians. *Cancer* 82(8):1476–81.

Corrigan JM, Nielsen DM. 1993. Toward the development of uniform reporting standards for managed care organizations: the Health Plan Employer Data and Information Set (Version 2.0). *Jt Comm J Qual Improv* 19(12):566–75.

Costanza ME, Hoople NE, Gaw VP, Stoddard AM. 1993. Cancer prevention practices and continuing education needs of primary care physicians. *Am J Prev Med* 9(2):107–12.

Costanza ME, Stoddard AM, Luckmann R, White MJ, Spitz Avrunin J, Clemow L. 2000. Promoting mammography: results of a randomized trial of telephone counseling and a medical practice intervention. *Am J Prev Med* 19(1):39–46.

Coughlin SS, Uhler RJ. 2000. Breast and cervical cancer screening practices among Asian and Pacific Islander women in the United States, 1994–1997. *Cancer Epidemiol Biomarkers Prev* 9(6):597–603.

Coughlin SS, Neaton JD, Sengupta A. 1996. Cigarette smoking as a predictor of death from prostate cancer in 348,874 men screened for the Multiple Risk Factor Intervention Trial. *Am J Epidemiol* 143(10):1002–6.

Coughlin SS, Uhler RJ, Blackman DK. 1999. Breast and cervical cancer screening practices among American Indian and Alaska Native women in the United States, 1992–1997. *Prev Med* 29(4):287–95.

Coultas DB, Klecan DA, Whitten RM, Obenshain SS, Rubin RH, Wiese WH, Wilson BE, Woodall GW, Stidley CA. 1994. Training medical students in smoking-cessation counseling. *Acad Med* 69(10 Suppl):S48–50.

Coulter A. 1997. Partnerships with patients: the pros and cons of shared clinical decision-making. *J Health Serv Res Policy* 2(2):112–21.

Cousins JH, Rubovits DS, Dunn JK, Reeves RS, Ramirez AG, Foreyt JP. 1992. Family versus individually oriented intervention for weight loss in Mexican American women. *Public Health Rep* 107(5):549–55.

Covey LS, Zang EA, Wynder EL. 1992. Cigarette smoking and occupational status: 1977 to 1990. *Am J Public Health* 82(9):1230–4.

Cox RH, Parker GG, Watson AC, Robinson SH, Simonson CJ, Elledge JC, Diggs S, Smith E. 1995. Dietary cancer risk of low-income women and change with intervention. *J Am Diet Assoc* 95(9):1031–4.

Crane LA, Leakey TA, Ehrsam G, Rimer BK, Warnecke RB. 2000. Effectiveness and cost-effectiveness of multiple outcalls to promote mammography among low-income women. *Cancer Epidemiol Biomarkers Prev* 9(9):923–31.

Cress RD, Morris CR, Wolfe BM. 2000. Cancer of the colon and rectum in California: trends in incidence by race/ethnicity, stage, and subsite. *Prev Med* 31(4):447–53.

Croghan IT, Offord KP, Evans RW, Schmidt S, Gomez-Dahl LC, Schroeder DR, Patten CA, Hurt RD. 1997. Cost-effectiveness of treating nicotine dependence: the Mayo Clinic experience. *Mayo Clin Proc* 72(10):917–24.

Cromwell J, Bartosch WJ, Fiore MC, Hasselblad V, Baker T. 1997. Cost-effectiveness of the clinical practice recommendations in the AHCPR guideline for smoking cessation. Agency for Health Care Policy and Research. *JAMA* 278(21):1759–66.

Croyle RT, Smith KR, Botkin JR, Baty B, Nash J. 1997. Psychological responses to BRCA1 mutation testing: preliminary findings. *Health Psychol* 16(1):63–72.

Crump SR, Mayberry RM, Taylor BD, Barefield KP, Thomas PE. 2000. Factors related to noncompliance with screening mammogram appointments among low-income African-American women. *J Natl Med Assoc* 92(5):237–46.

Cullen KW, Bartholomew LL, Parcel GS. 1997. Girl scouting: an effective channel for nutrition education. *Journal of Nutrition Education* 29:86–91.

Cummings DM, Whetstone L, Shende A, Weismiller D. 2000. Predictors of screening mammography: implications for office practice. *Arch Fam Med* 9(9):870–5.

Cummings SR, Coates TJ, Richard RJ, Hansen B, Zahnd EG, VanderMartin R, Duncan C, Gerbert B, Martin A, Stein MJ. 1989a. Training physicians in counseling about smoking cessation. A randomized trial of the "Quit for Life" program. *Ann Intern Med* 110(8): 640–7.

Cummings SR, Richard RJ, Duncan CL, Hansen B, Vander Martin R, Gerbert B, Coates TJ. 1989b. Training physicians about smoking cessation: a controlled trial in private practice. *J Gen Intern Med* 4(6):482–9.

Curry SJ. 1993. Self-help interventions for smoking cessation. *J Consult Clin Psychol* 61(5): 790–803.

Curry SJ. 1998. Building effective strategies to decrease tobacco use in a health maintenance organisation: Group Health Cooperative of Puget Sound. *Tob Control* 7(Suppl): S21–3.

Curry SJ, Wagner EH, Grothaus LC. 1991. Evaluation of intrinsic and extrinsic motivation interventions with a self-help smoking cessation program. *J Consult Clin Psychol* 59(2):318–24.

Curry SJ, Grothaus LC, McAfee T, Pabiniak C. 1998. Use and cost effectiveness of smoking-cessation services under four insurance plans in a health maintenance organization. *N Engl J Med* 339(10):673–9.

Daling JR, Madeleine MM, McKnight B, Carter JJ, Wipf GC, Ashley R, Schwartz SM, Beckmann AM, Hagensee ME, Mandelson MT, Galloway DA. 1996. The relationship of human papillomavirus-related cervical tumors to cigarette smoking, oral contraceptive use, and prior herpes simplex virus type 2 infection. *Cancer Epidemiol Biomarkers Prev* 5(7):541–8.

Daly MB, Balshem M, Sands C, James J, Workman S, Engstrom PF. 1993. Academic detailing: a model for in-office CME. *J Cancer Educ* 8(4):273–80.

Darby M. 1998. 12 ways to get physician buy-in to practice guidelines. *Quality Letter for Healthcare Leaders* 10(3):2–8.

Davis D, O'Brien MA, Freemantle N, Wolf FM, Mazmanian P, Taylor-Vaisey A. 1999. Impact of formal continuing medical education: do conferences, workshops, rounds, and other traditional continuing education activities change physician behavior or health care outcomes? *JAMA* 282(9):867–74.

Davis DA, Thomson MA, Oxman AD, Haynes RB. 1992. Evidence for the effectiveness of CME. A review of 50 randomized controlled trials. *JAMA* 268(9):1111–7.

Davis DA, Thomson MA, Oxman AD, Haynes RB. 1995a. Changing physician performance. A systematic review of the effect of continuing medical education strategies. *JAMA* 274(9):700–5.

Davis DT, Bustamante A, Brown CP, Wolde-Tsadik G, Savage EW, Cheng X, Howland L. 1994. The urban church and cancer control: a source of social influence in minority communities. *Public Health Rep* 109(4):500–6.

Davis NA, Lewis MJ, Rimer BK, Harvey CM, Koplan JP. 1997a. Evaluation of a phone intervention to promote mammography in a managed care plan. *Am J Health Promot* 11(4):247–9.

Davis NA, Nash E, Bailey C, Lewis MJ, Rimer BK, Koplan JP. 1997b. Evaluation of three methods for improving mammography rates in a managed care plan. *Am J Prev Med* 13(4):298–302.

Davis S, Lambert L, Gomez Y, Skipper B. 1995b. Southwest cardiovascular curriculum project: study findings for American Indian elementary students. *J Health Educ* 26:S72–81.

Dawson D. 2002. *A Guide to Helping Patients with Alcohol Problems*. National Institute on Alcohol Abuse and Alcoholism.

Deber RB, Kraetschmer N, Irvine J. 1996. What role do patients wish to play in treatment decision making? *Arch Intern Med* 156(13):1414–20.

Dee KE, Sickles EA. 2001. Medical audit of diagnostic mammography examinations: comparison with screening outcomes obtained concurrently. *Am J Roentgenol* 176(3):729–33.

Deen D, Karp R, Lowell B. 2000. A mini-fellowship in clinical nutrition for primary care physicians. *J Cancer Educ* 15(3):134–6.

De Koning HJ. 2000. Breast cancer screening: cost-effective in practice? *Eur J Radiol* 33(1):32–7.

Demark-Wahnefried W, Catoe KE, Paskett E, Robertson CN, Rimer BK. 1993. Characteristics of men reporting for prostate cancer screening. *Urology* 42(3):269–74.

Dennis TD. 2000. Cancer stage at diagnosis, treatment, and survival among American Indians and non-American Indians in Montana. *Cancer* 89(1):181–6.

Dershaw DD, Liberman L, Lippin BS. 1992. Mobile mammographic screening of self-referred women: results of 22,540 screenings. *Radiology* 184(2):415–9.

Desmond PM, Clark J, Thompson IM, Zeidman EJ, Mueller EJ. 1993. Morbidity with contemporary prostate biopsy. *J Urol* 150(5 Pt 1):1425–6.

Diederich S, Lenzen H, Windmann R, Puskas Z, Yelbuz TM, Henneken S, Klaiber T, Eameri M, Roos N, Peters PE. 1999. Pulmonary nodules: experimental and clinical studies at low-dose CT. *Radiology* 213(1):289–98.

Diefenbach PN, Ganz PA, Pawlow AJ, Guthrie D. 1996. Screening by the prostate-specific antigen test: what do the patients know? *J Cancer Educ* 11(1):39–44.

Dietrich AJ, O'Connor GT, Keller A, Carney PA, Levy D, Whaley FS. 1992. Cancer: improving early detection and prevention. A community practice randomised trial. *BMJ* 304(6828):687–91.

Dietrich AJ, Woodruff CB, Carney PA. 1994. Changing office routines to enhance preventive care. The preventive GAPS approach. *Arch Fam Med* 3(2):176–83.

Dietrich AJ, Tobin JN, Sox CH, Cassels AN, Negron F, Younge RG, Demby NA, Tosteson TD. 1998. Cancer early-detection services in community health centers for the underserved. A randomized controlled trial. *Arch Fam Med* 7(4):320–7; discussion 328.

Dignan M, Michielutte R, Blinson K, Wells HB, Case LD, Sharp P, Davis S, Konen J, McQuellon RP. 1996. Effectiveness of health education to increase screening for cervical cancer among Eastern Band Cherokee Indian women in North Carolina. *JNCI* 88:1670–6.

Dishman RK, Oldenburg B, O'Neal H, Shephard RJ. 1998. Worksite physical activity interventions. *Am J Prev Med* 15(4):344–61.

Ditschuneit HH, Flechtner-Mors M, Johnson TD, Adler G. 1999. Metabolic and weight-loss effects of a long-term dietary intervention in obese patients. *Am J Clin Nutr* 69(2):198–204.

Doescher MP, Saver BG. 2000. Physicians' advice to quit smoking. The glass remains half empty. *J Fam Pract* 49(6):543–7.

Dolan NC, McDermott MM, Morrow M, Venta L, Martin GJ. 1999. Impact of same-day screening mammography availability: results of a controlled clinical trial. *Arch Intern Med* 159(4):393–8.

Dolan TA, McGorray SP, Grinstead-Skigen CL, Mecklenburg R. 1997. Tobacco control activities in U.S. dental practices. *J Am Dent Assoc* 128(12):1669–79.

Doll R. 1997. One for the heart. *BMJ* 315(7123):1664–8.

Doll R, Peto R. 1981. The causes of cancer: quantitative estimates of avoidable risks of cancer in the United States today. *J Natl Cancer Inst* 66(6):1191–308.

Doll R, Peto R, Wheatley K, Gray R, Sutherland I. 1994. Mortality in relation to smoking: 40 years' observations on male British doctors. *BMJ* 309(6959):901–11.

Domel SB, Baranowski T, Davis H, Leonard SB, Riley P, Baranowski J. 1993. Measuring fruit and vegetable preferences among 4th- and 5th-grade students. *Prev Med* 22(6):866–79.

Donahue RP, Abbott RD, Reed DM, Yano K. 1986. Alcohol and hemorrhagic stroke. The Honolulu Heart Program. *JAMA* 255(17):2311–4.

Donnelly JE, Pronk NP, Jacobsen DJ, Pronk SJ, Jakicic JM. 1991. Effects of a very-low-calorie diet and physical-training regimens on body composition and resting metabolic rate in obese females. *Am J Clin Nutr* 54(1):56–61.

Donnelly JE, Jacobsen DJ, Whatley JE, Hill JO, Swift LL, Cherrington A, Polk B, Tran ZV, Reed G. 1996. Nutrition and physical activity program to attenuate obesity and promote physical and metabolic fitness in elementary school children. *Obes Res* 4(3):229–43.

Dorant E, van den Brandt PA, Goldbohm RA, Sturmans F. 1996. Consumption of onions and a reduced risk of stomach carcinoma. *Gastroenterology* 110(1):12–20.

Dressler WW. 1991. Social support, lifestyle incongruity, and arterial blood pressure in a southern black community. *Psychosom Med* 53(6):608–20.

Duan N, Fox SA, Derose KP, Carson S. 2000. Maintaining mammography adherence through telephone counseling in a church-based trial. *Am J Public Health* 90(9):1468–71.

Duffy SW, Tabar L. 2000. Screening mammography re-evaluated. *Lancet* 355(9205):747–8.

Duffy SW, Tabar L, Smith RA. 2001. Screening for breast cancer with mammography. *Lancet* 358(9299):2166; discussion 2167–8.

Duffy SW, Tabar L, Smith RA. 2002. The mammographic screening trials: commentary on the recent work by Olsen and Gotzsche. *CA Cancer J Clin* 52(2):68–71.

Dullum JR, Lewis EC, Mayer JA. 2000. Rates and correlates of discomfort associated with mammography. *Radiology* 214(2):547–52.

Dunn AL, Marcus BH, Kampert JB, Garcia ME, Kohl HW III, Blair SN. 1999. Comparison of lifestyle and structured interventions to increase physical activity and cardiorespiratory fitness: a randomized trial. *JAMA* 281(4):327–34.

Dunn AS, Shridharani KV, Lou W, Bernstein J, Horowitz CR. 2001. Physician-patient discussions of controversial cancer screening tests. *Am J Prev Med* 20(2):130–4.

Dunn J, Sprunt D. 1955. Uterine cancer case finding by vaginal cytology. *Public Health Rep* 70:341–6.

Eaton CB, Lapane KL, Garber CE, Gans KM, Lasater TM, Carleton RA. 1999. Effects of a community-based intervention on physical activity: the Pawtucket Heart Health Program. *Am J Public Health* 89(11):1741–4.

Ebeling K, Nischan P. 1987. Screening for lung cancer—results from a case-control study. *Int J Cancer* 40(2):141–4.

Eckstrom E, Hickam DH, Lessler DS, Buchner DM. 1999. Changing physician practice of physical activity counseling. *J Gen Intern Med* 14(6):376–8.

Eddy D. 1980a. ACS report on the cancer-related health checkup. *CA Cancer J Clin* 30(4): 193–240.

Eddy DM. 1980b. Screening for lung cancer. *Mayo Clin Proc* 55(10):653–4.

Eddy DM. 1981. The economics of cancer prevention and detection: getting more for less. *Cancer* 47(5 Suppl):1200–9.

Eddy DM. 1990a. Screening for colorectal cancer. *Ann Intern Med* 113(5):373–84.

Eddy DM. 1990b. Screening for lung cancer. *Ann Intern Med* 112(1):73–4.

Eisinger RA. 1971. Psychosocial predictors of smoking recidivism. *J Health Soc Behav* 12(4): 355–62.

Eisner MS, Lewis JH. 1991. Diagnostic yield of a positive fecal occult blood test found on digital rectal examination. Does the finger count? *Arch Intern Med* 151(11):2180–4.

Ekeh AP, Alleyne RS, Duncan AO. 2000. Role of mammography in diagnosis of breast cancer in an inner-city hospital. *J Natl Med Assoc* 92(8):372–4.

Elixhauser A. 1990. The costs of smoking and the cost effectiveness of smoking-cessation programs. *J Public Health Policy* 11(2):218–37.

Elmore JG, Barton MB, Moceri VM, Polk S, Arena PJ, Fletcher SW. 1998. Ten-year risk of false positive screening mammograms and clinical breast examinations. *N Engl J Med* 338(16):1089–96.

Eluf-Neto J, Booth M, Munoz N, Bosch FX, Meijer CJ, Walboomers JM. 1994. Human papillomavirus and invasive cervical cancer in Brazil. *Br J Cancer* 69(1):114–9.

Elwyn G, Edwards A, Kinnersley P. 1999. Shared decision-making in primary care: the neglected second half of the consultation. *Br J Gen Pract* 49(443):477–82.

Emery J, Hayflick S. 2001. The challenge of integrating genetic medicine into primary care. *BMJ* 322(7293):1027–30.

Emmons KM, Linnan LA, Shadel WG, Marcus B, Abrams DB. 1999. The Working Healthy Project: a worksite health-promotion trial targeting physical activity, diet, and smoking. *J Occup Environ Med* 41(7):545–55.

Entrekin NM, McMillan SC. 1993. Nurses' knowledge, beliefs, and practices related to cancer prevention and detection. *Cancer Nurs* 16(6):431–9.

Epstein JI, Carmichael M, Partin AW, Walsh PC. 1993. Is tumor volume an independent predictor of progression following radical prostatectomy? A multivariate analysis of 185 clinical stage B adenocarcinomas of the prostate with 5 years of followup. *J Urol* 149(6):1478–81.

Epstein JI, Walsh PC, Carmichael M, Brendler CB. 1994a. Pathologic and clinical findings to predict tumor extent of nonpalpable (stage T1c) prostate cancer. *JAMA* 271(5):368–74.

Epstein LH, Wing RR, Steranchak L, Dickson B, Michelson J. 1980. Comparison of family-based behavior modification and nutrition education for childhood obesity. *J Pediatr Psychol* 5(1):25–36.

Epstein LH, Wing RR, Koeske R, Andrasik F, Ossip DJ. 1981. Child and parent weight loss in family-based behavior modification programs. *J Consult Clin Psychol* 49(5):674–85.

Epstein LH, Wing RR, Koeske R, Valoski A. 1985. A comparison of lifestyle exercise, aerobic exercise, and calisthenics on weight loss in obese children. *Behavior Ther* 16(4):345–56.

Epstein LH, Valoski A, Koeske R, Wing RR. 1986. Family-based behavioral weight control in obese young children. *J Am Diet Assoc* 86(4):481–4.

Epstein LH, Valoski A, Wing RR, McCurley J. 1990. Ten-year follow-up of behavioral, family-based treatment for obese children. *JAMA* 264(19):2519–23.

Epstein LH, Valoski A, Wing RR, McCurley J. 1994b. Ten-year outcomes of behavioral family-based treatment for childhood obesity. *Health Psychol* 13(5):373–83.

Epstein LH, Valoski AM, Vara LS, McCurley J, Wisniewski L, Kalarchian MA, Klein KR, Shrager LR. 1995. Effects of decreasing sedentary behavior and increasing activity on weight change in obese children. *Health Psychol* 14(2):108–9.

Epstein LH, Myers MD, Raynor HA, Saelens BE. 1998. Treatment of pediatric obesity. *Pediatrics* 101:554–70.

Epstein SS, Swartz JB. 1981. Fallacies of lifestyle cancer theories. *Nature* 289(5794):127–30.

Erban S, Zapka J, Puleo E, Vickers-Lahti M. 2001. Colorectal cancer screening in Massachusetts: measuring compliance with current guidelines. *Eff Clin Pract* 4(1):10–7.

Ernster VL. 1997. Mammography screening for women aged 40 through 49—a guidelines saga and a clarion call for informed decision making. *Am J Public Health* 87(7):1103–6.

Ernster VL. 2002, February 14. Mammograms and Personal Choice. *The New York Times*. p. A35.

Ernster VL, Barclay J, Kerlikowske K, Grady D, Henderson C. 1996. Incidence of and treatment for ductal carcinoma in situ of the breast. *JAMA* 275(12):913–8.

Ernster VL, Barclay J, Kerlikowske K, Wilkie H, Ballard-Barbash R. 2000. Mortality among women with ductal carcinoma in situ of the breast in the population-based surveillance, epidemiology and end results program. *Arch Intern Med* 160(7):953–8.

Etzioni R, Cha R, Cowen ME. 1999a. Serial prostate specific antigen screening for prostate cancer: a computer model evaluates competing strategies. *J Urol* 162(3 Pt 1):741–8.

Etzioni R, Legler JM, Feuer EJ, Merrill RM, Cronin KA, Hankey BF. 1999b. Cancer surveillance series: interpreting trends in prostate cancer. Part III. Quantifying the link between population prostate-specific antigen testing and recent declines in prostate cancer mortality. *J Natl Cancer Inst* 91(12):1033–9.

Evans AT, Rogers LQ, Peden JG Jr, Seelig CB, Layne RD, Levine MA, Levin ML, Grossman RS, Darden PM, Jackson SM, Ammerman AS, Settle MB, Stritter FT, Fletcher SW. 1996. Teaching dietary counseling skills to residents: patient and physician outcomes. The CADRE Study Group. *Am J Prev Med* 12(4):259–65.

Evans D, Hibbard B, Jones J, et al. 1980. The Cardiff Cervical Cytology Study. *J Epidemiol Community Health* 34:9–13.

Evans JP, Skrzynia C, Burke W. 2001. The complexities of predictive genetic testing. *BMJ* 322(7293):1052–6.

Ewart RM. 2000. Primum non nocere and the quality of evidence: rethinking the ethics of screening. *J Am Board Fam Pract* 13(3):188–96.

Excerpts from Speech on Use of Mammograms. 2002, February 22. *The New York Times*. p. A22.

Facione NC, Katapodi M. 2000. Culture as an influence on breast cancer screening and early detection. *Semin Oncol Nurs* 16(3):238–47.

Fahs MC, Mandelblatt J, Schechter C, Muller C. 1992. Cost effectiveness of cervical cancer screening for the elderly. *Ann Intern Med* 117(6):520–7.

Fairfield KM, Hankinson SE, Rosner BA, Hunter DJ, Colditz GA, Willett WC. 2001. Risk of ovarian carcinoma and consumption of vitamins A, C, and E and specific carotenoids: a prospective analysis. *Cancer* 92(9):2318–26.

Farkas A, Schneider D, Perrotti M, Cummings KB, Ward WS. 1998. National trends in the epidemiology of prostate cancer, 1973 to 1994: evidence for the effectiveness of prostate-specific antigen screening. *Urology* 52(3):444–8.

Farkas AJ, Gilpin EA, White MM, Pierce JP. 2000. Association between household and workplace smoking restrictions and adolescent smoking. *JAMA* 284(6):717–22.

Farquhar JW, Fortmann SP, Maccoby N, Woods PD, Haskell WL, Taylor CB, Flora JA, Solomon DS, Togers T, Adler E, Breitrose P, Weiner L, Matarazzo JD, Weiss S.M., Herd J.A., Miller N.E. 1984. The Stanford Five City Project: an overview. In Matarazzo J.D., Weiss S.M., Herd J.A., Miller N.E. (eds.) *Behavioral Health: A Handbook of Health Enhancement and Disease Prevention*. New York: Wiley.

Farquhar JW, Fortmann SP, Flora JA, Taylor CB, Haskell WL, Williams PT, Maccoby N, Wood PD. 1990. Effects of communitywide education on cardiovascular disease risk factors. The Stanford Five-City Project. *JAMA* 264(3):359–65.

Fasouliotis SJ, Schenker JG. 2000. BRCA1 and BRCA2 gene mutations: decision-making dilemmas concerning testing and management. *Obstet Gynecol Surv* 55(6):373–84.

Feig SA. 1995. Estimation of currently attainable benefit from mammographic screening of women aged 40–49 years. *Cancer* 75(10):2412–9.

Feig SA. 1996. Strategies for improving sensitivity of screening mammography for women aged 40 to 49 years. *JAMA* 276(1):73–4.

Feig SA. 2000. Ductal carcinoma in situ. Implications for screening mammography. *Radiol Clin N Am* 38(4):653–68, vii.

Feig SA, Ehrlich SM. 1990. Estimation of radiation risk from screening mammography: recent trends and comparison with expected benefits. *Radiology* 174(3 Pt 1):638–47.

Feig SA, D'Orsi CJ, Hendrick RE, Jackson VP, Kopans DB, Monsees B, Sickles EA, Stelling CB, Zinninger M, Wilcox-Buchalla P. 1998. American College of Radiology guidelines for breast cancer screening. *Am J Roentgenol* 171(1):29–33.

Ferrini R, Woolf SH. 1998. American College of Preventive Medicine practice policy. Screening for prostate cancer in American men. *Am J Prev Med* 15(1):81–4.

Ferrini R, Mannino E, Ramsdell E, Hill L. 1996. Screening mammography for breast cancer: American College of Preventive Medicine practice policy statement. *Am J Prev Med* 12(5):340–1.

Ferry LH, Grissino LM, Runfola PS. 1999. Tobacco dependence curricula in U.S. undergraduate medical education. *JAMA* 282(9):825–9.

Feskanich D, Ziegler RG, Michaud DS, Giovannucci EL, Speizer FE, Willett WC, Colditz GA. 2000. Prospective study of fruit and vegetable consumption and risk of lung cancer among men and women. *J Natl Cancer Inst* 92(22):1812–23.

Feuer EJ, Merrill RM, Hankey BF. 1999. Cancer surveillance series: interpreting trends in prostate cancer. Part II. Cause of death misclassification and the recent rise and fall in prostate cancer mortality. *J Natl Cancer Inst* 91(12):1025–32.

Fichtenberg CM, Glantz SA. 2000. Association of the California Tobacco Control Program with declines in cigarette consumption and mortality from heart disease. *N Engl J Med* 343(24):1772–7.

Figueroa-Colon R, von Almen TK, Franklin FA, Schuftan C, Suskind RM. 1993. Comparison of two hypocaloric diets in obese children. *Am J Dis Child* 147(2):160–6.

Fiore M, Bailey W, et al. 1996. *Smoking Cessation: Clinical Practice Guideline No. 18*. U.S. Department of Health and Human Services, Public Health Service, Agency for Health Care Policy and Research. Rockville, MD: Agency for Healthcare Research and Quality.

Fiore MC. 1991. The new vital sign. Assessing and documenting smoking status. *JAMA* 266(22):3183–4.

Fiore MC, Epps RP, Manley MW. 1994. A missed opportunity. Teaching medical students to help their patients successfully quit smoking. *JAMA* 271(8):624–6.

Fiore MC, Jorenby DE, Schensky AE, Smith SS, Bauer RR, Baker TB. 1995. Smoking status as the new vital sign: effect on assessment and intervention in patients who smoke. *Mayo Clin Proc* 70(3):209–13.

Fishbein M, Ajzen I. 1975. *Belief, Attitude, Intention, and Behavior: An Introduction to Theory and Research*. Reading, MA: Addison-Wesley Publishing Company.

Fisher EB Jr. 1995. The results of the COMMIT trial. Community Intervention Trial for Smoking Cessation. *Am J Public Health* 85(2):159–60.

Fisher EB Jr, Auslander W, Sussman L, Owens N, Jackson-Thompson J. 1992. Community organization and health promotion in minority neighborhoods. *Ethn Dis* 2(3):252–72.

Fisher EB Jr, Bishop DB, Levitt-Gilmour T, Cappello MT, Ashenberg ZS, Newman E. 1994. Social support in worksite smoking cessation: qualitative analysis of the EASE project. *Am J Health Promot* 9(1):39–47, 75.

Fisher EB, Auslander WF, Munro JF, Arfken CL, Brownson RC, Owens NW. 1998. Neighbors for a smoke free north side: evaluation of a community organization approach to promoting smoking cessation among African Americans. *Am J Public Health* 88(11): 1658–63.

Fitzgibbon ML, Stolley MR, Avellone ME, Sugerman S, Chavez N. 1996. Involving parents in cancer risk reduction: a program for Hispanic American families. *Health Psychol* 15(6): 413–22.

Flay BR. 1987. Mass media and smoking cessation: a critical review. *Am J Public Health* 77(2):153–60.

Flechtner-Mors M, Ditschuneit HH, Johnson TD, Suchard MA, Adler G. 2000. Metabolic and weight loss effects of long-term dietary intervention in obese patients: four-year results. *Obes Res* 8(5):399–402.

Flegal KM, Carroll MD, Kuczmarski RJ, Johnson CL. 1998. Overweight and obesity in the United States: prevalence and trends, 1960–1994. *Int J Obes Relat Metab Disord* 22(1):39–47.

Flehinger BJ, Kimmel M. 1987. The natural history of lung cancer in a periodically screened population. *Biometrics* 43(1):127–44.

Flehinger BJ, Kimmel M, Polyak T, Melamed MR. 1993. Screening for lung cancer. The Mayo Lung Project revisited. *Cancer* 72(5):1573–80.

Fleming C, Wasson JH, Albertsen PC, Barry MJ, Wennberg JE. 1993. A decision analysis of alternative treatment strategies for clinically localized prostate cancer. Prostate Patient Outcomes Research Team. *JAMA* 269(20):2650–8.

Fletcher SW. 1997. Whither scientific deliberation in health policy recommendations? Alice in the Wonderland of breast-cancer screening. *N Engl J Med* 336(16):1180–3.

Fletcher SW, Black W, Harris R, Rimer BK, Shapiro S. 1993. Report of the International Workshop on Screening for Breast Cancer. *J Natl Cancer Inst* 85(20):1644–56.

Fletcher RH, Farraye FA. 1999. Screening flexible sigmoidoscopy: effectiveness is not enough. *Gastroenterology* 117(2):486–8.

Floch, MH. 1999. Will our healthcare system permit paramedical personnel to do endoscopy? *J Clin Gastroentero.* 28(2):95–6.

Flood AB, Wennberg JE, Nease RF Jr, Fowler FJ Jr, Ding J, Hynes LM. 1996. The importance of patient preference in the decision to screen for prostate cancer. Prostate Patient Outcomes Research Team. *J Gen Intern Med* 11(6):342–9.

Flores R. 1995. Dance for health: improving fitness in African American and Hispanic adolescents. *Public Health Rep* 110(2):189–93.

Floyd CE Jr, Lo JY, Tourassi GD. 2000. Case-based reasoning computer algorithm that uses mammographic findings for breast biopsy decisions. *Am J Roentgenol* 175(5):1347–52.

Foley EC, D'Amico F, Merenstein JH. 1995. Five-year follow-up of a nurse-initiated intervention to improve mammography recommendation. *J Am Board Fam Pract* 8(6):452–6.

Fontana RS, Sanderson DR, Miller WE, Woolner LB, Taylor WF, Uhlenhopp MA. 1972. The Mayo Lung Project: preliminary report of "early cancer detection" phase. *Cancer* 30(5): 1373–82.

Fontana RS, Sanderson DR, Woolner LB, Taylor WF, Miller WE, Muhm JR. 1986. Lung cancer screening: the Mayo program. *J Occup Med* 28(8):746–50.

Fontana RS, Sanderson DR, Woolner LB, Taylor WF, Miller WE, Muhm JR, Bernatz PE, Payne WS, Pairolero PC, Bergstralh EJ. 1991. Screening for lung cancer. A critique of the Mayo Lung Project. *Cancer* 67(4 Suppl):1155–64.

Foreyt JP, et al. 1982. Behavioral treatment of obesity: results and limitations. *Behav Ther* 13(2):153–61.

Foreyt JP, Goodrick GK. 1991. Factors common to successful therapy for the obese patient. *Med Sci Sports Exerc* 23(3):292–7.

Forrest AP, Alexander FE. 1995. A question that will not go away: at what age should mammographic screening begin? *J Natl Cancer Inst* 87(16):1195–7.

Fortmann SP, Winkleby MA, Flora JA, Haskell WL, Taylor CB. 1990. Effect of long-term community health education on blood pressure and hypertension control. The Stanford Five-City Project. *Am J Epidemiol* 132(4):629–46.

Foster GD, Wadden TA, Peterson FJ, Letizia KA, Bartlett SJ, Conill AM. 1992. A controlled comparison of three very-low-calorie diets: effects on weight, body composition, and symptoms. *Am J Clin Nutr* 55(4):811–7.

Fowler FJ Jr, McNaughton Collins M, Albertsen PC, Zietman A, Elliott DB, Barry MJ. 2000. Comparison of recommendations by urologists and radiation oncologists for treatment of clinically localized prostate cancer. *JAMA* 283(24):3217–22.

Fox S. General Electric Manager, CT Advance Applications. March 7, 2001.

Fox SA, Stein JA, Sockloskie RJ, Ory MG. 2001. Targeted mailed materials and the Medicare beneficiary: increasing mammogram screening among the elderly. *Am J Public Health* 1(1):5561.

Frame PS. 1992. Health maintenance in clinical practice: strategies and barriers. *Am Fam Physician* 45(3):1192–200.

Frame PS. 1995. The complete annual physical examination refuses to die. *J Fam Pract* 40(6):543–5.

Frame PS. 2000. Routine screening for lung cancer? Maybe someday, but not yet. *JAMA* 284(15):1980–3.

Frame PS, Frame JS. 1998. Determinants of cancer screening frequency: the example of screening for cervical cancer. *J Am Board Fam Pract* 11(2):87–95.

Frame PS, Werth PL. 1993. How primary health care providers can integrate cancer prevention into practice. *Cancer* 72(3 Suppl):1132–7.

Frank-Stromborg M, Rohan K. 1992. Nursing's involvement in the primary and secondary prevention of cancer. Nationally and internationally. *Cancer Nurs* 15(2):79–108.

Frank E, Winkleby MA, Altman DG, Rockhill B, Fortmann SP. 1991. Predictors of physician's smoking cessation advice. *JAMA* 266(22):3139–44.

Frazier AL, Colditz GA, Fuchs CS, Kuntz KM. 2000. Cost-effectiveness of screening for colorectal cancer in the general population. *JAMA* 284(15):1954–61.

Freedman MR, King J, Kennedy E. 2001. Popular diets: a scientific review. *Obes Res* 9(Suppl 1):1S–40S.

French SA, Jeffery RW, Story M, Hannan P, Snyder MP. 1997a. A pricing strategy to promote low-fat snack choices through vending machines. *Am J Public Health* 87(5):849–51.

French SA, Story M, Jeffery RW, Snyder P, Eisenberg M, Sidebottom A, Murray D. 1997b. Pricing strategy to promote fruit and vegetable purchasing in high school cafeterias. *J Am Diet Assoc* 97(9):1008–10.

Freudenheim JL, Graham S, Marshall JR, Haughey BP, Cholewinski S, Wilkinson G. 1991. Folate intake and carcinogenesis of the colon and rectum. *Int J Epidemiol* 20(2):368–74.

Friedman GD, Hiatt RA, Quesenberry CP Jr, Selby JV. 1991. Case-control study of screening for prostatic cancer by digital rectal examinations. *Lancet* 337(8756):1526–9.

Frisch RE, Wyshak G, Albright NL, Albright TE, Schiff I, Jones KP, Witschi J, Shiang E, Koff E, Marguglio M. 1985. Lower prevalence of breast cancer and cancers of the reproductive system among former college athletes compared to non-athletes. *Br J Cancer* 52(6): 885–91.

Frisell J, Lidbrink E. 1997. The Stockholm Mammographic Screening Trial: risks and benefits in age group 40–49 years. *J Natl Cancer Inst Monogr* (22):49–51.

Frosch DL, Kaplan RM. 1999. Shared decision making in clinical medicine: past research and future directions. *Am J Prev Med* 17(4):285–94.

Frost JK, Ball WC Jr, Levin ML, Tockman MS, Baker RR, Carter D, Eggleston JC, Erozan YS, Gupta PK, Khouri NF, et al. 1984. Early lung cancer detection: results of the initial (prevalence) radiologic and cytologic screening in the Johns Hopkins study. *Am Rev Respir Dis* 130(4):549–54.

Fuchs CS, Colditz GA, Stampfer MJ, Giovannucci EL, Hunter DJ, Rimm EB, Willett WC, Speizer FE. 1996. A prospective study of cigarette smoking and the risk of pancreatic cancer. *Arch Intern Med* 156(19):2255–60.

Fuchs CS, Giovannucci EL, Colditz GA, Hunter DJ, Stampfer MJ, Rosner B, Speizer FE, Willett WC. 1999. Dietary fiber and the risk of colorectal cancer and adenoma in women. *N Engl J Med* 340(3):169–76.

Fullmer CD. 1970. Pulmonary cytology and mass screening. *Acta Cytol* 14(3):121.

Gail M, Rimer B. 1998. Risk-based recommendations for mammographic screening for women in their forties. *J Clin Oncol* 16(9):3105–14.

Galanis DJ, Kolonel LN, Lee J, Nomura A. 1998. Intakes of selected foods and beverages and the incidence of gastric cancer among the Japanese residents of Hawaii: a prospective study. *Int J Epidemiol* 27(2):173–80.

Gallagher RE, Bakemeier RF, Chamberlain RM, Kupchella CE, O'Donnell JF, Parker JA, Hill GJ, Brooks CM. 1992. Instructional methods and the use of teaching resources in cancer education curricula. Cancer Education Survey II: cancer education in United States medical schools. *J Cancer Educ* 7(2):95–104.

Galuska DA, Will JC, Serdula MK, Ford ES. 1999. Are health care professionals advising obese patients to lose weight? *JAMA* 282(16):1576–8.

Gammon MD, Schoenberg JB, Britton JA, Kelsey JL, Coates RJ, Brogan D, Potischman N, Swanson CA, Daling JR, Stanford JL, Brinton LA. 1998. Recreational physical activity and breast cancer risk among women under age 45 years. *Am J Epidemiol* 147(3):273–80.

Gann PH, Hennekens CH, Stampfer MJ. 1995. A prospective evaluation of plasma prostate-specific antigen for detection of prostatic cancer. *JAMA* 273(4):289–94.

Gann PH, Hennekens CH, Ma J, Longcope C, Stampfer MJ. 1996. Prospective study of sex hormone levels and risk of prostate cancer. *J Natl Cancer Inst* 88(16):1118–26.

Garabrant DH, Peters JM, Mack TM, Bernstein L. 1984. Job activity and colon cancer risk. *Am J Epidemiol* 119(6):1005–14.

Garfinkel L, Boffetta P. 1990. Association between smoking and leukemia in two American Cancer Society prospective studies. *Cancer* 65(10):2356–60.

Garland M, Hunter DJ, Colditz GA, Spiegelman DL, Manson JE, Stampfer MJ, Willett WC. 1999. Alcohol consumption in relation to breast cancer risk in a cohort of United States women 25–42 years of age. *Cancer Epidemiol Biomarkers Prev* 8(11):1017–21.

Garr DR, Lackland DT, Wilson DB. 2000. Prevention education and evaluation in U.S. medical schools: a status report. *Acad Med* 75(7 Suppl):S14–21.

Garrow JS, Summerbell CD. 1995. Meta-analysis: effect of exercise, with or without dieting, on the body composition of overweight subjects. *Eur J Clin Nutr* 49(1):1–10.

Geiger WJ, Neuberger MJ, Bell GC. 1993. Implementing the US Preventive Services guidelines in a family practice residency. *Fam Med* 25(7):447–51.

Geller AC, Prout M, Sun T, Lew RA, Culbert AL, Koh HK. 1999. Medical students' knowledge, attitudes, skills, and practices of cancer prevention and detection. *J Cancer Educ* 14(2):72–7.

Gelmon KA, Olivotto I. 2002. The mammography screening debate: time to move on. *Lancet* 359(9310):904–5.

Gemson DH, Elinson J. 1986. Prevention in primary care: variability in physician practice patterns in New York City. *Am J Prev Med* 2(4):226–34.

Gemson DH, Sloan RP. 1995. Efficacy of computerized health risk appraisal as part of a periodic health examination at the worksite. *Am J Health Promot* 9(6):462–6.

Gemson DH, Dickey LL, Ganz ML, Ashford AR, Francis CK. 1996. Acceptance and use of Put Prevention into Practice materials at an inner-city hospital. *Am J Prev Med* 12(4):233–7.

Genovese L, Wholihan D. 1995. The "VANAC team": establishing a cancer prevention team. VA Nurses Against Cancer. *Cancer Nurs* 18(6):421–6.

Gerber GS, Thisted RA, Scardino PT, Frohmuller HG, Schroeder FH, Paulson DF, Middleton AW Jr, Rukstalis DB, Smith JA Jr, Schellhammer PF, Ohori M, Chodak GW. 1996. Results of radical prostatectomy in men with clinically localized prostate cancer. *JAMA* 276(8):615–9.

Gerhardsson de Verdier M, Steineck G, Hagman U, Rieger A, Norell SE. 1990. Physical activity and colon cancer: a case-referent study in Stockholm. *Int J Cancer* 46(6):985–9.

Gerhardsson de Verdier M, Hagman U, Peters RK, Steineck G, Overvik E. 1991. Meat, cooking methods and colorectal cancer: a case-referent study in Stockholm. *Int J Cancer* 49(4):520–5.

Gilbert FJ, Cordiner CM, Affleck IR, Hood DB, Mathieson D, Walker LG. 1998. Breast screening: the psychological sequelae of false-positive recall in women with and without a family history of breast cancer. *Eur J Cancer 34* (13):2010–4.

Gilbert JR, Wilson DM, Singer J, Lindsay EA, Willms DG, Best JA, Taylor DW. 1992. A family physician smoking cessation program: an evaluation of the role of follow-up visits. *Am J Prev Med* 8(2):91–5.

Giles JT, Kennedy DT, Dunn EC, Wallace WL, Meadows SL, Cafiero AC. 2001. Results of a community pharmacy-based breast cancer risk-assessment and education program. *Pharmacotherapy* 21(2):243–53.

Gilliland FD, Rosenberg RD, Hunt WC, Stauber P, Key CR. 2000. Patterns of mammography use among Hispanic, American Indian, and non-Hispanic white women in New Mexico, 1994–1997. *Am J Epidemiol* 152(5):432–7.

Gilpin EA, Pierce JP, Johnson M, Bal D. 1993. Physician advice to quit smoking: results from the 1990 California Tobacco Survey. *J Gen Intern Med* 8(10):549–53.

Giovannucci E. 1995a. Fat and colon cancer. *Cerin Symposium: Nutrition & Cancer*. Paris: Cerin.

Giovannucci E. 1995b. Insulin and colon cancer. *Cancer Causes Control* 6(2):164–79.

Giovannucci E. 1998. Dietary influences of 1,25dihydroxy vitamin D in relation to prostate cancer: a hypothesis. *Cancer Causes Control* 9(6):567–82.

Giovannucci E. 1999. Tomatoes, tomato-based products, lycopene, and cancer: review of the epidemiologic literature. *J Natl Cancer Inst* 91(4):317–31.

Giovannucci E, Goldin B. 1997. The role of fat, fatty acids, and total energy intake in the etiology of human colon cancer. *Am J Clin Nutr* 66(6 Suppl):1564S–71S.

Giovannucci E, Martinez ME. 1996. Tobacco, colorectal cancer, and adenomas: a review of the evidence. *J Natl Cancer Inst* 88(23):1717–30.

Giovannucci E, Willett WC. 1994. Dietary factors and risk of colon cancer. *Ann Med* 26(6): 443–52.

Giovannucci E, Rimm EB, Colditz GA, Stampfer MJ, Ascherio A, Chute CC, Willett WC. 1993a. A prospective study of dietary fat and risk of prostate cancer. *J Natl Cancer Inst* 85(19):1571–9.

Giovannucci E, Stampfer MJ, Colditz GA, Rimm EB, Trichopoulos D, Rosner BA, Speizer FE, Willett WC. 1993b. Folate, methionine, and alcohol intake and risk of colorectal adenoma. *J Natl Cancer Inst* 85(11):875–84.

Giovannucci E, Colditz GA, Stampfer MJ, Hunter D, Rosner BA, Willett WC, Speizer FE. 1994a. A prospective study of cigarette smoking and risk of colorectal adenoma and colorectal cancer in U.S. women. *J Natl Cancer Inst* 86(3):192–9.

Giovannucci E, Rimm EB, Chute CG, Kawachi I, Colditz GA, Stampfer MJ, Willett WC. 1994b. Obesity and benign prostatic hyperplasia. *Am J Epidemiol* 140(11):989–1002.

Giovannucci E, Ascherio A, Rimm EB, Colditz GA, Stampfer MJ, Willett WC. 1995a. Physical activity, obesity, and risk for colon cancer and adenoma in men. *Ann Intern Med* 122(5):327–34.

Giovannucci E, Rimm EB, Ascherio A, Stampfer MJ, Colditz GA, Willett WC. 1995b. Alcohol, low-methionine-low-folate diets, and risk of colon cancer in men. *J Natl Cancer Inst* 87(4):265–73.

Giovannucci E, Colditz GA, Stampfer MJ, Willett WC. 1996. Physical activity, obesity, and risk of colorectal adenoma in women (United States). *Cancer Causes Control* 7(2):253–63.

Giovannucci E, Leitzmann M, Spiegelman D, Rimm EB, Colditz GA, Stampfer MJ, Willett WC. 1998a. A prospective study of physical activity and prostate cancer in male health professionals. *Cancer Res* 58(22):5117–22.

Giovannucci E, Stampfer MJ, Colditz GA, Hunter DJ, Fuchs C, Rosner BA, Speizer FE, Willett WC. 1998b. Multivitamin use, folate, and colon cancer in women in the Nurses' Health Study. *Ann Intern Med* 129(7):517–24.

Giovannucci E, Rimm EB, Ascherio A, Colditz GA, Spiegelman D, Stampfer MJ, Willett WC. 1999. Smoking and risk of total and fatal prostate cancer in United States health professionals. *Cancer Epidemiol Biomarkers Prev* 8(4 Pt 1):277–82.

Giroux J, Welty TK, Oliver FK, Kaur JS, Leonardson G, Cobb N. 2000. Low national breast and cervical cancer-screening rates in American Indian and Alaska Native women with diabetes. *J Am Board Fam Pract* 13(4):239–45.

Glanz K, Tziraki C, Albright CL, Fernandes J. 1995. Nutrition assessment and counseling practices: attitudes and interests of primary care physicians. *J Gen Intern Med* 10(2):89–92.

Glasgow RE, Lichtenstein E. 1987. Long-term effects of behavioral smoking cessation interventions. *Behavior Therapy* 18(4):297–324.

Glasgow RE, Toobert DJ, Hampson SE. 1996. Effects of a brief office-based intervention to facilitate diabetes dietary self-management. *Diabetes Care* 19(8):835–42.

Glasgow RE, Whitlock EP, Valanis BG, Vogt TM. 2000. Barriers to mammography and Pap smear screening among women who recently had neither, one or both types of screening. *Ann Behav Med* 22(3):223–8.

Glass AG, La Chance PA, Vogt TM. 1996. Eighteen years of mammography experience in an HMO: 1975–1992. *HMO Pract* 10(4):184–9.

Glasziou P, Irwig L. 1997. The quality and interpretation of mammographic screening trials for women ages 40–49. *J Natl Cancer Inst Monogr* (22):73–7.

Glasziou PP, Woodward AJ, Mahon CM. 1995. Mammographic screening trials for women aged under 50. A quality assessment and meta-analysis. *Med J Aust* 162(12):625–9.

Gleim GW. 1993. Exercise is not an effective weight loss modality in women. *J Am Coll Nutr* 12(4):363–7.

Gnanadesigan N, Hirsch SH, Reuben DB. 2000. Preventive health behaviors and mammography use among urban older women. *Am J Health Promot* 14(6):343–6, ii.

Godin G., Shephard R. 1990. An evaluation of the potential role of physician in influencing community exercise behavior. *Am J Health Promotion* 4:225–9.

Gohagan JK, Prorok PC, Hayes RB, Kramer BS. 2000. The Prostate, Lung, Colorectal and Ovarian (PLCO) Cancer Screening Trial of the National Cancer Institute: history, organization, and status. *Control Clin Trials* 21(6 Suppl):251S–272S.

Gold MR, Siegel JE, Russell JB, Weinstein MC, eds. 1996. *Cost-Effectiveness in Health and Medicine*. New York: Oxford University Press.

Goldstein MG, Niaura R, Willey-Lessne C, DePue J, Eaton C, Rakowski W, Dube C. 1997. Physicians counseling smokers. A population-based survey of patients' perceptions of health care provider-delivered smoking cessation interventions. *Arch Intern Med* 157(12): 1313–9.

Golub ES. 1999. Heroic myths and probability: confronting the limits of screening. In Kramer BS, Prorok PC, Gohagan J (eds). *Cancer Screening: Theory and Practice,* Vol. 2. New York: Marcel Dekker, Inc.

Golub TR. 2001. Genome-wide views of cancer. *N Engl J Med* 344(8):601–2.

Gomel M, Oldenburg B, Simpson JM, Owen N. 1993. Work-site cardiovascular risk reduction: a randomized trial of health risk assessment, education, counseling, and incentives. *Am J Public Health* 83(9):1231–8.

Gomel MK, Oldenburg B, Simpson JM, Chilvers M, Owen N. 1997. Composite cardiovascular risk outcomes of a work-site intervention trial. *Am J Public Health* 87(4): 673–6.

Goodson P, Gottlieb NH, Smith MM. 1999. Put prevention into practice. Evaluation of program initiation in nine Texas clinical sites. *Am J Prev Med* 17(1):73–8.

Goodwin PJ. 2000. Management of familial breast cancer risk. *Breast Cancer Res Treat* 62(1):19–33.

Gordon NP, Rundall TG, Parker L. 1998. Type of health care coverage and the likelihood of being screened for cancer. *Med Care* 36(5):636–45.

Gordon T, Kannel WB. 1984. Drinking and mortality. The Framingham Study. *Am J Epidemiol* 120(1):97–107.

Gorman C. 2000. Katie's crusade. Colon cancer is one of the deadliest and most preventable malignancies. What you need to know about the disease—and the surprisingly painless test that could save your life. *Time* 155(10):70–6.

Gortmaker SL, Cheung LW, Peterson KE, Chomitz G, Cradle JH, Dart H, Fox MK, Bullock RB, Sobol AM, Colditz G, Field AE, Laird N. 1999a. Impact of a school-based interdisciplinary intervention on diet and physical activity among urban primary school children: eat well and keep moving. *Arch Pediatr Adolesc Med* 153(9):975–83.

Gortmaker SL, Peterson K, Wiecha J, Sobol AM, Dixit S, Fox MK, Laird N. 1999b. Reducing obesity via a school-based interdisciplinary intervention among youth: Planet Health. *Arch Pediatr Adolesc Med* 153(4):409–18.

Gotay CC, Banner RO, Matsunaga DS, Hedlund N, Enos R, Issell BF, DeCambra H. 2000. Impact of a culturally appropriate intervention on breast and cervical screening among native Hawaiian women. *Prev Med* 31(5):529–37.

Gøtzsche PC, Olsen O. 2000. Is screening for breast cancer with mammography justifiable? *Lancet* 355(9198):129–34.

Gøtzsche PC, Liberati A, Torri V, Rossetti L. 1996. Beware of surrogate outcome measures. *Int J Technol Assess Health Care* 12(2):238–46.

Goyder E, Barratt A, Irwig LM. 2000. Telling people about screening programmes and screening test results: how can we do it better? *J Med Screen* 7(3):123–6.

Gram IT, Lund E, Slenker SE. 1990. Quality of life following a false positive mammogram. *Br J Cancer* 62(6):1018–22.

Grann VR, Whang W, Jacobson JS, Heitjan DF, Antman KH, Neugut AI. 1999. Benefits and costs of screening Ashkenazi Jewish women for BRCA1 and BRCA2. *J Clin Oncol* 17(2):494–500.

Grantmakers in Health. 2000. *Prevention Strategies for All Ages: Findings from the Grantmakers in Health Resource Center*. Washington, DC: Grantmakers in Health

Graversen PH, Nielsen KT, Gasser TC, Corle DK, Madsen PO. 1990. Radical prostatectomy versus expectant primary treatment in stages I and II prostatic cancer. A fifteen-year follow-up. *Urology* 36(6):493–8.

Greenfield TK, Rogers JD. 1999. Who drinks most of the alcohol in the U.S.? The policy implications. *J Stud Alcohol* 60(1):78–89.

Greenlee RT, Murray T, Bolden S, Wingo PA. 2000. Cancer statistics, 2000. *CA Cancer J Clin* 50(1):7–33.

Greenlee RT, Hill-Harmon MB, Murray T, Thun M. 2001. Cancer statistics, 2001. *CA Cancer J Clin* 51(1):15–36.

Grol R. 1997. Personal paper. Beliefs and evidence in changing clinical practice. *BMJ* 315(7105): 418–21.

Guare JC, Wing RR, Marcus MD, Epstein LH, Burton LR, Gooding WE. 1989. Analysis of changes in eating behavior and weight loss in type II diabetic patients. Which behaviors to change. *Diabetes Care* 12(7):500–3.

Guo W, Blot WJ, Li JY, Taylor PR, Liu BQ, Wang W, Wu YP, Zheng W, Dawsey SM, Li B, et al. 1994. A nested case-control study of oesophageal and stomach cancers in the Linxian nutrition intervention trial. *Int J Epidemiol* 23(3):444–50.

Hackshaw AK, Law MR, Wald NJ. 1997. The accumulated evidence on lung cancer and environmental tobacco smoke. *BMJ* 315(7114):980–8.

Hahn RA, Teutsch SM, Rothenberg RB, Marks JS. 1990. Excess deaths from nine chronic diseases in the United States, 1986. *JAMA* 264(20):2654–9.

Haire-Joshu D, Auslander WF, Houston CA, Williams JH. 1999. Staging of dietary patterns among African American women. *Health Educ Behav* 26(1):90–102.

Halabi S, Skinner CS, Samsa GP, Strigo TS, Crawford YS, Rimer BK. 2000. Factors associated with repeat mammography screening. *J Fam Pract* 49(12):1104–12.

Halford JA, Wright RG, Ditchmen EJ. 1999. Prospective study of PAPNET: review of 25,656 Pap smears negative on manual screening and rapid rescreening. *Cytopathology* 10(5): 317–23.

Halpin Schauffler H, Mordavsky JK, McMenamin S. 2001. Adoption of the AHCPR Clinical Practice Guideline for Smoking Cessation: a survey of California's HMOs. *Am J Prev Med* 21(3):153–61.

Hamann HA, Croyle RT, Venne VL, Baty BJ, Smith KR, Botkin JR. 2000. Attitudes toward the genetic testing of children among adults in a Utah-based kindred tested for a BRCA1 mutation. *Am J Med Genet* 92(1):25–32.

Hamblin J, Connor PD. 1998. Cancer screening guideline preference surveys: physicians' perceptions of the American Cancer Society. *Tenn Med* 91(1):17–20.

Hamilton AS, Stanford JL, Gilliland FD, Albertsen PC, Stephenson RA, Hoffman RM, Eley JW, Harlan LC, Potosky AL. 2001. Health outcomes after external-beam radiation therapy for clinically localized prostate cancer: results from the Prostate Cancer Outcomes Study. *J Clin Oncol* 19(9):2517–26.

Hammerer P, Huland H. 1994. Systematic sextant biopsies in 651 patients referred for prostate evaluation. *J Urol* 151(1):99–102.

Hankey BF, Feuer EJ, Clegg LX, Hayes RB, Legler JM, Prorok PC, Ries LA, Merrill RM, Kaplan RS. 1999. Cancer surveillance series: interpreting trends in prostate cancer. Part I. Evidence of the effects of screening in recent prostate cancer incidence, mortality, and survival rates. *J Natl Cancer Inst* 91(12):1017–24.

Hankinson SE, Willett WC, Manson JE, Hunter DJ, Colditz GA, Stampfer MJ, Longcope C, Speizer FE. 1995. Alcohol, height, and adiposity in relation to estrogen and prolactin levels in postmenopausal women. *J Natl Cancer Inst* 87(17):1297–302.

Hanks GE, Hanlon A, Schultheiss T, Corn B, Shipley WU, Lee WR. 1994. Early prostate cancer: the national results of radiation treatment from the Patterns of Care and Radiation Therapy Oncology Group studies with prospects for improvement with conformal radiation and adjuvant androgen deprivation. *J Urol* 152(5 Pt 2):1775–80.

Hanlon P, McEwen J, Carey L, Gilmour H, Tannahill C, Tannahill A, Kelly M. 1995. Health checks and coronary risk: further evidence from a randomised controlled trial. *BMJ* 311(7020):1609–13.

Hardcastle JD, Chamberlain JO, Robinson MH, Moss SM, Amar SS, Balfour TW, James PD, Mangham CM. 1996. Randomised controlled trial of faecal-occult-blood screening for colorectal cancer. *Lancet* 348(9040):1472–7.

Harrell JS, McMurray RG, Bangdiwala SI, Frauman AC, Gansky SA, Bradley CB. 1996. Effects of a school-based intervention to reduce cardiovascular disease risk factors in elementary-school children: the Cardiovascular Health in Children (CHIC) study. *J Pediatr* 128(6):797–805.

Harrell JS, Gansky SA, McMurray RG, Bangdiwala SI, Frauman AC, Bradley CB. 1998. School-based interventions improve heart health in children with multiple cardiovascular disease risk factors. *Pediatrics* 102(2 Pt 1):371–80.

Harris JK, French SA, Jeffery RW, McGovern PG, Wing RR. 1994. Dietary and physical activity correlates of long-term weight loss. *Obesity Res* 2(4):307–13.

Harris R, Leininger L. 1995. Clinical strategies for breast cancer screening: weighing and using the evidence. *Ann Intern Med* 122(7):539–47.

Harris JR, Schauffler HH, Milstein A, Powers P, Hopkins DP. 2001. Expanding health insurance coverage for smoking cessation treatments: experience of the Pacific Business Group on Health. *Am J Health Promot* 15(5):350–6.

Hart AR, Eaden J, Barnett S, de Bono AM, Mayberry JF. 1998. Colorectal cancer prevention. An approach to increasing compliance in a faecal occult blood test screening programme. *J Epidemiol Community Health* 52(12):818–20.

Hartman TJ, McCarthy PR, Park RJ, Schuster E, Kushi LH. 1997. Results of a community-based low-literacy nutrition education program. *J Community Health* 22(5):325–41.

Harvard School of Public Health. 2001. *About the Health Professionals Follow-up Study*. [Online]. Available at: http://www.hsph.harvard.edu/hpfs/ (accessed March 2002).

Harvey EB, Schairer C, Brinton LA, Hoover RN, Fraumeni JF Jr. 1987. Alcohol consumption and breast cancer. *J Natl Cancer Inst* 78(4):657–61.

Harvey-Berino J. 1998. Changing health behavior via telecommunications technology: using interactive television to treat obesity. *Behav Ther* 29(3):505–19.

Hastreiter RJ, Bakdash B, Roesch MH, Walseth J. 1994. Use of tobacco prevention and cessation strategies and techniques in the dental office. *J Am Dent Assoc* 125(11):1475–84.

Hatch J, Derthick S. 1992. Empowering black churches for health promotion. *Health Values* 16(3):3–9.

Hatch J, Cunningham A, Woods W., Snipes F. 1986. The Fitness Through Churches project: description of a community-based cardiovascular health promotion intervention. *Hygie* 5(3):9–12.

Hatcher MB, Fallowfield L, A'Hern R. 2001. The psychosocial impact of bilateral prophylactic mastectomy: prospective study using questionnaires and semistructured interviews. *BMJ* 322(7278):76.

Hauptman J, Lucas C, Boldrin MN, Collins H, Segal KR. 2000. Orlistat in the long-term treatment of obesity in primary care settings. *Arch Fam Med* 9(2):160–7.

Havas S, Anliker J, Damron D, Langenberg P, Ballesteros M, Feldman R. 1998. Final results of the Maryland WIC 5-A-Day Promotion Program. *Am J Public Health* 88(8):1161–7.

Hawkes AP, Kronenberger CB, MacKenzie TD, Mardis AL, Palen TE, Schulter WW, Shah SA, Steele AW, Marine WM. 1996. Cervical cancer screening: American College of Preventive Medicine practice policy statement. *Am J Prev Med* 12(5):342–4.

Hayata Y, Funatsu H, Kato H, Saito Y, Sawamura K, Furose K. 1982. Results of lung cancer screening programs in Japan. *Recent Results Cancer Res* 82:163–73.

Hayek OR, Noble CB, de la Taille A, Bagiella E, Benson MC. 1999. The necessity of a second prostate biopsy cannot be predicted by PSA or PSA derivatives (density or free:total ratio) in men with prior negative prostatic biopsies. *Curr Opin Urol* 9(5):371–5.

Hayes C, Fitzpatrick P, Daly L, Buttimer J. 2000. Screening mammography re-evaluated. *Lancet* 355(9205):749.

Haynes RB, Davis DA, McKibbon A, Tugwell P. 1984. A critical appraisal of the efficacy of continuing medical education. *JAMA* 251(1):61–4.

Hays JT, Wolter TD, Eberman KM, Croghan IT, Offord KP, Hurt RD. 2001. Residential (inpatient) treatment compared with outpatient treatment for nicotine dependence. *Mayo Clin Proc* 76(2):124–33.

Health Care Financing Administration. 1997. Implementation of the Balanced Budget Act of 1997. *Federal Register* 62 (211):59047–83.

Health Care Financing Administration. 2000a. *State-Specific Estimates for Elderly Medicare Beneficiaries from the Behavioral Risk Factor Surveillance System, 1997*. Washington, DC: U.S. Department of Health and Human Services.

Health Care Financing Administration. 2000b. *1999 HCFA Statistics*. Washington, DC: U.S. Department of Health and Human Services.

Health Care Financing Administration. 2000c. *Medicare and You: Medicare Preventive Services. . . .To Help Keep You Healthy*. Washington, DC: U.S. Department of Health and Human Services.

Health Care Financing Administration. 2000d. *A Profile of Medicaid: Chartbook 2000*. Washington, DC: U.S. Department of Health and Human Services.

Health Care Financing Administration. 2001. *Active Projects Report: Research and Demonstrations in Health Care Financing*. Systems, Technical, and Analytic Resources Group. Washington, DC: U.S. Department of Health and Human Services.

Health Care Financing Administration. undated. *Evidence Report and Evidence-Based Recommendations: Interventions to Promote Smoking Cessation in the Medicare Population.* Washington, DC: U.S Department of Health and Human Services.

Health Resources and Services Administration. 2000a. *The Health Resources and Services Administration Cancer Action Plan, Recommendations, and Proposed Initiatives.* Rockville, MD: Health Services and Resource Administration.

Health Resources and Services Administration. 2000b. *FY 1999 Annual Report.* Rockville, MD: Health Services and Resource Administration.

Health Resources and Services Administration. 2001. *Experts with Experience, 1990–2000.* Rockville, MD: Bureau of Primary Health Care, Division of Community and Migrant Health, HRSA.

Hearn MD BT, Baranowski J, Doyle C, Smith M, Lin LS, Resnicow K. 1998. Environmental influences on dietary behavior among children: availability and accessibility of fruits and vegetables enable consumption. *J Health Educ* 29(1):26–32.

Hedegaard HB, Davidson AJ, Wright RA. 1996. Factors associated with screening mammography in low-income women. *Am J Prev Med* 12(1):51–6.

Heimburger DC, Waterbor J, Fish L, Brooks CM. 2000. Cancer Prevention and Control Training Program at the University of Alabama at Birmingham. *J Cancer Educ* 15(2):69–72.

Heimendinger J, Van Duyn MA, Chapelski D, Foerster S, Stables G. 1996. The national 5 a Day for Better Health Program: a large-scale nutrition intervention. *J Public Health Manage Pract* 2:27–35.

Heiskanen I, Luostarinen T, Jarvinen HJ. 2000. Impact of screening examinations on survival in familial adenomatous polyposis. *Scand J Gastroenterol* 35(12):1284–7.

Hellerstedt WL, Jeffery RW. 1997. The effects of a telephone-based intervention on weight loss. *Am J Health Promot* 11(3):177–82.

Henderson C. 2002, February 9. Regular mammograms remain a crucial tool. *The New York Times*. P. A19.

Hendrick RE, Smith RA, Rutledge JH III, Smart CR. 1997. Benefit of screening mammography in women aged 40–49: a new meta-analysis of randomized controlled trials. *J Natl Cancer Inst Monogr* (22):87–92.

Hennekens CH, Buring JE, Manson JE, Stampfer M, Rosner B, Cook NR, Belanger C, LaMotte F, Gaziano JM, Ridker PM, Willett W, Peto R. 1996. Lack of effect of long-term supplementation with beta carotene on the incidence of malignant neoplasms and cardiovascular disease. *N Engl J Med* 334(18):1145–9.

Hennrikus DJ, Jeffery RW. 1996. Worksite intervention for weight control: a review of the literature. *Am J Health Promot* 10(6):471–98.

Henschke CI, Yankelevitz DF. 2000. CT screening for lung cancer. *Radiol Clin N Am* 38(3):487–95, viii.

Henschke CI, McCauley DI, Yankelevitz DF, Naidich DP, McGuinness G, Miettinen OS, Libby DM, Pasmantier MW, Koizumi J, Altorki NK, Smith JP. 1999. Early Lung Cancer Action Project: overall design and findings from baseline screening. *Lancet* 354(9173): 99–105.

Henschke CI, Naidich DP, Yankelevitz DF, McGuinness G, McCauley DI, Smith JP, Libby D, Pasmantier M, Vazquez M, Koizumi J, Flieder D, Altorki N, Miettinen OS. 2001. Early Lung Cancer Action Project: initial findings on repeat screenings. *Cancer* 92(1):153–9.

Herl JL, Taren DL, Taylor AM, Bassford TL. 1999. Cancer prevention education in U.S. medical schools: a curricular assessment. *J Cancer Education* 14(4):214.

Heshka S, Greenway F, Anderson JW, Atkinson RL, Hill JO, Phinney SD, Miller-Kovach K, Xavier Pi-Sunyer F. 2000. Self-help weight loss versus a structured commercial program after 26 weeks: a randomized controlled study. *Am J Med* 109(4):282–7.

Hewitt M, Devesa S, Breen N. 2002. Papanicolaou test use among reproductive-age women at high risk for cervical cancer: analyses of the 1995 National Survey of Family Growth. *Am J Public Health* 92(4):666–9.

Hiatt RA, Rimer BK. 1999. A new strategy for cancer control research. *Cancer Epidemiol Biomarkers Prev* 8(11):957–64.

Hillerdal G. 1996. Long-term survival of patients with lung cancer from a defined geographical area before and after radiological screening. *Lung Cancer* 15(1):21–30.

Hirayama T. 1990. *Lifestyle and Mortality. A Large-Scale Census-Based Cohort Study in Japan*. New York: Karger Basel.

Hirst S, Mitchell H, Medley G. 1990. An evaluation of a campaign to increase cervical cancer screening in rural Victoria. *Community Health Stud* 14(3):263–8.

Hodgson CS, Wilkerson L, Go VL. 2000. Changes in nutrition knowledge among first- and second-year medical students following implementation of an integrated nutrition curriculum. *J Cancer Educ* 15(3):144–7.

Hoel DG, Davis DL, Miller AB, Sondik EJ, Swerdlow AJ. 1992. Trends in cancer mortality in 15 industrialized countries, 1969–1986. *Journal of the National Cancer Institute* 84(5): 313–20.

Holcomb JD, Lira J, Kingery PM, Smith DW, Lane D, Goodway J. 1998. Evaluation of Jump Into Action: a program to reduce the risk of non-insulin-dependent diabetes mellitus in school children on the Texas-Mexico border. *J School Health* 68(7):282–8.

Holden JH, Darga LL, Olson SM, Stettner DC, Ardito EA, Lucas CP. 1992. Long-term follow-up of patients attending a combination very-low calorie diet and behaviour therapy weight loss programme. *Int J Obes Relat Metab Disord* 16(8):605–13.

Holland BK, Foster JD, Louria DB. 1993. Cervical cancer and health care resources in Newark, New Jersey, 1970 to 1988. *Am J Public Health* 83(1):45–8.

Hollis JF, Lichtenstein E, Vogt TM, Stevens VJ, Biglan A. 1993. Nurse-assisted counseling for smokers in primary care. *Ann Intern Med* 118(7):521–5.

Holmberg H, Carlsson P, Lofman O, Varenhorst E. 1998. Economic evaluation of screening for prostate cancer: a randomized population based programme during a 10-year period in Sweden. *Health Policy* 45(2):133–47.

Holmes MM, Rovner DR, Rothert ML, Elstein AS, Holzman GB, Hoppe RB, Metheny WP, Ravitch MM. 1987. Women's and physicians' utilities for health outcomes in estrogen replacement therapy. *J Gen Intern Med* 2(3):178–82.

Hopkins DP, Briss PA, Ricard CJ, Husten CG, Carande-Kulis VG, Fielding JE, Alao MO, McKenna JW, Sharp DJ, Harris JR, Woollery TA, Harris KW. 2001a. Reviews of evidence regarding interventions to reduce tobacco use and exposure to environmental tobacco smoke. *Am J Prev Med* 20(2 Suppl):16–66.

Hopkins DP, Husten CG, Fielding JE, Rosenquist JN, Westphal LL. 2001b. Evidence reviews and recommendations on interventions to reduce tobacco use and exposure to environmental tobacco smoke: a summary of selected guidelines. *Am J Prev Med* 20(2 Suppl):67–87.

Hopper CA, Gruber MB, Munoz KD, Herb RA. 1992. Effect of including parents in a school-based exercise and nutrition program for children. *Res Q Exerc Sport* 63(3):315–21.

Hopper G, Gruber M, Munoz K, MacConnie S. 1996. School-based cardiovascular exercise and nutrition programs with parent participation. *J Health Educ* 27:32–9.

Howe GR, Burch JD. 1996. Nutrition and pancreatic cancer. *Cancer Causes Control* 7(1):69–82.

Howell SL, Nelson-Marten P, Krebs LU, Kaszyk L, Wold R. 1998. Promoting nurses' positive attitudes toward cancer prevention/screening. *J Cancer Educ* 13(2):76–84.

Hsia J, Kemper E, Kiefe C, Zapka J, Sofaer S, Pettinger M, Bowen D, Limacher M, Lillington L, Mason E. 2000. The importance of health insurance as a determinant of cancer screening: evidence from the Women's Health Initiative. *Prev Med* 31(3):261–70.

Hsing AW, McLaughlin JK, Hrubec Z, Blot WJ, Fraumeni JF Jr. 1990a. Cigarette smoking and liver cancer among U.S. veterans. *Cancer Causes Control* 1(3):217–21.

Hsing AW, McLaughlin JK, Schuman LM, Bjelke E, Gridley G, Wacholder S, Chien HT, Blot WJ. 1990b. Diet, tobacco use, and fatal prostate cancer: results from the Lutheran Brotherhood Cohort Study. *Cancer Res* 50(21):6836–40.

Hsing AW, McLaughlin JK, Hrubec Z, Blot WJ, Fraumeni JF Jr. 1991. Tobacco use and prostate cancer: 26-year follow-up of U.S. veterans. *Am J Epidemiol* 133(5):437–41.

Hu FB, Sigal RJ, Rich-Edwards JW, Colditz GA, Solomon CG, Willett WC, Speizer FE, Manson JE. 1999. Walking compared with vigorous physical activity and risk of type 2 diabetes in women: a prospective study. *JAMA* 282(15):1433–9.

Hu FB, Stampfer MJ, Colditz GA, Ascherio A, Rexrode KM, Willett WC, Manson JE. 2000. Physical activity and risk of stroke in women. *JAMA* 283(22):2961–7.

Huang Z, Hankinson SE, Colditz GA, Stampfer MJ, Hunter DJ, Manson JE, Hennekens CH, Rosner B, Speizer FE, Willett WC. 1997. Dual effects of weight and weight gain on breast cancer risk. *JAMA* 278(17):1407–11.

Hulka B. 1966. Motivational techniques in a cancer detection program. *Public Health Rep* 81:1009–14.

Hulka B. 1967. Motivational techniques in a cancer detection program: utilization of community resources. *Am J Public Health* 57:229–40.

Hulka BS. 1986. Screening for cancer: lessons learned. *J Occup Med* 28(8):687–91.

Hulscher ME, Wensing M, Grol RP, van der Weijden T, van Weel C. 1999. Interventions to improve the delivery of preventive services in primary care. *Am J Public Health* 89(5): 737–46.

Humphrey LL, Helfand M, Chan BKS, Woolf SH. 2002. Breast cancer screening with mammography. Summary of the Evidence for the U.S. Preventive Services Task Force. *Annals of Internal Medicine* 137(5 Part 1) E347–67.

Humphrey PA, Keetch DW, Smith DS, Shepherd DL, Catalona WJ. 1996. Prospective characterization of pathological features of prostatic carcinomas detected via serum prostate specific antigen based screening. *J Urol* 155(3):816–20.

Hunt JR, Kristal AR, White E, Lynch JC, Fries E. 1995. Physician recommendations for dietary change: their prevalence and impact in a population-based sample. *Am J Public Health* 85(5):722–6.

Hunt KA, Rosen EL, Sickles EA. 1999. Outcome analysis for women undergoing annual versus biennial screening mammography: a review of 24,211 examinations. *Am J Roentgenol* 173(2):285–9.

Hunter DJ, Willett WC. 1993. Diet, body size, and breast cancer. *Epidemiol Rev* 15(1):110–32.

Hunter DJ, Spiegelman D, Adami HO, Beeson L, Van den Brandt PA, Folsom AR, Fraser GE, Goldbohm RA, Graham S, Howe GR, Kushi LH, Marshall JR, McDermott A, Miller AB, Speizer FE, Wolk A, Yaun S-S, Willett W. 1996. Cohort studies of fat intake and the risk of breast cancer—a pooled analysis. *N Engl J Med* 334(6):356–61.

Hyndman JC, Holman CD, Dawes VP. 2000. Effect of distance and social disadvantage on the response to invitations to attend mammography screening. *J Med Screen* 7(3):141–5.

Imperiale TF, Wagner DR, Lin CY, Larkin GN, Rogge JD, Ransohoff DF. 2000. Risk of advanced proximal neoplasms in asymptomatic adults according to the distal colorectal findings. *N Engl J Med* 343(3):169–74.

Inciardi JF, Lee JG, Stijnen T. 2000. Incidence trends for colorectal cancer in California: implications for current screening practices. *Am J Med* 109(4):277–81.

Institute of Medicine. 1994. *Growing Up Tobacco Free: Preventing Nicotine Addiction in Children and Youths*. Washington, DC: National Academy Press.

Institute of Medicine. Field M, Tranquada R, Feasley J, eds. 1995a. *Health Services Research: Work Force and Educational Issues*. Washington, DC: National Academy Press.

Institute of Medicine. 1995b. *Weighing the Options. Criteria for Evaluating Weight-Management Programs*. Washington, DC: National Academy Press.

Institute of Medicine. 1998. *Taking Action to Reduce Tobacco Use*. Washington, DC: National Academy Press.

Institute of Medicine. 1999a. *The Role of Nutrition in Maintaining Health in the Nation's Elderly: Evaluating Coverage of Nutrition Services for the Medicare Population*. Washington, DC: National Academy Press.

Institute of Medicine. Haynes MA, Smedley BD, eds. 1999b. *The Unequal Burden of Cancer: An Assessment of NIH Research and Programs for Ethnic Minorities and the Medically Underserved*. Washington, DC: National Academy Press.

Institute of Medicine. 2000a. *State Programs Can Reduce Tobacco Use*. Washington, DC: National Academy Press.

Institute of Medicine. Smedley B, Syme SL, eds. 2000b. *Promoting Health: Intervention Strategies from Social and Behavioral Research*. Washington, DC: National Academy Press.

Institute of Medicine. Field M, Lawrence RL, Zwanziger L, eds. 2000c. *Extending Medicare Coverage for Preventive and Other Services*. Washington, DC: National Academy Press.

Institute of Medicine. Lewin ME, Altman S, eds. 2000d. *America's Health Care Safety Net: Intact but Endangered*. Washington D.C: National Academy Press.

Institute of Medicine. Kohn LT, Corrigan JM, Donaldson MS. 2000e. *To Err Is Human: Building a Safer Health System*. Washington, DC: National Academy Press.

Institute of Medicine. 2001a. *Health and Behavior: The Interplay of Biological, Behavioral, and Societal Influences*. Washington D.C: National Academy Press.

Institute of Medicine. 2001b. *Mammography and Beyond*. Washington, DC: National Academy Press.

Institute of Medicine. Committee on Quality of Health Care in America. 2001c. *Crossing the Quality Chasm: A New Health System for the 21st Century*. Washington, DC: National Academy Press.

Institute of Medicine. 2001d. *Improving Palliative Care for Cancer*. Washington, DC: National Academy Press.

Institute of Medicine. 2001e. *Clearing the Smoke: Assessing the Science Base for Tobacco Harm Reduction*. Washington, DC: National Academy Press.

Institute of Medicine. 2003. *The Future of the Public's Health in the 21st Century*. Washington DC: The National Academies Press.

Insull W Jr, Henderson MM, Prentice RL, Thompson DJ, Clifford C, Goldman S, Gorbach S, Moskowitz M, Thompson R, Woods M. 1990. Results of a randomized feasibility study of a low-fat diet. *Arch Intern Med* 150(2):421–7.

Interagency Board for Nutrition Monitoring and Related Research. 1993. *Nutrition Monitoring in the United States. Chartbook I. Selected Findings from the National Nutrition Monitoring and Related Research Program*. Hyattsville, MD: U.S. Public Health Service.

International Agency for Research on Cancer. Waterhouse J, Muir C, Correa P, Powell J. 1976. *Cancer Incidence in Five Continents*. IARC Pub. No. 15, Vol III. Lyon, France: IARC Press.

International Agency for Research on Cancer. 1988. Alcohol drinking. Biological data relevant to the evaluation of carcinogenic risk to humans. *IARC Monogr Eval Carcinog Risks Hum* 44:101–52.

International Agency for Research on Cancer. 2000. *The Role of Weight Control and Physical Activity in Cancer Prevention*. Lyon, France: IARC Press.

International Agency for Research on Cancer. 2002. *IARC Handbooks of Cancer Preventions: Weight Control and Physical Activity*. Lyon, France: IARC Press.

International Agency for Research on Cancer (IARC) Working Group on evaluation of cervical cancer screening programmes. 1986. Screening for squamous cervical cancer: duration of low risk after negative results of cervical cytology and its implication for screening policies. *Br Med J (Clin Res Ed)* 293(6548):659–64.

Intersociety Professional Nutrition Education Consortium. 1998. Bringing physician nutrition specialists into the mainstream: rationale for the Intersociety Professional Nutrition Education Consortium. *Am J Clin Nutr* 68(4):894–8.

Israel AC, Stolmaker L, Andrian CA. 1985. The effects of training parents in general child management skills on a behavioral weight loss program for children. *Behav Ther* 16(2): 169–80.

Jacobs DR Jr, Slavin J, Marquart L. 1995. Whole grain intake and cancer: a review of the literature. *Nutr Cancer* 24(3):221–9.

Jacobsen SJ, Bergstralh EJ, Guess HA, Katusic SK, Klee GG, Oesterling JE, Lieber MM. 1996. Predictive properties of serum-prostate-specific antigen testing in a community-based setting. *Arch Intern Med* 156(21):2462–8.

Jacobsen SJ, Bergstralh EJ, Katusic SK, Guess HA, Darby CH, Silverstein MD, Oesterling JE, Lieber MM. 1998. Screening digital rectal examination and prostate cancer mortality: a population-based case-control study. *Urology* 52(2):173–9.

Jadad A. 1998. *Randomised Controlled Trials*. London: BMJ Books.

Jaen CR. 1997. Primary-care physicians. *Tob Control* 6(Suppl 1):S34–6.

Jaen CR, Stange KC, Nutting PA. 1994. Competing demands of primary care: a model for the delivery of clinical preventive services. *J Fam Pract* 38(2):166–71.

Jaen CR, Stange KC, Tumiel LM, Nutting P. 1997b. Missed opportunities for prevention: smoking cessation counseling and the competing demands of practice. *J Fam Pract* 45(4):348–54.

Jaen CR, Crabtree BF, Zyzanski SJ, Goodwin MA, Stange KC. 1998. Making time for tobacco cessation counseling. *J Fam Pract* 46(5):425–8.

Jakicic JM, Wing RR. 1998. Differences in resting energy expenditure in African-American vs Caucasian overweight females. *Int J Obes Relat Metab Disord* 22(3):236–42.

Jakicic JM, Wing RR, Butler BA, Robertson RJ. 1995. Prescribing exercise in multiple short bouts versus one continuous bout: effects on adherence, cardiorespiratory fitness, and weight loss in overweight women. *Int J Obes Relat Metab Disord* 19(12):893–901.

Jakicic JM, Winters C, Lang W, Wing RR. 1999. Effects of intermittent exercise and use of home exercise equipment on adherence, weight loss, and fitness in overweight women: a randomized trial. *JAMA* 282(16):1554–60.

Janis IL, Mann L. 1977. *Decision Making: A Psychological Analysis of Conflict, Choice, and Commitment*. New York: Free Press.

Janz NK, Becker MH. 1984. The Health Belief Model: a decade later. *Health Educ Q* 11(1):1–47.

Janz NK, Becker MH, Kirscht JP, Eraker SA, Billi JE, Woolliscroft JO. 1987. Evaluation of a minimal-contact smoking cessation intervention in an outpatient setting. *Am J Public Health* 77(7):805–9.

Janz NK, Schottenfeld D, Doerr KM, Selig SM, Dunn RL, Strawderman M, Levine PA. 1997. A two-step intervention to increase mammography among women aged 65 and older. *Am J Public Health* 87(10):1683–6.

Jarvis KL, Friedman RH, Heeren T, Cullinane PM. 1997. Older women and physical activity: using the telephone to walk. *Womens Health Issues* 7(1):24–9.

Jaycox S, Baranowski T, Nader PR, Dworkin R, Vanderpool NA. 1983. Theory-based health education activities for third to sixth grade children. *J Sch Health* 53(10):584–8.

Jeffery RW. 1995. Community programs for obesity prevention: the Minnesota Heart Health Program. *Obes Res* 3(Suppl 2):283s–8s.

Jeffery RW, Forster JL, Snell MK. 1985. Promoting weight control at the worksite: a pilot program of self-motivation using payroll-based incentives. *Prev Med* 14(2):187–94.

Jeffery RW, Hellerstedt WL, Schmid TL. 1990. Correspondence programs for smoking cessation and weight control: a comparison of two strategies in the Minnesota Heart Health Program. *Health Psychol* 9(5):585–98.

Jeffery RW, Forster JL, French SA, Kelder SH, Lando HA, McGovern PG, Jacobs DR Jr, Baxter JE. 1993a. The Healthy Worker Project: a work-site intervention for weight control and smoking cessation. *Am J Public Health* 83(3):395–401.

Jeffery RW, Wing RR, Thorson C, Burton LR, Raether C, Harvey J, Mullen M. 1993b. Strengthening behavioral interventions for weight loss: a randomized trial of food provision and monetary incentives. *J Consult Clin Psychol* 61(6):1038–45.

Jeffery RW, French SA, Raether C, Baxter JE. 1994. An environmental intervention to increase fruit and salad purchases in a cafeteria. *Prev Med* 23(6):788–92.

Jeffery RW, Hellerstedt WL, French SA, Baxter JE. 1995. A randomized trial of counseling for fat restriction versus calorie restriction in the treatment of obesity. *Int J Obes Relat Metab Disord* 19(2):132–7.

Jeffery RW, Wing RR, Thorson C, Burton LC. 1998. Use of personal trainers and financial incentives to increase exercise in a behavioral weight-loss program. *Jl Consul Clin Psych* 66 (5):777–83.

Jencks SF, Cuerdon T, Burwen DR, Fleming B, Houck PM, Kussmaul AE, Nilasena DS, Ordin DL, Arday DR. 2000. Quality of medical care delivered to Medicare beneficiaries: A profile at state and national levels. *JAMA* 284(13):1670–6.

Jessor R, Donnovan JE, Costa FM. 1991. *Beyond Adolescence: Problem Behavior and Young Adult Development*. Cambridge, United Kingdom: Cambridge University Press.

Jhaveri FM, Zippe CD, Klein EA, Kupelian PA. 1999. Biochemical failure does not predict overall survival after radical prostatectomy for localized prostate cancer: 10-year results. *Urology* 54(5):884–90.

Ji BT, Chow WH, Yang G, McLaughlin JK, Gao RN, Zheng W, Shu XO, Jin F, Fraumeni JF Jr, Gao YT. 1997. Body mass index and the risk of cancers of the gastric cardia and distal stomach in Shanghai, China. *Cancer Epidemiol Biomarkers Prev* 6(7):481–5.

Jibaja ML, Kingery P, Neff NE, Smith Q, Bowman J, Holcomb JD. 2000. Tailored, interactive soap operas for breast cancer education of high-risk Hispanic women. *J Cancer Educ* 15(4):237–42.

Johansson JE. 1994. Expectant management of early stage prostatic cancer: Swedish experience. *J Urol* 152(5 Pt 2):1753–6.

Johansson JE, Holmberg L, Johansson S, Bergstrom R, Adami HO. 1997. Fifteen-year survival in prostate cancer. A prospective, population-based study in Sweden. *JAMA* 277(6): 467–71.

Johnson RK, Guthrie H, Smiciklas-Wright H, Wang MQ. 1994. Characterizing nutrient intakes of children by sociodemographic factors. *Public Health Rep* 109(3):414–20.

Johnstone PA, Gray C, Powell CR. 2000. Quality of life in T1-3N0 prostate cancer patients treated with radiation therapy with minimum 10-year follow-up. *Int J Radiat Oncol Biol Phys* 46(4):833–8.

Jones BA, Culler CS, Kasl SV, Calvocoressi L. 2001. Is variation in quality of mammographic services race linked? *J Health Care Poor Underserved* 12(1):113–26.

Jones RB. 2000. Tobacco or oral health: past progress, impending challenge. *J Am Dent Assoc* 131(8):1130–6.

Jonsson H, Tornberg S, Nystrom L, Lenner P. 2000. Service screening with mammography in Sweden—evaluation of effects of screening on breast cancer mortality in age group 40–49 years. *Acta Oncol* 39(5):617–23.

Jordan HS, Straus JH, Bailit MH. 1995. Reporting and using health plan performance information in Massachusetts. *Jt Comm J Qual Improv* 21(4):167–77.

Juon HS, Choi Y, Kim MT. 2000. Cancer screening behaviors among Korean-American women. *Cancer Detect Prev* 24(6):589–601.

Kagawa-Singer M, Pourat N. 2000. Asian American and Pacific Islander breast and cervical carcinoma screening rates and Healthy People 2000 objectives. *Cancer* 89(3): 696–705.

Kahn HA. 1966. The Dorn study of smoking and mortality among U.S. veterans: report on eight and one-half years of observation. *J Natl Cancer Inst Monogr* 19:1–125.

Kahn HS, Tatham LM, Thun MJ, Heath CW Jr. 1998. Risk factors for self-reported colon polyps. *J Gen Intern Med* 13(5):303–10.

Kalish LA, McKinlay JB. 1999. Serum prostate-specific antigen levels (PSA) in men without clinical evidence of prostate cancer: age-specific reference ranges for total PSA, free PSA, and percent free PSA. *Urology* 54(6):1022–7.

Kamimoto LA, Easton AN, Maurice E, Husten CG, Macera CA. 1999. Surveillance for five health risks among older adults—United States, 1993–1997. *Morb Mortal Wkly Rep CDC Surveill Summ* 48(8):89–130.

Kanazawa K, Kawata Y, Niki N, Satoh H, Ohmatsu H, Kakinuma R, Kaneko M, Moriyama N, Eguchi K. 1998. Computer-aided diagnosis for pulmonary nodules based on helical CT images. *Comput Med Imaging Graph* 22(2):157–67.

Kaneko M, Eguchi K, Ohmatsu H, Kakinuma R, Naruke T, Suemasu K, Moriyama N. 1996. Peripheral lung cancer: screening and detection with low-dose spiral CT versus radiography. *Radiology* 201(3):798–802.

Kassirer JP. 1994. Incorporating patients' preferences into medical decisions. *N Engl J Med* 330(26):1895–6.

Kassirer JP. 1997. Practicing medicine without a license—the new intrusions by Congress. *N Engl J Med* 336(24):1747.

Kassirer JP, Pauker SG. 1981. The toss-up. *N Engl J Med* 305(24):1467–9.

Kato I, Tominaga S, Matsumoto K. 1992. A prospective study of stomach cancer among a rural Japanese population: a 6-year survey. *Jpn J Cancer Res* 83(6):568–75.

Kayman S, Bruvold W, Stern JS. 1990. Maintenance and relapse after weight loss in women: behavioral aspects. *Am J Clin Nutr* 52(5):800–7.

Keemers-Gels ME, Groenendijk RP, van den Heuvel JH, Boetes C, Peer PG, Wobbes TH. 2000. Pain experienced by women attending breast cancer screening. *Breast Cancer Res Treat* 60(3):235–40.

Kelaher M, Stellman JM. 2000. The impact of medicare funding on the use of mammography among older women: implications for improving access to screening. *Prev Med* 31(6): 658–64.

Kendall A, Levitsky DA, Strupp BJ, Lissner L. 1991. Weight loss on a low-fat diet: consequence of the imprecision of the control of food intake in humans. *Am J Clin Nutr* 53(5):1124–9.

Kennedy TC, Miller Y, Prindiville S. 2000. Screening for lung cancer revisited and the role of sputum cytology and fluorescence bronchoscopy in a high-risk group. *Chest* 117(4 Suppl 1):72S–9S.

Kerins G, Gruman C, Schwartz R, Rauch EA, Curry L, Fogel D. 2000. Mammography utilization in a skilled nursing facility. *Conn Med* 64(10):595–9.

Kerlikowske K. 1997. Efficacy of screening mammography among women aged 40 to 49 years and 50 to 69 years: comparison of relative and absolute benefit. *J Natl Cancer Inst Monogr* (22):79–86.

Kerlikowske K, Grady D, Barclay J, Sickles EA, Eaton A, Ernster V. 1993. Positive predictive value of screening mammography by age and family history of breast cancer. *JAMA* 270(20):2444–50.

Kerlikowske K, Grady D, Rubin SM, Sandrock C, Ernster VL. 1995. Efficacy of screening mammography. A meta-analysis. *JAMA* 273(2):149–54.

Kerlikowske K, Grady D, Barclay J, Sickles EA, Ernster V. 1996. Effect of age, breast density, and family history on the sensitivity of first screening mammography. *JAMA* 276(1): 33–8.

Kerlikowske K, Grady D, Barclay J, Frankel SD, Ominsky SH, Sickles EA, Ernster V. 1998. Variability and accuracy in mammographic interpretation using the American College of Radiology Breast Imaging Reporting and Data System. *J Natl Cancer Inst* 90(23): 1801–9.

Kerlikowske K, Salzmann P, Phillips KA, Cauley JA, Cummings SR. 1999. Continuing screening mammography in women aged 70 to 79 years: impact on life expectancy and cost-effectiveness. *JAMA* 282(22):2156–63.

Kerlikowske K, Carney PA, Geller B, Mandelson MT, Taplin SH, Malvin K, Ernster V, Urban N, Cutter G, Rosenberg R, Ballard-Barbash R. 2000. Performance of screening mammography among women with and without a first-degree relative with breast cancer. *Ann Intern Med* 133(11):855–63.

Kessler HB, Rimer BK, Devine PJ, Gatenby RA, Engstrom PF. 1991. Corporate-sponsored breast cancer screening at the work site: results of a statewide program. *Radiology* 179(1):107–10.

Khandker RK, Dulski JD, Kilpatrick JB, Ellis RP, Mitchell JB, Baine WB. 2000. A decision model and cost-effectiveness analysis of colorectal cancer screening and surveillance guidelines for average-risk adults. *Int J Technol Assess Health Care* 16(3):799–810.

Khanna N, Phillips MD. 2001. Adherence to care plan in women with abnormal Papanicolaou smears: a review of barriers and interventions. *J Am Board Fam Pract* 14(2):123–30.

Kikano GE, Stange KC, Flocke SA, Zyzanski SJ. 1997. Put Prevention into Practice: outcomes in a family practice center. *Am J Prev Med* 13(5):352–4.

King AC. 1991. Community intervention for promotion of physical activity and fitness. *Exerc Sport Sci Rev* 19:211–59.

King AC, Taylor CB, Haskell WL, Debusk RF. 1988. Strategies for increasing early adherence to and long-term maintenance of home-based exercise training in healthy middle-aged men and women. *Am J Cardiol* 61(8):628–32.

King AC, Haskell WL, Taylor CB, Kraemer HC, DeBusk RF. 1991. Group- vs home-based exercise training in healthy older men and women. A community-based clinical trial. *JAMA* 266(11):1535–42.

King AC, Haskell WL, Young DR, Oka RK, Stefanick ML. 1995a. Long-term effects of varying intensities and formats of physical activity on participation rates, fitness, and lipoproteins in men and women aged 50 to 65 years. *Circulation* 91(10):2596–604.

King AC, Jeffery RW, Fridinger F, Dusenbury L, Provence S, Hedlund SA, Spangler K. 1995b. Environmental and policy approaches to cardiovascular disease prevention through physical activity: issues and opportunities. *Health Educ Q* 22(4):499–511.

King AC, Castro C, Wilcox S, Eyler AA, Sallis JF, Brownson RC. 2000. Personal and environmental factors associated with physical inactivity among different racial-ethnic groups of U.S. middle-aged and older-aged women. *Health Psychol* 19(4):354–64.

King E, Rimer BK, Balshem A, Ross E, Seay J. 1993a. Mammography-related beliefs of older women. A survey of an HMO population. *J Aging Health* 5(1):82–100.

King E, Rimer BK, Benincasa T, Harrop C, Amfoh K, Bonney G, Kornguth P, Demark-Wahnefried W, Strigo T, Engstrom P. 1998. Strategies to encourage mammography use among women in senior citizens' housing facilities. *J Cancer Educ* 13(2):108–15.

King ES, Rimer BK, Seay J, Balshem A, Engstrom PF. 1994. Promoting mammography use through progressive interventions: is it effective? *Am J Public Health* 84(1):104–6.

King G, Barry L, Carter DL. 1993b. Smoking prevalence among perinatal women: the role of socioeconomic status, race, and ethnicity. *Conn Med* 57(11):721–8.

King J, Fairbrother G, Thompson C, Morris DL. 1992. Colorectal cancer screening: optimal compliance with postal faecal occult blood test. *Aust N Z J Surg* 62(9):714–9.

Kinsinger LS, Harris R, Qaqish B, Strecher V, Kaluzny A. 1998. Using an office system intervention to increase breast cancer screening. *J Gen Intern Med* 13(8):507–14.

Kirby SBT, Reynolds K, Taylor G, Binkley D. 1995. Children's fruit and vegetable intake: socioeconomic adult child, regional, and urban-rural influences. *J Nutr Educ* 27:261–71.

Kirby SD, Ureda JR, Rose RL, Hussey J. 1998. Peripheral cues and involvement level: influences on acceptance of a mammography message. *J Health Commun* 3(2):119–35.

Kjaerheim K, Gaard M, Andersen A. 1998. The role of alcohol, tobacco, and dietary factors in upper aerogastric tract cancers: a prospective study of 10,900 Norwegian men. *Cancer Causes Control* 99–108.

Klatsky AL, Friedman GD, Siegelaub AB. 1981. Alcohol and mortality. A ten-year Kaiser-Permanente experience. *Ann Intern Med* 95(2):139–45.

Klem ML, Wing RR, McGuire MT, Seagle HM, Hill JO. 1997. A descriptive study of individuals successful at long-term maintenance of substantial weight loss. *Am J Clin Nutr* 66(2):239–46.

Knekt P, Hakama M, Jarvinen R, Pukkala E, Heliovaara M. 1998. Smoking and risk of colorectal cancer. *Br J Cancer* 78(1):136–9.

Knekt P, Jarvinen R, Teppo L, Aromaa A, Seppanen R. 1999. Role of various carotenoids in lung cancer prevention. *J Natl Cancer Inst* 91(2):182–4.

Kneller RW, McLaughlin JK, Bjelke E, Schuman LM, Blot WJ, Wacholder S, Gridley G, CoChien HT, Fraumeni JF Jr. 1991. A cohort study of stomach cancer in a high-risk American population. *Cancer* 68(3):672–8.

Knowler WC, Barrett-Connor E, Fowler SE, Hamman RF, Lachin JM, Walker EA, Nathan DM. 2002. Reduction in the incidence of type 2 diabetes with lifestyle intervention or metformin. *N Engl J Med* 346(6):393–403.

Knutsen SF, Knutsen R. 1991. The Tromso Survey: the Family Intervention study—the effect of intervention on some coronary risk factors and dietary habits, a 6-year follow-up. *Prev Med* 20(2):197–212.

Koenig BA, Greely HT, McConnell LM, Silverberg HL, Raffin TA. 1998. Genetic testing for BRCA1 and BRCA2: recommendations of the Stanford Program in Genomics, Ethics, and Society. Breast Cancer Working Group. *J Women's Health* 7(5):531–45.

Kohatsu ND, Cramer E, Bohnstedt M. 1994. Use of a clinician reminder system for screening mammography in a public health clinic. *Am J Prev Med* 10(6):348–52.

Kolata G. 2001a, December 9. Study Sets Off Debate over Mammograms' Value. *The New York Times*. P. A1.

Kolata G. 2001b, December 30. Questions Grow over Usefulness of Some Routine Cancer Tests. *The New York Times*. P. A1.

Kolata G. 2002a, January 24. Expert Panel Cites Doubts on Mammogram's Worth. *The New York Times*. P. A16.

Kolata G. 2002b, April 9. Breast Cancer: Mammography Finds More Tumors. Then the Debate Begins. *The New York Times*. P. F5.

Kolata G, Moss M. 2002, November. X-Ray Vision in Hindsight: Science Politics and the Mammogram. *The New York Times*. P. A18.

Kolonel LN. 1996. Nutrition and prostate cancer. *Cancer Causes Control* 7(1):83–44.

Komatsu K, Wehner N, Prestigiacomo AF, Chen Z, Stamey TA. 1996. Physiologic (intra-individual) variation of serum prostate-specific antigen in 814 men from a screening population. *Urology* 47(3):343–6.

Kono S, Honjo S, Todoroki I, Nishiwaki M, Hamada H, Nishikawa H, Koga H, Ogawa S, Nakagawa K. 1998. Glucose intolerance and adenomas of the sigmoid colon in Japanese men (Japan). *Cancer Causes Control* 9(4):441–6.

Kopans DB, Halpern E, Hulka CA. 1994. Statistical power in breast cancer screening trials and mortality reduction among women 40–49 years of age with particular emphasis on the National Breast Screening Study of Canada. *Cancer* 74(4):1196–203.

Korhonen HJ, Niemensivu H, Piha T, Koskela K, Wiio J, Johnson CA, Puska P. 1992. National TV smoking cessation program and contest in Finland. *Prev Med* 21(1):74–87.

Korte JE, Hertz-Picciotto I, Schulz MR, Ball LM, Duell EJ. 2000. The contribution of benzene to smoking-induced leukemia. *Environ Health Perspect* 108(4):333–9.

Kottke TE, Battista RN, DeFriese GH, Brekke ML. 1988. Attributes of successful smoking cessation interventions in medical practice. A meta-analysis of 39 controlled trials. *JAMA* 259(19):2883–9.

Kottke TE, Brekke ML, Solberg LI, Hughes JR. 1989. A randomized trial to increase smoking intervention by physicians. Doctors Helping Smokers, Round I. *JAMA* 261(14):2101–6.

Kottke TE, Brekke ML, Solberg LI. 1993. Making "time" for preventive services. *Mayo Clin Proc* 68(8):785–91.

Kottke TE, Solberg LI, Brekke ML, Cabrera A, Marquez MA. 1997. Delivery rates for preventive services in 44 Midwestern clinics. *Mayo Clin Proc* 72(6):515–23.

Krahn MD, Mahoney JE, Eckman MH, Trachtenberg J, Pauker SG, Detsky AS. 1994. Screening for prostate cancer. A decision analytic view. *JAMA* 272(10):773–80.

Krahn MD, Coombs A, Levy IG. 1999. Current and projected annual direct costs of screening asymptomatic men for prostate cancer using prostate-specific antigen. *Can Med Assoc J* 160(1):49–57.

Kramer BS, Brown ML, Prorok PC, Potosky AL, Gohagan JK. 1993. Prostate cancer screening: what we know and what we need to know. *Ann Intern Med* 119(9):914–23.

Krauss RM, Eckel RH, Howard B, Appel LJ, Daniels SR, Deckelbaum RJ, Erdman JW Jr, Kris-Etherton P, Goldberg IJ, Kotchen TA, Lichtenstein AH, Mitch WE, Mullis R, Robinson K, Wylie-Rosett J, St Jeor S, Suttie J, Tribble DL, Bazzarre TL. 2000. AHA Dietary Guidelines: revision 2000: a statement for healthcare professionals from the Nutrition Committee of the American Heart Association. *Circulation* 102(18):2284–99.

Krebs-Smith SM, Cook A, Subar AF, Cleveland L, Friday J. 1995a. U.S. adults' fruit and vegetable intakes, 1989 to 1991: a revised baseline for the Healthy People 2000 objective. *Am J Public Health* 85(12):1623–9.

Krebs-Smith SM, Heimendinger J, Patterson BH, Subar AF, Kessler R, Pivonka E. 1995b. Psychosocial factors associated with fruit and vegetable consumption. *Am J Health Promot* 10(2):98–104.

Kreuter MW, Scharff DP, Brennan LK, Lukwago SN. 1997. Physician recommendations for diet and physical activity: which patients get advised to change? *Prev Med* 26(6):825–33.

Kristal AR, Curry SJ, Shattuck AL, Feng Z, Li S. 2000a. A randomized trial of a tailored, self-help dietary intervention: the Puget Sound Eating Patterns study. *Prev Med* 31(4):380–9.

Kristal AR, Glanz K, Tilley BC, Li S. 2000b. Mediating factors in dietary change: understanding the impact of a worksite nutrition intervention. *Health Educ Behav* 27(1):112–25.

Kronborg O, Fenger C, Olsen J, Jorgensen OD, Sondergaard O. 1996. Randomised study of screening for colorectal cancer with faecal-occult-blood test. *Lancet* 348(9040):1467–71.

Krongrad A, Lai H, Lai S. 1997. Survival after radical prostatectomy. *JAMA* 278(1):44–6.

Kubik A, Haerting J. 1990. Survival and mortality in a randomized study of lung cancer detection. *Neoplasma* 37(4):467–75.

Kuhl CK, Schmutzler RK, Leutner CC, Kempe A, Wardelmann E, Hocke A, Maringa M, Pfeifer U, Krebs D, Schild HH. 2000. Breast MR imaging screening in 192 women proved or suspected to be carriers of a breast cancer susceptibility gene: preliminary results. *Radiology* 215(1):267–79.

Kuller LH, St. Jeor ST, Dwyer J, et al. 1993. *Report of the American Institute of Nutrition (AIN) Steering Committee on Healthy Weight*. Bethesda, MD: American Institute of Nutrition.

Kumanyika S. 2001. Minority populations. In Burke LE, Ockene IS (eds). *Compliance in Healthcare and Research*. Armonk, NY: Futra Publishing Company. Pp. 195–217.

Kumanyika SK, Charleston JB. 1992. Lose weight and win: a church-based weight loss program for blood pressure control among black women. *Patient Educ Couns* 19(1):19–32.

Kumanyika SK, Obarzanek E, Stevens VJ, Hebert PR, Whelton PK. 1991. Weight-loss experience of black and white participants in NHLBI-sponsored clinical trials. *Am J Clin Nutr* 53(6 Suppl):1631S–8S.

Kune GA, Kune S, Watson LF. 1990. Body weight and physical activity as predictors of colorectal cancer risk. *Nutr Cancer* 13(1–2):9–17.

Kushi LH, Mink PJ, Folsom AR, Anderson KE, Zheng W, Lazovich D, Sellers TA. 1999. Prospective study of diet and ovarian cancer. *Am J Epidemiol* 149(1):21–31.

Kushner RF. 1995. Barriers to providing nutrition counseling by physicians: a survey of primary care practitioners. *Prev Med* 24(6):546–52.

Kvåle G, Bjelke E, Gart JJ. 1983. Dietary habits and lung cancer risk. *Int J Cancer* 31(4):397–405.

Labrie F, Candas B, Cusan L, Gomez JL, Diamond P, Suburu R, Lemay M. 1996. Diagnosis of advanced or noncurable prostate cancer can be practically eliminated by prostate-specific antigen. *Urology* 47(2):212–7.

Labrie F, Candas B, Dupont A, Cusan L, Gomez JL, Suburu RE, Diamond P, Levesque J, Belanger A. 1999. Screening decreases prostate cancer death: first analysis of the 1988 Quebec prospective randomized controlled trial. *Prostate* 38(2):83–91.

Lacey L, Whitfield J, DeWhite W, Ansell D, Whitman S, Chen E, Phillips C. 1993. Referral adherence in an inner city breast and cervical cancer screening program. *Cancer* 72(3): 950–5.

Lallemand RC, Vakil PA, Pearson P, Box V. 1984. Screening for asymptomatic bowel cancer in general practice. *Br Med J (Clin Res Ed)* 288(6410):31–3.

Lam KC, Yu MC, Leung JW, Henderson BE. 1982. Hepatitis B virus and cigarette smoking: risk factors for hepatocellular carcinoma in Hong Kong. *Cancer Res* 42(12):5246–8.

Lam S, Kennedy T, Unger M, Miller YE, Gelmont D, Rusch V, Gipe B, Howard D, LeRiche JC, Coldman A, Gazdar AF. 1998. Localization of bronchial intraepithelial neoplastic lesions by fluorescence bronchoscopy. *Chest* 113(3):696–702.

Lancet. 1999. 16-year mortality from breast cancer in the U.K. Trial of Early Detection of Breast Cancer. *Lancet* 353(9168):1909–14.

Lane DS, Polednak AP, Burg MA. 1991. Effect of continuing medical education and cost reduction on physician compliance with mammography screening guidelines. *J Fam Pract* 33(4):359–68.

Lane DS, Zapka J, Breen N, Messina CR, Fotheringham DJ. 2000. A systems model of clinical preventive care: the case of breast cancer screening among older women. For the NCI Breast Cancer Screening Consortium. *Prev Med* 31(5):481–93.

Lang F. 2000. The evolving roles of patient and physician. *Arch Fam Med* 9(1):65–7.

Lange P, Nyboe J, Appleyard M, Jensen G, Schnohr P. 1992. Relationship of the type of tobacco and inhalation pattern to pulmonary and total mortality. *Eur Respir J* 5(9): 1111–7.

Lantz PM, Stencil D, Lippert MT, Beversdorf S, Jaros L, Remington PL. 1995. Breast and cervical cancer screening in a low-income managed care sample: the efficacy of physician letters and phone calls. *Am J Public Health* 85(6):834–6.

Lantz PM, Stencil D, Lippert MT, Jaros L, Eaker ED. 1996. Implementation issues and costs associated with a proven strategy for increasing breast and cervical cancer screening among low-income women. *J Public Health Manag Pract* 2(3):54–9.

Lantz PM, Jacobson PD, Warner KE, Wasserman J, Pollack HA, Berson J, Ahlstrom A. 2000. Investing in youth tobacco control: a review of smoking prevention and control strategies. *Tob Control* 9(1):47–63.

Larsson LG, Andersson I, Bjurstam N, Fagerberg G, Frisell J, Tabar L, Nystrom L. 1997. Updated overview of the Swedish Randomized Trials on Breast Cancer Screening with Mammography: age group 40–49 at randomization. *J Natl Cancer Inst Monogr* (22):57–61.

Lasater TM, Wells BL, Carleton RA, Elder JP. 1986. The role of churches in disease prevention research studies. *Public Health Rep* 101(2):125–31.

Last J (ed.). 1988. *A Dictionary of Epidemiology*, 2nd ed. New York: Oxford University Press.

Latner JD, Stunkard AJ, Wilson GT, Jackson ML, Zelitch DS, Labouvie E. 2000. Effective long-term treatment of obesity: a continuing care model. *Int J Obes Relat Metab Disord* 24(7):893–8.

Law J. 1993. Variations in individual radiation dose in a breast screening programme and consequences for the balance between associated risk and benefit. *Br J Radiol* 66(788): 691–8.

Law M, Hackshaw A, Wald N. 2000. Screening mammography re-evaluated. *Lancet* 355(9205): 749–50.

Lawrence VA, Streiner D, Hazuda HP, Naylor R, Levine M, Gafni A. 2000. A cross-cultural consumer-based decision aid for screening mammography. *Prev Med* 30(3):200–8.

Lean ME. 1997. Sibutramine—a review of clinical efficacy. *Int J Obes Relat Metab Disord* 21(Suppl 1):S30–6.

Leard LE, Savides TJ, Ganiats TG. 1997. Patient preferences for colorectal cancer screening. *J Fam Pract* 45(3):211–8.

Lee CY. 1991. A randomized controlled trial to motivate worksite fecal occult blood testing. *Yonsei Med J* 32(2):131–8.

Lee FI. 1983. Screening for colorectal cancer in a factory-based population with Fecatest. *Br J Cancer* 48(6):843–7.

Lee HP, Gourley L, Duffy SW, Esteve J, Lee J, Day NE. 1989. Colorectal cancer and diet in an Asian population—a case-control study among Singapore Chinese. *Int J Cancer* 43(6):1007–16.

Lee IM, Paffenbarger RS Jr. 1992. Change in body weight and longevity. *JAMA* 268(15): 2045–9.

Lee IM, Paffenbarger RS Jr, Hsieh C. 1991. Physical activity and risk of developing colorectal cancer among college alumni. *J Natl Cancer Inst* 83(18):1324–9.

Lee IM, Paffenbarger RS Jr, Hsieh CC. 1992. Physical activity and risk of prostatic cancer among college alumni. *Am J Epidemiol* 135(2):169–79.

Lee JH, Zuckerman D. 2001. Screening for breast cancer with mammography. *Lancet* 358(9299): 2164–5; discussion 2167–8.

Lee TH, Brennan TA. 2002. Direct-to-Consumer Marketing of High-Technology Screening Tests. *New England Journal of Medicine* 346(7):529–31.

Leermarkers EA, Jakicic JM, Viteri J, Wing RR. 1998. Clinic-based vs. home-based interventions for preventing weight gain in men. *Obes Res* 6(5):346–52.

Lehmann LS, Weeks JC, Klar N, Biener L, Garber JE. 2000. Disclosure of familial genetic information: perceptions of the duty to inform. *Am J Med* 109(9):705–11.

Leibel SA, Zelefsky MJ, Kutcher GJ, Burman CM, Kelson S, Fuks Z. 1994. Three-dimensional conformal radiation therapy in localized carcinoma of the prostate: interim report of a phase 1 dose-escalation study. *J Urol* 152(5 Pt 2):1792–8.

Leigh JP. 1996. Occupations, cigarette smoking, and lung cancer in the epidemiological follow-up to the NHANES I and the California Occupational Mortality Study. *Bull NY Acad Med* 73(2):370–97.

Leivo T, Sintonen H, Tuominen R, Hakama M, Pukkala E, Heinonen OP. 1999. The cost-effectiveness of nationwide breast carcinoma screening in Finland, 1987–1992. *Cancer* 86(4):638–46.

Le Marchand L, Kolonel LN, Wilkens LR, Myers BC, Hirohata T. 1994. Animal fat consumption and prostate cancer: a prospective study in Hawaii. *Epidemiology* 5(3):276–82.

Lerman C, Rimer BK. 1995. Psychosocial impact of cancer screening. In Croyle RT. (ed.). *Psychosocial Effects of Screening for Disease Prevention and Detection.* New York: Oxford University Press. Pp. 65–81.

Lerman C, Miller SM, Scarborough R, Hanjani P, Nolte S, Smith D. 1991a. Adverse psychologic consequences of positive cytologic cervical screening. *Am J Obstet Gynecol* 165(3): 658–62.

Lerman C, Trock B, Rimer BK, Boyce A, Jepson C, Engstrom PF. 1991b. Psychological and behavioral implications of abnormal mammograms. *Ann Intern Med* 114(8):657–61.

Lerman C, Hanjani P, Caputo C, Miller S, Delmoor E, Nolte S, Engstrom P. 1992. Telephone counseling improves adherence to colposcopy among lower-income minority women. *J Clin Oncol* 10(2):330–3.

Lerman C, Narod S, Schulman K, Hughes C, Gomez-Caminero A, Bonney G, Gold K, Trock B, Main D, Lynch J, Fulmore C, Snyder C, Lemon SJ, Conway T, Tonin P, Lenoir G, Lynch H. 1996. BRCA1 testing in families with hereditary breast-ovarian cancer. A prospective study of patient decision making and outcomes. *JAMA* 275(24):1885–92.

Lerman C, Hughes C, Lemon SJ, Main D, Snyder C, Durham C, Narod S, Lynch HT. 1998. What you don't know can hurt you: adverse psychologic effects in members of BRCA1-linked and BRCA2-linked families who decline genetic testing. *J Clin Oncol* 16(5):1650–4.

Lerman C, Hughes C, Croyle RT, Main D, Durham C, Snyder C, Bonney A, Lynch JF, Narod SA, Lynch HT. 2000. Prophylactic surgery decisions and surveillance practices one year following BRCA1/2 testing. *Prev Med* 31(1):75–80.

Lerner BH. 2002, March 5. Screening for Cancer: A Downside. *The New York Times*. p. D6.

Lerner SE, Blute ML, Zincke H. 1995. Extended experience with radical prostatectomy for clinical stage T3 prostate cancer: outcome and contemporary morbidity. *J Urol* 154(4): 1447–52.

Leslie NS. 1995. Role of the nurse practitioner in breast and cervical cancer prevention. *Cancer Nurs* 18(4):251–7.

Levin A. 1999. Nutrition and policy. 5: Who should teach patients about nutrition? *Ann Intern Med* 131(4):317–8.

Levy S, Dowling P, Boult L, Monroe A, McQuade W. 1992. The effect of physician and patient gender on preventive medicine practices in patients older than fifty. *Fam Med* 24(1):58–61.

Lewin JM, Hendrick RE, D'Orsi CJ, Isaacs PK, Moss LJ, Karellas A, Sisney GA, Kuni CC, Cutter GR. 2001. Comparison of full-field digital mammography with screen-film mammography for cancer detection: results of 4,945 paired examinations. *Radiology* 218(3): 873–80.

Lewis BS, Lynch WD. 1993. The effect of physician advice on exercise behavior. *Prev Med* 22(1):110–21.

Lewis JD, Asch DA. 1999. Barriers to office-based screening sigmoidoscopy: does reimbursement cover costs? *Ann Intern Med* 130(6):525–30.

Lewis PC, Harrell JS, Bradley C, Deng S. 2001. Cigarette use in adolescents: the Cardiovascular Health in Children and Youth Study. *Res Nurs Health* 24(1):27–37.

Li R, Serdula M, Bland S, Mokdad A, Bowman B, Nelson D. 2000. Trends in fruit and vegetable consumption among adults in 16 U.S. states: Behavioral Risk Factor Surveillance System, 1990–1996. *Am J Public Health* 90(5):777–81.

Lichtenstein E, Glasgow RE. 1992. Smoking cessation: what have we learned over the past decade? *J Consult Clin Psychol* 60(4):518–27.

Lichtenstein E, Green SB, Lynn WR, Corle DK, Ockene JK, Giffen CA, Cummings M, Freedman LS, Gail MH, The COMMIT Research Group. 1995. Community Intervention Trial for Smoking Cessation (COMMIT): I. cohort results from a four-year community intervention. *Am J Public Health* 85(2):183–92.

Lichtenstein E, Glasgow RE, Lando HA, Ossip-Klein DJ, Boles SM. 1996. Telephone counseling for smoking cessation: rationales and meta-analytic review of evidence. *Health Educ Res* 11(2):243–57.

Lieberman DA, Weiss DG, Bond JH, Ahnen DJ, Garewal H, Chejfec G. 2000. Use of colonoscopy to screen asymptomatic adults for colorectal cancer. Veterans Affairs Cooperative Study Group 380. *N Engl J Med* 343(3):162–8.

Lilienfeld A. 1966. An evaluation of radiologic and cytologic screening for the early detection of lung cancer: a cooperative pilot study of the American Cancer Society and the Veterans Administration. *Cancer Res* 26(10):2083–121.

Lillie-Blanton M, Parsons PE, Gayle H, Dievler A. 1996. Racial differences in health: not just black and white, but shades of gray. *Annu Rev Public Health* 17:411–48.

Lillquist PP. 2001. Breast cancer policy as a paradigm for other health prevention issues: analysis of the Breast and Cervical Cancer Mortality Prevention Act of 1990. *J Health Soc Policy* 12(3):17–32.

Lindblad P, Wolk A, Bergstrom R, Adami HO. 1997. Diet and risk of renal cell cancer: a population-based case-control study. *Cancer Epidemiol Biomarkers Prev* 6(4):215–23.

Lindert KA, Kabalin JN, Terris MK. 2000. Bacteremia and bacteriuria after transrectal ultrasound guided prostate biopsy. *J Urol* 164(1):76–80.

Lindholm LH, Ekbom T, Dash C, Eriksson M, Tibblin G, Schersten B. 1995. The impact of health care advice given in primary care on cardiovascular risk. CELL Study Group. *BMJ* 310(6987):1105–9.

Lindsay EA, Ockene JK, Hymowitz N, Giffen C, Berger L, Pomrehn P. 1994. Physicians and smoking cessation. A survey of office procedures and practices in the Community Intervention Trial for Smoking Cessation. *Arch Fam Med* 3(4):341–8.

Linenger JM, Chesson CV II, Nice DS. 1991. Physical fitness gains following simple environmental change. *Am J Prev Med* 7(5):298–310.

Linver MN, Paster SB. 1997. Mammography outcomes in a practice setting by age: prognostic factors, sensitivity, and positive biopsy rate. *J Natl Cancer Inst Monogr* (22):113–7.

Lipkus IM, Rimer BK, Lyna PR, Pradhan AA, Conaway M, Woods-Powell CT. 1996. Colorectal screening patterns and perceptions of risk among African-American users of a community health center. *J Community Health* 21(6):409–27.

Lipkus IM, Lyna PR, Rimer BK. 1999. Using tailored interventions to enhance smoking cessation among African-Americans at a community health center. *Nicotine Tob Res* 1(1):77–85.

Lipkus IM, Halabi S, Strigo TS, Rimer BK. 2000a. The impact of abnormal mammograms on psychosocial outcomes and subsequent screening. *Psychooncology* 9(5):402–10.

Lipkus IM, Rimer BK, Halabi S, Strigo TS. 2000b. Can tailored interventions increase mammography use among HMO women? *Am J Prev Med* 18(1):1–10.

Littrup PJ. 1997. Future benefits and cost-effectiveness of prostate carcinoma screening. American Cancer Society. *Cancer* 80(9):1864–70.

Litwin MS, Hays RD, Fink A, Ganz PA, Leake B, Leach GE, Brook RH. 1995. Quality-of-life outcomes in men treated for localized prostate cancer. *JAMA* 273(2):129–35.

Litzelman DK, Dittus RS, Miller ME, Tierney WM. 1993. Requiring physicians to respond to computerized reminders improves their compliance with preventive care protocols. *J Gen Intern Med* 8(6):311–7.

Liu S, Willett WC, Stampfer MJ, Hu FB, Franz M, Sampson L, Hennekens CH, Manson JE. 2000. A prospective study of dietary glycemic load, carbohydrate intake, and risk of coronary heart disease in U.S. women. *Am J Clin Nutr* 71(6):1455–61.

Lo C. 2000. Integrating nutrition as a theme throughout the medical school curriculum. *Am J Clin Nutr* 72(3 Suppl):882S–9S.

Lockwood JH, Danoff D, Whitcomb ME. 2000. The AAMC's 2000 graduation questionnaire. Association of American Medical Colleges. *JAMA* 284(9):1080.

Logan-Young W. 2000. The breast imaging center. Successful management in today's environment. *Radiol Clin N Am* 38(4):853–60.
Logsdon DN, Lazaro CM, Meier RV. 1989. The feasibility of behavioral risk reduction in primary medical care. *Am J Prev Med* 5(5):249–56.
Lombard DN, Lombard TN, Winett RA. 1995. Walking to meet health guidelines: the effect of prompting frequency and prompt structure. *Health Psychol* 14(2):164–70.
Long BJ, Calfas KJ, Wooten W, Sallis JF, Patrick K, Goldstein M, Marcus BH, Schwenk TL, Chenoweth J, Carter R, Torres T, Palinkas LA, Heath G. 1996. A multisite field test of the acceptability of physical activity counseling in primary care: project PACE. *Am J Prev Med* 12(2):73–81.
Longnecker MP, Berlin JA, Orza MJ, Chalmers TC. 1988. A meta-analysis of alcohol consumption in relation to risk of breast cancer. *JAMA* 260(5):652–6.
Love RR. 1993. Cancer CME: too often off target. *J Cancer Educ* 8(4):269–72.
Love RR, Fryback DG, Kimbrough SR. 1985. A cost-effectiveness analysis of screening for carcinoma of the prostate by digital examination. *Med Decis Making* 5(3):263–78.
Lowe JB, Balanda KP, Del Mar C, Hawes E. 1999. Psychologic distress in women with abnormal findings in mass mammography screening. *Cancer* 85(5):1114–8.
Lowe MR, Miller-Kovach K, Phelan S. 2001. Weight-loss maintenance in overweight individuals one to five years following successful completion of a commercial weight loss program. *Int J Obes Relat Metab Disord* 25(3):325–31.
Lowry R, Kann L, Collins JL, Kolbe LJ. 1996. The effect of socioeconomic status on chronic disease risk behaviors among U.S. adolescents. *JAMA* 276(10):792–7.
Ludman EJ, Curry SJ, Meyer D, Taplin SH. 1999. Implementation of outreach telephone counseling to promote mammography participation. *Health Educ Behav* 26(5):689–702.
Luepker RV, Murray DM, Jacobs DR Jr, Mittelmark MB, Bracht N, Carlaw R, Crow R, Elmer P, Finnegan J, Folsom AR, et al. 1994. Community education for cardiovascular disease prevention: risk factor changes in the Minnesota Heart Health Program. *Am J Public Health* 84(9):1383–93.
Luepker RV, Perry CL, McKinlay SM, Nader PR, Parcel GS, Stone EJ, Webber LS, Elder JP, Feldman HA, Johnson CC, Kelder S, Wu M. 1996. Outcomes of a field trial to improve children's dietary patterns and physical activity. The Child and Adolescent Trial for Cardiovascular Health. CATCH collaborative group. *JAMA* 275(10):768–76.
Luke DA, Stamatakis KA, Brownson RC. 2000. State youth-access tobacco control policies and youth smoking behavior in the United States. *Am J Prev Med* 19(3):180–7.
Lutz SF, Ammerman AS, Atwood JR, Campbell MK, DeVellis RF, Rosamond WD. 1999. Innovative newsletter interventions improve fruit and vegetable consumption in healthy adults. *J Am Diet Assoc* 99(6):705–9.
Lu-Yao GL, Greenberg ER. 1994. Changes in prostate cancer incidence and treatment in U.S.A. *Lancet* 343(8892):251–4.
Lu-Yao GL, McLerran D, Wasson J, Wennberg JE. 1993. An assessment of radical prostatectomy. Time trends, geographic variation, and outcomes. The Prostate Patient Outcomes Research Team. *JAMA* 269(20):2633–6.
Ma J, Pollak MN, Giovannucci E, Chan JM, Tao Y, Hennekens CH, Stampfer MJ. 1999. Prospective study of colorectal cancer risk in men and plasma levels of insulin-like growth factor (IGF)-I and IGF-binding protein-3. *J Natl Cancer Inst* 91(7): 620–5.
MacDowell NM, Nitz-Weiss M, Short A. 2000. The role of physician communication in improving compliance with mammography screening among women ages 50–79 in a commercial HMO. *Manag Care Q* 8(4):11–9.
Madlon-Kay DJ, Harper PG, Reif CJ. 1994. Health promotion counseling in residency training. *J Gen Intern Med* 9(8):465–7.

Mahmoodian S. 1997. Cervical and breast cancer screening rates in Sioux Indian women. *South Med J* 90(3):316–20.

Makuc D, Freid V, Parsons P. 1994. *Health Insurance and Cancer Screening Among Women*. Hyattsville, MD: National Center for Health Statistics.

Malin JL, Kahn K, Dulai G, Farmer MM, Rideout J, Simon LP, Ganz PA. 2000. Organizational systems used by California capitated medical groups and independent practice associations to increase cancer screening. *Cancer* 88(12):2824–31.

Mandel JS, Bond JH, Church TR, Snover DC, Bradley GM, Schuman LM, Ederer F. 1993. Reducing mortality from colorectal cancer by screening for fecal occult blood. Minnesota Colon Cancer Control Study. *N Engl J Med* 328(19):1365–71.

Mandel JS, Church TR, Ederer F, Bond JH. 1999. Colorectal cancer mortality: effectiveness of biennial screening for fecal occult blood. *J Natl Cancer Inst* 91(5):434–7.

Mandel JS, Church TR, Bond JH, Ederer F, Geisser MS, Mongin SJ, Snover DC, Schuman LM. 2000. The effect of fecal occult-blood screening on the incidence of colorectal cancer. *N Engl J Med* 343(22):1603–7.

Mandelblatt J, Yabroff KR, Lawrence W, Yi B, Orosz G, Bloom HG, Schecther CB, Extermann M, Balducci L, Satadano W, Fox S, Silliman RA, Fahs MC, Muening P. 2000. Screening mammography in elderly women. Research on Breast Cancer in Older Women Consortium. *JAMA* 283(24):3202–3.

Mandelblatt JS, Yabroff KR. 1999. Effectiveness of interventions designed to increase mammography use: a meta-analysis of provider-targeted strategies. *Cancer Epidemiol Biomarkers Prev* 8(9):759–67.

Mandelblatt JS, Yabroff KR. 2000. Breast and cervical cancer screening for older women: recommendations and challenges for the 21st century. *J Am Med Women's Assoc* 55(4): 210–5.

Mandelblatt JS, Wheat ME, Monane M, Moshief RD, Hollenberg JP, Tang J. 1992. Breast cancer screening for elderly women with and without comorbid conditions. A decision analysis model. *Ann Intern Med* 116(9):722–30.

Mandelblatt JS, Yabroff KR, Kerner JF. 1999. Equitable access to cancer services: a review of barriers to quality care. *Cancer* 86(11):2378–90.

Mandelson MT, Curry SJ, Anderson LA, Nadel MR, Lee NC, Rutter CM, LaCroix AZ. 2000. Colorectal cancer screening participation by older women. *Am J Prev Med* 19(3): 149–54.

Manfredi C, Czaja R, Freels S, Trubitt M, Warnecke R, Lacey L. 1998. Prescribe for health. Improving cancer screening in physician practices serving low-income and minority populations. *Arch Fam Med* 7(4):329–37.

Manley M, Epps RP, Husten C, Glynn T, Shopland D. 1991. Clinical interventions in tobacco control. A National Cancer Institute training program for physicians. *JAMA* 266(22): 3172–3.

Manley MW, Epps RP, Glynn TJ. 1992. The clinician's role in promoting smoking cessation among clinic patients. *Med Clin N Am* 76(2):477–94.

Manson JE, Hu FB, Rich-Edwards JW, Colditz GA, Stampfer MJ, Willett WC, Speizer FE, Hennekens CH. 1999. A prospective study of walking as compared with vigorous exercise in the prevention of coronary heart disease in women. *N Engl J Med* 341(9): 650–8.

Mant D, Fitzpatrick R, Hogg A, Fuller A, Farmer A, Verne J, Northover J. 1990. Experiences of patients with false positive results from colorectal cancer screening. *Br J Gen Pract* 40(339):423–5.

Marcus AC, Crane LA. 1998. A review of cervical cancer screening intervention research: implications for public health programs and future research. *Prev Med* 27(1):13–31.

Marcus AC, Garrett KM, Cella D, Wenzel LB, Brady MJ, Crane LA, McClatchey MW, Kluhsman BC, Pate-Willig M. 1998a. Telephone counseling of breast cancer patients after treatment: a description of a randomized clinical trial. *Psychooncology* 7(6):470–82.

Marcus AC, Heimendinger J, Wolfe P, Rimer BK, Morra M, Cox D, Lang PJ, Stengle W, Van Herle MP, Wagner D, Fairclough D, Hamilton L. 1998b. Increasing fruit and vegetable consumption among callers to the CIS: results from a randomized trial. *Prev Med* 27(5 Pt 2):S16–28.

Marcus AC, Morra M, Rimer BK, Stricker M, Heimendinger J, Wolfe P, Darrow SL, Hamilton L, Cox DS, Miller N, Perocchia RS. 1998c. A feasibility test of a brief educational intervention to increase fruit and vegetable consumption among callers to the Cancer Information Service. *Prev Med* 27(2):250–61.

Marcus BH, Goldstein MG, Jette A, Simkin-Silverman L, Pinto BM, Milan F, Washburn R, Smith K, Rakowski W, Dube CE. 1997. Training physicians to conduct physical activity counseling. *Prev Med* 26(3):382–8.

Marcus BH, Owen N, Forsyth LH, Cavill NA, Fridinger F. 1998d. Physical activity interventions using mass media, print media, and information technology. *Am J Prev Med* 15(4):362–78.

Margetts BM, Thompson RL, Speller V, McVey D. 1998. Factors which influence 'healthy' eating patterns: results from the 1993 Health Education Authority health and lifestyle survey in England. *Public Health Nutr* 1(3):193–8.

Margolis KL, Lurie N, McGovern PG, Tyrrell M, Slater JS. 1998. Increasing breast and cervical cancer screening in low-income women. *J Gen Intern Med* 13(8):515–21.

Mark DH. 1994. Mortality of patients after radical prostatectomy: analysis of recent Medicare claims. *J Urol* 152(3):896–8.

Marrett LD, Theis B, Ashbury FD. 2000. Workshop report: physical activity and cancer prevention. *Chronic Dis Can* 21(4):143–9.

Martin LM, Bouquot JE, Wingo PA, Heath CW Jr. 1996. Cancer prevention in the dental practice: oral cancer screening and tobacco cessation advice. *J Public Health Dent* 56(6):336–40.

Martinez ME, Giovannucci E, Spiegelman D, Hunter DJ, Willett WC, Colditz GA. 1997. Leisure-time physical activity, body size, and colon cancer in women. Nurses' Health Study Research Group. *J Natl Cancer Inst* 89(13):948–55.

Martinez ME, Heddens D, Earnest DL, Bogert CL, Roe D, Einspahr J, Marshall JR, Alberts DS. 1999. Physical activity, body mass index, and prostaglandin E2 levels in rectal mucosa. *J Natl Cancer Inst* 91(11):950–3.

Mattsson A, Leitz W, Rutqvist LE. 2000. Radiation risk and mammographic screening of women from 40 to 49 years of age: effect on breast cancer rates and years of life. *Br J Cancer* 82(1):220–6.

Maule WF. 1994. Screening for colorectal cancer by nurse endoscopists. *N Engl J Med* 330(3):183–7.

Mausner JS, Kramer S. 1985. *Epidemiology—An Introductory Text.* Philadelphia: W.B. Saunders Company.

May DS, Kiefe CI, Funkhouser E, Fouad MN. 1999. Compliance with mammography guidelines: physician recommendation and patient adherence. *Prev Med* 28(4):386–94.

Mayer JA, Lewis EC, Slymen DJ, Dullum J, Kurata H, Holbrook A, Elder JP, Williams SJ. 2000. Patient reminder letters to promote annual mammograms: a randomized controlled trial. *Prev Med* 31(4):315–22.

Mayo RM, Ureda JR, Parker VG. 2001. Importance of fatalism in understanding mammography screening in rural elderly women. *J Women Aging* 13(1):57–72.

Mazur DJ, Merz JF. 1996. How older patients' treatment preferences are influenced by disclosures about therapeutic uncertainty: surgery versus expectant management for localized prostate cancer. *J Am Geriatr Soc* 44(8):934–7.

McAfee TA. 2000. Managed care and the state tobacco settlements. *Tob Control* 9(Suppl 1):I17.

McBride PE, Plane MB, Underbakke G, Brown RL, Solberg LI. 1997. Smoking screening and management in primary care practices. *Arch Fam Med* 6(2):165–72.

McCarron DA, Oparil S, Chait A, Haynes RB, Kris-Etherton P, Stern JS, Resnick LM, Clark S, Morris CD, Hatton DC, Metz JA, McMahon M, Holcomb S, Snyder GW, Pi-Sunyer FX. 1997. Nutritional management of cardiovascular risk factors. A randomized clinical trial. *Arch Intern Med* 157(2):169–77.

McCarthy BD, Yood MU, Janz NK, Boohaker EA, Ward RE, Johnson CC. 1996. Evaluation of factors potentially associated with inadequate follow-up of mammographic abnormalities. *Cancer* 77(10):2070–6.

McGinnis JM, Foege WH. 1993. Actual causes of death in the United States. *JAMA* 270(18): 2207–12.

McGuire MT, Wing RR, Klem ML, Lang W, Hill JO. 1999. What predicts weight regain in a group of successful weight losers? *J Consult Clin Psychol* 67(2):177–85.

McIlvain HE, Susman JL, Manners MA, Davis CM, Gilbert CS. 1992. Improving smoking cessation counseling by family practice residents. *J Fam Pract* 34(6):745–9.

McIsaac WJ, Fuller-Thomson E, Talbot Y. 2001. Does having regular care by a family physician improve preventive care? *Can Fam Physician* 47:70–6.

McKee MD, Lurio J, Marantz P, Burton W, Mulvihill M. 1999. Barriers to follow-up of abnormal Papanicolaou smears in an urban community health center. *Arch Fam Med* 8(2):129–34.

McKenzie TL, Nader PR, Strikmiller PK, Yang M, Stone EJ, Perry CL, Taylor WC, Epping JN, Feldman HA, Luepker RV, Kelder SH. 1996. School physical education: effect of the Child and Adolescent Trial for Cardiovascular Health. *Prev Med* 25(4):423–31.

McKeown-Eyssen G. 1994. Epidemiology of colorectal cancer revisited: are serum triglycerides and/or plasma glucose associated with risk? *Cancer Epidemiol Biomarkers Prev* 3(8):687–95.

McKnight JT, Tietze PH, Adcock BB, Maxwell AJ, Smith WO, Nagy MC. 1996. Screening for prostate cancer: a comparison of urologists and primary care physicians. *South Med J* 89(9):885–8.

McLaren DB, McKenzie M, Duncan G, Pickles T. 1998. Watchful waiting or watchful progression? prostate specific antigen doubling times and clinical behavior in patients with early untreated prostate carcinoma. *Cancer* 82(2):342–8.

McLaughlin JK, Hrubec Z, Blot WJ, Fraumeni JF Jr. 1995a. Smoking and cancer mortality among U.S. veterans: a 26-year follow-up. *Int J Cancer* 60(2):190–3.

McLaughlin JK, Lindblad P, Mellemgaard A, McCredie M, Mandel JS, Schlehofer B, Pommer W, Adami HO. 1995b. International renal-cell cancer study. I. Tobacco use. *Int J Cancer* 60(2):194–8.

McLaughlin JW, Blot W, et al. 1996. Renal Cancer. Schottenfeld D, Fraumeni J, Jr. *Cancer Epidemiology and Prevention.* Oxford: Oxford University Press. Pp. 1142–55.

McLeroy KR, Bibeau D, Steckler A, Glanz K. 1988. An ecological perspective on health promotion programs. *Health Educ Q* 15(4):351–77.

McNabb WL, Quinn MT, Rosing L. 1993. Weight loss program for inner-city black women with non-insulin-dependent diabetes mellitus: PATHWAYS. *J Am Diet Assoc* 93(1): 75–7.

McNaughton Collins M, Stafford RS, Barry MJ. 2000. Age-specific patterns of prostate-specific antigen testing among primary care physician visits. *J Fam Pract* 49(2):169–72.

McNeal JE, Bostwick DG, Kindrachuk RA, Redwine EA, Freiha FS, Stamey TA. 1986. Patterns of progression in prostate cancer. *Lancet* 1(8472):60–3.

McPhee SJ, Bird JA, Fordham D, Rodnick JE, Osborn EH. 1991. Promoting cancer prevention activities by primary care physicians. Results of a randomized, controlled trial. *JAMA* 266(4):538–44.

McPhillips-Tangum C. 1998. Results from the first annual survey on addressing tobacco in managed care. *Tob Control* 7 Suppl:S11–3.

McTiernan A, Ulrich C, Slate S, Potter J. 1998. Physical activity and cancer etiology: associations and mechanisms. *Cancer Causes Control* 9(5):487–509.

Medder J, Susman JL, Gilbert C, Crabtree BF, McIlvain HE, McVea K, Davis CM, Hawver M. 1997. Dissemination and implementation of Put Prevention into Family Practice. *Am J Prev Med* 13(5):345–51.

Meerding WJ, Doornewaard H, van Ballegooijen M, Bos A, van der Graaf Y, van den Tweel JG, van der Schouw YT, Habbema JD. 2001. Cost analysis of PAPNET-assisted vs. conventional Pap smear evaluation in primary screening of cervical smears. *Acta Cytol* 45(1):28–35.

Meijers-Heijboer EJ, Verhoog LC, Brekelmans CT, Seynaeve C, Tilanus-Linthorst MM, Wagner A, Dukel L, Devilee P, van den Ouweland AM, van Geel AN, Klijn JG. 2000. Presymptomatic DNA testing and prophylactic surgery in families with a BRCA1 or BRCA2 mutation. *Lancet* 355(9220):2015–20.

Melamed MR, Flehinger BJ, Zaman MB, Heelan RT, Perchick WA, Martini N. 1984. Screening for early lung cancer. Results of the Memorial Sloan-Kettering study in New York. *Chest* 86(1):44–53.

Mellemgaard A, McLaughlin JK, Overvad K, Olsen JH. 1996. Dietary risk factors for renal cell carcinoma in Denmark. *Eur J Cancer* 32A(4):673–82.

Metcalfe KA, Liede A, Hoodfar E, Scott A, Foulkes WD, Narod SA. 2000. An evaluation of needs of female BRCA1 and BRCA2 carriers undergoing genetic counselling. *J Med Genet* 37(11):866–74.

Mettlin CJ, Black B, Lee F, Littrup PJ, DuPont A, Babaian R. 1993. Workgroup #2: Screening and detection. Reference range/clinical issues of PSA. *Cancer* 71(8):2679–80.

Mettlin C, Murphy GP, Lee F, Littrup PJ, Chesley A, Babaian R, Badalament R, Kane RA, Mostofi FK. 1994. Characteristics of prostate cancer detected in the American Cancer Society-National Prostate Cancer Detection Project. *J Urol* 152(5 Pt 2):1737–40.

Mettlin CJ, Murphy GP, Rosenthal DS, Menck HR. 1998. The National Cancer Data Base report on prostate carcinoma after the peak in incidence rates in the U.S. The American College of Surgeons Commission on Cancer and the American Cancer Society. *Cancer* 83(8):1679–84.

Metz JA, Stern JS, Kris-Etherton P, Reusser ME, Morris CD, Hatton DC, Oparil S, Haynes RB, Resnick LM, Pi-Sunyer FX, Clark S, Chester L, McMahon M, Snyder GW, McCarron DA. 2000. A randomized trial of improved weight loss with a prepared meal plan in overweight and obese patients: impact on cardiovascular risk reduction. *Arch Intern Med* 160(14):2150–8.

Meyer F, Moore L, Bairati I, Fradet Y. 1999. Downward trend in prostate cancer mortality in Quebec and Canada. *J Urol* 161(4):1189–91.

Meyer JS, Terayama Y, Konno S, Akiyama H, Margishvili GM, Mortel KF. 1998. Risk factors for cerebral degenerative changes and dementia. *Eur Neurol* 39(Suppl 1):7–16.

Meyers AW, Graves TJ, Whelan JP, Barclay DR. 1996. An evaluation of a television-delivered behavioral weight loss program: are the ratings acceptable? *J Consult Clin Psychol* 64(1):172–8.

Michaelson JS, Halpern E, Kopans DB. 1999. Breast cancer: computer simulation method for estimating optimal intervals for screening. *Radiology* 212(2):551–60.

Michalek AM, Mahoney MC, Burhansstipanov L, Tenney M, Cobb N. 1996. Urban-based Native American cancer-control activities: services and perceptions. *J Cancer Educ* 11(3):159–63.

Michaud CM, Murray CJ, Bloom BR. 2001. Burden of disease—implications for future research. *JAMA* 285(5):535–9.

Michels KB, Giovannucci E, Joshipura KJ, Rosner BA, Stampfer MJ, Fuchs CS, Colditz GA, Speizer FE, Willett WC. 2000. Prospective study of fruit and vegetable consumption and incidence of colon and rectal cancers. *J Natl Cancer Inst* 92(21):1740–52.

Miesfeldt S, Jones SM, Cohn WF. 2000. Informed consent for BRCA1 and BRCA2 testing: what clinicians should know about the process and content. *J Am Med Women's Assoc* 55(5):275–9.

Miles BJ, Kattan MW, Giesler RB, Cowen M. 1995. Screening for prostate cancer. *JAMA* 273(15):1173–4.

Miller AB. 2001. Screening for breast cancer with mammography. *Lancet* 358(9299):2164; discussion 2167–8.

Miller AB, Baines CJ, To T, Wall C. 1992a. Canadian National Breast Screening Study. 1. Breast cancer detection and death rates among women aged 40 to 49 years. *Can Med Assoc J* 147(10):1459–76.

Miller AB, Baines CJ, To T, Wall C. 1992b. Canadian National Breast Screening Study. 2. Breast cancer detection and death rates among women aged 50 to 59 years. *Can Med Assoc J* 147(10):1477–88.

Miller AB, To T, Baines CJ, Wall C. 2000. Canadian National Breast Screening Study. 2: 13-year results of a randomized trial in women aged 50–59 years. *J Natl Cancer Inst* 92(18):1490–9.

Miller AB, To T, Baines CJ, Wall C. 2002. The Canadian National Breast Screening Study. 1: Breast Cancer Mortality after 11 to 16 years of follow-up: a randomized screening trial of mammography in women aged 40–49 years. *Annals of Internal Medicine* 137(5, Part 1):E305–15.

Miller BA, Kolonel LN, Bernstein L, Young Jr. JL, Swanson GM , West D, Key CR, Liff JM, Glover CS, Alexander GA, et al. 1996. Racial/Ethnic Patterns of Cancer in the United States 1988–1992. NIH Pub. 96-4104. Bethesda, MD: National Cancer Institute.

Miller SM, Siejak KK, Schroeder CM, Lerman C, Hernandez E, Helm CW. 1997. Enhancing adherence following abnormal Pap smears among low-income minority women: a preventive telephone counseling strategy. *J Natl Cancer Inst* 89(10):703–8.

Miller WR, Rollnick S. 1991. *Motivational Interviewing: Preparing People to Change Addictive Behaviors*. New York: Guilford Press.

Minkler M, Wallerstein N. 1997. Improving health through community organization and community building. In *Health Behavior and Health Education: Theory, Research & Practice*. Glantz K, Lewis F, Rimer B, eds. 2nd ed. San Francisco: Jossey-Bass.

Mitchell-Beren ME, Dodds ME, Choi KL, Waskerwitz TR. 1989. A colorectal cancer prevention, screening, and evaluation program in community black churches. *CA Cancer J Clin* 39(2):115–8.

Moberg K, Grundstrom H, Lundquist H, Svane G, Havervall E, Muren C. 2000. Radiological review of incidence breast cancers. *J Med Screen* 7(4):177–83.

Mohler PJ. 1995. Enhancing compliance with screening mammography recommendations: a clinical trial in a primary care office. *Fam Med* 27(2):117–21.

Mold JW, Holtgrave DR, Bisonni RS, Marley DS, Wright RA, Spann SJ. 1992. The evaluation and treatment of men with asymptomatic prostate nodules in primary care: a decision analysis. *J Fam Pract* 34(5):561–8.

Monsees BS. 2000. The Mammography Quality Standards Act. An overview of the regulations and guidance. *Radiol Clin N Am* 38(4):759–72.

Monson RR, Christiani DC. 1997. Summary of the evidence: occupation and environment and cancer. *Cancer Causes Control* 8(3):529–31.

Montano DE, Thompson B, Taylor VM, Mahloch J. 1997. Understanding mammography intention and utilization among women in an inner city public hospital clinic. *Prev Med* 26(6):817–24.

Montano DE, Phillips WR, Kasprzyk D. 2000. Explaining physician rates of providing flexible sigmoidoscopy. *Cancer Epidemiol Biomarkers Prev* 9(7):665–9.

Moran WP, Cohen SJ, Preisser JS, Wofford JL, Shelton BJ, McClatchey MW. 2000. Factors influencing use of the prostate-specific antigen screening test in primary care. *Am J Manag Care* 6(3):315–24.

Morgan TO, Jacobsen SJ, McCarthy WF, Jacobson DJ, McLeod DG, Moul JW. 1996. Age-specific reference ranges for prostate-specific antigen in black men. *N Engl J Med* 335(5):304–10.

Mori M, Hariharan M, Anandakumar M, Tsutsumi M, Ishikawa O, Konishi Y, Chellam VG, John M, Praseeda I, Priya R, Narendranathan M. 1999. A case-control study on risk factors for pancreatic diseases in Kerala, India. *Hepatogastroenterology* 46(25):25–30.

Morris K. 1997. U.K. experts advise against prostate cancer screening. *Lancet* 349(9050):477.

Morrison AB. 2002. Counteracting cigarette advertising. JAMA 287(22):3001–3.

Morrow M, Schnitt SJ. 2000. Treatment selection in ductal carcinoma in situ. JAMA 283(4): 453–5.

Moskowitz M. 1986. Breast cancer: age-specific growth rates and screening strategies. *Radiology* 161(1):37–41.

Moss S. 1999. A trial to study the effect on breast cancer mortality of annual mammographic screening in women starting at age 40. Trial Steering Group. *J Med Screen* 6(3):144–8.

Moss S, Blanks R, Quinn MJ. 2000. Screening mammography re-evaluated. *Lancet* 355(9205): 748.

Mullen P, Zapka J. 1982. *Guidelines for Health Promotion and Education Services in HMOs*. Washington, DC: U.S. Government Printing Office.

Muller AD, Sonnenberg A. 1995. Protection by endoscopy against death from colorectal cancer. A case-control study among veterans. *Arch Intern Med* 155(16):1741–8.

Muller S (Chairman). 1984. Physicians for the twenty-first century. Report of the Project Panel on the General Professional Education of the Physician and College Preparation for Medicine. *J Med Educ* 59(11 Pt 2):1-208.

Mundt MH. 1996. Public education programs in the nursing curriculum. *Nurse Educ* 21(2): 31–4.

Muñoz N, Bosch FX, de Sanjose S, Vergara A, del Moral A, Munoz MT, Tafur L, Gili M, Izarzugaza I, Viladiu P, et al. 1993. Risk factors for cervical intraepithelial neoplasia grade III/carcinoma in situ in Spain and Colombia. *Cancer Epidemiol Biomarkers Prev* 2(5):423–31.

Murphy GP, Mettlin C, Menck H, Winchester DP, Davidson AM. 1994. National patterns of prostate cancer treatment by radical prostatectomy: results of a survey by the American College of Surgeons Commission on Cancer. *J Urol* 152(5 Pt 2):1817–9.

Mushlin AI, Kouides RW, Shapiro DE. 1998. Estimating the accuracy of screening mammography: a meta-analysis. *Am J Prev Med* 14(2):143–53.

Myers RE, Ross EA, Wolf TA, Balshem A, Jepson C, Millner L. 1991. Behavioral interventions to increase adherence in colorectal cancer screening. *Med Care* 29(10):1039–50.

Myers RE, Ross E, Jepson C, Wolf T, Balshem A, Millner L, Leventhal H. 1994. Modeling adherence to colorectal cancer screening. *Prev Med* 23(2):142–51.

Nader PR, Baranowski T, Vanderpool NA, Dunn K, Dworkin R, Ray L. 1983. The family health project: cardiovascular risk reduction education for children and parents. *J Dev Behav Pediatr* 4(1):3–10.

Nader PR, Sallis JF, Patterson TL, Abramson IS, Rupp JW, Senn KL, Atkins CJ, Roppe BE, Morris JA, Wallace JP, et al. 1989. A family approach to cardiovascular risk reduction: results from the San Diego Family Health Project. *Health Educ Q* 16(2):229–44.

Nader PR, Stone EJ, Lytle LA, Perry CL, Osganian SK, Kelder S, Webber LS, Elder JP, Montgomery D, Feldman HA, Wu M, Johnson C, Parcel GS, Luepker RV. 1999. Three-year maintenance of improved diet and physical activity: the CATCH cohort. Child and Adolescent Trial for Cardiovascular Health. *Arch Pediatr Adolesc Med* 153(7):695–704.

Naidich DP, Marshall CH, Gribbin C, Arams RS, McCauley DI. 1990. Low-dose CT of the lungs: preliminary observations. *Radiology* 175(3):729–31.

Najman JM, Lanyon A, Andersen M, Williams G, Bor W, O'Callaghan M. 1998. Socioeconomic status and maternal cigarette smoking before, during and after a pregnancy. *Aust NZ J Public Health* 22(1):60–6.

Nash FA, Morgan JM, Tomkins JG. 1968. South London Lung Cancer Study. *Br Med J* 2(607):715–21.

National Cancer Institute. Division of Cancer Prevention and Control. 1986. *Cancer control. Objectives for the nation: 1985–2000.* NCI Monogr (2):1–93.

National Cancer Institute. 2000a. *State Cancer Legislative Database Program.* Bethesda, MD: National Cancer Institute.

National Cancer Institute. 2000b. *The Nation's Investment in Cancer Research: A Plan and Budget Proposal for Fiscal Year 2002.*

National Cancer Institute. 2001. *Cancer Progress Report.* Bethesda, MD: U.S. Department of Health and Human Services, Public Health Service, National Institutes of Health, National Cancer Institute.

National Cancer Institute and American Cancer Society. 2001. *Lung Cancer Early Detection Workshop.* Rockville, MD: National Cancer Institute and American Cancer Society.

National Center for Health Statistics. Pamuk E, Makuc D, Heck K, Reuben C, Lochner K. 1998. *Health, United States, 1998 with Socioeconomic Status and Health Chartbook.* Hyattsville, MD: U.S. Department of Health and Human Services, National Center for Health Statistics.

National Center for Health Statistics. MacKay AP, Fingerhut LA, Duran CR. 2000. *Health, United States, 2000 with Adolescent Health Chartbook.* Hyattsville, MD: U.S. Department of Health and Human Services.

National Center for Health Statistics. Eberhardt MS, Ingram DD/Makuc DM, et al. 2001. *Health, United States, 2001 with Urban and Rural Health Chartbook.* Hyattsville, MD: U.S. Department of Health and Human Services.

National Committee for Quality Assurance. 2001. *The State of Managed Care Quality.* Washington, DC: National Committee for Quality Assurance.

National Conference of State Legislatures. 2001. *State Management and Allocation of Tobacco Settlement Revenue—1999 to 2001.* Washington, DC: National Center of State Legislatures.

National Governors Association. *NGA Center for Best Practices Online.* [Online]. Available at: http://www.nga.org/special/1,1260,C_MINI_WEB_SITE^D_365,00.html.

National Heart, Lung, and Blood Institute. 1998. Obesity Education Initiative Expert Panel on the Identification and Treatment of Overweight and Obesity in Adults. *Clinical Guidelines on the Identification, Evaluation, and Treatment of Overweight and Obesity in Adults.* Bethesda, MD: National Heart, Lung, and Blood Institute, National Institutes of Health.

National Institutes of Health. 1994. *Ovarian Cancer: Screening, Treatment, and Follow-up.* National Institutes of Health Consensus Conference Statement. Bethesda, MD: National Institutes of Health.

National Institutes of Health. 1996. *Cervical Cancer.* National Institutes of Health Consensus Conference Statement. Bethesda, MD: National Institutes of Health.

National Institutes of Health. 1997. *Breast Cancer Screening for Women Ages 40–49.* National Institutes of Health Consensus Conference Statement. Bethesda, MD: National Institutes of Health.

National Institutes of Health. 1998. *Key Facts and History of Funding: FY 1988–FY 1997.* Bethesda, MD: NIH.

National Institutes of Health Consensus Development Panel on Physical Activity and Cardiovascular Health. 1996. Physical activity and cardiovascular health. *JAMA* 276(3): 241–6.

National League for Nursing. 1997. *Nursing Datasource, Vol 1.* Washington, DC: American Nurses Association.

National Library of Medicine. 2001. *Medical Subject Headings-Annotated Alphabetic List: 2001.* Bethesda, MD, National Library of Medicine.

National Research Council. 1985. *Nutrition Education in U.S. Medical Schools.* Committee on Nutrition in Education. Washington, DC: National Academy Press.

National Task Force on the Prevention and Treatment of Obesity. 1993. Very low-calorie diets. *Journal of the American Medical Association* 270(8):967–74.

Naughton CK, Miller DC, Mager DE, Ornstein DK, Catalona WJ. 2000a. A prospective randomized trial comparing 6 versus 12 prostate biopsy cores: impact on cancer detection. *J Urol* 164(2):388–92.

Naughton CK, Ornstein DK, Smith DS, Catalona WJ. 2000b. Pain and morbidity of transrectal ultrasound guided prostate biopsy: a prospective randomized trial of 6 versus 12 cores. *J Urol* 163(1):168–71.

Naughton CK, Miller DC, Yan Y. 2001. Impact of transrectal ultrasound guided prostate biopsy on quality of life: a prospective randomized trial comparing 6 versus 12 cores. *J Urol* 165(1):100–3.

Navarro AM, Senn KL, McNicholas LJ, Kaplan RM, Roppe B, Campo MC. 1998. Por La Vida model intervention enhances use of cancer screening tests among Latinas. *Am J Prev Med* 15(1):32–41.

Nelson DE, Emont SL, Brackbill RM, Cameron LL, Peddicord J, Fiore MC. 1994. Cigarette smoking prevalence by occupation in the United States. A comparison between 1978 to 1980 and 1987 to 1990. *J Occup Med* 36(5):516–25.

Nelson DE, Tomar SL, Mowery P, Siegel PZ. 1996. Trends in smokeless tobacco use among men in four states, 1988 through 1993. *Am J Public Health* 86(9):1300–3.

Ness RB, Nelson DB, Kumanyika SK, Grisso JA. 1997. Evaluating minority recruitment into clinical studies: how good are the data? *Ann Epidemiol* 7(7):472–8.

Newcomb PA, Norfleet RG, Storer BE, Surawicz TS, Marcus PM. 1992. Screening sigmoidoscopy and colorectal cancer mortality. *J Natl Cancer Inst* 84(20):1572–5.

Newman L. 2001. Panel examines impact of public figures on cancer awareness. *J Natl Cancer Inst* 93(1):8–9.

Newschaffer CJ, Otani K, McDonald MK, Penberthy LT. 2000. Causes of death in elderly prostate cancer patients and in a comparison nonprostate cancer cohort. *J Natl Cancer Inst* 92(8):613–21.

Nguyen BH, Nguyen KP, McPhee SJ, Nguyen AT, Tran DQ, Jenkins CN. 2000. Promoting cancer prevention activities among Vietnamese physicians in California. *J Cancer Educ* 15(2):82–5.

Nichols S, Koch E, Lallemand RC, Heald RJ, Izzard L, Machin D, Mullee MA. 1986. Randomised trial of compliance with screening for colorectal cancer. *Br Med J (Clin Res Ed)* 293(6539):107–10.

Nicklas TA, Johnson CC, Myers L, Farris RP, Cunningham A. 1998. Outcomes of a high school program to increase fruit and vegetable consumption: Gimme 5—a fresh nutrition concept for students. *J Sch Health* 68(6):248–53.

Nitta N, Takahashi M, Murata K, Morita R. 1998. Ultra low-dose helical CT of the chest. *Am J Roentgenol* 171(2):383–5.

Nitta N, Takahashi M, Murata K, Morita R. 1999. Ultra low-dose helical CT of the chest: evaluation in clinical cases. *Radiation Medicine* 17(1):1–7.

Nomura A, Grove JS, Stemmermann GN, Severson RK. 1990. A prospective study of stomach cancer and its relation to diet, cigarettes, and alcohol consumption. *Cancer Res* 50(3):627–31.

Norton R, Batey R, Dwyer T, MacMahon S. 1987. Alcohol consumption and the risk of alcohol related cirrhosis in women. *Br Med J (Clin Res Ed)* 295(6590):80–2.

Norton SA and Lipson DJ. 1998. *Portraits of the Safety Net: The Market Policy Environment, and Safety Net Response.* Washington, DC: The Urban Institute.

Nyström L. 2000. Screening mammography re-evaluated. *Lancet* 355(9205):748–9.

Nyström L, Rutqvist LE, Wall S, Lindgren A, Lindqvist M, Ryden S, Andersson I, Bjurstam N, Fagerberg G, Frisell J, et al. 1993. Breast cancer screening with mammography: overview of Swedish randomised trials. *Lancet* 341(8851):973–8.

Nyström L, Andersson I, Bjurstam N, Frisell J, Nordenskjold B, Rutqvist LE. 2002. Long-term effects of mammography screening: updated overview of the Swedish randomised trials. *Lancet 359* (9310):909–19.

Ockene I, Ockene JE. 1992. *Prevention of Coronary Heart Disease*. Boston, MA: Little, Brown & Company.

Ockene IS, Hebert JR, Ockene JK, Merriam PA, Hurley TG, Saperia GM. 1996. Effect of training and a structured office practice on physician-delivered nutrition counseling: the Worcester-Area Trial for Counseling in Hyperlipidemia (WATCH). *Am J Prev Med* 12(4):252–8.

Ockene IS, Hebert JR, Ockene JK, Saperia GM, Stanek E, Nicolosi R, Merriam PA, Hurley TG. 1999. Effect of physician-delivered nutrition counseling training and an office-support program on saturated fat intake, weight, and serum lipid measurements in a hyperlipidemic population: Worcester Area Trial for Counseling in Hyperlipidemia (WATCH). *Arch Intern Med* 159(7):725–31.

Ockene JK. 1987. Physician-delivered interventions for smoking cessation: strategies for increasing effectiveness. *Prev Med* 16(5):723–37.

Ockene JK, Zapka J. 1997. Changing provider behaviour: provider education and training. *Tob Control* 6(Suppl 1):S63–7.

Ockene JK, Zapka JG. 2000. Provider education to promote implementation of clinical practice guidelines. *Chest* 118(2 Suppl):33S–9S.

Ockene JK, Quirk ME, Goldberg RJ, Kristeller JL, Donnelly G, Kalan KL, Gould B, Greene HL, Harrison-Atlas R, Pease J, et al. 1988. A residents' training program for the development of smoking intervention skills. *Arch Intern Med* 148(5):1039–45.

Ockene, JK; Ockene, IS; Kabat-Zinn, J; Greene, HL, and Frid, D. 1990. Teaching risk-factor counseling skills to medical students, house staff, and fellows. *Am J Prev Med*. 6(2 Suppl):35–42.

Ockene JK, Hymowitz N, Lagus J, Shaten BJ. 1991a. Comparison of smoking behavior change for SI and UC study groups. MRFIT Research Group. *Prev Med* 20(5):564–73.

Ockene JK, Kristeller J, Goldberg R, Amick TL, Pekow PS, Hosmer D, Quirk M, Kalan K. 1991b. Increasing the efficacy of physician-delivered smoking interventions: a randomized clinical trial. *J Gen Intern Med* 6(1):1–8.

Ockene JK, Zapka JG. 1997. Physician-based smoking intervention: a rededication to a five-step strategy to smoking research. *Addict Behav* 22(6):835–48.

O'Connor AM, Rostom A, Fiset V, Tetroe J, Entwistle V, Llewellyn-Thomas H, Holmes-Rovner M, Barry M, Jones J. 1999. Decision aids for patients facing health treatment or screening decisions: systematic review. *BMJ* 319(7212):731–4.

O'Donnell JF, Bakemeier RF, Chamberlain RM, Gallagher RE, Kupchella CE, Parker JA, Hill GJ, Brooks CM. 1992. Changing the cancer curriculum: a curriculum committee's response to the results of the AACE Cancer Education Survey II. Cancer education in United States medical schools. *J Cancer Educ* 7(2):115–24.

Oesterling JE. 1991. Prostate specific antigen: a critical assessment of the most useful tumor marker for adenocarcinoma of the prostate. *J Urol* 145(5):907–23.

Oesterling JE, Jacobsen SJ, Chute CG, Guess HA, Girman CJ, Panser LA, Lieber MM. 1993. Serum prostate-specific antigen in a community-based population of healthy men. Establishment of age-specific reference ranges. *JAMA* 270(7):860–4.

Ohba S, Nishi M, Miyake H. 1996. Eating habits and pancreas cancer. *Int J Pancreatol* 20(1):37–42.

Okamoto N, Suzuki T, Hasegawa H, Gotoh T, Hagiwara S, Sekimoto M, Kaneko M. 1999. Evaluation of a clinic-based screening program for lung cancer with a case-control design in Kanagawa, Japan. *Lung Cancer* 25(2):77–85.

Oliveria SA, Kohl HW III, Trichopoulos D, Blair SN. 1996. The association between cardiorespiratory fitness and prostate cancer. *Med Sci Sports Exerc* 28(1):97–104.

Olsen SJ, Frank-Stromborg M. 1994. Cancer prevention and screening activities reported by African-American nurses. *Oncol Nurs Forum* 21(3):487–94.

Olsen O, Gøtzsche PC. 2001. Screening for breast cancer with mammography (Cochrane Review). *Cochrane Database Syst Rev* 4:CD001877.

Olsson P, Armelius K, Nordahl G, Lenner P, Westman G. 1999. Women with false positive screening mammograms: how do they cope? *J Med Screen* 6(2):89–93.

O'Malley MS, Earp JA, Hawley ST, Schell MJ, Mathews HF, Mitchell J. 2001. The association of race/ethnicity, socioeconomic status, and physician recommendation for mammography: who gets the message about breast cancer screening? *Am J Public Health* 91(1):49–54.

Omenn GS, Goodman GE, Thornquist MD, Balmes J, Cullen MR, Glass A, Keogh JP, Meyskens FL, Valanis B, Williams JH, Barnhart S, Hammar S. 1996. Effects of a combination of beta carotene and vitamin A on lung cancer and cardiovascular disease. *N Engl J Med* 334(18): 1150–5.

Oncology Nursing Society. 1995. *Standards of Oncology Nursing Education: Generalist and Advanced Practice Levels*. Pittsburgh, PA: Oncology Nursing Society.

Oncology Nursing Society. 1996. *Statement on the Scope and Standards of Oncology Nursing Practice*. Washington, DC: Oncology Nursing Society, American Nurses Association.

Optenberg SA, Wojcik BE, Thompson IM. 1995. Morbidity and mortality following radical prostatectomy: a national analysis of Civilian Health and Medical Program of the Uniformed Services beneficiaries. *J Urol* 153(6):1870–2.

Orel SG. 2000. MR imaging of the breast. *Radiol Clin N Am* 38(4):899–913.

Orleans CT, George LK, Houpt JL, Brodie KH. 1985. Health promotion in primary care: a survey of U.S. family practitioners. *Prev Med* 14(5):636–47.

Ornstein SM, Garr DR, Jenkins RG, Musham C, Hamadeh G, Lancaster C. 1995. Implementation and evaluation of a computer-based preventive services system. *Fam Med* 27(4): 260–6.

Paffenbarger RS Jr, Hyde RT, Wing AL. 1987. Physical activity and incidence of cancer in diverse populations: a preliminary report. *Am J Clin Nutr* 45(1 Suppl):312–7.

Paffenbarger RS Jr, Lee IM, Wing AL. 1992. The influence of physical activity on the incidence of site-specific cancers in college alumni. *Adv Exp Med Biol* 322:7–15.

Paffenbarger RS Jr, Hyde RT, Wing AL, Lee IM, Jung DL, Kampert JB. 1993. The association of changes in physical-activity level and other lifestyle characteristics with mortality among men. *N Engl J Med* 328(8):538–45.

Page DL, Dupont WD, Rogers LW, Jensen RA, Schuyler PA. 1995. Continued local recurrence of carcinoma 15–25 years after a diagnosis of low grade ductal carcinoma in situ of the breast treated only by biopsy. *Cancer* 76(7):1197–200.

Palitz AM, Selby JV, Grossman S, Finkler LJ, Bevc M, Kehr C, Conell CA. 1997. The Colon Cancer Prevention Program (CoCaP): rationale, implementation, and preliminary results. *HMO Pract* 11(1):5–12.

Palmisano WA, Divine KK, Saccomanno G, Gilliland FD, Baylin SB, Herman JG, Belinsky SA. 2000. Predicting lung cancer by detecting aberrant promoter methylation in sputum. *Cancer Res* 60(21):5954–8.

Pandey M, Mathew A, Nair MK. 1999. Global Perspective of Tobacco Habits and Lung Cancer: a Lesson for Third World Countries. [Review] [58 Refs]. *European Journal of Cancer Prevention* 8(4):271–9.

Paquette D, Snider J, Bouchard F, Olivotto I, Bryant H, Decker K, Doyle G. 2000. Performance of screening mammography in organized programs in Canada in 1996. The Database Management Subcommittee to the National Committee for the Canadian Breast Cancer Screening Initiative. *Can Med Assoc J* 163(9):1133–8.

Parcel GS, Simons-Morton B, O'Hara NM, Baranowski T, Wilson B. 1989. School promotion of healthful diet and physical activity: impact on learning outcomes and self-reported behavior. *Health Educ Q* 16(2):181–99.

Parkes C, Wald NJ, Murphy P, George L, Watt HC, Kirby R, Knekt P, Helzlsouer KJ, Tuomilehto J. 1995. Prospective observational study to assess value of prostate specific antigen as screening test for prostate cancer. *BMJ* 311(7016):1340–3.

Parkin DM, Muir CS, Whelan SL, Gao YT, Ferlay J, Powell J. 1992. *Cancer Incidence in Five Continents*, Vol. 6. IARC Scientific Publication No. 120: Lyon, France: International Agency for Research on Cancer.

Parkin M, Whelan SL, Ferlay J, Raymond L, Young J. 1997. *Cancer in Five Continents*, Vol. VII. IARC Publication No. 143. Lyon, France: International Agency for Research on Cancer.

Parkin DM, Pisani P, Ferlay J. 1999. Global Cancer Statistics. *Ca: A Cancer Journal for Clinicians* 49(1):33–64, 1.

Parnes BL, Smith PC, Conry CM, Domke H. 2001. When should we stop mamography screening for breast cancer in elderly women? *J Fam Pract* 50(2):110–1.

Partin AW, Catalona WJ, Finlay JA, Darte C, Tindall DJ, Young CY, Klee GG, Chan DW, Rittenhouse HG, Wolfert RL, Woodrum DL. 1999. Use of human glandular kallikrein 2 for the detection of prostate cancer: preliminary analysis. *Urology* 54(5):839–45.

Partnership for Prevention. 1997. *Why Invest in Disease Prevention?* Washington, DC: Partnership for Prevention.

Pascale RW, Wing RR, Butler BA, Mullen M, Bononi P. 1995. Effects of a behavioral weight loss program stressing calorie restriction versus calorie plus fat restriction in obese individuals with NIDDM or a family history of diabetes. *Diabetes Care* 18(9):1241–8.

Paskett ED, Rushing J, D'Agostino R Jr, Tatum C, Velez R. 1997. Cancer screening behaviors of low-income women: the impact of race. *Women's Health* 3(3–4):203–26.

Paskett ED, McMahon K, Tatum C, Velez R, Shelton B, Case LD, Wofford J, Moran W, Wymer A. 1998. Clinic-based interventions to promote breast and cervical cancer screening. *Prev Med* 27(1):120–8.

Pate RR, Pratt M, Blair SN, Haskell WL, Macera CA, Bouchard C, Buchner D, Ettinger W, Heath GW, King AC, et al. 1995a. Physical activity and public health. A recommendation from the Centers for Disease Control and Prevention and the American College of Sports Medicine. *JAMA* 273(5):402–7.

Pate RR, Small ML, Ross JG, Young JC, Flint KH, Warren CW. 1995b. School physical education. *J Sch Health* 65(8):312–8.

Patterson B, Domanik R, Wernke P, Gombrich M. 2001. Molecular biomarker-based screening for early detection of cervical cancer. *Acta Cytol* 45(1):36–47.

Patz EF Jr, Goodman PC, Bepler G. 2000a. Screening for lung cancer. *N Engl J Med* 343(22): 1627–33.

Patz EF Jr, Rossi S, Harpole DH Jr, Herndon JE, Goodman PC. 2000b. Correlation of tumor size and survival in patients with stage IA non-small cell lung cancer. *Chest* 117(6):1568–71.

Pauker SG, Kassirer JP. 1997. Contentious screening decisions: does the choice matter? *N Engl J Med* 336(17):1243–4.

Pbert L, Ockene JK, Ewy BM, Leicher ES, Warner D. 2000. Development of a state wide tobacco treatment specialist training and certification programme for Massachusetts. *Tob Control* 9(4):372–81.

Pearl R. 1926. *Alcohol and Longevity*. New York: Alfred A Knopf.

Pearlman DN, Rakowski W, Clark MA, Ehrich B, Rimer BK, Goldstein MG, Woolverton H III, Dube CE. 1997. Why do women's attitudes toward mammography change over time? Implications for physician-patient communication. *Cancer Epidemiol Biomarkers Prev* 6(6):451–7.

Perri MG, McAllister DA, Gange JJ, Jordan RC, McAdoo G, Nezu AM. 1988. Effects of four maintenance programs on the long-term management of obesity. *J Consult Clin Psychol* 56(4):529–34.

Perri MG, Martin AD, Leermakers EA, Sears SF, Notelovitz M. 1997. Effects of group-versus home-based exercise in the treatment of obesity. *J Consult Clin Psychol* 65(2):278–85.

Perry C, Killen J, Telch M, Slinkard LA, Danaher BG. 1980. Modifying smoking behavior of teenagers: a school-based intervention. *Am J Public Health* 70(7):722–5.

Perry CL, Lytle LA, Feldman H, et al. 1998a. Effects of the Child and Adolescent Trial for Cardiovascular Health (CATCH) on fruit and vegetable intake. *J Nutr Educ* 30(6):354.

Perry CL, Bishop DB, Taylor G, Murray DM, Mays RW, Dudovitz BS, Smyth M, Story M. 1998b. Changing fruit and vegetable consumption among children: the 5-a-Day Power Plus program in St. Paul, Minnesota. *Am J Public Health* 88(4):603–9.

Peterson AV Jr, Kealey KA, Mann SL, Marek PM, Sarason IG. 2000. Hutchinson Smoking Prevention Project: long-term randomized trial in school-based tobacco use prevention—results on smoking. *J Natl Cancer Inst* 92(24):1979–91.

Peterson AV Jr, Kealey KA, Mann SL, Marek PM, Sarason IG. 2001. Re: Hutchinson Smoking Prevention Project: long-term randomized trial in school-based tobacco use prevention—results on smoking. *J Natl Cancer Inst* 93(16):1269-70.

Peterson TR, Aldana SG. 1999. Improving exercise behavior: an application of the stages of change model in a worksite setting. *Am J Health Promot* 13(4):229–32, iii.

Peticolas A. 2000. Women's attitudes to false positive mammography results. People in the United States may ignore harms of screening. *BMJ* 321(7273):1410.

Peto R, Darby S, Deo H, Silcocks P, Whitley E, Doll R. 2000. Smoking, smoking cessation, and lung cancer in the U.K. since 1950: combination of national statistics with two case-control studies. *BMJ* 321(7257):323–9.

Phillips KA, Fernyak S, Potosky AL, Schauffler HH, Egorin M. 2000. Use of preventive services by managed care enrollees: an updated perspective. *Health Aff (Millwood)* 19(1):102–16.

Phillips RL, Snowdon DA. 1985. Dietary relationships with fatal colorectal cancer among Seventh-Day Adventists. *J Natl Cancer Inst* 74(2):307–17.

Piasecki TM, Baker TB. 2001. Any further progress in smoking cessation treatment? *Nicotine Tob Res* 3(4):311–23.

Pickett KE, Abrams B, Schauffler HH, Savage J, Brandt P, Kalkbrenner A, Chapman SA. 2001. Coverage of tobacco dependence treatments for pregnant smokers in health maintenance organizations. *Am J Public Health* 91(9):1393–4.

Pierce J, Gilpin EA. 1994. *Trends in Physicians' Smoking Behavior and Patterns of Advice to Quit*. Washington, DC: National Cancer Institute.

Pierce JP, Faerber S, Wright FA, Newman V, Flatt SW, Kealey S, Rock CL, Hryniuk W, Greenberg ER. 1997. Feasibility of a randomized trial of a high-vegetable diet to prevent breast cancer recurrence. *Nutr Cancer* 28(3):282–8.

Pierce JP, Gilpin EA, Emery SL, White MM, Rosbrook B, Berry CC, Farkas AJ. 1998. Has the California tobacco control program reduced smoking? *JAMA* 280(10):893–9.

Pignone M, Bucholtz D, Harris R. 1999. Patient preferences for colon cancer screening. *J Gen Intern Med* 14(7):432–7.

Pignone M, Harris R, Kinsinger L. 2000. Videotape-based decision aid for colon cancer screening. A randomized, controlled trial. *Ann Intern Med* 133(10):761–9.

Pinto BM, Goldstein MG, DePue JD, Milan FB. 1998. Acceptability and feasibility of physician-based activity counseling. The PAL project. *Am J Prev Med* 15(2):95–102.

Pisano ED, Burns CB, Washburn D. 1998a. Educational outreach to mammography facility staff to assist with compliance with the Mammography Quality Standards Act in rural North Carolina. *Acad Radiol* 5(7):485–90.

Pisano ED, Earp JA, Gallant TL. 1998b. Screening mammography behavior after a false positive mammogram. *Cancer Detect Prev* 22(2):161–7.

Plaisted CS, Kohlmeier M, Cooksey K, Zeisel SH. 2000. The development of "Nutrition in Medicine" interactive CD-ROM programs for medical nutrition education. *J Cancer Educ* 15(3):140–3.

Podl TR, Goodwin MA, Kikano GE, Stange KC. 1999. Direct observation of exercise counseling in community family practice. *Am J Prev Med* 17(3):207–10.

Podolsky DK. 2000. Going the distance—the case for true colorectal-cancer screening. *N Engl J Med* 343(3):207–8.

Polednak AP, Flannery JT. 1994. Late-stage breast cancer in Connecticut's three largest cities. *Conn Med* 58(5):261–4.

Pollack ES, Nomura AM, Heilbrun LK, Stemmermann GN, Green SB. 1984. Prospective study of alcohol consumption and cancer. *N Engl J Med* 310(10):617–21.

Pomrehn PR, Davis MV, Chen DW, Barker W. 2000. Prevention for the 21st century: setting the context through undergraduate medical education. *Acad Med* 75(7 Suppl):S5–13.

Popkin BM, Siega-Riz AM, Haines PS. 1996. A comparison of dietary trends among racial and socioeconomic groups in the United States. *N Engl J Med* 335(10):716–20.

Poplack SP, Tosteson AN, Grove MR, Wells WA, Carney PA. 2000. Mammography in 53,803 women from the New Hampshire mammography network. *Radiology* 217(3):832–40.

Post-White J, Carter M, Anglim MA. 1993. Cancer prevention and early detection: nursing students' knowledge, attitudes, personal practices, and teaching. *Oncol Nurs Forum* 20(5):743–9.

Poteat HT, Chen P, Loughlin KR, Winkelman JW, Allada R, Ma'luf N, Tanasijevic MJ, Bates DW. 2000. Appropriateness of prostate-specific antigen testing. *Am J Clin Pathol* 113(3): 421–8.

Potischman N, Brinton LA. 1996. Nutrition and cervical neoplasia. *Cancer Causes Control* 7(1):113–26.

Potosky AL, Miller BA, Albertsen PC, Kramer BS. 1995. The role of increasing detection in the rising incidence of prostate cancer. *JAMA* 273(7):548–52.

Potosky AL, Breen N, Graubard BI, Parsons PE. 1998. The association between health care coverage and the use of cancer screening tests. Results from the 1992 National Health Interview Survey. *Med Care* 36(3):257–70.

Potosky AL, Legler J, Albertsen PC, Stanford JL, Gilliland FD, Hamilton AS, Eley JW, Stephenson RA, Harlan LC. 2000. Health outcomes after prostatectomy or radiotherapy for prostate cancer: results from the Prostate Cancer Outcomes Study. *J Natl Cancer Inst* 92(19):1582–92.

Potter JD, Sellers TA, Folsom AR, McGovern PG. 1992. Alcohol, beer, and lung cancer in postmenopausal women. The Iowa Women's Health Study. *Ann Epidemiol* 2(5): 587–95.

Potter SJ, Mauldin PD, Hill HA. 1996. Access to and participation in breast cancer screening: a review of recent literature. *Clin Perform Qual Health Care* 4(2):74–85.

President's Advisory Commission on Consumer Protection and Quality in the Health Care Industry. 1998. *Quality First: Better Health Care for All Americans*. Washington D.C.: U.S. Government Printing Office.

President's Cancer Panel. 1994. *Avoidable Causes of Cancer*. April 7, 1994 Meeting Summary. Bethesda, MD.

President's Cancer Panel. 1998. *Cancer Prevention and Control Research in the 21st Century*. November 18, 1998 Meeting Summary. Tuscon, AZ.

Prochaska JO, DiClemente CC. 1982. Transtheoretical therapy: Towards a more integrative model of change. *Psychotherapy: Theory, Research and Practice* 20:161–173.

Prochaska JO, DiClemente CC, Velicer WF, Rossi JS. 1993. Standardized, individualized, interactive, and personalized self-help programs for smoking cessation. *Health Psychol* 12(5):399–405.

Prochaska JO, Velicer WF, Fava JL, Ruggiero L, Laforge RG, Rossi JS, Johnson SS, Lee PA. 2001. Counselor and stimulus control enhancements of a stage-matched expert system intervention for smokers in a managed care setting. *Prev Med* 32(1): 23–32.

Professional Assisted Cessation Therapy (PACT). 2001. *Reimbursement for Smoking Cessation Therapy: A Healthcare Practitioner's Guide*. Oradell, NJ: RSi Communications.

Pronk NP, Wing RR. 1994. Physical activity and long-term maintenance of weight loss. *Obes Res* 2:587–99.

Puska P, Nissinen A, Tuomilehto J, Salonen JT, Koskela K, McAlister A, Kottke TE, Maccoby N, Farquhar JW. 1985. The community-based strategy to prevent coronary heart disease: conclusions from the ten years of the North Karelia project. *Annu Rev Public Health* 6:147–93.

Qureshi M, Thacker HL, Litaker DG, Kippes C. 2000. Differences in breast cancer screening rates: an issue of ethnicity or socioeconomics? *J Women's Health Gend Based Med* 9(9):1025–31.

Rafferty M. 1998. Prevention services in primary care: taking time, setting priorities. *West J Med* 169(5):269–75.

Ramirez AG, Suarez L, Laufman L, Barroso C, Chalela P. 2000a. Hispanic women's breast and cervical cancer knowledge, attitudes, and screening behaviors. *Am J Health Promot* 14(5):292–300.

Ramirez AG, Talavera GA, Villarreal R, Suarez L, McAlister A, Trapido E, Perez-Stable E, Marti J. 2000b. Breast cancer screening in regional Hispanic populations. *Health Educ Res* 15(5):559–68.

Rankin KV, Burznski NJ, Silverman S, Scheetz JP. 1999. Cancer curricula in U.S. dental schools. *J Cancer Educ* 14(1):8–12.

Ransdell LB. 1995. Church-based health promotion: an untapped resource for women 65 and older. *Am J Health Promot* 9(5):333–6.

Ransohoff DF, Harris RP. 1997. Lessons from the mammography screening controversy: can we improve the debate? *Ann Intern Med* 127(11):1029–34.

Ransohoff DF, Lang CA. 1997. Screening for colorectal cancer with the fecal occult blood test: a background paper. American College of Physicians. *Ann Intern Med* 126(10):811–22.

Rasmussen M, Kronborg O, Fenger C, Jorgensen OD. 1999. Possible advantages and drawbacks of adding flexible sigmoidoscopy to Hemoccult-II in screening for colorectal cancer. A randomized study. *Scand J Gastroenterol* 34(1):73–8.

Rathore SS, McGreevey JD III, Schulman KA, Atkins D. 2000. Mandated coverage for cancer-screening services: whose guidelines do states follow? *Am J Prev Med* 19(2):71–8.

Reed CA, Selleck CS. 1996. The role of midlevel providers in cancer screening. *Med Clin North Am* 80(1):135–44.

Regan J, Lefkowitz B, Gaston MH. 1999. Cancer screening among community health center women: eliminating the gaps. *J Ambulatory Care Manage* 22(4):45–52.

Reich JM. 1995. More on lung cancer screening. *Chest* 108(1):294–5.

Reichman ME, Judd JT, Longcope C, Schatzkin A, Clevidence BA, Nair PP, Campbell WS, Taylor PR. 1993. Effects of alcohol consumption on plasma and urinary hormone concentrations in premenopausal women. *J Natl Cancer Inst* 85(9):722–7.

Reifel J, Bastani R, Ganz PA. 1998. Controversy about mammography screening guidelines and physician practices at a university medical center. *J Cancer Educ* 13(3):145–51.

Rembacken BJ, Fujii T, Cairns A, Dixon MF, Yoshida S, Chalmers DM, Axon AT. 2000. Flat and depressed colonic neoplasms: a prospective study of 1000 colonoscopies in the UK. *Lancet* 355(9211):1211–4.

Rembold CM. 1998. Number needed to screen: development of a statistic for disease screening. *BMJ* 317(7154):307–12.

Ren JJ, Peer PG. 2000. A study on effectiveness of screening mammograms. *Int J Epidemiol* 29(5):803–6.

Renneker M, Saner H. 1995. Low-cost flexible sigmoidoscopy screening: a community demonstration and education project. *J Cancer Educ* 10(1):25–30.

Resnicow K, Cohn L, Reinhardt J, Cross D, Futterman R, Kirschner E, Wynder EL, Allegrante JP. 1992. A three-year evaluation of the Know Your Body program in inner-city schoolchildren. *Health Educ Q* 19(4):463–80.

Resnicow K, Davis M, Smith M, Baranowski T, Lin LS, Baranowski J, Doyle C, Wang DT. 1998. Results of the TeachWell worksite wellness program. *Am J Public Health* 88(2): 250–7.

Resnicow K, Yaroch AL, Davis A, Wang DT, Carter S, Slaughter L, Coleman D, Baranowski T. 2000. GO GIRLS! results from a nutrition and physical activity program for low-income, overweight African American adolescent females. *Health Educ Behav* 27(5): 616–31.

Rex DK, Cutler CS, Lemmel GT, Rahmani EY, Clark DW, Helper DJ, Lehman GA, Mark DG. 1997a. Colonoscopic miss rates of adenomas determined by back-to-back colonoscopies. *Gastroenterology* 112(1):24–8.

Rex DK, Rahmani EY, Haseman JH, Lemmel GT, Kaster S, Buckley JS. 1997b. Relative sensitivity of colonoscopy and barium enema for detection of colorectal cancer in clinical practice. *Gastroenterology* 112(1):17–23.

Rex DK, Johnson DA, Lieberman DA, Burt RW, Sonnenberg A. 2000. Colorectal cancer prevention 2000: screening recommendations of the American College of Gastroenterology. American College of Gastroenterology. *Am J Gastroenterol* 95(4):868–77.

Richardson ML, Norris TE. 1997. On-line delivery of continuing medical education over the World-Wide Web: an on-line needs assessment. *Am J Roentgenol* 168(5):1161–4.

Richert-Boe KE, Humphrey LL, Glass AG, Weiss NS. 1998. Screening digital rectal examination and prostate cancer mortality: a case-control study. *J Med Screen* 5(2):99–103.

Ries LAG, Eisner MP, Kosary CL, Hankey BF, Miller BA, Clegg L, Edwards BK, eds. 2000a. *SEER Cancer Statistics Review, 1973–1997*. Bethesda, MD: National Cancer Institute.

Ries LA, Wingo PA, Miller DS, Howe HL, Weir HK, Rosenberg HM, Vernon SW, Cronin K, Edwards BK. 2000b. The annual report to the nation on the status of cancer, 1973–1997, with a special section on colorectal cancer. *Cancer* 88(10):2398–424.

Ries LAG, Eisner MP, Kosary CL, Hankey BF, Miller BA, Clegg L, Edwards BK, eds. 2002. *SEER Cancer Statistics Review, 1973–1999*. Bethesda, MD: National Cancer Institute.

Rietbergen JB, Hoedemaeker RF, Kruger AE, Kirkels WJ, Schroder FH. 1999. The changing pattern of prostate cancer at the time of diagnosis: characteristics of screen detected prostate cancer in a population based screening study. *J Urol* 161(4):1192–8.

Rimer BK. 1994. Interventions to increase breast screening. Lifespan and ethnicity issues. *Cancer* 74(1 Suppl):323–8.

Rimer BK. 1997. Current use and how to increase mammography screening in women. *Surg Oncol Clin N Am* 6(2):203–11.

Rimer BK, Conaway MR, Lyna PR, Rakowski W, Woods-Powell CT, Tessaro I, Yarnall KS, Barber LT. 1996a. Cancer screening practices among women in a community health center population. *Am J Prev Med* 12(5):351–7.

Rimer BK, Schildkraut JM, Lerman C, Lin TH, Audrain J. 1996b. Participation in a women's breast cancer risk counseling trial. Who participates? Who declines? High Risk Breast Cancer Consortium. *Cancer* 77(11):2348–55.

Rimer BK, Halabi S, Strigo TS, Crawford Y, Lipkus IM. 1999. Confusion About Mammography: Prevalence and Consequences. *J Women's Health Gend Med*8(4):509–20.

Rimer BK, Halabi S, Skinner CS, Kaplan EB, Crawford Y, Samsa GP, Strigo TS, Lipkus IM. 2001. The short-term impact of tailored mammography decision-making interventions. *Patient Educ Couns* 43(3):271–87.

Rimm EB, Stampfer MJ, Giovannucci E, Ascherio A, Spiegelman D, Colditz GA, Willett WC. 1995. Body size and fat distribution as predictors of coronary heart disease among middle-aged and older U.S. men. *Am J Epidemiol* 141(12):1117–27.

Risch HA, Jain M, Marrett LD, Howe GR. 1994. Dietary fat intake and risk of epithelial ovarian cancer. *J Natl Cancer Inst* 86(18):1409–15.

Risendal B, Dezapien J, Fowler B, Papenfuss M, Giuliano A. 1999a. Cancer prevention among urban southwestern American Indian women: comparison to selected Year 2000 national health objectives. *Ann Epidemiol* 9(6):383–90.

Risendal B, Roe D, DeZapien J, Papenfuss M, Giuliano A. 1999b. Influence of health care, cost, and culture on breast cancer screening: issues facing urban American Indian women. *Prev Med* 29(6 Pt 1):501–9.

Roberts K, Dench S, Minten J, York C. 1989. *Community Response to Leisure Centre Provision in Belfast.* London: Sports Council.

Roberts RO, Bergstralh EJ, Katusic SK, Lieber MM, Jacobsen SJ. 1999. Decline in prostate cancer mortality from 1980 to 1997, and an update on incidence trends in Olmsted County, Minnesota. *J Urol* 161(2):529–33.

Robinson MD, Laurent SL, Little JM Jr. 1995. Including smoking status as a new vital sign: it works! *J Fam Pract* 40(6):556–61.

Robinson MH, Pye G, Thomas WM, Hardcastle JD, Mangham CM. 1994. Haemoccult screening for colorectal cancer: the effect of dietary restriction on compliance. *Eur J Surg Oncol* 20(5):545–8.

Robinson MH, Hardcastle JD, Moss SM, Amar SS, Chamberlain JO, Armitage NC, Scholefield JH, Mangham CM. 1999. The risks of screening: data from the Nottingham randomised controlled trial of faecal occult blood screening for colorectal cancer. *Gut* 45(4):588–92.

Robinson TN. 1999. Reducing children's television viewing to prevent obesity: a randomized controlled trial. *JAMA* 282(16):1561–7.

Rockhill B, Newman B, Weinberg C. 1998. Use and misuse of population attributable fractions. *Am J Public Health* 88(1):15–9.

Rodgers AB, Kessler LG, Portnoy B, Potosky AL, Patterson B, Tenney J, Thompson FE, Krebs-Smith SM, Breen N, Mathews O, et al. 1994. "Eat for Health": a supermarket intervention for nutrition and cancer risk reduction. *Am J Public Health* 84(1):72–6.

Rodriguez C, Tatham LM, Thun MJ, Calle EE, Heath CW Jr. 1997. Smoking and fatal prostate cancer in a large cohort of adult men. *Am J Epidemiol* 145(5):466–75.

Rogers E. 1993. *Diffusion of Innovations.* London: The Free Press.

Rogers J. 2000. Clinical preventive medicine: primum non nocere? *J Fam Pract* 49(5):442–5.

Rogers LQ, Johnson KC, Young ZM, Graney M. 1997. Demographic bias in physician smoking cessation counseling. *Am J Med Sci* 313(3):153–8.

Rogot E, Murray JL. 1980. Smoking and causes of death among U.S. veterans: 16 years of observation. *Public Health Rep* 95(3):213–22.

Rollnick S, Heather N, Bell A. 1992. Negotiating behavior change in medical settings: The development of brief motivational interviewing. *Jl Men Health* 1:25–37.

Rose G. 1992. (ital.) *The Strategy of Preventive Medicine.* New York: Oxford University Press.

Rose G, Hamilton PJ. 1978. A randomised controlled trial of the effect on middle-aged men of advice to stop smoking. *J Epidemiol Community Health* 32(4):275–81.

Rosen MA, Logsdon DN, Demak MM. 1984. Prevention and health promotion in primary care: baseline results on physicians from the INSURE Project on Lifecycle Preventive Health Services. *Prev Med* 13(5):535–48.

Rosenbaum P, O'Shea R. 1992. Large-scale study of freedom from smoking clinics—factors in quitting. *Public Health Rep* 107(2):150–5.

Rosenquist CJ, Lindfors KK. 1998. Screening mammography beginning at age 40 years: a reappraisal of cost-effectiveness. *Cancer* 82(11):2235–40.

Rosenstock IM. 1974. Historical Origins of the Health Belief Model. *Health Educ Monogr* 2:328–35.

Ross CE. 2000. Walking, exercising, and smoking: does neighborhood matter? *Soc Sci Med* 51(2):265–74.

Ross KS, Carter HB, Pearson JD, Guess HA. 2000. Comparative efficiency of prostate-specific antigen screening strategies for prostate cancer detection. *JAMA* 284(11):1399–405.

Ruffin MT. 1999. Screening for prostate cancer. *J Fam Pract* 48(8):581–2.

Russell LB. 2000. Cost-effectiveness analysis and screening tests for women. *J Am Med Women's Assoc* 55(4):207–9.

Russell MA, Wilson C, Taylor G. 1979. Effects of general practitioners' advice against smoking. *BMJ* 188:231–35.

Russell NK, Roter DL. 1993. Health promotion counseling of chronic-disease patients during primary care visits. *Am J Public Health* 83(7):979–82.

Russell WD, Dzewaltowski DA, Ryan GJ. 1999. The effectiveness of a point-of-decision prompt in deterring sedentary behavior. *Am J Health Promot* 13(5):257–9, ii.

Saccomanno G, Archer VE, Auerbach O, Saunders RP, Brennan LM. 1974. Development of carcinoma of the lung as reflected in exfoliated cells. *Cancer* 33(1):256–70.

Sachs DP. 1986. Cigarette smoking. Health effects and cessation strategies. *Clin Geriatr Med* 2(2):337–62.

Sallis JF, Bauman A, Pratt M. 1998. Environmental and policy interventions to promote physical activity. *Am J Prev Med* 15(4):379–97.

Salmeron J, Ascherio A, Rimm EB, Colditz GA, Spiegelman D, Jenkins DJ, Stampfer MJ, Wing AL, Willett WC. 1997a. Dietary fiber, glycemic load, and risk of NIDDM in men. *Diabetes Care* 20(4):545–50.

Salmeron J, Manson JE, Stampfer MJ, Colditz GA, Wing AL, Willett WC. 1997b. Dietary fiber, glycemic load, and risk of non-insulin-dependent diabetes mellitus in women. *JAMA* 277(6):472–7.

Salzmann P, Kerlikowske K, Phillips K. 1997. Cost-effectiveness of extending screening mammography guidelines to include women 40 to 49 years of age. *Ann Intern Med* 127(11): 955–65.

Samet JM, Howard CA, Coultas DB, Skipper BJ. 1992. Acculturation, education, and income as determinants of cigarette smoking in New Mexico Hispanics. *Cancer Epidemiol Biomarkers Prev* 1(3):235–40.

Sampson NH. 1995. The Health Resources and Services Administration: a partner in public health practice. *Am J Prev Med* 11(3 Suppl):6.

Sanderson D, Fontana R. 1982. Results of Mayo Lung Project: an interim report. *Recent Results Cancer Res* 82:179–86.

Sarna LP, Brown JK, Lillington L, Rose M, Wewers ME, Brecht ML. 2000. Tobacco interventions by oncology nurses in clinical practice: report from a national survey. *Cancer* 89(4):881–9.

Satariano W, Schwartz A, Swanson G. 1982. *Screening for Cervical Cancer: Results from Several Intervention Strategies*. New York: Alan R. Liss.

Satariano WA, Ragland KE, Van Den Eeden SK. 1998. Cause of death in men diagnosed with prostate carcinoma. *Cancer* 83(6):1180–8.

Sawaya GF, Grimes DA. 1999. New technologies in cervical cytology screening: a word of caution. *Obstet Gynecol* 94(2):307–10.

Sawaya GF, Grady D, Kerlikowske K, Valleur JL, Barnabei VM, Bass K, Snyder TE, Pickar JH, Agarwal SK, Mandelblatt J. 2000a. The positive predictive value of cervical smears in previously screened postmenopausal women: the Heart and Estrogen/Progestin Replacement Study (HERS). *Ann Intern Med* 133(12):942–50.

Sawaya GF, Kerlikowske K, Lee NC, Gildengorin G, Washington AE. 2000b. Frequency of cervical smear abnormalities within 3 years of normal cytology. *Obstet Gynecol* 96(2): 219–23.

Saywell RM Jr, Champion VL, Skinner CS, McQuillen D, Martin D, Maraj M. 1999. Cost-effectiveness comparison of five interventions to increase mammography screening. *Prev Med* 29(5):374–82.

Scaletscky R, Koch MO, Eckstein CW, Bicknell SL, Gray GF Jr, Smith JA Jr. 1994. Tumor volume and stage in carcinoma of the prostate detected by elevations in prostate specific antigen. *J Urol* 152(1):129–31.

Scardino PT. 1989. Early detection of prostate cancer. *Urol Clin N Am* 16(4):635–55.

Scardino PT, Beck JR, Miles BJ. 1994. Conservative management of prostate cancer. *N Engl J Med* 330(25):1831.

Schapira MM, VanRuiswyk J. 2000. The effect of an illustrated pamphlet decision-aid on the use of prostate cancer screening tests. *J Fam Pract* 49(5):418–24.

Schatzkin A, Lanza E, Corle D, Lance P, Iber F, Caan B, Shike M, Weissfeld J, Burt R, Cooper MR, Kikendall JW, Cahill J. 2000. Lack of effect of a low-fat, high-fiber diet on the recurrence of colorectal adenomas. Polyp Prevention Trial Study Group. *N Engl J Med* 342(16):1149–55.

Schauffer H, Brown E. 2000. *The State of Health Insurance in California, 1999*. Berkeley: University of California.

Schauffler HH. 1993. Disease prevention policy under Medicare: a historical and political analysis. *Am J Prev Med* 9(2):71–7.

Schauffler HH, Parkinson MD. 1993. Health insurance coverage for smoking cessation services. *Health Educ Q* 20(2):185–206.

Schauffler HH, Rodriguez T. 1996. Exercising purchasing power for preventive care. *Health Aff (Millwood)* 15(1):73–85.

Schauffler HH, Brown C, Milstein A. 1999. Raising the bar: the use of performance guarantees by the Pacific Business Group on Health. *Health Aff (Millwood)* 18(2):134–42.

Schauffler HH, Barker DC, Orleans CT. 2001a. Medicaid coverage for tobacco-dependence treatments. *Health Aff (Millwood)* 20(1):298–303.

Schauffler HH, McMenamin S, Olson K, Boyce-Smith G, Rideout JA, Kamil J. 2001b. Variations in treatment benefits influence smoking cessation: results of a randomised controlled trial. *Tob Control* 10(2):175–80.

Schiffman MH, Andrews AW, Van Tassell RL, Smith L, Daniel J, Robinson A, Hoover RN, Rosenthal J, Weil R, Nair PP, et al. 1989. Case-control study of colorectal cancer and fecal mutagenicity. *Cancer Res* 49(12):3420–4.

Schlundt DG, Hill JO, Pope-Cordle J, Arnold D, Virts KL, Katahn M. 1993. Randomized evaluation of a low fat ad libitum carbohydrate diet for weight reduction. *Int J Obes Relat Metab Disord* 17(11):623–9.

Schmid TL, Pratt M, Howze E. 1995. Policy as intervention: environmental and policy approaches to the prevention of cardiovascular disease. *Am J Public Health* 85(9):1207–11.

Schmitz KH, Jeffery RW. 2002. Prevention of obesity. In Wadden TA, Stunkard AJ (eds.). *Handbook of Obesity*. New York: Guilford Press.

Schoenfeld P. 1999. Flexible sigmoidoscopy by paramedical personnel. *J Clin Gastroenterol* 28(2):110–6.

Schoenfeld P, Lipscomb S, Crook J, Dominguez J, Butler J, Holmes L, Cruess D, Rex D. 1999. Accuracy of polyp detection by gastroenterologists and nurse endoscopists during flexible sigmoidoscopy: a randomized trial. *Gastroenterology* 117(2):312–8.

Schonfeld-Warden N, Warden CH. 1997. Pediatric obesity. An overview of etiology and treatment. *Pediatr Clin N Am* 44(2):339–61.

Schootman M, Myers-Geadelmann J, Fuortes L. 2000. Factors associated with adequacy of diagnostic workup after abnormal breast cancer screening results. *J Am Board Fam Pract* 13(2):94–100.

Schottenfeld D, Fraumeni JF Jr., eds. 1996. *Cancer Epidemiology and Prevention*. New York: Oxford University Press.

Schrammel P, Griffiths RI, Griffiths CB. 1998. A workplace breast cancer screening program. Costs and components. *AAOHN J* 46(11):523–9.

Schroder FH, Denis LJ, Kirkels W, de Koning HJ, Standaert B. 1995. European randomized study of screening for prostate cancer. Progress report of Antwerp and Rotterdam pilot studies. *Cancer* 76(1):129–34.

Schroder FH, van der Cruijsen-Koeter I, de Koning HJ, Vis AN, Hoedemaeker RF, Kranse R. 2000. Prostate cancer detection at low prostate specific antigen. *J Urol* 163(3):806–12.

Schroy PC, Heeren T, Bliss CM, Pincus J, Wilson S, Prout M. 1999. Implementation of on-site screening sigmoidoscopy positively influences utilization by primary care providers. *Gastroenterology* 117(2):304–11.

Schultz SJ. 1993. Educational and behavioral strategies related to knowledge of and participation in an exercise program after cardiac positron emission tomography. *Patient Educ Couns* 22(1):47–57.

Schuurman AG, van den Brandt PA, Dorant E, Goldbohm RA. 1999. Animal products, calcium and protein and prostate cancer risk in The Netherlands Cohort Study. *Br J Cancer* 80(7):1107–13.

Schwartz LM, Woloshin S, Black WC, Welch HG. 1997. The role of numeracy in understanding the benefit of screening mammography. *Ann Intern Med* 127(11):966–72.

Schwartz LM, Woloshin S, Sox HC, Fischhoff B, Welch HG. 2000. U.S. women's attitudes to false-positive mammography results and detection of ductal carcinoma in situ: cross-sectional survey. *West J Med* 173(5):307–12.

Scott CS, Neighbor WE, Brock DM. 1992. Physicians' attitudes toward preventive care services: a seven-year prospective cohort study. *Am J Prev Med* 8(4):241–8.

Secker-Walker RH, Flynn BS, Solomon LJ, Skelly JM, Dorwaldt AL, Ashikaga T. 2000. Helping women quit smoking: results of a community intervention program. *Am J Public Health* 90(6):940–6.

Selby JV, Friedman GD, Quesenberry CP Jr, Weiss NS. 1992. A case-control study of screening sigmoidoscopy and mortality from colorectal cancer. *N Engl J Med* 326(10):653–7.

Semiglazov VF, Moiseenko VM, Manikhas AG, Protsenko SA, Kharikova RS, Popova RT, Migmanova NS, Orlov AA, Barash NI, Ivanova OA, Ivanov VG. 1999. Interim results of a prospective randomized study of self-examination for early detection of breast cancer (Russia/St. Petersburg/WHO). *Vopr Onkol* 45(3):265–71. (In Russian.)

Senn S. 2001. Screening for breast cancer with mammography. *Lancet* 358(9299):2165; discussion 2167–8.

Sershon PD, Barry MJ, Oesterling JE. 1994. Serum prostate-specific antigen discriminates weakly between men with benign prostatic hyperplasia and patients with organ-confined prostate cancer. *Eur Urol* 25(4):281–7.

Sesink AL, Termont DS, Kleibeuker JH, Van der Meer R. 1999. Red meat and colon cancer: the cytotoxic and hyperproliferative effects of dietary heme. *Cancer Res* 59(22):5704–9.

Sesink AL, Termont DS, Kleibeuker JH, Van Der Meer R. 2000. Red meat and colon cancer: dietary haem, but not fat, has cytotoxic and hyperproliferative effects on rat colonic epithelium. *Carcinogenesis* 21(10):1909–15.

Sesney JW, Kreher NE, Hickner JM, Webb S. 1997. Smoking cessation interventions in rural family practices: an UPRNet study. *J Fam Pract* 44(6):578–85.

Severson RK, Nomura AM, Grove JS, Stemmermann GN. 1989. A prospective study of demographics, diet, and prostate cancer among men of Japanese ancestry in Hawaii. *Cancer Res* 49(7):1857–60.

Severson HH, Andrews JA, Lichtenstein E, Gordon JS, Barckley MF. 1998. Using the hygiene visit to deliver a tobacco cessation program: results of a randomized clinical trial. *J Am Dent Assoc* 129(7):993–9.

Shannon BM, Tershakovec AM, Martel JK, Achterberg CL, Cortner JA, Smiciklas-Wright HS, Stallings VA, Stolley PD. 1994. Reduction of elevated LDL-cholesterol levels of 4-

to 10-year-old children through home-based dietary education. *Pediatrics* 94(6 Pt 1): 923–7.

Shapiro JA, Jacobs EJ, Thun MJ. 2000. Cigar smoking in men and risk of death from tobacco-related cancers. *J Natl Cancer Inst* 92(4):333–7.

Shapiro S. 1988. *Periodic Screening for Breast Cancer. The Health Insurance Plan Project and Its Sequelae, 1963–1986.* Baltimore: Johns Hopkins University Press.

Shapiro S. 1997. Periodic Screening for Breast Cancer: the HIP Randomized Controlled Trial. Health Insurance Plan. *Journal of the National Cancer Institute* Monographs(22): 27–30.

Shapiro S, Venet W, Strax P, Venet L, Roeser R. 1982. Ten- to fourteen-year effect of screening on breast cancer mortality. *J Natl Cancer Inst* 69(2):349–55.

Sheinfeld Gorin S, Gemson D, Ashford A, Bloch S, Lantigua R, Ahsan H, Neugut A. 2000. Cancer education among primary care physicians in an underserved community. *Am J Prev Med* 19(1):53–8.

Shephard RJ. 1996. Worksite fitness and exercise programs: a review of methodology and health impact. *Am J Health Promot* 10(6):436–52.

Shields HM, Weiner MS, Henry DR, Lloyd JA, Ransil BJ, Lamphier DA, Gallagher DW, Antonioli DA, Rosner BA. 2001. Factors that influence the decision to do an adequate evaluation of a patient with a positive stool for occult blood. *Am J Gastroenterol* 96(1):196–203.

Shiffman S, Paty JA, Rohay JM, Di Marino ME, Gitchell J. 2000. The efficacy of computer-tailored smoking cessation material as a supplement to nicotine polacrilex gum therapy. *Arch Intern Med* 160(11):1675–81.

Shipley WU, Thames HD, Sandler HM, Hanks GE, Zietman AL, Perez CA, Kuban DA, Hancock SL, Smith CD. 1999. Radiation therapy for clinically localized prostate cancer: a multi-institutional pooled analysis. *JAMA* 281(17):1598–604.

Shortell SM, Levin DZ, O'Brien JL, Hughes EF. 1995. Assessing the evidence on CQI: is the glass half empty or half full? *Hosp Health Serv Admin* 40(1):4–24.

Shrader-Bogen CL, Kjellberg JL, McPherson CP, Murray CL. 1997. Quality of life and treatment outcomes: prostate carcinoma patients' perspectives after prostatectomy or radiation therapy. *Cancer* 79(10):1977–86.

Sickles EA. 2000a. Breast imaging: from 1965 to the present. *Radiology* 215(1):1–16.

Sickles EA. 2000b. Successful methods to reduce false-positive mammography interpretations. *Radiol Clin N Am* 38(4):693–700.

Siegel M, Biener L, Rigotti NA. 1999. The effect of local tobacco sales laws on adolescent smoking initiation. *Prev Med* 29(5):334–42.

Siegel M, Mowery PD, Pechacek TP, Strauss WJ, Schooley MW, Merritt RK, Novotny TE, Giovino GA, Eriksen MP. 2000. Trends in adult cigarette smoking in California compared with the rest of the United States, 1978–1994. *Am J Public Health* 90(3):372–9.

Siegel MJ, Evens RG. 1999. Advances in the use of computed tomography. *JAMA* 281(14): 1252–4.

Silagy C, Ketteridge S. 1998. *Physician Advice for Smoking Cessation.* Oxford: The Cochrane Library.

Silverman DT, Hartge P, Morrison AS, Devesa SS. 1992. Epidemiology of bladder cancer. *Hematol Oncol Clin N Am* 6(1):1–30.

Simkin-Silverman L, Wing RR, Hansen DH, Klem ML, Pasagian-Macaulay AP, Meilahn EN, Kuller LH. 1995. Prevention of cardiovascular risk factor elevations in healthy premenopausal women. *Prev Med* 24(5):509–17.

Simmang CL, Senatore P, Lowry A, Hicks T, Burnstein M, Dentsman F, Fazio V, Glennon E, Hyman N, Kerner B, Kilkenny J, Moore R, Peters W, Ross T, Savoca P, Vernava A, Wong WD. 1999. Practice parameters for detection of colorectal neoplasms. The Standards Committee, The American Society of Colon and Rectal Surgeons. *Dis Colon Rectum* 42(9):1123–9.

Simmons D, Fleming C, Voyle J, Fou F, Feo S, Gatland B. 1998. A pilot urban church-based programme to reduce risk factors for diabetes among Western Samoans in New Zealand. *Diabet Med* 15(2):136–42.

Simon MS, Gimotty PA, Coombs J, McBride S, Moncrease A, Burack RC. 1998. Factors affecting participation in a mammography screening program among members of an urban Detroit health maintenance organization. *Cancer Detect Prev* 22(1):30–8.

Simons-Morton BG, Parcel GS, Baranowski T, Forthofer R, O'Hara NM. 1991. Promoting physical activity and a healthful diet among children: results of a school-based intervention study. *Am J Public Health* 81(8):986–91.

Simons-Morton DG, Calfas KJ, Oldenburg B, Burton NW. 1998. Effects of interventions in health care settings on physical activity or cardiorespiratory fitness. *Am J Prev Med* 15(4):413–30.

Simpson NK, Johnson CC, Ogden SL, Gamito E, Trocky N, McGuire C, Martin J, Barrow S, Lamerato L, Flickinger LM, Broski KG, Engelhard D, Hilke C, Bonk J, Gahagan B, Gren LH, Childs J, Lappe K, Fouad M, Thompson J, Sullivan D. 2000. Recruitment strategies in the Prostate, Lung, Colorectal and Ovarian (PLCO) Cancer Screening Trial: the first six years. *Control Clin Trials* 21(6 Suppl):356S–78S.

Sin JP, St Leger AS. 1999. Interventions to increase breast screening uptake: do they make any difference? *J Med Screen* 6(4):170–81.

Singh PN, Fraser GE. 1998. Dietary risk factors for colon cancer in a low-risk population. *Am J Epidemiol* 148(8):761–74.

Sjostrom L, Rissanen A, Andersen T, Boldrin M, Golay A, Koppeschaar HP, Krempf M. 1998. Randomised placebo-controlled trial of orlistat for weight loss and prevention of weight regain in obese patients. European Multicentre Orlistat Study Group. *Lancet* 352(9123):167–72.

Skarsgard D, Tonita J. 2000. Prostate cancer in Saskatchewan Canada, before and during the PSA era. *Cancer Causes Control* 11(1):79–88.

Skinner CS, Arfken CL, Waterman B. 2000. Outcomes of the Learn, Share & Live breast cancer education program for older urban women. *Am J Public Health* 90(8):1229–34.

Slater JS, Ha CN, Malone ME, McGovern P, Madigan SD, Finnegan JR, Casey-Paal AL, Margolis KL, Lurie N. 1998. A randomized community trial to increase mammography utilization among low-income women living in public housing. *Prev Med* 27(6):862–70.

Slattery ML, Schumacher MC, Smith KR, West DW, Abd-Elghany N. 1988. Physical activity, diet, and risk of colon cancer in Utah. *Am J Epidemiol* 128(5):989–99.

Smart CR, Hendrick RE, Rutledge JH III, Smith RA. 1995. Benefit of mammography screening in women ages 40 to 49 years. Current evidence from randomized controlled trials. *Cancer* 75(7):1619–26.

Smith DL. 1998. Screening for prostate cancer. *Am Fam Physician* 57(11):2618, 2624, 2627.

Smith DS, Catalona WJ. 1994. The nature of prostate cancer detected through prostate specific antigen based screening. *J Urol* 152(5 Pt 2):1732–6.

Smith DS, Catalona WJ, Herschman JD. 1996a. Longitudinal screening for prostate cancer with prostate-specific antigen. *JAMA* 276(16):1309–15.

Smith DS, Carvalhal GF, Schneider K, Krygiel J, Yan Y, Catalona WJ. 2000. Quality-of-life outcomes for men with prostate carcinoma detected by screening. *Cancer* 88(6):1454–63.

Smith I. 2001. Executive physical: there's a whole battery of new high-tech scans for those who can afford them. Are they worth it? *Time* January 22:86.

Smith RA. 2000. Breast cancer screening among women younger than age 50: a current assessment of the issues. *CA Cancer J Clin* 50(5):312–36.

Smith RA, von Eschenbach AC, Wender R, Levin B, Byers T, Rothenberger D, Brooks D, Creasman W, Cohen C, Runowicz C, Saslow D, Cokkinides V, Eyre H. 2001. American Cancer Society guidelines for the early detection of cancer: update of early detection guidelines for prostate, colorectal, and endometrial cancers. *CA Cancer J Clin* 51(1):38–75.

Smith RA, Cokkinides V, von E, Levin B, Cohen C, Runowicz CD, Sener S, Saslow D, Eyre HJ. 2002. American Cancer Society guidelines for the early detection of cancer. *CA Cancer J Clin* 52(1):8–22.

Smith WA, Ekdahl SS, Henley CE. 1985. Use of Health Hazard Appraisal in counseling for reduction of risk factors. *J Am Osteopath Assoc* 85(12):809–14.

Smith-Bindman R, Kerlikowske K, Gebretsadik T, Newman J. 2000. Is screening mammography effective in elderly women? *Am J Med* 108(2):112–9.

Smith-Warner SA, Spiegelman D, Yaun SS, van den Brandt PA, Folsom AR, Goldbohm RA, Graham S, Holmberg L, Howe GR, Marshall JR, Miller AB, Potter JD, Speizer FE, Willett WC, Wolk A, Hunter DJ. 1998. Alcohol and breast cancer in women: a pooled analysis of cohort studies. *JAMA* 279(7):535–40.

Smith-Warner SA, Spiegelman D, Yaun SS, Adami HO, Beeson WL, van den Brandt PA, Folsom AR, Fraser GE, Freudenheim JL, Goldbohm RA, Graham S, Miller AB, Potter JD, Rohan TE, Speizer FE, Toniolo P, Willett WC, Wolk A, Zeleniuch-Jacquotte A, Hunter DJ. 2001. Intake of fruits and vegetables and risk of breast cancer: a pooled analysis of cohort studies. *JAMA* 285(6):769–76.

Snowdon DA, Phillips RL, Choi W. 1984. Diet, obesity, and risk of fatal prostate cancer. *Am J Epidemiol* 120(2):244–50.

Sobue T, Suzuki T, Matsuda M, Horai T, Kajita A, Kuriyama K, Fukuoka M, Kusunoki Y, Kikui M, Ryu S et al. 1991. Sensitivity and specificity of lung cancer screening in Osaka, Japan. *Jpn J Cancer Res* 82(10):1069–76.

Sobue T, Suzuki T, Matsuda M, Kuroishi T, Ikeda S, Naruke T. 1992a. Survival for clinical stage I lung cancer not surgically treated. Comparison between screen-detected and symptom-detected cases. The Japanese Lung Cancer Screening Research Group. *Cancer* 69(3):685–92.

Sobue T, Suzuki T, Naruke T. 1992b. A case-control study for evaluating lung-cancer screening in Japan. Japanese Lung-Cancer-Screening Research Group. *Int J Cancer* 50(2):230–7.

Sobue T, Moriyama N, Kaneko M, Kusumoto M, Kobayashi T, Tsuchiya R, Kakinuma R, Ohmatsu H, Nagai K, Nishiyama H, Matsui E, Eguchi K. 2002. Screening for lung cancer with low-dose helical computed tomography: Anti-Lung Cancer Association Project. *J Clin Oncol* 20(4):911–20.

Solanki G, Schauffler HH. 1999. Cost-sharing and the utilization of clinical preventive services. *Am J Prev Med* 17(2):127–33.

Solanki G, Schauffler HH, Miller LS. 2000. The Direct and Indirect Effects of Cost-Sharing on the Use of Preventive Services. *Health Services Research* 34(6):1331–50.

Solberg LI, Maxwell PL, Kottke TE, Gepner GJ, Brekke ML. 1990. A systematic primary care office-based smoking cessation program. *J Fam Pract* 30(6):647–54.

Solberg LI, Brekke ML, Kottke TE. 1997a. Are physicians less likely to recommend preventive services to low-SES patients? *Prev Med* 26(3):350–7.

Solberg LI, Brekke ML, Kottke TE. 1997b. How important are clinician and nurse attitudes to the delivery of clinical preventive services? *J Fam Pract* 44(5):451–61.

Solberg LI, Kottke TE, Brekke ML. 1998. Will primary care clinics organize themselves to improve the delivery of preventive services? A randomized controlled trial. *Prev Med* 27(4):623–31.

Solberg LI, Kottke TE, Brekke ML, Magnan S, Davidson G, Calomeni CA, Conn SA, Amundson GM, Nelson AF. 2000. Failure of a continuous quality improvement intervention to increase the delivery of preventive services. A randomized trial. *Effect Clin Pract* 3(3): 105–15.

Sone S, Takashima S, Li F, Yang Z, Honda T, Maruyama Y, Hasegawa M, Yamanda T, Kubo K, Hanamura K, Asakura K. 1998. Mass screening for lung cancer with mobile spiral computed tomography scanner. *Lancet* 351(9111):1242–5.

Sone S, Li F, Yang ZG, Takashima S, Maruyama Y, Hasegawa M, Wang JC, Kawakami S, Honda T. 2000. Characteristics of small lung cancers invisible on conventional chest radiography and detected by population based screening using spiral CT. *Br J Radiol* 73(866):137–45.

Sone S, Li F, Yang ZG, Honda T, Maruyama Y, Takashima S, Hasegawa M, Kawakami S, Kubo K, Haniuda M, Yamanda T. 2001. Results of three-year mass screening programme for lung cancer using mobile low-dose spiral computed tomography scanner. *Br J Cancer* 84(1):25–32.

Sonnenberg A, Delco F, Inadomi JM. 2000. Cost-effectiveness of colonoscopy in screening for colorectal cancer. *Ann Intern Med* 133(8):573–84.

Sopko G, Leon AS, Jacobs DR Jr, Foster N, Moy J, Kuba K, Anderson JT, Casal D, McNally C, Frantz I. 1985. The effects of exercise and weight loss on plasma lipids in young obese men. *Metabolism* 34(3):227–36.

Sorensen G, Morris DM, Hunt MK, Hebert JR, Harris DR, Stoddard A, Ockene JK. 1992. Work-site nutrition intervention and employees' dietary habits: the Treatwell program. *Am J Public Health* 82(6):877–80.

Sorensen G, Thompson B, Glanz K, Feng Z, Kinne S, DiClemente C, Emmons K, Heimendinger J, Probart C, Lichtenstein E. 1996. Work site-based cancer prevention: primary results from the Working Well Trial. *Am J Public Health* 86(7):939–47.

Sorsensen G, Rigotti N, Rosen A, Pinney J, Prible R. 1991. Effects of a worksite nonsmoking policy: evidence for increased cessation. *Am J Public Health* 81(2):202–4.

Southwick PC, Catalona WJ, Partin AW, Slawin KM, Brawer MK, Flanigan RC, Patel A, Richie JP, Walsh PC, Scardino PT, Lange PH, Gasior GH, Parson RE, Loveland KG. 1999. Prediction of post-radical prostatectomy pathological outcome for stage T1c prostate cancer with percent free prostate specific antigen: a prospective multicenter clinical trial. *J Urol* 162(4):1346–51.

Sowden A, Arblaster L. 2000a. *Community Interventions for Preventing Smoking in Young People*. Pub. CD00129: Cochrane Database of Systematic Reviews. Oxford: Update Software.

Sowden AJ, Arblaster L. 2000b. *Mass Media Interventions for Preventing Smoking in Young People*. Pub. CD001006: Cochrane Database of Systematic Reviews. Oxford: Update Software.

Spapen SJ, Damhuis RA, Kirkels WJ. 2000. Trends in the curative treatment of localized prostate cancer after the introduction of prostate-specific antigen: data from the Rotterdam Cancer Registry. *Br J Urol Int* 85(4):474–80.

Spitz MR, Chamberlain RM, Sider JG, Fueger JJ. 1992. Cancer prevention practices among Texas primary care physicians. *J Cancer Educ* 7(1):55–60.

Stamey TA, Prestigiacomo A, Komatsu K. 1995. Physiological variation of serum prostate specific antigen (PSA) from a screening population in the range of 4–10 ng/mL using the Hybritech Tandem-R PSA assay. *J Urol* 153(Suppl):420A.

Stanford JL, Feng Z, Hamilton AS, Gilliland FD, Stephenson RA, Eley JW, Albertsen PC, Harlan LC, Potosky AL. 2000. Urinary and sexual function after radical prostatectomy for clinically localized prostate cancer: the Prostate Cancer Outcomes Study. *JAMA* 283(3):354–60.

Stange KC, Kelly R, Chao J, Zyzanski SJ, Shank JC, Jaen CR, Melnikow J, Flocke S. 1992. Physician agreement with U.S. Preventive Services Task Force recommendations. *J Fam Pract* 34(4):409–16.

Stange KC, Fedirko T, Zyzanski SJ, Jaen CR. 1994. How do family physicians prioritize delivery of multiple preventive services? *J Fam Pract* 38(3):231–7.

Stange KC, Zyzanski SJ, Smith TF, Kelly R, Langa DM, Flocke SA, Jaen CR. 1998. How valid are medical records and patient questionnaires for physician profiling and health services research? A comparison with direct observation of patients visits. *Med Care* 36(6):851–67.

Stange KC, Flocke SA, Goodwin MA, Kelly RB, Zyzanski SJ. 2000. Direct observation of rates of preventive service delivery in community family practice. *Prev Med* 31(2 Pt 1):167–76.

Stead MJ, Wallis MG, Wheaton ME. 1998. Improving uptake in non-attenders of breast screening: selective use of second appointment. *J Med Screen* 5(2):69–72.

Steinmaus CM, Nunez S, Smith AH. 2000. Diet and bladder cancer: a meta-analysis of six dietary variables. *Am J Epidemiol* 151(7):693–702.

Steinmetz KA, Potter JD. 1991. Vegetables, fruit, and cancer. II. Mechanisms. *Cancer Causes Control* 2(6):427–42.

Steinmetz KA, Kushi LH, Bostick RM, Folsom AR, Potter JD. 1994. Vegetables, fruit, and colon cancer in the Iowa Women's Health Study. *Am J Epidemiol* 139(1):1–15.

Stern MP, Farquhar JW, McCoby N, Russell SH. 1976. Results of a two-year health education campaign on dietary behavior. The Stanford Three Community Study. *Circulation* 54(5):826–33.

Stevens VJ, Hollis JF. 1989. Preventing smoking relapse, using an individually tailored skills-training technique. *J Consult Clin Psychol* 57(3):420–4.

Stewart-Brown S, Farmer A. 1997. Screening could seriously damage your health. *BMJ* 314(7080):533–4.

Stoler MH, Schiffman M. 2001. Interobserver reproducibility of cervical cytologic and histologic interpretations: realistic estimates from the ASCUS-LSIL Triage Study. *JAMA* 285(11):1500–5.

Stolley MR, Fitzgibbon ML. 1997. Effects of an obesity prevention program on the eating behavior of African American mothers and daughters. *Health Educ Behav* 24(2): 152–64.

Stone EJ, Osganian SK, McKinlay SM, Wu MC, Webber LS, Luepker RV, Perry CL, Parcel GS, Elder JP. 1996. Operational design and quality control in the CATCH multicenter trial. *Prev Med* 25(4):384–99.

Stone EJ, McKenzie TL, Welk GJ, Booth ML. 1998. Effects of physical activity interventions in youth. Review and synthesis. *Am J Prev Med* 15(4):298–315.

Stormont TJ, Farrow GM, Myers RP, Blute ML, Zincke H, Wilson TM, Oesterling JE. 1993. Clinical stage B0 or T1c prostate cancer: nonpalpable disease identified by elevated serum prostate-specific antigen concentration. *Urology* 41(1):3–8.

Strauss GM, Gleason RE, Sugarbaker DJ. 1995. Chest X-ray screening improves outcome in lung cancer. A reappraisal of randomized trials on lung cancer screening. *Chest* 107(6 Suppl):270S–9S.

Strauss KF, Mokdad A, Ballew C, Mendlein JM, Will JC, Goldberg HI, White L, Serdula MK. 1997. The health of Navajo women: findings from the Navajo Health and Nutrition Survey, 1991–1992. *J Nutr* 127(10 Suppl):2128S–33S.

Strecher VJ, O'Malley MS, Villagra VG, Campbell EE, Gonzalez JJ, Irons TG, Kenney RD, Turner RC, Rogers CS, Lyles MF, et al. 1991. Can residents be trained to counsel patients about quitting smoking? Results from a randomized trial. *J Gen Intern Med* 6(1):9–17.

Strecher VJ, Kreuter M, Den Boer DJ, Kobrin S, Hospers HJ, Skinner CS. 1994. The effects of computer-tailored smoking cessation messages in family practice settings. *J Fam Pract* 39(3):262–70.

Strull WM, Lo B, Charles G. 1984. Do patients want to participate in medical decision making? *JAMA* 252(21):2990–4.

Strychar IM, Champagne F, Ghadirian P, Bonin A, Jenicek M, Lasater TM. 1998. Impact of receiving blood cholesterol test results on dietary change. *Am J Prev Med* 14(2): 103–10.

Suarez L, Ramirez AG, Villarreal R, Marti J, McAlister A, Talavera GA, Trapido E, Perez-Stable EJ. 2000. Social networks and cancer screening in four U.S. Hispanic groups. *Am J Prev Med* 19(1):47–52.

Subar AF, Heimendinger J, Patterson BH, Krebs-Smith SM, Pivonka E, Kessler R. 1995. Fruit and vegetable intake in the United States: the baseline survey of the Five A Day for Better Health Program. *Am J Health Promot* 9(5):352–60.

Sugarman JR, Dennis LK, White E. 1994. Cancer survival among American Indians in western Washington state (United States). *Cancer Causes Control* 5(5):440–8.

Sugarman JR, Holliday M, Ross A, Castorina J, Hui Y. 1996. Improving American Indian cancer data in the Washington State Cancer Registry using linkages with the Indian Health Service and tribal records. *Cancer* 78(7 Suppl):1564–8.

Sullivan MA, Covey LS. 2002. Current perspectives on smoking cessation among substance abusers. *Curr Psychiatry Rep* 4(5):388–96.

Summnex SK, Schiller EL, Marr ER, Thompson DI. 1986. A weight control and nutrition education program for insurance company employees. *J Nutr Educ* 18:S60–62.

Sussman S, Dent CW. 2000. One-year prospective prediction of drug use from stress-related variables. *Subst Use Misuse* 35(5):717–35.

Sussman S, Hansen WB, Flay BR, Botvin GJ. 2001. Re: Hutchinson Smoking Prevention Project: long-term randomized trial in school-based tobacco use prevention—results on smoking. *J Natl Cancer Inst* 93(16):1267.

Swedish Cancer Society and the Swedish National Board of Health and Welfare. 1996. Breast-cancer screening with mammography in women aged 40–49 years. 1996. *Int J Cancer* 68(6):693–9.

Swedish Council on Technology Assessment in Health Care. 1996. Mass screening for prostate cancer. *Int J Cancer Suppl* 9:1–72.

Swensen SJ, Jett JR, Sloan JA, Midthun DE, Hartman TE, Sykes AM, Aughenbaugh GL, Zink FE, Hillman SL, Noetzel GR, Marks RS, Clayton AC, Pairolero PC. 2002. Screening for lung cancer with low-dose spiral computed tomography. *Am J Respir Crit Care Med* 165(4):508–12.

Tabàr L, Fagerberg G, Chen HH, Duffy SW, Smart CR, Gad A, Smith RA. 1995. Efficacy of breast cancer screening by age. New results from the Swedish Two-County Trial. *Cancer* 75(10):2507–17.

Tabàr L, Vitak B, Chen HH, Prevost TC, Duffy SW. 1999. Update of the Swedish Two-County Trial of breast cancer screening: histologic grade-specific and age-specific results. *Swiss Surg* 5(5):199–204.

Tabàr L, Vitak B, Chen HH, Duffy SW, Yen MF, Chiang CF, Krusemo UB, Tot T, Smith RA. 2000. The Swedish Two-County Trial twenty years later. Updated mortality results and new insights from long-term follow-up. *Radiol Clin N Am* 38(4):625–51.

Taira DA, Safran DG, Seto TB, Rogers WH, Tarlov AR. 1997. The relationship between patient income and physician discussion of health risk behaviors. *JAMA* 278(17):1412–7.

Takakuwa KM, Ernst AA, Weiss SJ, Nick TG. 2000. Breast cancer knowledge and preventive behaviors: an urban emergency department-based survey. *Acad Emerg Med* 7(12):1393–8.

Talcott JA, Rieker P, Propert KJ, Clark JA, Wishnow KI, Loughlin KR, Richie JP, Kantoff PW. 1997. Patient-reported impotence and incontinence after nerve-sparing radical prostatectomy. *J Natl Cancer Inst* 89(15):1117–23.

Tanaka K, Hirohata T, Takeshita S, Hirohata I, Koga S, Sugimachi K, Kanematsu T, Ohryohji F, Ishibashi H. 1992. Hepatitis B virus, cigarette smoking and alcohol consumption in the development of hepatocellular carcinoma: a case-control study in Fukuoka, Japan. *Int J Cancer* 51(4):509–14.

Tang TS, Solomon LJ, McCracken LM. 2000. Cultural barriers to mammography, clinical breast exam, and breast self-exam among Chinese-American women 60 and older. *Prev Med* 31(5):575–83.

Taplin SH, Montano DE. 1993. Attitudes, age, and participation in mammographic screening: a prospective analysis. *J Am Board Fam Pract* 6(1):13–23.

Taplin SH, Anderman C, Grothaus L, Curry S, Montano D. 1994. Using physician correspondence and postcard reminders to promote mammography use. *Am J Public Health* 84(4):571–4.

Taplin SH, Mandelson MT, Anderman C, White E, Thompson RS, Timlin D, Wagner EH. 1997a. Mammography diffusion and trends in late-stage breast cancer: Evaluating outcomes in a population. *Cancer Epidemio, Biomarkers Prev* 6(8):625–31.

Taplin SH, Urban N, Taylor VM, Savarino J. 1997b. Conflicting national recommendations and the use of screening mammography: Does the physician's recommendation matter? *J Am Board Fam Prac* 10(2):88–95.

Taplin SH, Barlow WE, Ludman E, MacLehos R, Meyer DM, Seger D, Herta D, Chin C, Curry S. 2000. Testing reminder and motivational telephone calls to increase screening mammography: a randomized study. *J Natl Cancer Inst* 92(3):233–42.

Tarone RE. 1995. The excess of patients with advanced breast cancer in young women screened with mammography in the Canadian National Breast Screening Study. *Cancer* 75(4):997–1003.

Tarone RE, Chu KC, Brawley OW. 2000. Implications of stage-specific survival rates in assessing recent declines in prostate cancer mortality rates. *Epidemiology* 11(2): 167–70.

Task Force on Community Preventive Services. 2001. Recommendations regarding interventions to reduce tobacco use and exposure to environmental tobacco smoke. *Am J Prev Med* 20(2 Suppl):10–5.

Tate DF, Wing RR, Winett RA. 2001. Using Internet technology to deliver a behavioral weight loss program. *JAMA* 285(9):1172–7.

Taubes G. 1997. The breast-screening brawl. *Science* 275(5303):1056–9.

Taylor CB, Agras WS, Losch M, Plante TG, et al. 1991a. Improving the effectiveness of computer-assisted weight loss. *Behav Ther* 22(2):229–36.

Taylor CB, Fortmann SP, Flora J, Kayman S, Barrett DC, Jatulis D, Farquhar JW. 1991b. Effect of long-term community health education on body mass index. The Stanford Five-City Project. *Am J Epidemiol* 134(3):235–49.

Taylor VM, Thompson B, Montano DE, Mahloch J, Johnson K, Li S. 1998. Mammography use among women attending an inner-city clinic. *J Cancer Educ* 13(2):96–101.

Tefilli MV, Gheiler EL, Tiguert R, Banerjee M, Sakr W, Grignon D, Wood DP Jr, Pontes JE. 1999. Role of radical prostatectomy in patients with prostate cancer of high Gleason score. *Prostate* 39(1):60–6.

Terry P, Nyren O, Yuen J. 1998. Protective effect of fruits and vegetables on stomach cancer in a cohort of Swedish twins. *Int J Cancer* 76(1):35–7.

Terry P, Baron JA, Weiderpass E, Yuen J, Lichtenstein P, Nyren O. 1999. Lifestyle and endometrial cancer risk: a cohort study from the Swedish Twin Registry. *Int J Cancer* 82(1):38–42.

Tessaro I, Lyna PR, Rimer BK, Heisler J, Woods-Powell CT, Yarnall KS, Barber LT. 1997. Readiness to change smoking behavior in a community health center population. *J Community Health* 22(1):15–31.

Tessaro IA, Herman CJ, Shaw JE, Giese EA. 1996. Cancer prevention knowledge, attitudes, and clinical practice of nurse practitioners in local public health departments in North Carolina. *Cancer Nurs* 19(4):269–74.

Theuer CP, Wagner JL, Taylor TH, Brewster WR, Tran D, McLaren CE, Anton-Culver H. 2001. Racial and ethnic colorectal cancer patterns affect the cost-effectiveness of colorectal cancer screening in the United States. *Gastroenterology* 120(4):848–56.

Thomas DB, Gao DL, Self SG, Allison CJ, Tao Y, Mahloch J, Ray R, Qin Q, Presley R, Porter P. 1997. Randomized trial of breast self-examination in Shanghai: methodology and preliminary results. *J Natl Cancer Inst* 89(5):355–65.

Thompson B, Demark-Wahnefried W, Taylor G, McClelland JW, Stables G, Havas S, Feng Z, Topor M, Heimendinger J, Reynolds KD, Cohen N. 1999. Baseline fruit and vegetable intake among adults in seven 5 a day study centers located in diverse geographic areas. *J Am Diet Assoc* 99(10):1241–8.

Thompson IM, Rounder JB, Teague JL, Peek M, Spence CR. 1987. Impact of routine screening for adenocarcinoma of the prostate on stage distribution. *J Urol* 137(3):424–6.

Thompson RS, Taplin SH, McAfee TA, Mandelson MT, Smith AE. 1995. Primary and secondary prevention services in clinical practice. Twenty years' experience in development, implementation, and evaluation. *JAMA* 273(14):1130–5.

Thomson CA, Taren D, Koff N, Marian M, Canfield L, Bassford T, Ritenbaugh C. 2000. An integrated nutrition curriculum in medical education. *J Cancer Educ* 15(3):127–9.

Thorndike AN, Rigotti NA, Stafford RS, Singer DE. 1998. National patterns in the treatment of smokers by physicians. *JAMA* 279(8):604–8.

Thun MJ, Calle EE, Namboodiri MM, Flanders WD, Coates RJ, Byers T, Boffetta P, Garfinkel L, Heath CW Jr. 1992. Risk factors for fatal colon cancer in a large prospective study. *J Natl Cancer Inst* 84(19):1491–500.

Thun M, Dally-Lally C et al. 1997. Trends in tobacco smoking and mortality from cigarette use in Cancer Prevention Studies I (1959 through 1965) and II (1982 through 1988). In *Changes in Cigarette-related Disease Risk and their Implications for Prevention and Control.* D Burns, L Garfinkel and J Samet. Washington DC, NIH Publication No 97-4213:305–33.

Thun MJ, Peto R, Lopez AD, Monaco JH, Henley SJ, Heath CW Jr, Doll R. 1997. Alcohol consumption and mortality among middle-aged and elderly U.S. adults. *N Engl J Med* 337(24):1705–14.

Thune I, Lund E. 1997. The influence of physical activity on lung-cancer risk: a prospective study of 81,516 men and women. *Int J Cancer* 70(1):57–62.

Tibblin G, Welin L, Bergstrom R, Ronquist G, Norlen BJ, Adami HO. 1995. The value of prostate specific antigen in early diagnosis of prostate cancer: the study of men born in 1913. *J Urol* 154(4):1386–9.

Tilanus-Linthorst MM, Obdeijn IM, Bartels KC, de Koning HJ, Oudkerk M. 2000. First experiences in screening women at high risk for breast cancer with MR imaging. *Breast Cancer Res Treat* 63(1):53–60.

Tilley BC, Glanz K, Kristal AR, Hirst K, Li S, Vernon SW, Myers R. 1999a. Nutrition intervention for high-risk auto workers: results of the Next Step Trial. *Prev Med* 28(3): 284–92.

Tilley BC, Vernon SW, Myers R, Glanz K, Lu M, Hirst K, Kristal AR. 1999b. The Next Step Trial: impact of a worksite colorectal cancer screening promotion program. *Prev Med* 28(3):276–83.

Tockman MS. 1986. Survival and mortality from lung cancer in a screened population: The Johns Hopkins Study. *Chest.* 89(4 Suppl):324S–6S.

Tockman MS. 2000. Advances in sputum analysis for screening and early detection of lung cancer. *Cancer Control* 7(1):19–24.

Tomar SL, Husten CG, Manley MW. 1996. Do dentists and physicians advise tobacco users to quit? *J Am Dent Assoc* 127(2):259–65.

Tomeo CA, Colditz GA, Willett WC, Giovannucci E, Platz E, Rockhill B, Dart H, Hunter DJ. 1999. Harvard Report on Cancer Prevention. Volume 3: prevention of colon cancer in the United States. *Cancer Causes Control* 10(3):167–80.

Tornberg SA, Carstensen JM. 1994. Relationship between Quetelet's index and cancer of breast and female genital tract in 47,000 women followed for 25 years. *Br J Cancer* 69(2):358–61.

Tornblom M, Norming U, Adolfsson J, Becker C, Abrahamsson PA, Lilja H, Gustafsson O. 1999. Diagnostic value of percent free prostate-specific antigen: retrospective analysis of a population-based screening study with emphasis on men with PSA levels less than 3.0 ng/mL. *Urology* 53(5):945–50.

Tortolero-Luna G, Glober GA, Villarreal R, Palos G, Linares A. 1995. Screening practices and knowledge, attitudes, and beliefs about cancer among Hispanic and non-Hispanic white women 35 years old or older in Nueces County, Texas. *J Natl Cancer Inst Monogr* (18):49–56.

Traverso G, Shuber A, Levin B, Johnson C, Olsson L, Schoetz DJ Jr, Hamilton SR, Boynton K, Kinzler KW, Vogelstein B. 2002. Detection of APC mutations in fecal DNA from patients with colorectal tumors. *N Engl J Med* 346(5):311–20.

Travis WD, Travis LB, Devesa SS. 1995. Lung Cancer. [Erratum Appears in *Cancer* 1995 Jun 15;75(12):2979.]. *Cancer* 75(1 Suppl):191–202.

Tredaniel J, Boffetta P, Buiatti E, Saracci R, Hirsch A. 1997. Tobacco smoking and gastric cancer: review and meta-analysis. *Int J Cancer* 72(4):565–73.

Trichopoulos D, MacMahon B, Sparros L, Merikas G. 1980. Smoking and hepatitis B-negative primary hepatocellular carcinoma. *J Natl Cancer Inst* 65(1):111–4.

Trichopoulos D, Day NE, Kaklamani E, Tzonou A, Munoz N, Zavitsanos X, Koumantaki Y, Trichopoulou A. 1987. Hepatitis B virus, tobacco smoking and ethanol consumption in the etiology of hepatocellular carcinoma. *Int J Cancer* 39(1):45–9.

Trnka YM, Henderson CA. 1997. Flexible sigmoidoscopy screening: patient acceptance. *HMO Pract* 11(3):130–3.

Troni GM, Cipparrone I, Cariaggi MP, Ciatto S, Miccinesi G, Zappa M, Confortini M. 2000. Detection of false-negative Pap smears using the PAPNET system. *Tumor* 86(6):455–7.

Tseng DS, Cox E, Plane MB, Hla KM. 2001. Efficacy of patient letter reminders on cervical cancer screening: a meta-analysis. *J Gen Intern Med*16(8):563–8.

Tu JT, Gao RN, Zhang DH, Gu BC. 1985. Hepatitis B virus and primary liver cancer on Chongming Island, People's Republic of China. *J Natl Cancer Inst Monogr* 69:213–5.

Tu SP, Yasui Y, Kuniyuki A, Thompson B, Schwartz SM, Jackson JC, Taylor VM. 2000. Breast cancer screening among Cambodian American women. *Cancer Detect Prev* 24(6): 549–63.

Tudor-Smith C, Nutbeam D, Moore L, Catford J. 1998. Effects of the Heartbeat Wales programme over five years on behavioural risks for cardiovascular disease: quasi-experimental comparison of results from Wales and a matched reference area. *BMJ* 316(7134): 818–22.

Turnin MC, Beddok RH, Clottes JP, Martini PF, Abadie RG, Buisson JC, Soule-Dupuy C, Bonneu M, Camare R, Anton JP, et al. 1992. Telematic expert system Diabeto. New tool for diet self-monitoring for diabetic patients. *Diabetes Care* 15(2):204–12.

Tziraki C, Graubard BI, Manley M, Kosary C, Moler JE, Edwards BK. 2000. Effect of training on adoption of cancer prevention nutrition-related activities by primary care practices: results of a randomized, controlled study. *J Gen Intern Med* 15(3):155–62.

Ulcickas Yood M, McCarthy BD, Lee NC, Jacobsen G, Johnson CC. 1999. Patterns and characteristics of repeat mammography among women 50 years and older. *Cancer Epidemiol Biomarkers Prev* 8(7):595–9.

Underwood SM. 1999. Development of a cancer prevention and early detection program for nurses working with African Americans. *J Contin Educ Nurs* 30(1):30–6.

Unger JB, Rohrbach LA, Ribisl KM. 2001. Are adolescents attempting to buy cigarettes on the Internet? *Tob Control* 10(4):360–3.

Urban N, Taplin SH, Taylor VM, Peacock S, Anderson G, Conrad D, Etzioni R, White E, Montano DE, Mahloch J, et al. 1995. Community organization to promote breast cancer screening among women ages 50–75. *Prev Med* 24(5):477–84.

U.S. Census Bureau. Bergman M. 2002. Health Insurance in America: Numbers of Americans With and Without Health Insurance Rise. [Online]. Available at: www.census.gov/Press-Release/www/2002/cb02-127.html. Washington, DC: U.S. Census Bureau, Public Information Office.

U.S. Congress. 1995. *Costs and Effectiveness of Prostate Cancer Screening in Elderly Men.* Office of Technology Assessment Publication No. OTA-BP-H-145. Washington, DC: U.S. Government Printing Office.

U.S. Department of Agriculture. 1992. The Food Guide Pyramid. In *USDA Home and Garden Bulletin No. 252.* Washington, DC: U.S. Department of Agriculture.

U.S. Department of Agriculture, E. R. S., Food and Rural Economics Division. 1999. America's Eating Habits: Changes and Consequences. In *Agriculture Information Bulletin* No. 750, p. 784. Washington, DC: U.S. Department of Agriculture.

U.S. Department of Agriculture and U. S. Department of Health and Human Services (USDHHS). 1995. *Nutrition and Your Health: Dietary Guidelines for Americans.* Washington, DC: U.S. Government Printing Office.

U.S. Department of Agriculture and U.S. Department of Health and Human Services. 2000. Dietary Guidelines for Americans. In *USDA Home and Garden Bulletin No. 232.* Washington, DC: U.S. Department of Agriculture.

U.S. Department of Health, Education, and Welfare. 1964. *Smoking and Health.* Report of the Advisory Committee to the Surgeon General. DHEW Publication No. [PHS] 1103. Washington, DC: U.S. Department of Health, Education and Welfare, Public Health Service.

US DHHS (U.S. Department of Health and Human Services). 1982. *The Health Consequences of Smoking: Cancer. A Report of the Surgeon General.* Rockville, MD: U.S. Department of Health and Human Services, Public Health Service, Centers for Disease Control, Center for Health Promotion and Education, Office on Smoking and Health.

US DHHS. 1986. *The Health Consequences of Involuntary Smoking: A Report of the Surgeon General.* Rockville, MD: U.S. Department of Health and Human Services, Public Health Service, Centers for Disease Control, Center for Health Promotion and Education, Office on Smoking and Health.

US DHHS. 1988. *The Health Consequences of Smoking: Nicotine Addiction. A Report of the Surgeon General.* DHHS Publication No. (CDC) 88-8406. Rockville, MD: U.S. Department of Health and Human Services, Public Health Service, Centers for Disease Control, Center for Health Promotion and Education, Office on Smoking and Health.

US DHHS. 1989. *Reducing the Health Consequences of Smoking: 25 Years of Progress. A Report of the Surgeon General.* DHHS Publication No. (CDC) 89-8411. Rockville, MD: U.S. Department of Health and Human Services, Public Health Service, Centers for Disease Control, Center for Chronic Disease Prevention and Health Promotion, Office on Smoking and Health.

US DHHS. 1990. *The Health Benefits of Smoking Cessation. A Report of the Surgeon General.* Rockville, MD: U.S. Department of Health and Human Services, Public Health Service, Centers for Disease Control, Center for Chronic Disease Prevention and Health Promotion, Office on Smoking and Health.

US DHHS. 1991. *Healthy People 2000: National Health Promotion and Disease Prevention Objectives.* Rockville, MD: U.S. Department of Health and Human Services, Public Health Service.

US DHHS. 1994. *Preventing Tobacco Use Among Young People: A Report of the Surgeon General.* Washington, DC: U.S. Department of Health and Human Services, Public Health Service, Centers for Disease Control, Center for Chronic Disease Prevention and Health Promotion, Office on Smoking and Health.

US DHHS. 1996. *Physical Activity and Health: A Report of the Surgeon General.* Atlanta: U.S. Department of Health and Human Services, Centers for Disease Control and Prevention, National Center for Chronic Disease Prevention and Health Promotion.

US DHHS. 1998. *Tobacco Use Among U.S. Racial/Ethnic Minority Groups: African Americans, American Indians and Alaska Natives, Asian Americans and Pacific Islanders, and Hispanics. A Report of the Surgeon General.* Washington, DC: U.S. Department of Health and Human Services.

US DHHS. Fiore M, Bailey W, Cohen SJ, Dorfman SF, Goldstein MG, Gritz E, Heyman RB, Jaen C, Kottke TE, Lando HA, Mecklenburg R, Mullen P, Nett L, Robinon L, Stitzer M, Tommasello A, Villejo L, Wewers ME. 2000a. *Treating Tobacco Use and Dependence.* Rockville, MD: U.S. Department of Health and Human Services, U.S. Public Health Service.

US DHHS. 2000b. *Reducing Tobacco Use: A Report of the Surgeon General.* Atlanta: U.S. Department of Health and Human Services, Centers for Disease Control and Prevention, National Center for Chronic Disease Prevention and Health Promotion, Office of Smoking and Health.

US DHHS. 2001a. *Women and Smoking: A Report of the Surgeon General.* Rockville, MD: U.S. Department of Health and Human Services, Centers for Disease Control and Prevention, National Center for Chronic Disease Prevention and Health Promotion, Office on Smoking and Health.

US DHHS. 2001b. *The Surgeon General's Call to Action to Prevent and Decrease Overweight and Obesity, 2001.* Rockville, MD: U.S. Department of Health and Human Services, Public Health Service, Office of the Surgeon General.

US DHHS. Expected. *Smoking and Health.* Rockville, MD: U.S. Department of Health and Human Services, Centers for Disease Control and Prevention, National Center for Chronic Disease Prevention and Health Promotion, Office on Smoking and Health.

US DHHS and Office of Disease Prevention and Health Promotion. 2000. *Healthy People 2010: Understanding and Improving Health and Objectives for Improving Health.* Washington, DC: U.S. Department of Health and Human Services.

U.S. Department of Labor, Bureau of Labor Statistics 1999a. *Employee Benefits in Small Private Establishments, 1996.* Bulletin 2507, April. Washington DC: U.S. Bureau of Labor Statistics.

U.S. Department of Labor, Bureau of Labor Statistics. 1999b. *Employee Benefits in Medium and Large Private Establishments, 1997.* Bulletin 2517, September. Washington DC: U.S. Bureau of Labor Statistics.

U.S. Department of Labor, Bureau of Labor Statistics. 2000. *Employee Benefits in State and Local Governments, 1998.* Bulletin 2531, December. Washington, DC: U.S. Department of Labor.

US General Accounting Office. 2000. Medicare: Few Beneficiaries Use Colorectal Cancer Screening and Diagnostic Services. (Pub no. T-HEHS-00-68). Washington, DC: General Accounting Office.

U.S. Preventive Services Task Force. 1989. *Guide to Clinical Preventive Services: An Assessment of the Effectiveness of 169 Interventions.* Baltimore: Williams & Wilkins.

U.S. Preventive Services Task Force. 1990. Screening for lung cancer. *Am Fam Physician* 41(6):1763–6.

U.S. Preventive Services Task Force. 1996. *Guide to Clinical Preventive Services: Report of the U.S. Preventive Services Task Force.* Washington, DC: Office of Disease Prevention and Health Promotion.

U.S. Preventive Services Task Force. 2001a. *Guide to Clinical Preventive Services. An Assessment of the Effectiveness of 169 Interventions.* Baltimore: Williams & Williams.

U.S. Preventive Services Task Force. 2001b. Screening for skin cancer: recommendations and rationale. *Am J Prev Med* 20(3 Suppl):44–6.

U.S. Preventive Services Task Force. 2002. Screening for breast cancer: recommendations and rationale. Rockville, MD: U.S Department of Health and Human Services, Agency for Healthcare Research and Quality.

Valdini A, Cargill LC. 1997. Access and barriers to mammography in New England community health centers. J Fam Pract 45(3):243–9.

Valoski A, Epstein LH. 1990. Nutrient intake of obese children in a family-based behavioral weight control program. *Int J Obes* 14(8):667–77.

Vaughan TL, Davis S, Kristal A, Thomas DB. 1995. Obesity, alcohol, and tobacco as risk factors for cancers of the esophagus and gastric cardia: adenocarcinoma versus squamous cell carcinoma. *Cancer Epidemiol Biomarkers Prev* 4(2):85–92.

Velicer WF, Prochaska JO, Fava JL, Laforge RG, Rossi JS. 1999. Interactive versus non-interactive interventions and dose-response relationships for stage-matched smoking cessation programs in a managed care setting. *Health Psychol* 18(1):21–8.

Vernon SW. 1995. Adherence to colorectal cancer screening. A brief overview. *Ann NY Acad Sci* 768:292–5.

Vernon SW. 1997. Participation in colorectal cancer screening: a review. *J Natl Cancer Inst* 89(19):1406–22.

Veterans Administration Office of Research and Development, Health Services Research and Development Service. 2000. *QUERI Factsheet*Washington DC: U.S. Department of Veterans Affairs.

Veterans Administration Office of Research and Development, Health Services Research and Development Service. 2001. *QUERI Colorectal Cancer (CRC) Factsheet*. Washington DC: U.S. Department of Veterans Affairs.

Veterans Health Administration. 1999. *VHA Handbook 1120.2 Health Promotion and Disease Prevention Program*. Washington, DC: Department of Veterans Affairs.

Vineis P, Caporaso N. 1995. Tobacco and cancer: epidemiology and the laboratory. *Environ Health Perspect* 103(2):156–60.

Volk RJ, Spann SJ. 2000. Decision-aids for prostate cancer screening. *J Fam Pract* 49(5):425–7.

Volk RJ, Cass AR, Spann SJ. 1999. A randomized controlled trial of shared decision making for prostate cancer screening. *Arch Fam Med* 8(4):333–40.

Voorhees CC, Stillman FA, Swank RT, Heagerty PJ, Levine DM, Becker DM. 1996. Heart, body, and soul: impact of church-based smoking cessation interventions on readiness to quit. *Prev Med* 25(3):277–85.

Voorrips LE, Goldbohm RA, van Poppel G, Sturmans F, Hermus RJ, van den Brandt PA. 2000a. Vegetable and fruit consumption and risks of colon and rectal cancer in a prospective cohort study: The Netherlands Cohort Study on Diet and Cancer. *Am J Epidemiol* 152(11):1081–92.

Voorrips LE, Goldbohm RA, Verhoeven DT, van Poppel GA, Sturmans F, Hermus RJ, van den Brandt PA. 2000b. Vegetable and fruit consumption and lung cancer risk in The Netherlands Cohort Study on diet and cancer. *Cancer Causes Control* 11(2):101–15.

Vuori IM, Oja P, Paronen O. 1994. Physically active commuting to work—testing its potential for exercise promotion. *Med Sci Sports Exerc* 26(7):844–50.

Wadden T, Berkowitz R. 2001. Very-Low-Calorie Diets. In Fairburn CG, Brownell K (eds.). *Eating Disorders and Obesity*. New York: Guilford. Pp. 534–38.

Wadden TA. 1993. The treatment of obesity: an overview. In Stunkard AJ, Wadden TA (eds.). *Obesity Theory and Therapy*, Vol. 2, limited ed. New York: Raven Press. Pp. 197–218.

Wadden TA, Bell ST. 1990. Obesity. In Bellack AS, Hersen M, Kazdin A. (eds.). *International Handbook of Behavior Modification and Therapy*, Vol. II. New York: Plenum Press. Pp. 449–72.

Wadden TA, Sternberg JA, Letizia KA, Stunkard AJ, Foster GD. 1989. Treatment of obesity by very low calorie diet, behavior therapy, and their combination: a five-year perspective. *Int J Obes* 13(Suppl 2):39–46.

Wadden TA, Foster GD, Letizia KA. 1994. One-year behavioral treatment of obesity: comparison of moderate and severe caloric restriction and the effects of weight maintenance therapy. *J Consult Clin Psychol* 62(1):165–71.

Wadden TA, Vogt RA, Foster GD, Anderson DA. 1998. Exercise and the maintenance of weight loss: 1-year follow-up of a controlled clinical trial. *J Consult Clin Psychol* 66(2):429–33.

Wagner Jr. H, Ruckdeschel JC. 1996. Cost-effectiveness of colorectal cancer screening in average-risk adults. In Young G, Rozen P, Levin B (eds). *Prevention and Early Detection of Colorectal Cancer*. London: Saunders. Pp. 321–56.

Wagner TH. 1998. The effectiveness of mailed patient reminders on mammography screening: a meta-analysis. *Am J Prev Med* 14(1):64–70.

Wagner TH, Hu TW, Duenas GV, Pasick RJ. 2000. Willingness to pay for mammography: item development and testing among five ethnic groups. *Health Policy* 53(2):105–21.

Wakefield M, Chaloupka F. 2000. Effectiveness of comprehensive tobacco control programmes in reducing teenage smoking in the U.S.A. *Tob Control* 9(2):177–86.

Wald N. 2000. Populist instead of professional. *J Med Screen* 7(1):1.

Wald NJ, Watt HC, George L, Knekt P, Helzlsouer KJ, Tuomilehto J. 2000. Adding free to total prostate-specific antigen levels in trials of prostate cancer screening. *Br J Cancer* 82(3):731–6.

Walsh JM, Swangard DM, Davis T, McPhee SJ. 1999. Exercise counseling by primary care physicians in the era of managed care. *Am J Prev Med* 16(4):307–13.

Walsh PC. 1993. A decision analysis of alternative treatment strategies for clinically localized prostate cancer. *J Urol* 150(4):1330–2.

Walsh PC, Brooks JD. 1997. The Swedish prostate cancer paradox. *JAMA* 277(6):497–8.

Walter HJ, Hofman A, Vaughan RD, Wynder EL. 1988. Modification of risk factors for coronary heart disease. Five-year results of a school-based intervention trial. *N Engl J Med* 318(17):1093–100.

Walter SD, Kubik A, Parkin DM, Reissigova J, Adamec M, Khlat M. 1992. The natural history of lung cancer estimated from the results of a randomized trial of screening. *Cancer Causes Control* 3(2):115–23.

Wan H, Karesen R, Hervik A, Thoresen SO. 2001. Mammography screening in Norway: results from the first screening round in four counties and cost-effectiveness of a modeled nationwide screening. *Cancer Causes Control* 12(1):39–45.

Ward JE, Proude EM. 1999. Evaluation of doctors' reminders in emergency departments to encourage cervical screening. *Aust NZ J Public Health* 23(1):95–8.

Wardle J, Pope R. 1992. The psychological costs of screening for cancer. *J Psychosom Res* 36(7):609–24.

Warnecke RB, Langenberg P, Wong SC, Flay BR, Cook TD. 1992. The second Chicago televised smoking cessation program: a 24-month follow-up. *Am J Public Health* 82(6): 835–40.

Warner E, Heisey RE, Goel V, Carroll JC, McCready DR. 1999. Hereditary breast cancer. Risk assessment of patients with a family history of breast cancer. *Can Fam Physician* 45:104–12.

Warner J, Whitmore WF Jr. 1994. Expectant management of clinically localized prostatic cancer. *J Urol* 152(5 Pt 2):1761–5.

Warner KE. 1997. Cost effectiveness of smoking-cessation therapies. Interpretation of the evidence and implications for coverage. *Pharmacoeconomics* 11(6):538–49.

Warner KE. 1998. Smoking out the incentives for tobacco control in managed care settings. *Tob Control* 7(Suppl):S50–4.

Warner KE. 2000. The need for, and value of, a multi-level approach to disease prevention: the case of tobacco control. In Institute of Medicine, Smedley B, Syme SL (eds). *Promoting Health: Intervention Strategies from Social and Behavioral Research*. Washington, DC: National Academy Press. Pp. 417–49.

Wasserman MP. 2001. Guide to community preventive services: state and local opportunities for tobacco use reduction. *Am J Prev Med* 20(Suppl 2):8–9.

Wasson JH, Cushman CC, Bruskewitz RC, Littenberg B, Mulley AG Jr, Wennberg JE. 1993. A structured literature review of treatment for localized prostate cancer. Prostate Disease Patient Outcome Research Team. *Arch Fam Med* 2(5):487–93.

Weber BE, Reilly BM. 1997. Enhancing mammography use in the inner city. A randomized trial of intensive case management. *Arch Intern Med* 157(20):2345–9.

Wee CC, McCarthy EP, Davis RB, Phillips RS. 1999. Physician counseling about exercise. *JAMA* 282(16):1583–8.

Wegman DH. 1992. The potential impact of epidemiology on the prevention of occupational disease. *Am J Public Health* 82(7):944–54.

Weingarten S. 1999. Using practice guideline compendiums to provide better preventive care. *Ann Intern Med* 130(5):454–8.

Weinick RM, Beauregard KM. 1997. Women's use of preventive screening services: a comparison of HMO versus fee-for-service enrollees. *Med Care Res Rev* 54(2):176–99.

Weiss NS, Friedman GD, van den Eeden S. 1999. Digital rectal examination and mortality from prostate cancer. *Urology* 53(4):863–4.

Weiss W, Boucot KR, Seidman H. 1982. The Philadelphia Pulmonary Neoplasms Research Project. *Clin Chest Med* 3(2):243–56.

Weissman NJ. 2001. Appetite suppressants and valvular heart disease. *Am J Med Sci* 321(4): 285–91.

Weitzman ER, Zapka J, Estabrook B, Goins KV. 2001. Risk and reluctance: understanding impediments to colorectal cancer screening. *Prev Med* 32(6):502–13.

Welch HG, Fisher ES. 1998. Diagnostic testing following screening mammography in the elderly. *J Natl Cancer Inst* 90(18):1389–92.

Welch HG, Schwartz LM, Woloshin S. 2000. Are increasing 5-year survival rates evidence of success against cancer? *JAMA* 283(22):2975–8.

Wells KB, Lewis CE, Leake B, Schleiter MK, Brook RH. 1986. The practices of general and subspecialty internists in counseling about smoking and exercise. *Am J Public Health* 76(8):1009–13.

White E, Lee CY, Kristal AR. 1990. Evaluation of the increase in breast cancer incidence in relation to mammography use. *J Natl Cancer Inst* 82(19):1546–52.

White E, Shattuck AL, Kristal AR, Urban N, Prentice RL, Henderson MM, Insull W Jr, Moskowitz M, Goldman S, Woods MN. 1992. Maintenance of a low-fat diet: follow-up of the Women's Health Trial. *Cancer Epidemiol Biomarkers Prev* 1(4):315–23.

Whitlock EP, Vogt TM, Hollis JF, Lichtenstein E. 1997a. Does gender affect response to a brief clinic-based smoking intervention? *Am J Prev Med* 13(3):159–66.

Whitlock G, MacMahon S, Vander Hoorn S, Davis P, Jackson R, Norton R. 1997b. Socioeconomic distribution of smoking in a population of 10,529 New Zealanders. *NZ Med J* 110(1051):327–30.

Whitmore WF Jr. 1988. Consensus Development Conference on the Management of Clinically Localized Prostate Cancer. Overview: historical and contemporary. *J Natl Can Inst Monogr* (7):7–11.

Whittemore AS, Wu-Williams AH, Lee M, Zheng S, Gallagher RP, Jiao DA, Zhou L, Wang XH, Chen K, Jung D, et al. 1990. Diet, physical activity, and colorectal cancer among Chinese in North America and China. *J Natl Cancer Inst* 82(11):915–26.

Wilde J. 1989. A 10 year follow-up of semi-annual screening for early detection of lung cancer in the Erfurt County, GDR. *Eur Respir J* 2(7):656–62.

Wilfond BS, Rothenberg KH, Thomson EJ, Lerman C. 1997. Cancer genetic susceptibility testing: ethical and policy implications for future research and clinical practice. Cancer Genetic Studies Consortium, National Institutes of Health. *J Law Med Ethics* 25(4):243–51, 230.

Wilkins EG, Lowery JC, Hamill JB. 1999. The impact of shared decision-making in prostate-specific antigen (PSA) screening. *Med Decis Making* 19:525.

Willemsen MC, De Zwart WM. 1999. The effectiveness of policy and health education strategies for reducing adolescent smoking: a review of the evidence. *J Adolesc* 22(5):587–99.

Willett W, Rockhill B., et al. 2000. Epidemiology and assessing and managing risk. In Harris JR (ed.). *Diseases of the Breast*, 2nd ed. Philadelphia: Lippincott Williams & Wilkins.

Willett WC. 1995. Diet, nutrition, and avoidable cancer. *Environ Health Perspect* 103(Suppl 8):165–70.

Willett WC. 1998. Nutritional epidemiology. in Rothman KJ, Greenland S (eds.). *Modern Epidemiology*. Philadelphia: Lippincott-Raven Publishers. Pp. 623–6.

Willett WC. 1999. Dietary fat and breast cancer. *Toxicol Sci* 52(2 Suppl):127–46.

Willett WC. 2000. Diet and cancer. *Oncologist* 5(5):393–404.

Willett WC, Trichopoulos D. 1996. Nutrition and cancer: a summary of the evidence. *Cancer Causes Control* 7(1):178–80.

Willett WC, Manson JE, Stampfer MJ, Colditz GA, Rosner B, Speizer FE, Hennekens CH. 1995. Weight, weight change, and coronary heart disease in women. Risk within the 'normal' weight range. *JAMA* 273(6):461–5.

Willett WC, Colditz GA, Mueller NE. 1996. Strategies for minimizing cancer risk. *Sci Am* 275(3):88–91, 94–5.

Williams PT, Eckert G, Epstein A, Mourad L, Helmick F. 1994. In-office cancer-screening education of primary care physicians. *J Cancer Educ* 9(2):90–5.

Williams RB, Boles M, Johnson RE. 1998. A patient-initiated system for preventive health care. A randomized trial in community-based primary care practices. *Arch Fam Med* 7(4):338–45.

Wilson DM, Taylor DW, Gilbert JR, Best JA, Lindsay EA, Willms DG, Singer J. 1988. A randomized trial of a family physician intervention for smoking cessation. *JAMA* 260(11): 1570–4.

Wilt TJ, Brawer MK. 1994. The Prostate Cancer Intervention Versus Observation Trial: a randomized trial comparing radical prostatectomy versus expectant management for the treatment of clinically localized prostate cancer. *J Urol* 152(5 Pt 2):1910–4.

Wilt TJ, Cowper DC, Gammack JK, Going DR, Nugent S, Borowsky SJ. 1999. An evaluation of radical prostatectomy at Veterans Affairs medical centers: time trends and geographic variation in utilization and outcomes. *Med Care* 37(10):1046–56.

Winawer SJ, Flehinger BJ, Schottenfeld D, Miller DG. 1993a. Screening for colorectal cancer with fecal occult blood testing and sigmoidoscopy. *J Natl Cancer Inst* 85(16):1311–8.

Winawer SJ, Zauber AG, Ho MN, O'Brien MJ, Gottlieb LS, Sternberg SS, Waye JD, Schapiro M, Bond JH, Panish JF, et al. 1993b. Prevention of colorectal cancer by colonoscopic polypectomy. The National Polyp Study Workgroup. *N Engl J Med* 329(27):1977–81.

Winawer SJ, Fletcher RH, Miller L, Godlee F, Stolar MH, Mulrow CD, Woolf SH, Glick SN, Ganiats TG, Bond JH, Rosen L, Zapka JG, Olsen SJ, Giardiello FM, Sisk JE, Van Antwerp R, Brown-Davis C, Marciniak DA, Mayer RJ. 1997. Colorectal cancer screening: clinical guidelines and rationale. *Gastroenterology* 112(2):594–642.

Winawer SJ, Stewart ET, Zauber AG, Bond JH, Ansel H, Waye JD, Hall D, Hamlin JA, Schapiro M, O'Brien MJ, Sternberg SS, Gottlieb LS. 2000. A comparison of colonoscopy and double-contrast barium enema for surveillance after polypectomy. National Polyp Study Work Group. *N Engl J Med* 342(24):1766–72.

Winchester DP, Jeske JM, Goldschmidt RA. 2000. The diagnosis and management of ductal carcinoma in-situ of the breast. *CA Cancer J Clin* 50(3):184–200.

Winett RA, King AC, Altman DG. 1989. *Health Psychology and Public Health: An Integrative Approach*. New York: Pergamon Press.

Winett RA, Moore JF, Wagner JL, Hite LA, Leahy M, Neubauer TE, Walberg JL, Walker WB, Lombard D, Geller ES, et al. 1991. Altering shoppers' supermarket purchases to fit nutritional guidelines: an interactive information system. *J Appl Behav Anal* 24(1):95–105.

Wing RR. 1996. Behavioral approaches to the treatment of obesity. *Curr Opin Endocrinol Diab* 3:74–79.

Wing RR. 1999. Behavioral strategies to improve long-term weight loss and maintenance. *Med Health R I* 82(4):123.

Wing RR, Anglin K. 1992. Effectiveness of a behavioral weight control program for blacks and whites with NIDDM. *Diabetes Care* 15(5):409–13.

Wing RR, Blair E, Marcus M, Epstein LH, Harvey J. 1994. Year-long weight loss treatment for obese patients with type II diabetes: does including an intermittent very-low-calorie diet improve outcome? *Am J Med* 97(4):354–62.

Wing RR, Jeffery RW, Burton LR, Thorson C, Nissinoff KS, Baxter JE. 1996a. Food provision vs structured meal plans in the behavioral treatment of obesity. *Int J Obes Relat Metab Disord* 20(1):56–62.

Wing RR, Jeffery RW, Hellerstedt WL, Burton LR. 1996b. Effect of frequent phone contacts and optional food provision on maintenance of weight loss. *Ann Behav Med* 18(3):172–6.

Wingo PA, Ries LA, Giovino GA, Miller DS, Rosenberg HM, Shopland DR, Thun MJ, Edwards BK. 1999. Annual report to the nation on the status of cancer, 1973–1996, with a special section on lung cancer and tobacco smoking. *J Natl Cancer Inst* 91(8): 675–90.

Wolf AM, Schorling JB. 2000. Does informed consent alter elderly patients' preferences for colorectal cancer screening? Results of a randomized trial. *J Gen Intern Med* 15(1): 24–30.

Wolk A, Gridley G, Niwa S, Lindblad P, McCredie M, Mellemgaard A, Mandel JS, Wahrendorf J, McLaughlin JK, Adami HO. 1996. International renal cell cancer study. VII. Role of diet. *Int J Cancer* 65(1):67–73.

Wolk A, Gridley G, Svensson M, Nyren O, McLaughlin JK, Fraumeni JF, Adam HO. 2001. A prospective study of obesity and cancer risk (Sweden). *Cancer Causes Control* 12(1): 13–21.

Woloshin, S; Schwartz, LM; Byram, SJ; Sox, HC; Fischhoff, B, and Welch, HG. 2000. Women's understanding of the mammography screening debate. (ital.) *Arch Intern Med* 160(10):1434–40.

Woodson K, Albanes D, Tangrea JA, Rautalahti M, Virtamo J, Taylor PR. 1999. Association between alcohol and lung cancer in the alpha-tocopherol, beta-carotene cancer prevention study in Finland. *Cancer Causes Control* 10(3):219–26.

Woolf SH. 1995. Screening for prostate cancer with prostate-specific antigen. An examination of the evidence. *N Engl J Med* 333(21):1401–5.

Woolf SH. 1997a. Shared decision-making: the case for letting patients decide which choice is best. *J Fam Pract* 45(3):205–8.

Woolf SH. 1997b. Should we screen for prostate cancer? *BMJ* 314(7086):989–90.

Woolf SH. 1999. The need for perspective in evidence-based medicine. *JAMA* 282(24): 2358–65.

Woolf SH. 2000a. The best screening test for colorectal cancer—a personal choice. *N Engl J Med* 343(22):1641–3.

Woolf SH. 2000b. Taking critical appraisal to extremes. The need for balance in the evaluation of evidence. *J Fam Pract* 49(12):1081–5.

Woolf SH. 2001. The logic and limits of shared decision making. *J Urol* 166(1):244–5.

Woolf SH, Dickey LL. 1999. Differing perspectives on preventive care guidelines: a new look at the mammography controversy. *Am J Prev Med* 17(4):260–8.

Woolf SH, George JN. 2000. Evidence-based medicine. Interpreting studies and setting policy. *Hematol Oncol Clin N Am* 14(4):761–84.

Woolf SH, Lawrence RS. 1997. Preserving scientific debate and patient choice: lessons from the Consensus Panel on Mammography Screening, National Institutes of Health. *JAMA* 278(23):2105–8.

Woolf SH, Rothemich SF. 1999. Screening for prostate cancer: the roles of science, policy, and opinion in determining what is best for patients. *Annu Rev Med* 50:207–21.

Woolf SH, DiGuiseppi CG, Atkins D, Kamerow DB. 1996. Developing evidence-based clinical practice guidelines: lessons learned by the US Preventive Services Task Force. *Annu Rev Public Health* 17:511–38.

World Cancer Research Fund and American Institute for Cancer Research. 1997. *Food, Nutrition and the Prevention of Cancer: A Global Perspective*. Washington, DC: American Institute for Cancer Research.

World Health Organization. 1995. *Physical Status: The Use and Interpretation of Anthropometry*. Report of a WHO Expert Committee, WHO Technical Report Series No. 854. Geneva: World Health Organization.

World Health Organization. 1998. *Obesity: Preventing and Managing the Global Epidemic*. Report of a WHO Consultation on Obesity, Geneva, June 3–5, 1997. Geneva: World Health Organization.

World Health Organization. 1999. *The World Health Report 1999: Making a Difference*. Geneva: World Health Organization.

Wu JT. 1994. Assay for prostate specific antigen (PSA): problems and possible solutions. *J Clin Lab Anal* 8(1):51–62.

Yabroff KR, Mandelblatt JS. 1999. Interventions targeted toward patients to increase mammography use. *Cancer Epidemiol Biomarkers Prev* 8(9):749–57.

Yabroff KR, Kerner JF, Mandelblatt JS. 2000. Effectiveness of interventions to improve follow-up after abnormal cervical cancer screening. *Prev Med* 31(4):429–39.

Yanovitzky I, Blitz CL. 2000. Effect of media coverage and physician advice on utilization of breast cancer screening by women 40 years and older. *J Health Commun* 5(2):117–34.

Yanovski SZ, Gormally JF, Leser MS, Gwirtsman HE, Yanovski JA. 1994. Binge eating disorder affects outcome of comprehensive very-low-calorie diet treatment. *Obes Res* 2:205–12.

Yarnall KS, Rimer BK, Hynes D, Watson G, Lyna PR, Woods-Powell CT, Terrenoire J, Barber LT. 1998. Computerized prompts for cancer screening in a community health center. *J Am Board Fam Pract* 11(2):96–104.

Yip JK, Hay JL, Ostroff JS, Stewart RK, Cruz GD. 2000. Dental students' attitudes toward smoking cessation guidelines. *J Dent Educ* 64(9):641–50.

Ylitalo N, Sorensen P, Josefsson A, Frisch M, Sparen P, Ponten J, Gyllensten U, Melbye M, Adami HO. 1999. Smoking and oral contraceptives as risk factors for cervical carcinoma in situ. *Int J Cancer* 81(3):357–65.

Yong LC, Brown CC, Schatzkin A, Dresser CM, Slesinski MJ, Cox CS, Taylor PR. 1997. Intake of vitamins E, C, and A and risk of lung cancer. The NHANES I epidemiologic followup study. First National Health and Nutrition Examination Survey. *Am J Epidemiol* 146(3):231–43.

Young DR, Haskell WL, Taylor CB, Fortmann SP. 1996. Effect of community health education on physical activity knowledge, attitudes, and behavior. The Stanford Five-City Project. *Am J Epidemiol* 144(3):264–74.

Young TB. 1989. A case-control study of breast cancer and alcohol consumption habits. *Cancer* 64(2):552–8.

Yuan JM, Gago-Dominguez M, Castelao JE, Hankin JH, Ross RK, Yu MC. 1998. Cruciferous vegetables in relation to renal cell carcinoma. *Int J Cancer* 77(2):211–6.

Zapka JG. 1994. Promoting participation in breast cancer screening. *Am J Public Health* 84(1):12–3.

Zapka JG, Harris DR, Hosmer D, Costanza ME, Mas E, Barth R. 1993. Effect of a community health center intervention on breast cancer screening among Hispanic American women. *Health Serv Res* 28(2):223–35.

Zapka JG, Merriam P, Ockene J. 1997. Smoking cessation benefits in HMOs. *HMO Pract* 11(1):27–33.

Zapka JG, Luckmann R, Sulsky SI, Goins KV, Bigelow C, Mazor K, Quirk M. 2000a. Cancer control knowledge, attitudes, and perceived skills among medical students. *J Cancer Educ* 15(2):73–8.

Zapka JG, Pbert L, Stoddard AM, Ockene JK, Goins KV, Bonollo D. 2000b. Smoking cessation counseling with pregnant and postpartum women: a survey of community health center providers. *Am J Public Health* 90(1):78–84.

Zappa M, Ciatto S, Bonardi R, Mazzotta A. 1998. Overdiagnosis of prostate carcinoma by screening: an estimate based on the results of the Florence Screening Pilot Study. *Ann Oncol* 9(12):1297–300.

Zhang S, Hunter DJ, Forman MR, Rosner BA, Speizer FE, Colditz GA, Manson JE, Hankinson SE, Willett WC. 1999a. Dietary carotenoids and vitamins A, C, and E and risk of breast cancer. *J Natl Cancer Inst* 91(6):547–56.

Zhang S, Hunter DJ, Rosner BA, Colditz GA, Fuchs CS, Speizer FE, Willett WC. 1999b. Dietary fat and protein in relation to risk of non-Hodgkin's lymphoma among women. *J Natl Cancer Inst* 91(20):1751–8.

Zheng W, McLaughlin JK, Gridley G, Bjelke E, Schuman LM, Silverman DT, Wacholder S, Co-Chien HT, Blot WJ, Fraumeni JF Jr. 1993. A cohort study of smoking, alcohol consumption, and dietary factors for pancreatic cancer (United States). *Cancer Causes Control* 4(5):477–82.

Zheng W, Sellers TA, Doyle TJ, Kushi LH, Potter JD, Folsom AR. 1995. Retinol, antioxidant vitamins, and cancers of the upper digestive tract in a prospective cohort study of postmenopausal women. *Am J Epidemiol* 142(9):955–60.

Zhu BP, Liu M, Shelton D, Liu S, Giovino GA. 1996. Cigarette smoking and its risk factors among elementary school students in Beijing. *Am J Public Health* 86(3):368–75.

Zincke H, Oesterling JE, Blute ML, Bergstralh EJ, Myers RP, Barrett DM. 1994. Long-term (15 years) results after radical prostatectomy for clinically localized (stage T2c or lower) prostate cancer. *J Urol* 152(5 Pt 2):1850–7.

Zyzanski SJ, Stange KC, Kelly R, Flocke S, Shank JC, Chao J, Jaen CR, Smith CK. 1994. Family physicians' disagreements with the U.S. Preventive Services Task Force recommendations. *J Fam Pract* 39(2):140–7.

Glossary

Accuracy—the degree to which a test measures the true value of the attribute it is testing.

Adiposity—the quality or state of being fat: obesity.

Ambulatory care—the use of outpatient facilities—doctors' offices, home care, outpatient hospital clinics, and day-care facilities—to provide medical care without the need for hospitalization. Often refers to any care outside a hospital.

Beta-carotene—an antioxidant which protects cells against oxidation damage that can lead to cancer. Beta carotene is converted, as needed, to vitamin A.

Bias—in general, any factor that distorts the true nature of an event or observation. In clinical investigations, a bias is any systematic factor other than the intervention of interest that affects the magnitude of (i.e., tends to increase or decrease) an observed difference in the outcomes of a treatment group and a control group.

Biopsy—refers to a procedure that involves obtaining a tissue specimen for microscopic analysis to establish a precise diagnosis.

BRCA1—gene located on the short arm of chromosome 17; when damaged (mutated), a woman is at greater risk of developing breast and/or ovarian cancer compared to women who do not have the mutation.

BRCA2—mutation of this gene, located on chromosome 13, is associated with increased risk of breast cancer.

Bupropion—a unicyclic, aminoketone antidepressant. The mechanism of its therapeutic actions is not well understood, but it does appear to block dopamine uptake. It is effective in the treatment of major depression and has some beneficial effects in children and adults with attention deficit disorder.

Cancer—a general term for more than 100 diseases that are characterized by uncontrolled, abnormal growth of cells. Cancer cells can spread locally or through the bloodstream and lymphatic system to other parts of the body.

Carcinogenesis—the generation of cancer, uncontrolled, abnormal growth, from normal cells; correctly the formation of a carcinoma from epithelial cells, but often used synonymously with transformation, tumorigenesis.

Case-control study—a retrospective observational study in which investigators identify a group of patients with a specified outcome (cases) and a group of patients without the specified outcome (controls). Investigators then compare the histories of the cases and the controls to determine the extent to which each was exposed to the intervention of interest.

Case report—a description of a single case, typically describing the manifestations, clinical course, and prognosis of that case.

Case series—a descriptive, observational study of a series of cases, typically describing the manifestations, clinical course, and prognosis of a condition.

Chemoprevention—the use of natural or laboratory-made substances to prevent cancer.

Chemoprophylaxis—drug treatment designed to prevent future occurrences of disease.

Chemotherapy—the treatment of disease by means of chemicals that have a specific toxic effect upon the disease producing microorganisms (antibiotics) or that selectively destroy cancerous tissue (anticancer therapy).

Cohort study—an observational study in which outcomes in a group of patients that received an intervention are compared with outcomes in a similar group, that is, the cohort, either contemporary or historical, of patients that did not receive the intervention. In an adjusted- (or matched-) cohort study, investigators identify (or make statistical adjustments to provide) a cohort group that has characteristics (e.g., age, gender, disease severity) that are as similar as possible to the group that experienced the intervention.

Colonoscopy—an endoscopic (fiberoptic) examination of the large intestine (colon).

Computed tomography—a special radiographic technique that uses a computer to assimilate multiple X-ray images into a two-dimensional, cross-sectional image. This can reveal many soft tissue structures not shown by conventional radiography.

Confidence interval—a range within which an estimate is deemed to fall with specified statistical confidence.

Confounding factors—factors for which data adjustment is needed because they are entangled with other factors related to the disease or condition of interest.

Controlled observational studies—studies that compare outcomes among those who do or do not receive screening.

Cost-benefit analysis—a comparison of alternative interventions in which costs and outcomes are quantified in common monetary units.

Cost-effectiveness analysis—a comparison of alternative interventions in which costs are measured in monetary units and outcomes are measured in non-monetary units, for example, reduced mortality or morbidity.

Cross-sectional comparison—an observational study in which both risk factor(s) and disease are ascertained at the same time.

Cytological screening—examination of cells for changes indicative of a disease or risk of disease, for example, Papanicolaou test.

Diagnostic testing—the evaluation of patients with signs or symptoms associated with a disease.

DNA (deoxyribonucleic acid)—the genetic material of all cells and many viruses that is a polymer of nucleotides. The monomer consists of phosphorylated 2-deoxyribose N-glycosidically linked to one of four bases: adenine, cytosine, guanine or thymine. The sequence of these bases encodes genetic information.

Dose-response—the relation between the dose of a drug or other chemical and the degree of response it produces, as measured by the percentage of the exposed population showing a defined, often quantal, effect.

Dosimetry—measurement of the amount of X-rays and radioactivity absorbed.

Ductal carcinoma in situ—a very early form of breast cancer confined to cells lining the breast ducts.

Etiology—the science and study of the causes of disease and their mode of operation.
Exercise—a subset of physical activity that is planned, structured, and repetitive.

False-negative result—relating to or being an individual or a test result that is erroneously classified in a negative category (as of diagnosis) because of imperfect testing methods or procedures.
False-positive result—relating to or being an individual or a test result that is erroneously classified in a positive category (as of diagnosis) because of imperfect testing methods or procedures.

Genotype—the genetic constitution of an organism or cell, as distinct from its expressed features or phenotype.

Health Maintenance Organization (HMO)—organized system for providing comprehensive prepaid health care that has five basic attributes: 1) provides care in a defined geographic area; 2) provides or ensures delivery of an agreed-upon set of basic and supplemental health maintenance and treatment services; 3) provides care to a voluntarily enrolled group of persons; 4) requires their enrollees to use the services of designated providers; and 5) receives reimbursement through a predetermined, fixed, periodic prepayment made by the enrollee without regard to the degree of services provided.
Health services research—a multidisciplinary field of inquiry, both basic and applied, that examines the use, costs, quality, accessibility, delivery, organization, financing, and outcomes of health care services to increase knowledge and understand the structure, processes, and effects of health services for individuals and populations.
Human papillomavirus—any of numerous papillomaviruses that cause various human warts (as the common warts of the extremities, plantar warts, and genital warts) including some associated with the production of cancer; called also *HPV.*
Hyperplasia—A condition in which there is an increase in the number of normal cells in a tissue or organ.

Incidence—the number of new cases of a disease that occur in the population per unit of time.
Indemnity plan—traditional health insurance plans that pay for all or a share of the cost of covered services, regardless of which doctor, hospital, or other licensed health care provider is used. Members choose when and where to get health care services. In exchange for the premiums that members pay, the indemnity plan either pays the provider directly or reimburses members when they file claims.
Intermediate outcomes—findings that are not health outcomes in themselves (e.g., cellular atypia) but that precede or that are thought to increase the risk of such outcomes.

Lead-time bias—overestimation of survival time because of the backward shift in the starting point for the measurement of survival as a result of early detection.
Length bias—the tendency of screening to detect slowly growing lesions more readily than aggressive cancers.
Lifetime probability—the probability of being diagnosed with a specified cancer during an individual's lifetime, expressed as percent. It is derived by summing all cancer cases from age 0 through 95+ and dividing by 100,000 × 100 (expressed as percent).

Mammography—the practice of taking diagnostic X-ray pictures of breasts to produce a mammogram.
Managed care —any system that manages healthcare delivery to control costs.
Meta-analysis—systematic methods that use statistical techniques for combining results from different studies to obtain a quantitative estimate of the overall effect of a particular

intervention or variable on a defined outcome. This combination may produce a stronger conclusion than can be provided by any individual study (also known as data synthesis or quantitative overview).

Metabolism—the sum of all the physical and chemical processes by which living organized substance is produced and maintained (anabolism) and also the transformation by which energy is made available for the uses of the organism (catabolism).

Metaplasia—the change in the type of adult cells in a tissue to a form which is not normal for that tissue.

Molecular epidemiology—a science that focuses on the contribution of potential genetic and environmental risk factors, identified at the molecular level, to the etiology, distribution, and prevention of disease within families and across populations.

Morbidity—a diseased condition or state, the incidence of a disease or of all diseases in a population.

Mortality rate—expresses the number of deaths in a unit of population within a prescribed time and may be expressed as crude death rates or as death rates specific for diseases and, sometimes, for age, sex, or other attributes.

Nulliparity—condition of not having given birth to a child.

Observational studies—follow-up studies where clinical interventions are not specified by protocol.

Odds ratio—a comparison of the presence of a risk factor for disease in a sample of diseased subjects and non-diseased controls.

Oncology—the study of diseases that cause cancer.

Pap smear—a cytological test developed by George N. Papanicolaou for the detection of cervical cancer.

Pharmacotherapy—treatment or therapy using drugs.

Phenotype—the observable characteristic of an organism, the expression of the gene alleles (genotype) as an observable physical or biological trait.

Physical activity—any bodily movement produced by skeletal muscles that results in energy expenditure.

Population attributable risk—the proportion of all cancers in the population due to a particular risk factor. Its calculation relies on estimates of relative risk, which is the ratio of the cancer incidence rate among those exposed to a risk factor divided by the rate among those not exposed and the proportion of the population exposed to that risk factor.

Positive predictive value—the probability that an abnormal result correctly indicates cancer.

Prevalence—the number of cases of disease, infected persons, or persons with some other attribute, present at a particular time and in relation to the size of the population from which drawn.

Primary cancer prevention—prevention of acquisition of cancer.

Prophylaxis—the prevention of disease, preventive treatment.

PSA (prostate-specific antigen) testing—used to screen for cancer of the prostate and to monitor treatment by measuring the amount of PSA in the blood. PSA is a protein produced in the bloodstream.

p-value—the probability that an outcome as large as or larger than that observed would occur in a properly designed, executed, and analyzed analytical study if in reality there was no difference between the groups.

Randomized controlled trial—a true prospective experiment in which investigators randomly assign an eligible sample of patients to one or more treatment groups and a control group and follow patients' outcomes (also known as randomized clinical trial).

Relative risk—the proportion of diseased people among those exposed to the relevant risk factor divided by the proportion of diseased people among those not exposed to the risk factor. This statistic should be used in those cohort studies where those with and without disease are followed to observe which individuals become diseased.

Reliability—the consistency of the result when a test is repeated.

Screening—early detection of cancer or premalignant disease in persons without signs or symptoms suggestive of the target condition (the type of cancer that the test seeks to detect).

Secondary cancer—cancer that has spread from the site where it first appeared to another site.

Sigmoidoscopy—a procedure in which a scope is used to view the sigmoid flexure.

Specificity—the proportion of persons without disease who correctly test negative.

Spiral computed tomography—a detailed cross-sectional picture of areas inside the body. The images are created by a computer linked to an X-ray machine that scans the body in a spiral path. Also called helical computed tomography.

Squamous cell carcinoma—a malignant growth originating from a squamous cell. This form of cancer can be seen on the skin, lips, and inside the mouth, throat, or esophagus.

Statistical power—the likelihood that a study will find a particular effect if the effect exists.

Surrogate outcomes—indicators that correlate with, but that are not themselves, health outcomes (e.g., length of hospital stay).

Surveillance—close and continuous observation, screening, and testing of those at risk for a disease.

Survival—average period of time from diagnosis to death.

Translational research—the research needed to move the fruits of research into provider and community practice.

Tumor—an abnormal mass of tissue that results from excessive cell division that is uncontrolled and progressive, also called a neoplasm. Tumors perform no useful body function. They may be either benign (not cancerous) or malignant.

Venipuncture—the puncture of a vein (usually in the arm) with a hollow bore needle for the purpose of obtaining a blood specimen.

X-ray—a type of irradiation used for imaging purposes that uses energy beams of very short wavelengths (0.1 to 1000 angstroms) that can penetrate most substances except heavy metals.

Index*

*Page numbers followed by *t* refer to tables. Page numbers followed by *f* refer to figures.

B

D

E

G

H

I

M

N

Q

R

S

T

U

V

W

Y